Taylor's Handbook of Clinical Nursing Skills

Pamela Lynn, MSN, RN
Instructor
School of Nursing
Gwynedd-Mercy College
Gwynedd Valley, Pennsylvania

Wolters Kluwer | Lippincott Williams & Wilkins
Health
Philadelphia · Baltimore · New York · London
Buenos Aires · Hong Kong · Sydney · Tokyo

Executive Acquisitions Editor: Carrie Brandon
Product Manager: Michelle Clarke
Editorial Assistant: Amanda Jordan
Design Coordinator: Holly Reid McLaughlin
Art Director, Illustration: Brett MacNaughton
Manufacturing Coordinator: Karin Duffield
Production Services: Aptara, Inc.

9 8 7 6 5 4 3 2 1

Printed in China

Library of Congress Cataloging-in-Publication Data

Lynn, Pamela Barbara, 1961-
  Taylor's handbook of clinical nursing skills / Pamela Lynn. — 1st ed.
  p. ; cm.
  Other title: Handbook of clinical nursing skills
  Abridgement of: Taylor's clinical nursing skills / Pamela Lynn. 3rd ed.
© 2011.
  ISBN 978-1-58255-735-9 (alk. paper)
  1. Nursing—Handbooks, manuals, etc. I. Taylor, Carol, CSFN. II. Lynn,
Pamela Barbara, 1961- Taylor's clinical nursing skills.
III. Title. IV. Title: Handbook of clinical nursing skills.
  [DNLM: 1. Nursing Process—Handbooks. 2. Clinical
Medicine—methods—Handbooks. 3. Nursing Care—methods—Handbooks. WY 49]
  RT51.L96 2011
  610.73—dc22

                                                      2010032323

Care has been taken to confirm the accuracy of the information presented and to describe
generally accepted practices. However, the authors, editors, and publisher are not responsible
for errors or omissions or for any consequences from the application of the information in this
book and make no warranty, express or implied, with respect to the content of the publication.
  The authors, editors, and publisher have exerted every effort to ensure that drug selection
and dosage set forth in this text are in accordance with the current recommendations and
practice at the time of publication. However, in view of ongoing research, changes in govern-
ment regulations, and the constant flow of information relating to drug therapy and drug reactions, the reader is urged to check the package insert for each drug for any change in
indications and dosage and for added warnings and precautions. This is particularly important when the recommended agent is a new or infrequently employed drug.
  Some drugs and medical devices presented in this publication have U.S. Food and Drug
Administration (FDA) clearance for limited use in restricted research settings. It is the responsibility of the healthcare provider to ascertain the FDA status of each drug or device
planned for use in his or her clinical practice.

LWW.com

To John, Jenn, and Anna:
The best support system anyone could ask for.

Contributors and Reviewers

CONTRIBUTORS

Lynn Burbank, RN, CPNP, MSN
Learning Resource Coordinator
Dixon School of Nursing
Abington Memorial Hospital
Abington, Pennsylvania
Medications

REVIEWERS

Rose A. Harding, MSN, RN
Instructor
Lamar University
JoAnne Gay Dishman
     Department of Nursing
Beaumont, Texas

Patti Simmons, RN, MN, CHPN
Assistant Professor of Nursing
North Georgia College and State
     University
Dahlonega, Georgia

Diane E. Witt, RN, PhD, CNP
Assistant Professor
School of Nursing
Minnesota State University
Mankato, Minnesota

Preface

Taylor's Handbook of Clinical Nursing Skills is a quick-reference guide to basic and advanced nursing skills. It outlines step-by-step instructions and reinforces the cognitive and technical knowledge needed to perform skills safely and effectively. The convenient handbook format is helpful for student review in the lab or clinical setting and as a reference for graduate nurses in practice.

LEARNING EXPERIENCE

This text and the entire Taylor Suite have been created with the student's experience in mind. Care has been taken to appeal to all learning styles. The student-friendly writing style ensures that students will comprehend and retain information. The extensive art program enhances understanding of important actions. In addition, each element of the Taylor Suite, which is described later in the preface, coordinates the information to provide a consistent and cohesive learning experience.

ORGANIZATION

In general, the content of this book provides streamlined skills consistent with those in *Taylor's Clinical Nursing Skills*, *3rd Edition*. Skills are organized alphabetically, based on the main word(s) of the skill, allowing the user to access the information about the desired skill quickly and easily.

FEATURES

- **Step-by-Step Skills.** Each skill is presented in a concise, straight-forward, and simplified two-column format to facilitate competent performance of nursing skills.
- The **nursing process** framework is used to integrate related nursing responsibilities for each of the five steps.
- **Scientific rationales** accompany each nursing action to promote a deeper understanding of the basic principles supporting nursing care.
- **Hand hygiene** icons alert you to this crucial step that is the best way to prevent the spread of microorganisms.

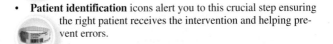

- **Patient identification** icons alert you to this crucial step ensuring the right patient receives the intervention and helping prevent errors.

- **Documentation guidelines** direct students and graduate nurses in accurate documentation of the skill and their findings.
- **General considerations** appear throughout to explain the varying needs of patients across the lifespan and in various settings.
- **Photos.** Key steps are clarified and reinforced with pictures.

TAYLOR SUITE RESOURCES

From traditional texts to video and interactive products, the Taylor Fundamentals/Skills Suite is tailored to fit every learning style. This integrated suite of products offers students a seamless learning experience you will not find anywhere else. The following products accompany *Taylor's Handbook of Clinical Nursing Skills:*

- *Fundamentals of Nursing: The Art and Science of Nursing Care,* **7th Edition**, by Carol Taylor, Carol Lillis, Priscilla LeMone, and Pamela Lynn. This traditional **fundamentals** text promotes nursing as an evolving art and science, directed to human health and well-being. It challenges students to focus on the four blended skills of nursing care, which prepare students to combine the highest level of scientific knowledge and technologic skill with responsible, caring practice. The text includes engaging features to promote critical thinking and comprehension.

- *Taylor's Clinical Nursing Skills,* **3rd Edition**, by Pamela Lynn, MSN, RN. This text covers all of the *Skills* and *Guidelines for Nursing Care* identified in *Fundamentals of Nursing,* as well as additional skills, at the basic, intermediate, and advanced levels. Each Skill follows the nursing process format. Features include Fundamentals Review displays, which reinforce important concepts; Skill Variations, which present alternate techniques; Documentation Guidelines and Samples; Unexpected Situations and Associated Interventions; and Special Considerations. A new feature for the third edition, Evidence for Practice, highlights available best practice guidelines and/or research-based evidence to support the skills as available.

- *Taylor's Video Guide to Clinical Nursing Skills,* **2nd Edition.** From reinforcing fundamental nursing skills to troubleshooting clinical problems on the fly, this dynamic video series follows nursing students and their instructors as they perform and discuss a range of essential nursing procedures. The second edition of these videos is updated with tons of brand new footage to reflect the most current best practice, to address changes in medication administration and equipment, and to include even more skills. Ideal as a stand-alone learning tool or as a companion to this book, these videos parallel the text and are organized into topical modules for easy reference. The videos are available in DVD/DVD-ROM or video streaming versions for purchase by schools. Student versions of the videos are available on DVD/DVD-ROM or online through thePoint.

Contact your sales representative or check out LWW.com/Nursing for more details and ordering information.

Pamela Lynn, MSN, RN

*Material related to nursing diagnoses from *Nursing Diagnoses—Definitions and Classification 2009–2011.* Copyright © 2009, 2007, 2005, 2003, 2001, 1998, 1996, 1994 by NANDA International. Used by arrangement with Wiley-Blackwell Publishing, a company of John Wiley & Sons, Inc. In order to make safe and effective judgments using NANDA-I nursing diagnoses, it is essential that nurses refer to the definitions and defining characteristics of the diagnoses listed in this work.

Acknowledgments

This edition is the work of many talented people. I would like to acknowledge the hard work of all who have contributed to the completion of this project. Thanks to Carol Taylor, Carol Lillis, and Priscilla LeMone for offering generous support and encouragement. You have been excellent mentors.

The work of this book was skillfully coordinated by my dedicated Product Manager, Michelle Clarke, in the Nursing Education division of Lippincott Williams & Wilkins. I am grateful to you for your patience, support, unending encouragement, and total commitment. My thanks to Jean Rodenberger, Executive Acquisitions Editor, for her hard work and guidance throughout most of the project. Thank you to the members of the production department, who patiently pulled everything together to form a completed book: Helen Ewan, Director of Nursing Production; Cindy Rudy, Vendor Manager; Holly Reid McLaughlin, Design Coordinator; and Brett MacNaughton, Illustration Coordinator.

A special thanks to my colleagues at Gwynedd-Mercy College, who offer unending support and professional guidance.

Finally, I would like to gratefully acknowledge my family, for their love, understanding, and encouragement. Their support was essential during the long hours of research and writing.

Pamela Lynn, MSN, RN

Contents

Skill · 1   Assisting a Patient with Ambulation

Walking exercises most of the body's muscles and increases joint flexibility. It improves respiratory and gastrointestinal function. Ambulating also reduces the risk for complications of immobility. However, even a short period of immobility can decrease a person's tolerance for ambulating. If necessary, make use of appropriate equipment and assistive devices to aid in patient movement and handling.

EQUIPMENT
- Gait belt, as necessary
- Nonskid shoes or slippers
- Nonsterile gloves and/or other PPE, as indicated
- Stand-assist device, as necessary, if available
- Additional staff for assistance, as needed

ASSESSMENT GUIDELINES
- Assess the patient's ability to walk and the need for assistance. Review the patient's record for conditions that may affect ambulation.
- Perform a pain assessment before the time for the activity. If the patient reports pain, administer the prescribed medication in sufficient time to allow for the full effect of the analgesic.
- Take vital signs and assess the patient for dizziness or lightheadedness with position changes.

NURSING DIAGNOSES
- Impaired Physical Mobility
- Impaired Walking
- Deficient Knowledge
- Impaired Bed Mobility
- Acute Pain
- Activity Intolerance
- Chronic Pain
- Fatigue

OUTCOME IDENTIFICATION AND PLANNING
Expected outcomes may include:
- The patient ambulates safely, without falls or injury.
- The patient improves or maintains muscle strength.
- The patient's level of independence increases.
- The patient remains free of complications of immobility.

IMPLEMENTATION

ACTION	RATIONALE

1. Review the medical record and nursing plan of care for conditions that may influence the patient's ability to move and ambulate. Assess for tubes, IV lines, incisions, or equipment that may alter the procedure for ambulation. Identify any movement limitations.

   Reviewing the medical record and plan of care validates the correct patient and correct procedure. Checking for equipment and limitations reduces the risk for patient injury.

2. Perform hand hygiene. Put on PPE as indicated.

   Hand hygiene and PPE prevent the spread of microorganisms. PPE is required based on transmission precautions.

3. Identify the patient. Explain the procedure to the patient. Ask the patient to report any feelings of dizziness, weakness, or shortness of breath while walking. Decide how far to walk.

   Patient identification validates the correct patient and correct procedure. Discussion and explanation help allay anxiety and prepare the patient for what to expect.

4. Place the bed in the lowest position.

   Proper bed height ensures safety when getting the patient out of bed.

5. Encourage the patient to make use of a stand-assist aid, either free-standing or attached to the side of the bed, if available, to move to the side of the bed. Assist the patient to the side of the bed, if necessary.

   Encourages independence, reduces strain for staff, and decreases risk for patient injury.

6. Have the patient sit on the side of the bed for several minutes and assess for dizziness or lightheadedness. Have the patient stay sitting until he or she feels secure.

   Having the patient sit at the side of the bed minimizes the risk for blood pressure changes (orthostatic hypotension) that can occur with position change. Allowing the patient to sit until he or she feels secure reduces anxiety and helps prevent injury.

ACTION	RATIONALE
7. Assist the patient to put on footwear and a robe, if desired.	Doing so ensures safety and patient warmth.
8. Wrap the gait belt around the patient's waist, based on assessed need and facility policy.	Gait belts improve the caregiver's grasp, reducing the risk of musculoskeletal injuries to staff and the patient. The belt also provides a firmer grasp for the caregiver if the patient should lose his or her balance.
9. Encourage the patient to make use of the stand-assist device. Assist the patient to stand, using the gait belt, if necessary. Assess the patient's balance and leg strength. If the patient is weak or unsteady, return the patient to bed or assist to a chair.	Use of gait belt prevents injury to nurse and patient. Assessing balance and strength helps to identify need for additional assistance to prevent falling.
10. If you are the only nurse assisting, position yourself to the side and slightly behind the patient. Support the patient by the waist or transfer belt (FIGURE 1).	Positioning to the side and slightly behind the patient encourages the patient to stand and walk erect. It also places the nurse in a safe position if the patient should lose his or her balance or begin to fall.

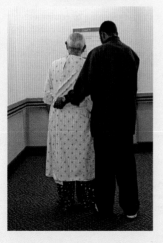

FIGURE 1 Nurse positioned to the side and slightly behind the patient while walking, supporting the patient by the gait belt or waist.

ACTION	RATIONALE
When two nurses assist, position yourself to the side and slightly behind the patient, supporting the patient by the waist or gait belt. Have the other nurse carry or manage equipment or provide additional support from the other side.	Gait belts improve the caregiver's grasp, reducing the risk of musculoskeletal injuries to staff and the patient, and allow for a firmer grasp for the caregiver if patient should lose his or her balance.
Alternatively, when two nurses assist, stand at the patient's sides (one nurse on each side) with near hands grasping the gait belt and far hands holding the patient's lower arm or hand.	Gait belts improve the caregiver's grasp, reducing the risk of musculoskeletal injuries to staff and the patient, and allow for a firmer grasp for the caregiver if patient should lose his or her balance.
11. Take several steps forward with the patient. Continue to assess the patient's strength and balance. Remind the patient to stand erect.	Taking several steps with the patient and standing erect promote good balance and stability. Continued assessment helps maintain patient safety.
12. Continue with ambulation for the planned distance and time. Return the patient to the bed or chair, based on the patient's tolerance and condition.	Ambulation as prescribed promotes activity and prevents fatigue.
13. Remove gait belt. Clean transfer aids, per facility policy, if not indicated for single patient use. Remove gloves and any other PPE, if used. Perform hand hygiene.	Proper cleaning of equipment between patient use prevents the spread of microorganisms. Removing PPE properly reduces the risk for infection transmission and contamination of other items. Hand hygiene prevents the spread of microorganisms.

EVALUATION

• The patient ambulates safely for the prescribed distance and time and remains free from falls or injury.
• The patient exhibits increasing muscle strength, joint mobility.
• The patient exhibits increasing independence.
• The patient remains free of any signs and symptoms of immobility.

DOCUMENTATION

- Document the activity, any observations, the patient's tolerance of the procedure, and the distance walked. Document the use of transfer aids and number of staff required for transfer.

GENERAL CONSIDERATIONS

- Secure all equipment, such as indwelling urinary catheters, drains, or IV infusions, to a pole for ambulation.
- Do not carry equipment while helping the patient. Your hands should be free to provide support.

Skill · 2   Assisting a Patient with Ambulation Using a Cane

Canes are useful for patients who can bear weight but need support for balance. They are also useful for patients who have decreased strength in one leg. Canes provide an additional point of support during ambulation. Canes are made of wood or metal and often have a rubberized cap on the tip to prevent slipping. Canes come in three variations: single-ended canes with half-circle handles (recommended for patients requiring minimal support and for those who will be using stairs frequently); single-ended canes with straight handles (recommended for patients with hand weakness because the handgrip is easier to hold, but not recommended for patients with poor balance); canes with three (tripod) or four prongs (quad cane) or legs to provide a wide base of support (recommended for patients with poor balance). The cane should rise from the floor to the height of the person's waist, and the elbow should be flexed about 30 degrees when holding the cane. The patient holds the cane in the hand opposite the weak or injured leg.

EQUIPMENT

- Cane of appropriate size with rubber tip
- Nonskid shoes or slippers
- Nonsterile gloves and/or other PPE, as indicated
- Stand-assist aid, if necessary and available
- Gait belt, based on assessment

ASSESSMENT GUIDELINES

- Assess the patient's upper body strength, ability to bear weight, ability to walk, and the need for assistance. Review the patient's record for conditions that may affect ambulation.
- Perform a pain assessment before the time for the activity. If the patient reports pain, administer the prescribed medication in sufficient time to allow for the full effect of the analgesic.

- Take vital signs and assess the patient for dizziness or light-headedness with position changes.
- Assess for muscle strength in the legs and arms.
- Assess the patient's knowledge regarding the use of a cane.

NURSING DIAGNOSES

- Impaired Walking
- Deficient Knowledge
- Acute Pain
- Activity Intolerance
- Chronic Pain
- Risk for Falls

OUTCOME IDENTIFICATION AND PLANNING

Expected outcomes may include:
- The patient ambulates safely without falls or injury.
- The patient demonstrates proper use of the cane.
- The patient demonstrates increased muscle strength and joint mobility.
- The patient demonstrates increased independence.

IMPLEMENTATION

ACTION	RATIONALE
1. Review the medical record and nursing plan of care for conditions that may influence the patient's ability to move and ambulate. Assess for tubes, IV lines, incisions, or equipment that may alter the procedure for ambulation.	Review of the medical record and plan of care validates the correct patient and correct procedure. Identification of equipment and limitations helps reduce the risk for injury.
2. Perform hand hygiene. Put on PPE, as indicated.	Hand hygiene and PPE prevent the spread of microorganisms. PPE is required based on transmission precautions.
3. Identify the patient. Explain the procedure to the patient. Tell the patient to report any feelings of dizziness, weakness, or shortness of breath while walking. Decide how far to walk.	Patient identification validates the correct patient and correct procedure. Discussion and explanation help allay anxiety and prepare the patient for what to expect.

ACTION	RATIONALE
4. Encourage the patient to make use of a stand-assist aid, either free standing or attached to the side of the bed, if available, to move to and sit on the side of the bed.	Encourages independence, reduces strain for staff, and decreases risk for patient injury.
5. Wrap the gait belt around the patient's waist, based on assessed need and facility policy.	Gait belts improve the caregiver's grasp, reducing the risk of musculoskeletal injuries to staff and the patient and provide firmer grasp for the caregiver if patient should lose his or her balance.
6. Encourage the patient to make use of the stand-assist device to stand with weight evenly distributed between the feet and the cane.	A stand-assist device reduces strain for caregiver and decreases the risk for patient injury. Evenly distributed weight provides a broad base of support and balance.
7. Have the patient hold the cane on his or her stronger side, close to the body, while you stand to the side and slightly behind the patient. (FIGURE 1).	Holding the cane on the stronger side helps to distribute the patient's weight away from the involved side and prevents leaning. Positioning to the side and slightly behind the patient encourages the patient to stand and walk erect. It also places the nurse in a safe position if the patient should lose his or her balance or begin to fall.

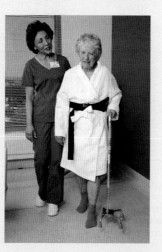

FIGURE 1 The nurse stands slightly behind the patient. The cane is held on the patient's stronger side close to the body.

ACTION	RATIONALE
8. Tell the patient to advance the cane 4 to 12 inches (10 to 30 cm) and then, while supporting his or her weight on the stronger leg and the cane, advance the weaker foot forward, parallel with the cane.	Moving in this manner provides support and balance.
9. While supporting his or her weight on the weaker leg and the cane, have the patient advance the stronger leg forward ahead of the cane (heel slightly beyond the tip of the cane).	Moving in this manner provides support and balance.
10. Tell the patient to move the weaker leg forward until it is even with the stronger leg, and then advance the cane again.	This motion provides support and balance.
11. Continue with ambulation for the planned distance and time. Return the patient to the bed or chair, based on the patient's tolerance and condition, ensuring the patient's comfort. Make sure call bell and other necessary items are within easy reach.	Continued ambulation promotes activity. Adhering to the planned distance and patient's tolerance prevents the patient from becoming fatigued.
12. Clean the transfer aids, per facility policy, if not indicated for single patient use. Remove PPE, if used. Perform hand hygiene.	Proper cleaning of equipment between patient use prevents the spread of microorganisms. Removing PPE properly reduces the risk for infection transmission and contamination of other items. Hand hygiene prevents the spread of microorganisms.

EVALUATION

• The patient uses the cane to ambulate safely and is free from falls or injury.
• The patient demonstrates proper use of the cane.
• The patient exhibits increased muscle strength, joint mobility, and independence.

DOCUMENTATION

• Document the activity, any observations, the patient's ability to use the cane, the patient's tolerance of the procedure, and the distance walked. Document the use of transfer aids and the number of staff required for transfer.

GENERAL CONSIDERATIONS

• Patients with bilateral weakness should not use a cane. Crutches or a walker would be more appropriate.
• To climb stairs, the patient should advance the stronger leg up the stair first, followed by the cane and weaker leg. To descend, reverse the process.
• When less support is required from the cane, the patient can advance the cane and weaker leg forward simultaneously while the stronger leg supports the patient's weight.
• Teach patients to position their canes within easy reach when they sit down so that they can rise easily.

| Skill · 3 | Assisting a Patient with Ambulation Using Crutches |

Crutches enable a patient to walk and remove weight from one or both legs. The patient uses the arms to support the body weight. Crutches can be used for the short or the long term. This section discusses short-term crutch use. Crutches must be fitted to each person. Have the patient stand up straight with the palm of the hand pressed against the body under the arm. The hand should fit between the top of the crutches and the armpit. When using crutches, the elbow should be slightly bent at about 30 degrees and the hands, not the armpits, should support the patient's weight. Weight on the armpits can cause nerve damage. If anything needs to be carried, it is best to use a backpack (University of Iowa, 2006). The procedure for crutch walking is usually taught by a physical therapist, but it is important for the nurse to be knowledgeable about the patient's progress and the gait being taught. Be prepared to guide the patient at home or in the hospital after the initial teaching is completed. Remind the patient that the support of body weight should come primarily on the hands and arms while using the crutches. There are a number of different ways to walk using crutches, based on how much weight the patient is allowed to bear on one or both legs.

EQUIPMENT

• Crutches with axillary pads, hand grips, and rubber suction tips
• Nonskid shoes or slippers
• Nonsterile gloves and/or other PPE, as indicated
• Stand-assist device, as necessary, if available

ASSESSMENT GUIDELINES

• Review the patient's record and nursing plan of care to determine the reason for using crutches and instructions for weight-bearing. Check for specific instructions from Physical Therapy.
• Perform a pain assessment before the time for the activity. If the patient reports pain, administer the prescribed medication in sufficient time to allow for the full effect of the analgesic.
• Determine the patient's knowledge regarding the use of crutches and assess the patient's ability to balance on the crutches.
• Assess for muscle strength in the legs and arms.
• Determine the appropriate gait for the patient to use.

NURSING DIAGNOSES

• Impaired Walking
• Deficient Knowledge
• Acute Pain
• Activity Intolerance
• Chronic Pain
• Risk for Falls

OUTCOME IDENTIFICATION AND PLANNING

Expected outcomes may include:
• The patient ambulates safely with the crutches and is free from falls or injury.
• The patient demonstrates proper crutch-walking technique.
• The patient demonstrates increased muscle strength and joint mobility.

IMPLEMENTATION

ACTION	RATIONALE
1. Review the medical record and nursing plan of care for conditions that may influence the patient's ability to move and ambulate. Assess for tubes, IV lines, incisions, or equipment that may alter the procedure for ambulation. Assess the patient's knowledge and previous experience regarding the use of crutches. Determine that the appropriate size crutch has been obtained.	Reviewing the medical record and plan of care validates the correct patient and correct procedure. Assessment helps identify problem areas to minimize the risk for injury.

ACTION	RATIONALE
2. Perform hand hygiene. Put on PPE, if indicated.	Hand hygiene and PPE prevent the spread of microorganisms. PPE is required based on transmission precautions.
3. Identify the patient. Explain the procedure to the patient. Tell the patient to report any feelings of dizziness, weakness, or shortness of breath while walking. Decide how far to walk.	Patient identification validates the correct patient and correct procedure. Discussion and explanation help allay anxiety and prepare the patient for what to expect.
4. **Encourage the patient to make use of the stand-assist device, if available.** Assist the patient to stand erect, face forward in the tripod position (FIGURE 1). This means the patient holds the crutches 12 inches in front of and 12 inches to the side of each foot.	Stand-assist device reduces caregiver strain and decreases risk of patient injury. Positioning the crutches in this manner provides a wide base of support to increase stability and balance.

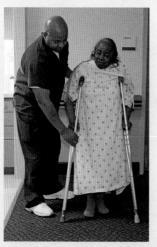

FIGURE 1 Assisting the patient to stand erect facing forward in the tripod position.

ACTION	RATIONALE
5. For the four-point gait:	This movement ensures stability and safety.
a. Have the patient move the right crutch forward 12 inches and then move the left foot forward to the level of the right crutch.	
b. Then have the patient move the left crutch forward 12 inches and then move the right foot forward to the level of the left crutch.	
6. For the three-point gait:	Patient bears weight on the stronger leg.
a. Have the patient move the affected leg and both crutches forward about 12 inches.	
b. Have the patient move the stronger leg forward to the level of the crutches.	
7. For the two-point gait:	Patient bears partial weight on both feet.
a. Have the patient move the left crutch and the right foot forward about 12 inches at the same time.	
b. Have the patient move the right crutch and left leg forward to the level of the left crutch at the same time.	
8. For the swing-to gait:	Swing-to gait provides mobility for patients with weakness or paralysis of the hips or legs.
a. Have the patient move both crutches forward about 12 inches.	
b. Have the patient lift the legs and swing them to the crutches, supporting his or her body weight on the crutches.	
9. Continue with ambulation for the planned distance and time. Return the patient to the bed or chair based on the	Continued ambulation promotes activity. Adhering to the planned distance and time prevents the patient from becoming fatigued.

ACTION	RATIONALE

patient's tolerance and condition, ensuring that the patient is comfortable and that the call light is within reach.

10. Remove PPE, if used. Perform hand hygiene.

Removing PPE properly reduces the risk for infection transmission and contamination of other items. Hand hygiene prevents the spread of microorganisms.

EVALUATION
- The patient demonstrates correct use of crutches to ambulate safely and without injury.
- The patient demonstrates increased muscle strength and joint mobility.

DOCUMENTATION
- Document the activity, any observations, the patient's ability to use the crutches, the patient's tolerance of the procedure, and the distance walked. Document the use of transfer aids and number of staff required for transfer.

GENERAL CONSIDERATIONS
- Crutches can be used when climbing stairs. The patient grasps both crutches as one on one side of the body and uses the stair railing. Have the patient stand in the tripod position facing the stairs. The patient transfers his or her weight to the crutches and holds the railing. The patient places the unaffected leg on the first stair tread. The patient then transfers his or her weight to the unaffected leg, moving up onto the stair tread. The patient moves the crutches and affected leg up to the stair tread and continues to the top of the stairs. Using this process, the crutches always support the affected leg.
- Long-term use of the swing-to gait can lead to atrophy of the hips and legs. Include appropriate exercises in the patient's plan of care to avoid this complication.
- Patients should not lean on the crutches. Prolonged pressure on the axillae can damage the brachial nerves, causing brachial nerve palsy, with resulting loss of sensation and inability to move the upper extremities.
- Patients using crutches should perform arm- and shoulder-strengthening exercises to aid with crutch walking.

| Skill · 4 | **Assisting a Patient with Ambulation Using a Walker** |

A walker is a lightweight metal frame with four legs. Walkers provide stability and security for patients with insufficient strength and balance to use other ambulatory aids. There are several kinds of walkers; the choice of which to use is based on the patient's arm strength and balance. Regardless of the type used, the patient stands between the back legs of the walker with arms relaxed at the side; the top of the walker should line up with the crease on the inside of the patient's wrist. When the patient's hands are placed on the grips, elbows should be flexed about 30 degrees (Mayo Clinic, 2007). Usually, the legs of the walker can be adjusted to the appropriate height.

EQUIPMENT

- Walker, adjusted to the appropriate height
- Nonskid shoes or slippers
- Nonsterile gloves and/or other PPE, as indicated
- Additional staff for assistance, as needed
- Stand-assist device, as necessary, if available
- Gait belt

ASSESSMENT GUIDELINES

- Assess the patient's ability to walk and the need for assistance. Review the patient's record for conditions that may affect ambulation.
- Perform a pain assessment before the time for the activity. If the patient reports pain, administer the prescribed medication in sufficient time to allow for the full effect of the analgesic.
- Take vital signs and assess the patient for dizziness or lightheadedness with position changes.
- Assess the patient's knowledge regarding the use of a walker. Ensure that the walker is at the appropriate height for the patient.

NURSING DIAGNOSES

- Risk for Falls
- Impaired Walking
- Deficient Knowledge
- Risk for Injury
- Activity Intolerance
- Acute Pain
- Chronic Pain
- Fatigue

OUTCOME IDENTIFICATION AND PLANNING

Expected outcomes may include:
- The patient ambulates safely with the walker and is free from falls or injury.

- The patient demonstrates proper use of the walker and states the need for the walker.
- The patient's level of independence increases.
- The patient demonstrates increasing muscle strength and joint mobility.
- The patient remains free of complications of immobility.

IMPLEMENTATION

ACTION	RATIONALE
1. Review the medical record and nursing plan of care for conditions that may influence the patient's ability to move and ambulate, and for specific instructions for ambulation, such as distance. Assess for tubes, IV lines, incisions, or equipment that may alter the procedure for ambulation. Assess the patient's knowledge and previous experience regarding the use of a walker. Identify any movement limitations.	Reviewing the medical record and plan of care validates the correct patient and correct procedure. Checking for equipment and limitations helps minimize the risk for injury.
2. Perform hand hygiene. Put on PPE, if indicated.	Hand hygiene and PPE prevent the spread of microorganisms. PPE is required based on Transmission Precautions.
3. Identify the patient. Explain the procedure to the patient. Tell the patient to report any feelings of dizziness, weakness, or shortness of breath while walking. Decide how far to walk.	Patient identification validates the correct patient and correct procedure. Discussion and explanation help allay anxiety and prepare the patient for what to expect.
4. Place the bed in the lowest position, if the patient is in bed.	Proper bed height ensures safety when getting the patient out of bed.
5. **Encourage the patient to make use of a stand-assist aid, either free standing or attached to the side of the bed, if available, to move to the side of the bed.**	Use of assistive devices encourages independence, reduces strain for staff, and decreases risk for patient injury.

ACTION	RATIONALE
6. Assist the patient to the side of the bed, if necessary. Have the patient sit on the side of the bed. Assess for dizziness or lightheadedness. Have the patient stay seated until he or she feels secure.	Having the patient sit on the side of the bed minimizes the risk for blood pressure changes (orthostatic hypotension) that can occur with position change. Assessing patient complaints helps prevent injury.
7. Assist the patient to put on footwear and a robe, if desired.	Doing so ensures safety and warmth.
8. Wrap the gait belt around the patient's waist, based on assessed need and facility policy.	Gait belts improve the caregiver's grasp, reducing the risk of musculoskeletal injuries to staff and the patient and provide for a firmer grasp if patient should lose his or her balance.
9. **Place the walker directly in front of the patient.** Ask the patient to push himself or herself off the bed or chair; make use of the stand-assist device or assist the patient to stand. Once the patient is standing, have him or her hold the walker's hand grips firmly and equally. Stand slightly behind the patient, on one side.	Proper positioning with the walker ensures balance. Standing within the walker and holding the hand grips firmly provide stability when moving the walker and helps ensure safety. Positioning to the side and slightly behind the patient encourages the patient to stand and walk erect. It also places the nurse in a safe position if the patient should lose his or her balance or begin to fall.
10. Have the patient move the walker forward 6 to 8 inches and set it down, making sure all four feet of the walker stay on the floor. Then, tell the patient to step forward with either foot into the walker, supporting himself or herself on his or her arms. Follow through with the other leg.	Having all four feet of the walker on the floor provides a broad base of support. Moving the walker and stepping forward moves the center of gravity toward the walker, ensuring balance and preventing tipping of the walker.
11. Move the walker forward again, and continue the same pattern. Continue with ambulation for the planned distance and time (FIGURE 1). Return the patient to the bed or chair	Moving the walker promotes activity. Continuing for the planned distance and time prevents the patient from becoming fatigued.

ACTION	RATIONALE

based on the patient's tolerance and condition, ensuring that the patient is comfortable and the call bell is within reach.

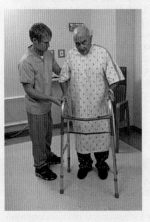

FIGURE 1 Assisting the patient to walk with the walker.

12. Remove the gait belt, if used. Clean transfer aids, per facility policy, if not indicated for single patient use. Remove gloves and any other PPE, if used. Perform hand hygiene.

Proper cleaning of equipment between patient use prevents the spread of microorganisms. Removing PPE properly reduces the risk for infection transmission and contamination of other items. Hand hygiene prevents the spread of microorganisms.

EVALUATION
- The patient uses the walker to ambulate safely and remains free of injury.
- The patient exhibits increasing muscle strength and joint mobility.
- The patient exhibits increasing independence.
- The patient remains free from complications of immobility.

DOCUMENTATION
- Document the activity, any observations, the patient's ability to use the walker, the patient's tolerance of the procedure, and the distance walked. Document the use of transfer aids and number of staff required for transfer.

GENERAL CONSIDERATIONS

- Never use a walker on the stairs.
- The patient should wear nonskid shoes or slippers.
- Some walkers have wheels on the front legs. These walkers are best for patients with a gait that is too fast for a walker without wheels and for patients who have difficulty lifting a walker. This type of walker is rolled forward while the patient walks as normally as possible. Because lifting repeatedly is not required, energy expenditure and stress to the back and upper extremities is lower than with a standard walker (Mincer, 2007).
- Keep in mind, walkers often prove to be difficult to maneuver through doorways and congested areas.
- Advise the patient to check the walker before use for signs of damage, frame deformity, or loose or missing parts.
- Teach patients to use the arms of the chair or a stand-assist device for leverage when getting up from a chair. Explain to patients that they should not pull on the walker to get up; the walker could tip or become unbalanced.

Skill · 5 | **Applying and Removing Antiembolism Stockings**

Antiembolism stockings are often used for patients at risk for deep-vein thrombosis and pulmonary embolism, and to help prevent phlebitis. They are made of elastic material and are available in either knee-high or thigh-high length. By applying pressure, antiembolism stockings increase the velocity of blood flow in the superficial and deep veins and improve venous valve function in the legs, promoting venous return to the heart. A medical order is required for their use. Be prepared to apply the stockings in the morning before the patient is out of bed and while the patient is supine. If the patient is sitting or has been up and about, have the patient lie down with legs and feet elevated for at least 15 minutes before applying the stockings. Otherwise, the leg vessels are congested with blood, reducing the effectiveness of the stockings.

EQUIPMENT

- Elastic antiembolism stockings in ordered length in correct size. See Assessment for appropriate measurement procedure.
- Measuring tape
- Talcum powder (optional)
- Skin cleanser, basin, towel
- Nonsterile gloves
- Additional PPE as indicated

ASSESSMENT GUIDELINES

- Assess the skin condition and neurovascular status of the legs. Report any abnormalities before continuing with the application of the

stockings. Assess patient's legs for any redness, swelling, warmth, tenderness, or pain that may indicate a deep-vein thrombosis. If any of these symptoms are noted, notify the primary care provider before applying the stockings.
- Measure the patient's legs to obtain the correct size stocking. For knee-high length: Measure around the widest part of the calf and the leg length from the bottom of the heel to the back of the knee, at the bend. For thigh-high length: Measure around the widest part of the calf and the thigh. Measure the length from the bottom of the heel to the gluteal fold. Follow the manufacturer's specifications to select the correct sized stockings. Each leg should have a correct fitting stocking; if measurements are different, then two different sizes of stocking need to be ordered to ensure correct fitting on each leg (Walker & Lamont, 2008).

NURSING DIAGNOSES
- Ineffective Peripheral Tissue Perfusion
- Risk for Impaired Skin Integrity
- Excess Fluid Volume
- Risk for Injury

OUTCOME IDENTIFICATION AND PLANNING
Expected outcomes may include:
- The stockings will be applied and removed with minimal discomfort to the patient.
- Edema will decrease in the lower extremities.
- The patient will verbalize an understanding of the rationale for stocking application.
- The patient will remain free of deep-vein thrombosis.

IMPLEMENTATION

ACTION	RATIONALE
1. Review the medical record and medical orders to determine the need for antiembolism stockings.	Reviewing the medical record and order validates the correct patient and correct procedure.
2. Perform hand hygiene. Put on PPE, as indicated.	Hand hygiene and PPE prevent the spread of microorganisms. PPE is required based on transmission precautions.
3. Identify the patient. Explain what you are going to do and the rationale for the use of elastic stockings.	Patient identification validates the correct patient and correct procedure. Discussion and explanation allay anxiety and prepare the patient for what to expect.

ACTION	RATIONALE
4. Close curtains around bed and close the door to the room, if possible.	This ensures the patient's privacy.
5. Adjust the bed to a comfortable working height, usually elbow height of the caregiver (VISN 8 Patient Safety Center, 2009).	Having the bed at the proper height prevents back and muscle strain.
6. Assist the patient to a supine position. If patient has been sitting or walking, have him or her lie down with legs and feet well elevated for at least 15 minutes before applying stockings.	Dependent position of legs encourages blood to pool in the veins, reducing the effectiveness of the stockings if they are applied to congested blood vessels.
7. Expose legs one at a time. Wash and dry legs, if necessary. Powder the leg lightly unless the patient has a breathing problem, dry skin, or sensitivity to the powder. If the skin is dry, a lotion may be used. Powders and lotions are not recommended by some manufacturers; check the package material for manufacturer specifications.	Helps maintain patient's privacy. Powder and lotion reduce friction and make application of stockings easier.
8. Stand at the foot of the bed. Place hand inside stocking and grasp heel area securely. Turn stocking inside-out to the heel area, leaving the foot inside the stocking leg.	Inside-out technique provides for easier application; bunched elastic material can compromise extremity circulation.
9. With the heel pocket down, ease the stocking foot over the patient's foot and heel (FIGURE 1). Check that the patient's heel is centered in heel pocket of stocking.	Wrinkles and improper fit interfere with circulation.
10. Using your fingers and thumbs, carefully grasp the stocking edge and pull it up smoothly over the ankle and	Easing the stocking carefully into position ensures the stocking fits properly to the contour of the leg. Even distribution prevents interference with circulation.

ACTION RATIONALE

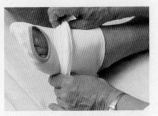

FIGURE 1 Putting foot of stocking onto patient.

calf, toward the knee. Make sure it is distributed evenly.

11. Pull forward slightly on toe section. If the stocking has a toe window, make sure it is properly positioned. Adjust, if necessary, to ensure material is smooth.

Ensures toe comfort and prevents interference with circulation.

12. If the stockings are knee-length, make sure each stocking top is 1 to 2 inches below the patella. Make sure the stocking does not roll down.

Prevents pressure and interference with circulation. Rolling stockings may have a constricting effect on veins.

13. If applying thigh-length stocking, continue the application. Flex the patient's leg. Stretch the stocking over the knee.

This ensures even distribution.

14. Pull the stocking over the thigh until the top is 1 to 3 inches below the gluteal fold (FIGURE 2). Adjust the stocking, as necessary, to distribute the fabric evenly. Make sure the stocking does not roll down.

Prevents excessive pressure and interference with circulation. Rolling stockings may have a constricting effect on veins.

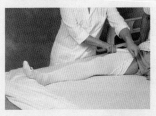

FIGURE 2 Pulling the stocking up over the thigh.

ACTION	RATIONALE
15. Remove equipment and return the patient to a position of comfort. Remove your gloves. Raise side rail and lower bed.	Promotes patient comfort and safety. Removing gloves properly reduces the risk for infection transmission and contamination of other items.
16. Remove any other PPE, if used. Perform hand hygiene.	Removing PPE properly reduces the risk for infection transmission and contamination of other items. Hand hygiene prevents the spread of microorganisms.

Removing Stockings

17. To remove stocking, grasp top of stocking with your thumb and fingers and smoothly pull stocking off inside-out to heel. Support foot and ease stocking over it.	This preserves the elasticity and contour of the stocking. It allows assessment of circulatory status and condition of skin on lower extremity and for skin care.

EVALUATION

- The stockings are applied and removed as indicated.
- The patient exhibits a decrease in peripheral edema.
- The patient can state the reason for using the stockings.

DOCUMENTATION

- Document the patient's leg measurements as a baseline. Document the application of the stockings, size stocking applied, skin and leg assessment, and neurovascular assessment.

GENERAL CONSIDERATIONS

- Remove stockings once every shift for 20 to 30 minutes. Wash and air-dry, as necessary, according to manufacturer's directions.
- Assess at least every shift for skin color, temperature, sensation, swelling, and the ability to move. If complications are evident, remove the stockings and notify the physician or primary care provider.
- Evaluate stockings to ensure the top or toe opening does not roll with movement. Rolled stocking edges can cause excessive pressure and interfere with circulation.
- Despite the use of elastic stockings, a patient may develop deep-vein thrombosis or phlebitis. Unilateral swelling, redness, tenderness, pain, and warmth are possible indicators of these complications. Notify the primary care provider of the presence of any symptoms.

Skill · 6   Removing Arterial and Femoral Lines

Arterial and femoral lines are used for intensive and continuous cardiac monitoring and intraarterial access. Once the lines are no longer necessary or have become ineffective, they need to be removed. Consult facility policy to determine whether nurses are permitted to perform this procedure. Two nurses should be at the bedside until bleeding is controlled, and are available to give emergency medications, if necessary. The patient should be kept NPO until catheter is removed in case of nausea with a vasovagal response.

EQUIPMENT
- Sterile gloves
- Clean gloves
- Goggles or face shield
- Sterile gauze pads
- Waterproof protective pad
- Sterile suture removal set
- Transparent dressing
- Alcohol pads
- Hypoallergenic tape
- For femoral line: small sandbag (5 to 10 pounds), wrapped in towel or pillowcase
- Emergency medications (e.g., atropine, for a vasovagal response with femoral line removal) for emergency response, per facility policy and guidelines
- Indelible pen

ASSESSMENT GUIDELINES
- Review the patient's medical record and plan of care for information about discontinuation of the arterial or femoral line.
- Assess the patient's coagulation status, including laboratory studies, to reduce the risk of complications secondary to impaired clotting ability.
- Assess the patient's understanding of the procedure.
- Inspect the site for leakage, bleeding, or hematoma.
- Assess skin color and temperature and assess distal pulses for strength and quality. Mark distal pulses with an 'X' for easy identification after the procedure.
- Assess patient's blood pressure; systolic blood pressure should be less than 180 mm Hg before catheter is removed.

NURSING DIAGNOSES
- Risk for Injury
- Risk for Infection
- Impaired Skin Integrity
- Anxiety

OUTCOME IDENTIFICATION AND PLANNING
Expected outcomes may include:
- Line is removed intact and without injury to the patient.
- Site remains clean and dry, without evidence of infection, bleeding, or hematoma.

IMPLEMENTATION

ACTION	RATIONALE

1. Verify the order for removal of arterial or femoral line in the patient's medical record.

This ensures that the correct intervention is performed on the correct patient.

2. Gather all equipment and bring to bedside.

Having equipment available saves time and facilitates accomplishment of procedure.

3. Perform hand hygiene and put on PPE, if indicated.

Hand hygiene and PPE prevent the spread of microorganisms. PPE is required based on transmission precautions.

4. Identify the patient.

Identifying the patient ensures the right patient receives the intervention and helps prevent errors.

5. Close curtains around bed and close the door to the room, if possible. Explain the procedure to the patient.

This ensures the patient's privacy. Explanation relieves anxiety and facilitates cooperation.

6. Ask patient to empty bladder. Maintain an IV infusion of normal saline via another venous access during procedure, as per medical orders or facility guidelines.

Emptying the bladder ensures patient comfort. IV access may be needed in case of hypotension or bradycardia.

7. If bed is adjustable, raise bed to comfortable working height, usually elbow height of the caregiver (VISN 8 Patient Safety Center, 2009).

Having the bed at the proper height prevents back and muscle strain.

8. Put on clean gloves, goggles, and gown.

These prevent contact with blood and body fluids.

9. If line being removed is in a femoral site, use Doppler ultrasound to locate the femoral artery 1 to 2 inches above the entrance site of the femoral line. Mark with 'X' using indelible marker.

This ensures accurate location of femoral artery.

10. Turn off the monitor alarms and then turn off the flow

These measures help prepare for withdrawal of the line.

ACTION	RATIONALE
clamp to the flush solution. Carefully remove the dressing over the insertion site. Remove any sutures using the suture removal kit; make sure all sutures have been removed.	
11. **Withdraw the catheter using a gentle, steady motion. Keep the catheter parallel to the blood vessel during withdrawal. Watch for hematoma formation during catheter removal by gently palpating surrounding tissue. If hematoma starts to form, reposition hands until optimal pressure is obtained to prevent further leakage of blood.**	Using a gentle, steady motion parallel to the blood vessel reduces the risk for traumatic injury.
12. **Immediately after withdrawing the catheter, apply pressure 1 or 2 inches above the site at the previously marked spot with a sterile 4 × 4 gauze pad. Maintain pressure for at least 10 minutes, or per facility policy (longer if bleeding or oozing persists). Apply additional pressure to a femoral site if the patient has coagulopathy or is receiving anticoagulants.**	If sufficient pressure is not applied, a large, painful hematoma may form.
13. **Assess distal pulses every 3 to 5 minutes while pressure is being applied. Note: Dorsalis pedis and posterior tibial pulses should be markedly weaker from baseline if sufficient pressure is applied to the femoral artery.**	Assessment of distal pulses determines blood flow to the extremity. Pulses should return to baseline after pressure is released.
14. **Cover the site with an appropriate dressing and secure the dressing with tape. If**	Sufficient pressure is needed to prevent continued bleeding and hematoma formation.

ACTION	RATIONALE
stipulated by facility policy, make a pressure dressing for a femoral site by folding four sterile 4 × 4 gauze pads in half, and apply the dressing.	
15. Cover the dressing with a tight adhesive bandage, per policy, and then cover the femoral bandage with a sandbag. Remove gloves. Maintain the patient on bed rest, with the head of the bed elevated less than 30 degrees, for 6 hours with the sandbag in place. Lower bed height. Remind the patient not to lift his or her head while on bed rest.	Sufficient pressure is needed to prevent continued bleeding and hematoma formation. Removing gloves properly reduces the risk for infection transmission and contamination of other items. Raising head of the bed increases intraabdominal pressure, which could lead to bleeding from site.
16. Remove additional PPE. Perform hand hygiene. Send specimens to the laboratory immediately.	Removing PPE properly reduces the risk for infection transmission and contamination of other items. Hand hygiene prevents transmission of microorganisms. Specimens must be processed in a timely manner to ensure accuracy.
17. Observe the site for bleeding. Assess circulation in the extremity distal to the site by evaluating color, pulses, and sensation. Repeat this assessment every 15 minutes for the first 1 hour, every 30 minutes for the next 2 hours, hourly for the next 2 hours, then every 4 hours, or according to facility policy. Use log roll to assist patient in using bedpan, if needed.	Continued assessment allows for early detection and prompt intervention should problems arise.

EVALUATION

• Patient exhibits an arterial or femoral line site that is clean and dry without evidence of injury, infection, bleeding, or hematoma.
• Patient demonstrates intact peripheral circulation and verbalizes a reduction in anxiety.

DOCUMENTATION

- Document the time the line was removed and how long pressure was applied.
- Document site assessment every 5 minutes while pressure is being applied (second nurse can do this).
- Document assessment of peripheral circulation, appearance of site, type of dressing applied, the timed assessments, patient's response, and any medications given.

GENERAL CONSIDERATIONS

- Sometimes, a culture of the catheter tip is ordered to aid in identifying the source of infection. If ordered, place the catheter tip on a 4 × 4 sterile gauze pad. After the bleeding is under control and the dressing is secure, hold the catheter over the sterile container. Cut the tip of the catheter with sterile scissors and allow it to fall into the sterile container. Label the specimen and send it to the laboratory.

Skill · 7   Giving a Back Massage

Massage has many benefits, including general relaxation and increased circulation. Massage can help alleviate pain (The Joint Commission, 2008). A back massage can be incorporated into the patient's bath, as part of care before bedtime, or at any time to promote increased patient comfort. Some nurses do not always give back massages to patients because they do not think they have enough time. However, giving a back massage provides an opportunity for the nurse to observe the skin for signs of breakdown. It improves circulation; decreases pain, symptom distress, and anxiety; improves sleep quality; and also provides a means of communicating with the patient through the use of touch. A back massage also provides cutaneous stimulation as a method of pain relief.

Because some patients consider the back massage a luxury and may be reluctant to accept it, communicate its importance and value to the patient. An effective back massage should take 4 to 6 minutes to complete. A lotion is usually used; warm it before applying to the back. Be aware of the patient's medical diagnosis when considering giving a back massage. A back massage is contraindicated, for example, when the patient has had back surgery or has fractured ribs. Position the patient on the abdomen or, if this is contraindicated, on the side for a back massage.

EQUIPMENT

- Massage lubricant or lotion, warmed
- Pain assessment tool and/or scale
- Powder, if not contraindicated
- Bath blanket
- Towel
- Nonsterile gloves, if indicated
- Additional PPE, as indicated

ASSESSMENT GUIDELINES

- Review the patient's medical record and plan of care for information about the patient's status and contraindications to back massage. Question the patient about any conditions that might require modifications or that might contraindicate a massage. Inquire about any allergies, such as to lotions or scents.
- Ask if the patient has any preferences for lotion or has his or her own lotion.
- Assess the patient's level of pain.
- Check the patient's medication administration record for the time an analgesic was last administered. If appropriate, administer an analgesic early enough so that it has time to take effect.

NURSING DIAGNOSES

- Acute Pain
- Deficient Knowledge
- Chronic Pain
- Anxiety
- Disturbed Sleep Pattern
- Risk for Impaired Skin Integrity
- Activity Intolerance

OUTCOME IDENTIFICATION AND PLANNING

Expected outcomes may include:
- Patient reports increased comfort and/or decreased pain.
- Patient displays decreased anxiety and improved relaxation.
- Patient is free of skin breakdown.
- Patient verbalizes an understanding of the reasons for back massage.

IMPLEMENTATION

ACTION	RATIONALE
1. Perform hand hygiene and put on PPE, if indicated.	Hand hygiene and PPE prevent the spread of microorganisms. PPE is required based on transmission precautions.
2. Identify the patient.	Identifying the patient ensures the right patient receives the intervention and helps prevent errors.
3. Offer a back massage to the patient and explain the procedure.	Explanation encourages patient understanding and cooperation and reduces apprehension.

ACTION	RATIONALE
4. Put on gloves, if indicated.	Gloves are not usually necessary. Gloves prevent contact with blood and body fluid.
5. Close room door or curtain.	Closing the door or curtain provides privacy, promotes relaxation, and reduces noise and stimuli that may aggravate pain and reduce comfort.
6. Assess the patient's pain, using an appropriate assessment tool and measurement scale.	Accurate assessment is necessary to guide treatment/relief interventions and to evaluate the effectiveness of pain control measures.
7. Raise bed to a comfortable working position, usually elbow height of the caregiver (VISN 8, Patient Safety Center, 2009), and lower the side rail.	Having the bed at the proper height prevents back and muscle strain.
8. Assist the patient to a comfortable position, preferably the prone or side-lying position. Remove the covers and move the patient's gown just enough to expose the patient's back from the shoulders to the sacral area. Drape the patient, as needed, with the bath blanket.	This position exposes an adequate area for massage. Draping the patient provides privacy and warmth.
9. Warm the lubricant or lotion in the palm of your hand, or place the container in small basin of warm water. **During massage, observe the patient's skin for reddened or open areas. Pay particular attention to the skin over bony prominences.**	Cold lotion causes chilling and discomfort. Pressure may interfere with circulation and lead to pressure ulcers.
10. Using light gliding strokes (*effleurage*), apply lotion to the patient's shoulders, back, and sacral area (FIGURE 1).	Effleurage relaxes the patient and lessens tension.
11. Place your hands beside each other at the base of the patient's spine and stroke upward to the shoulders and back downward to the	Continuous contact is soothing and stimulates circulation and muscle relaxation.

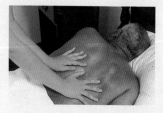

FIGURE 1 Using effleurage on a patient's back.

buttocks in slow, continuous strokes. Continue for several minutes.

12. Massage the patient's shoulder, entire back, areas over iliac crests, and sacrum with circular stroking motions. **Keep your hands in contact with the patient's skin.** Continue for several minutes, applying additional lotion, as necessary.

A firm stroke with continuous contact promotes relaxation.

13. Knead the patient's skin by gently alternating grasping and compression motions (*pétrissage*) (FIGURE 2).

Kneading increases blood circulation.

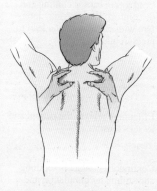

FIGURE 2 Using pétrissage.

14. Complete the massage with additional long stroking

Long, stroking motions are soothing and promote relaxation;

ACTION	RATIONALE

movements that eventually become lighter in pressure.

continued stroking with gradual lightening of pressure helps extend the feeling of relaxation.

15. Use the towel to pat the patient dry and to remove excess lotion.

Drying provides comfort and reduces the feeling of moisture on the back.

16. Remove gloves, if worn. Reposition patient's gown and covers. Raise side rail and lower the bed. Assist patient to a position of comfort.

Repositioning bedclothes, linens, and the patient helps to promote patient comfort and safety.

17. Remove additional PPE, if used. Perform hand hygiene.

Removing PPE properly reduces the risk for infection transmission and contamination of other items. Hand hygiene prevents transmission of microorganisms.

18. Evaluate the patient's response to interventions. Reassess level of discomfort or pain using original assessment tools. Reassess and alter plan of care, as appropriate.

Reassessment allows for individualization of plan of care and promotes optimal patient comfort.

EVALUATION

- Patient reports increased comfort and/or decreased pain.
- Patient displays decreased anxiety and improved relaxation.
- Patient's skin is without evidence of breakdown.
- Patient verbalizes an understanding of the reasons for back massage.

DOCUMENTATION

- Document pain assessment and other significant assessments. Document the use of, and length of time of, massage, and patient response. Record alternative treatments to consider, if appropriate.

GENERAL CONSIDERATIONS

- Before giving a back massage, assess the patient's body structure and skin condition, and tailor the duration and intensity of the massage accordingly. If you are giving a back massage at bedtime, have the patient ready for bed beforehand so the massage can help him or her fall asleep.

- If the patient has oily skin, substitute a talcum powder or lotion of the patient's choice. However, to avoid aspiration, do not use powder if the patient has an endotracheal or tracheal tube in place. Avoid using powder and lotion together because this may lead to skin maceration.
- When massaging the patient's back, stand with one foot slightly forward and your knees slightly bent to allow effective use of your arm and shoulder muscles.

Skill · 8   Giving a Bed Bath

A bed bath may be considered a partial bed bath if the patient is well enough to perform most of the bath, and the nurse needs to assist with washing areas that the patient cannot reach easily. A partial bath may also refer to bathing only those body parts that absolutely have to be cleaned, such as the perineal area and any soiled body parts. Many of the bedside skin-cleaning products available today do not require rinsing. After cleaning the body part, dry it thoroughly. Refer to the accompanying skill variations for the procedures related to perineal cleansing and a bath using a disposable self-contained bathing system.

EQUIPMENT

- Washbasin and warm water
- Personal hygiene supplies (deodorant, lotion)
- Skin-cleaning agent
- Emollient and skin barrier, as indicated
- Towels (2)
- Washcloths (2)
- Bath blanket
- Gown or pajamas
- Bedpan or urinal
- Laundry bag
- Nonsterile gloves; other PPE as indicated

ASSESSMENT GUIDELINES

- Assess the patient's knowledge of hygiene practices and bathing preferences—frequency, time of day, and type of hygiene products.
- Assess for any physical-activity limitations. Assess the patient's ability to bathe himself or herself. Allow the patient to do any part of the bath that he or she can do. For example, the patient may be able to wash his or her face, while the nurse does the rest.
- Assess the patient's skin for dryness, redness, or areas of breakdown, and gather any other appropriate supplies that may be needed as a result.

NURSING DIAGNOSES

- Bathing Self-Care Deficit
- Risk for Infection

- Disturbed Body Image
- Risk for Impaired Skin Integrity
- Impaired Skin Integrity
- Deficient Knowledge
- Ineffective Coping

OUTCOME IDENTIFICATION AND PLANNING

Expected outcomes may include:
- The patient will be clean and fresh.
- The patient regains feelings of control by assisting with the bath.
- The patient verbalizes positive body image.
- The patient demonstrates an understanding about the need for cleanliness.

IMPLEMENTATION

ACTION	RATIONALE
1. Review chart for any limitations in physical activity.	Identifying limitations prevents patient discomfort and injury.
2. Bring necessary equipment to the bedside stand or over-bed table.	Bringing everything to the bedside conserves time and energy. Arranging items nearby is convenient, saves time, and avoids unnecessary stretching and twisting of muscles on the part of the nurse.
3. Perform hand hygiene and put on gloves and/or other PPE, if indicated.	Hand hygiene and PPE prevent the spread of microorganisms. PPE is required based on transmission precautions.
4. Identify the patient. Discuss the procedure with the patient and assess his or her ability to assist in the bathing process, as well as personal hygiene preferences.	Identifying the patient ensures the right patient receives the intervention and helps prevent errors. Discussion promotes reassurance and provides knowledge about the procedure. Dialogue encourages patient participation and allows for individualized nursing care.
5. Close curtains around bed and close the door to the room, if possible. Adjust the room temperature, if necessary.	This ensures the patient's privacy and lessens the risk for loss of body heat during the bath.

ACTION	RATIONALE
6. Remove sequential compression devices and antiembolism stockings from lower extremities according to agency protocol.	Most manufacturers and agencies recommend removal of these devices before the bath to allow for assessment.
7. Offer the patient bedpan or urinal.	Voiding or defecating before the bath lessens the likelihood that the bath will be interrupted, because warm bath water may stimulate the urge to void.
8. Remove gloves and perform hand hygiene.	Hand hygiene deters the spread of microorganisms.
9. Adjust the bed to a comfortable working height, usually elbow height of the caregiver (VISN 8 Patient Safety Center, 2009).	Having the bed at the proper height prevents back and muscle strain.
10. Put on gloves. Lower side rail nearer to you and assist patient to side of bed where you will work. Have patient lie on his or her back.	Gloves prevent transmission of microorganisms. Having the patient positioned near the nurse and lowering the side rail prevent unnecessary stretching and twisting of muscles on the part of the nurse.
11. Loosen top covers and remove all except the top sheet. Place bath blanket over the patient and then remove the top sheet while the patient holds the bath blanket in place. If linen is to be reused, fold it over a chair. Place soiled linen in laundry bag. Take care to prevent linen from coming in contact with your clothing.	The patient is not exposed unnecessarily, and warmth is maintained. If a bath blanket is unavailable, the top sheet may be used in place of the bath blanket.
12. Remove the patient's gown and keep the bath blanket in place. If the patient has an IV line and is not wearing a gown with snap sleeves, remove the gown from other arm first.	This provides uncluttered access during the bath and maintains warmth of the patient. IV fluids must be maintained at the prescribed rate.

ACTION	RATIONALE
Lower the IV container and pass the gown over the tubing and the container. Rehang the container and check the drip rate.	
13. **Raise side rail.** Fill basin with a sufficient amount of comfortably warm water (110ºF to 115ºF). Add the skin cleanser, if appropriate, according to manufacturer's directions. Change as necessary throughout the bath. Lower side rail closer to you when you return to the bedside to begin the bath.	Side rails maintain patient safety. Warm water is comfortable and relaxing for the patient. It also stimulates circulation and provides for more effective cleansing.
14. Put on gloves, if necessary. Fold the washcloth like a mitt on your hand so that there are no loose ends.	Gloves are necessary if there is potential contact with blood or body fluids. Having loose ends of cloth drag across the patient's skin is uncomfortable. Loose ends cool quickly and feel cold to the patient.
15. Lay a towel across patient's chest and on top of bath blanket.	This prevents chilling and keeps the bath blanket dry.
16. **With no cleanser on the washcloth, wipe one eye from the inner part of the eye, near the nose, to the outer part. Rinse or turn the cloth before washing the other eye.**	Soap is irritating to the eyes. Moving from the inner to the outer aspect of the eye prevents carrying debris toward the nasolacrimal duct. Rinsing or turning the washcloth prevents spreading organisms from one eye to the other.
17. Bathe patient's face, neck, and ears. Apply appropriate emollient.	Use of emollients is recommended to restore and maintain skin integrity (Voegeli, 2008a; Watkins, 2008; Brown & Butcher, 2005).
18. Expose the patient's far arm and place the towel lengthwise under it. Using firm strokes, wash hand, arm, and axilla, lifting the arm as necessary to access axillary	The towel helps to keep the bed dry. Washing the far side first eliminates contaminating a clean area once it is washed. Gentle friction stimulates circulation and muscles and helps remove

ACTION	RATIONALE
region. Rinse, if necessary, and dry. Apply appropriate emollient.	dirt, oil, and organisms. Long, firm strokes are relaxing and more comfortable than short, uneven strokes. Rinsing is necessary when using some cleansing products. Use of emollients is recommended to restore and maintain skin integrity (Voegeli, 2008a; Watkins, 2008; Brown & Butcher, 2005).
19. Place a folded towel on the bed next to the patient's hand and put basin on it. Soak the patient's hand in the basin. Wash, rinse if necessary, and dry hand. Apply appropriate emollient.	Placing the hand in the basin of water is an additional comfort measure for the patient. It facilitates thorough washing of the hands and between the fingers and aids in removing debris from under the skin. Use of emollients is recommended to restore and maintain skin integrity (Voegeli, 2008a; Watkins, 2008; Brown & Butcher, 2005).
20. Repeat Actions 15 and 16 for the arm nearer you. An option for the shorter nurse or one susceptible to back strain might be to bathe one side of the patient and move to the other side of the bed to complete the bath.	
21. Spread a towel across the patient's chest. Lower the bath blanket to the patient's umbilical area. Wash, rinse, if necessary, and dry chest. Keep chest covered with towel between the wash and rinse. Pay special attention to skin folds under the breasts.	Exposing, washing, rinsing, and drying one part of the body at a time avoids unnecessary exposure and chilling. Skin-fold areas may be sources of odor and skin breakdown if not cleaned and dried properly.
22. Lower the bath blanket to the perineal area. Place a towel over the patient's chest.	Keeping the bath blanket and towel in place avoids exposure and chilling.
23. Wash, rinse, if necessary, and dry the abdomen. Carefully inspect and clean the umbilical	Skin-fold areas may be sources of odor and skin breakdown if not cleaned and dried properly.

ACTION	RATIONALE
area and any abdominal folds or creases.	
24. Return the bath blanket to its original position and expose the far leg. Place towel under the far leg. Using firm strokes, wash, rinse, if necessary, and dry the leg from ankle to knee and knee to groin. Apply appropriate emollient.	The towel protects linens and prevents the patient from feeling uncomfortable from a damp or wet bed. Washing from ankle to groin with firm strokes promotes venous return. Use of emollients is recommended to restore and maintain skin integrity (Voegeli, 2008a; Watkins, 2008; Brown & Butcher, 2005).
25. Wash, rinse if necessary, and dry the foot. Pay particular attention to the areas between toes. Apply appropriate emollient.	Drying of the feet is important to prevent irritation, possible skin breakdown, and infections (NIA, 2009). Use of emollients is recommended to restore and maintain skin integrity (Voegeli, 2008a; Watkins, 2008; Brown & Butcher, 2005).
26. Repeat Actions 21 and 22 for the other leg and foot.	
27. Make sure the patient is covered with the bath blanket. Change water and washcloth at this point, or earlier, if necessary.	The bath blanket maintains warmth and privacy. Clean, warm water prevents chilling and maintains patient comfort.
28. Assist patient to prone or side-lying position. Put on gloves, if not applied earlier. Position bath blanket and towel to expose only the back and buttocks.	Positioning the towel and bath blanket protects the patient's privacy and provides warmth. Gloves prevent contact with body fluids.
29. Wash, rinse, if necessary, and dry back and buttocks area. **Pay particular attention to cleansing between gluteal folds, and observe for any redness or skin breakdown in the sacral area.**	Fecal material near the anus may be a source of microorganisms. Prolonged pressure on the sacral area or other bony prominences may compromise circulation and lead to development of decubitus ulcer.
30. If not contraindicated, give patient a backrub. Back massage may be given also after perineal care. Apply	A backrub improves circulation to the tissues and is an aid to relaxation. A backrub may be contraindicated in patients with

ACTION	RATIONALE
appropriate emollient and/or skin barrier product.	cardiovascular disease or musculoskeletal injuries. Use of emollients is recommended to restore and maintain skin integrity (Voegeli, 2008a; Watkins, 2008; Brown & Butcher, 2005). Skin barriers protect the skin from damage caused by excessive exposure to water and irritants, such as urine and feces (Voegeli, 2008a).
31. Raise the side rail. Refill basin with clean water. Discard washcloth and towel. Remove gloves and put on clean gloves.	The washcloth, towel, and water are contaminated after washing the patient's gluteal area. Changing to clean supplies decreases the spread of organisms from the anal area to the genitals.
32. Clean perineal area or set up patient so that he or she can complete perineal self-care. If the patient is unable, lower the side rail and complete perineal care, following guidelines in the accompanying Skill Variation. Apply skin barrier, as indicated. Raise side rail, remove gloves, and perform hand hygiene.	Providing perineal self-care may decrease embarrassment for the patient. Effective perineal care reduces odor and decreases the risk for infection through contamination. Skin barriers protect the skin from damage caused by excessive exposure to water and irritants, such as urine and feces (Voegeli, 2008a).
33. Help patient put on a clean gown and assist with the use of other personal toiletries, such as deodorant or cosmetics.	This provides for the patient's warmth and comfort.
34. Protect pillow with towel and groom patient's hair.	
35. When finished, make sure the patient is comfortable, with the side rails up and the bed in the lowest position.	Proper positioning with raised side rails and proper bed height provide for patient comfort and safety.

ACTION	RATIONALE
36. Change bed linens. Dispose of soiled linens according to agency policy. Remove gloves and any other PPE, if used. Perform hand hygiene.	Removing PPE properly reduces the risk for infection transmission and contamination of other items. Hand hygiene prevents the spread of microorganisms.

EVALUATION

- The patient is clean.
- The patient demonstrates some feeling of control in his or her care.
- The patient verbalizes an improved body image.
- The patient verbalizes the importance of cleanliness.

DOCUMENTATION

- Record any significant observations and communication on the patient's chart. Document the condition of the patient's skin. Record the procedure, amount of assistance given, and patient participation. Document the application of skin care products, such as a skin barrier.

GENERAL CONSIDERATIONS

- To remove the gown from a patient with an IV line, take the gown off the uninvolved arm first and then thread the IV tubing and bottle or bag through the arm of the gown. To replace the gown, place the clean gown on the unaffected arm first and thread the IV tubing and bottle or bag from inside the arm of the gown on the involved side. Never disconnect IV tubing to change a gown, because this causes a break in a sterile system and could introduce infection.
- Lying flat in bed during the bed bath may be contraindicated for certain patients. The position may have to be modified to accommodate their needs.
- Incontinent patients require special attention to perineal care. Patients with urinary or fecal incontinence are at risk for perineal skin damage. This damage is related to moisture, changes in the pH of the skin, overgrowth of bacteria and infection of the skin, and erosion of perineal skin from friction on moist skin. Skin care for these patients should include measures to reduce overhydration (excess exposure to moisture), reduce contact with ammonia and bacteria, and reduce friction. Remove soil and irritants from the skin during routine hygiene, as well as cleansing when the skin becomes exposed to irritants. Avoid using soap and excessive force for cleaning. The use of perineal skin cleansers, moisturizers, and moisture barriers are recommended for skin care for the incontinent patient. These products help promote healing and prevent further skin damage.

• If the patient has an indwelling catheter and the agency recommends daily care for the catheter, this is usually done after perineal care. Agency policy may recommend use of an antiseptic cleaning agent or plain soap and water on a clean washcloth. Put on clean gloves before cleaning the catheter. Clean 6 to 8 inches of the catheter, moving from the meatus downward. Be careful not to pull or tug on the catheter during the cleaning motion. Also inspect the meatus for drainage and note the characteristics of the urine.

Skill Variation | **Performing Perineal Cleansing**

Perineal care may be carried out while the patient remains in bed. When performing perineal care, follow these guidelines:

1. Assemble supplies and provide for privacy.
2. Explain the procedure to the patient, perform hand hygiene, and put on disposable gloves.
3. Wash and rinse the groin area (both male and female patients).
   • **For a female patient,** spread the labia and move the washcloth from the pubic area toward the anal area to prevent carrying organisms from the anal area back over the genital area (FIGURE A). Always

proceed from the least contaminated area to the most contaminated area. Use a clean portion of the washcloth for each stroke. Rinse the washed areas well with plain water.
   • **For a male patient,** clean the tip of the penis first, moving the washcloth in a circular motion from the meatus outward. Wash the shaft of the penis using downward strokes toward the pubic area (FIGURE B). Always proceed from the least contaminated area to the most contaminated area. Rinse the washed areas well with plain water. In an *uncircumcised male patient* (teenage or older),

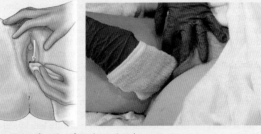

FIGURE A Performing female perineal care.

(continued on page 41)

Performing Perineal Cleansing *continued*

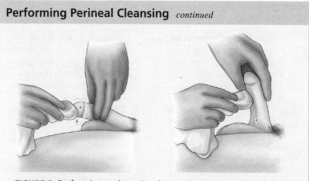

FIGURE B Performing male perineal care.

retract the foreskin (prepuce) while washing the penis. Pull the *uncircumcised male patient's* foreskin back into place over the glans penis to prevent constriction of the penis, which may result in edema and tissue injury. It is not recommended to retract the foreskin for cleaning during infancy and childhood, because injury and scarring could occur (MedlinePlus, 2007b). Wash and rinse the male patient's scrotum. Handle the scrotum, which houses the testicles, with care because the area is sensitive.

4. Dry the cleaned areas and apply an emollient, as indicated. Avoid the use of powder. Powder may become a medium for the growth of bacteria.

5. Turn the patient on his or her side and continue cleansing the anal area. Continue in the direction of least contaminated to most contaminated area. In the female patient, cleanse from the vagina toward the anus. In both female and male patients, change the washcloth with each stroke until the area is clean. Rinse and dry the area.

6. Remove gloves and perform hand hygiene. Continue with additional care, as necessary.

Skill Variation **Giving a Bath Using a Disposable Self-contained Bathing System**

This product is packaged with 8 to 10 premoistened, disposable washcloths. If more than eight cloths are available in package, use a separate cloth for hands and feet. When giving a bath with a disposable system, follow these guidelines:

1. Warm the unopened package in the microwave, according

(continued on page 42)

Giving a Bath Using a Disposable Self-contained Bathing System *continued*

to manufacturer's directions or remove the package from storage warmer.

2. Provide for privacy.

3. Explain the procedure to the patient; perform hand hygiene and put on disposable gloves and/or other PPE, as indicated.

4. Cover the patient with a bath blanket and remove top linens. Remove the patient's gown and keep the bath blanket in place.

5. Remove first cloth from package. Wipe one eye from the inner part of the eye, near the nose, to the outer part. Use a different part of the cloth for the other eye.

6. Bathe the face, neck, and ears. Allow the skin to air dry for approximately 30 seconds, according to manufacturer's directions. Air drying allows the emollient ingredient of the cleanser to remain on the skin. Alternately, dry the skin with a towel, based on the product used. Apply appropriate emollient. Dispose of cloth in trash receptacle.

7. Expose the patient's far arm. Remove another cloth. Using firm strokes, wash hand, arm, and axilla. Allow the skin to air dry for approximately 30 seconds, according to manufacturer's directions. Air drying allows the emollient ingredient of the cleanser to remain on the skin.

Alternately, dry the skin with a towel, based on the product used. Apply appropriate emollient. Dispose of cloth in trash receptacle. Cover arm with blanket.

8. Repeat for nearer arm with a new cloth. Cover arm with blanket.

9. Expose the patient's chest. Remove new cloth and cleanse chest. Allow the skin to air dry for approximately 30 seconds, according to manufacturer's directions. Cover chest with a towel. Expose patient's abdomen. Cleanse abdomen. Allow the skin to air dry for approximately 30 seconds, according to manufacturer's directions. Air drying allows the emollient ingredient of the cleanser to remain on the skin. Alternately, dry the skin with a towel, based on the product used. Apply appropriate emollient. Dispose of cloth in trash receptacle. Cover the patient's body with blanket.

10. Expose far leg. Remove new cloth and cleanse leg and foot. Allow the skin to air dry for approximately 30 seconds, according to manufacturer's directions. Air drying allows the emollient ingredient of the cleanser to remain on the skin. Alternately, dry the skin with a towel, based on the product used. Apply appropriate emollient. Dispose of cloth in trash

(continued on page 43)

Giving a Bath Using a Disposable Self-contained Bathing System   *continued*

receptacle. Cover the patient's leg with blanket.

11. Repeat for nearer leg with a new cloth. Cover leg with blanket.

12. Assist patient to prone or side-lying position. Put on gloves, if not applied earlier. Position blanket to expose back and buttocks. Remove a new cloth and cleanse back and buttocks area. Allow the skin to air dry for approximately 30 seconds, according to manufacturer's directions. Air drying allows the emollient ingredient of the cleanser to remain on the skin. Alternately, dry the skin with a towel, based on the product used. Apply appropriate emollient. Dispose of cloth in trash recep-

tacle. If not contraindicated, give the patient a back massage. Apply skin barrier, as indicated. Cover the patient with blanket.

13. Remove gloves and put on clean gloves. Remove last cloth and cleanse the perineal area. Dispose of cloth in trash receptacle. Apply skin barrier, as indicated.

14. Remove gloves. Assist patient to put on clean gown. Assist with the use of other personal toiletries.

15. Change bed linens.

16. Remove gloves and perform hand hygiene. Dispose of soiled linens according to facility policy.

Skill Variation   **Meeting the Bathing Needs of Patients with Dementia**

1. Shift the focus of the interaction from the "task of bathing" to the needs and abilities of the patient. Focus on comfort, safety, autonomy, and self-esteem, in addition to cleanliness.

2. Individualize patient care. Consult the patient, the patient's record, family members, and other caregivers to determine patient preferences.

3. Consider what can be learned from the behaviors associated with dementia about the needs and preferences of the patient. A

patient's behavior may be an expression of unmet needs; unwillingness to participate may be a response to uncomfortable water temperatures or levels of sound or light in the room.

4. Consider other methods for bathing. Showers and tub baths are not the only options in bathing. Towel baths, washing under clothes, and bathing "body sections" one day at a time are other possible options.

5. Maintain a relaxed demeanor. Use calming language. Try to

(continued on page 44)

**Meeting the Bathing Needs of Patients
with Dementia** *continued*

determine phrases and terms
the patient understands in
relation to bathing and make
use of them. Offer frequent
reassurance.

6. Explore the need for routine analgesia before bathing. Move limbs carefully
and be aware of signs of

discomfort during
bathing.

7. Wash the face and hair at the
end of the bath or at a separate
time. Water dripping in the
face and having a wet head are
often the most upsetting parts
of the bathing process for people with dementia.

Adapted from Flori, L. (2007). Don't throw in the towel: Tips for bathing a
patient who has dementia. *Nursing*, 37(7), 22–23; and Rader, J., Barrick, A.,
Hoeffer, B., et al. (2006). The bathing of older adults with dementia: Easing
the unnecessarily unpleasant aspects of assisted bathing. *American Journal of
Nursing*, 106(4), 40–49.

Skill · 9   Assisting with a Sitz Bath

A sitz bath can help relieve pain and discomfort in the perineal area, such
as after childbirth or surgery, and can increase circulation to the tissues,
promoting healing.

EQUIPMENT
- Clean gloves
- Additional PPE, as indicated
- Towel
- Adjustable IV pole
- Disposable sitz bath bowl with
  water bag

ASSESSMENT GUIDELINES
- Review any orders related to the sitz bath.
- Determine patient's ability to ambulate to the bathroom and maintain
  sitting position for 15 to 20 minutes.
- Assess patient's perineal/rectal area for swelling, drainage, redness,
  warmth, and tenderness.
- Assess bladder fullness and encourage the patient to void before sitz bath.

NURSING DIAGNOSES
- Acute Pain
- Risk for Infection
- Risk for Hypothermia
- Impaired Tissue Integrity

OUTCOME IDENTIFICATION AND PLANNING

Expected outcomes may include:
• Patient verbalizes an increase in comfort.
• Patient experiences a decrease in healing time, maintains normal body temperature, remains free of any signs and symptoms of infection, and exhibits signs and symptoms of healing.

IMPLEMENTATION

ACTION	RATIONALE
1. Review the medical order for the application of a sitz bath, including frequency, and length of time for the application.	Reviewing the order and plan of care validates the correct patient and correct procedure.
2. Gather the necessary supplies and bring to the bedside stand or overbed table.	Preparation promotes efficient time management and an organized approach to the task. Bringing everything to the bedside conserves time and energy. Arranging items nearby is convenient, saves time, and avoids unnecessary stretching and twisting of muscles on the part of the nurse.
3. Perform hand hygiene and put on PPE, if indicated.	Hand hygiene and PPE prevent the spread of microorganisms. PPE is required based on transmission precautions.
4. Identify the patient.	Identifying the patient ensures the right patient receives the intervention and helps prevent errors.
5. Close curtains around bed and close door to the room, if possible.	This ensures the patient's privacy.
6. Put on gloves. Assemble equipment, at the bedside if using a bedside commode, or in the bathroom.	Gloves prevent exposure to blood and body fluids. Organization facilitates performance of the task.
7. Raise lid of toilet or commode. Place bowl of sitz bath,	Sitz bath will not drain appropriately if placed in toilet backward.

ACTION	RATIONALE
with drainage ports to rear and infusion port in front, in the toilet. Fill bowl of sitz bath about halfway full with tepid to warm water (37°C to 46°C [98°F to 115°F]).	Tepid water can promote relaxation and help with edema; warm water can help with circulation.
8. Clamp tubing on bag. Fill bag with same temperature water as mentioned above. Hang bag above patient's shoulder height on the IV pole.	If bag is hung lower, the rate of flow will not be sufficient and water may cool too quickly.
9. Assist patient to sit on toilet or commode and provide any extra draping if needed. Insert tubing into infusion port of sitz bath. Slowly unclamp tubing and allow sitz bath to fill.	If tubing is placed into sitz bath before the patient sits on the toilet, the patient may trip over the tubing. Filling the sitz bath ensures that the tissue is submerged in water.
10. Clamp tubing once the sitz bath is full. Instruct the patient to open the clamp when the water in the bowl becomes cool. **Ensure that the call bell is within reach. Instruct the patient to call if he or she feels light-headed or dizzy or has any problems. Instruct the patient not to try standing without assistance.**	Cool water may produce hypothermia. Patient may become light-headed due to vasodilation, so call bell should be within reach.
11. Remove gloves and perform hand hygiene.	Hand hygiene deters the spread of microorganisms.
12. When patient is finished (in about 15 to 20 minutes, or prescribed time), put on clean gloves. Assist the patient to stand and gently pat perineal area dry. Remove gloves. Assist the patient to the bed or chair. Ensure that the call bell is within reach.	Gloves prevent contact with blood and body fluids. Patient may be light-headed and dizzy due to vasodilation. Patient should not stand alone, and bending over to dry self may cause patient to fall.

ACTION	RATIONALE
13. Put on gloves. Empty and disinfect the sitz bath bowl according to agency policy.	Proper equipment cleaning deters the spread of microorganisms.
14. Remove gloves and any additional PPE, if used. Perform hand hygiene.	Removing PPE properly reduces the risk for infection transmission and contamination of other items. Hand hygiene prevents the spread of microorganisms.

EVALUATION

* Patient verbalizes a decrease in pain or discomfort.
* Patient tolerates sitz bath without incident.
* Patient demonstrates signs of healing.

DOCUMENTATION

* Document administration of the sitz bath, including water temperature and duration. Document patient response, and assessment of perineum before and after administration.

Skill · 10   Making an Occupied Bed

If the patient cannot get out of bed, the linens may need to be changed with the patient still in the bed. This is termed an "occupied" bed. The following procedure explains how to make the bed using a fitted bottom sheet. Some facilities do not provide fitted bottom sheets, or sometimes a fitted bottom sheet may not be available. If this is the case, refer to the Skill Variation at the end of Skill 11, for using a flat bottom sheet instead of a fitted sheet.

EQUIPMENT

* One large flat sheet
* One fitted sheet
* Drawsheet (optional)
* Blankets
* Bedspread
* Pillowcases

* Linen hamper or bag
* Bedside chair
* Waterproof protective pad (optional)
* Disposable gloves
* Additional PPE, as indicated

ASSESSMENT GUIDELINES

- Assess the patient's preferences regarding linen changes.
- Assess for any precautions or activity restrictions for the patient.
- Check for any patient belongings that may have accidentally been placed in the bed linens, such as eyeglasses or prayer cloths.
- Note the presence and position of any tubes or drains that the patient may have.

NURSING DIAGNOSES

- Risk for Impaired Skin Integrity
- Risk for Activity Intolerance
- Impaired Physical Mobility
- Impaired Bed Mobility
- Impaired Transfer Ability

OUTCOME IDENTIFICATION AND PLANNING

Expected outcomes may include:
- The bed linens will be changed without injury to the nurse or patient.
- The patient verbalizes feelings of increased comfort.

IMPLEMENTATION

ACTION	RATIONALE
1. Check chart for limitations on the patient's physical activity.	This facilitates patient cooperation, determines level of activity, and promotes patient safety.
2. Assemble equipment and arrange on bedside chair in the order the items will be used.	Organization facilitates performance of the task.
3. Perform hand hygiene. Put on PPE, as indicated.	Hand hygiene and PPE prevent the spread of microorganisms. PPE is required based on transmission precautions.
4. Identify the patient. Explain what you are going to do.	Patient identification validates the correct patient and correct procedure. Discussion and explanation allay anxiety and prepare the patient for what to expect.

ACTION	RATIONALE
5. Close curtains around bed and close the door to the room, if possible.	This ensures the patient's privacy.
6. Adjust the bed to a comfortable working height, usually elbow height of the caregiver (VISN 8 Patient Safety Center, 2009).	Having the bed at the proper height prevents back and muscle strain.
7. Lower side rail nearest you, leaving the opposite side rail up. Place bed in flat position unless contraindicated.	Having the mattress flat makes it easier to prepare a wrinkle-free bed.
8. Put on gloves. Check bed linens for patient's personal items. **Disconnect the call bell or any tubes/drains from bed linens.**	Gloves prevent the spread of microorganisms. It is costly and inconvenient when personal items are lost. Disconnecting tubes from linens prevents discomfort and accidental dislodging of the tubes.
9. Place a bath blanket over the patient. Have patient hold on to bath blanket while you reach under it and remove top linens. Leave the top sheet in place if a bath blanket is not used. Fold linen that is to be reused over the back of a chair. Discard soiled linen in laundry bag or hamper. **Do not place on floor or furniture. Do not hold soiled linens against your uniform.**	The blanket provides warmth and privacy. Placing linens directly into the hamper helps prevent the spread of microorganisms. The floor is heavily contaminated; soiled linen will further contaminate furniture. Soiled linen contaminates the nurse's uniform, and this may spread organisms to another patient.
10. If possible, and another person is available to assist, grasp the mattress securely and shift it up to the head of the bed.	This allows more foot room for the patient.
11. Assist the patient to turn toward the opposite side of the bed, and reposition the pillow under the patient's head.	This allows the bed to be made on the vacant side.

ACTION	RATIONALE
12. Loosen all bottom linens from head, foot, and side of bed.	This facilitates removal of linens.
13. Fan-fold soiled linens as close to the patient as possible.	This makes it easier to remove linens when the patient turns to the other side.
14. Use clean linen and make the near side of the bed. Place the bottom sheet with its center fold in the center of the bed. Open the sheet and fan-fold to the center, positioning it under the old linens. Pull the bottom sheet over the corners at the head and foot of the mattress.	Opening linens on the bed reduces strain on the nurse's arms and diminishes the spread of microorganisms. Centering the sheet ensures sufficient coverage for both sides of the mattress. Positioning under the old linens makes it easier to remove linens.
15. If using, place the drawsheet with its center fold in the center of the bed and positioned so it will be located under the patient's midsection. Open the drawsheet and fan-fold to the center of the mattress. Tuck the drawsheet securely under the mattress. If a protective pad is used, place it over the drawsheet in the proper area and open to the center fold. Not all agencies use drawsheets routinely. The nurse may decide to use one.	If the patient soils the bed, drawsheet and pad can be changed without the bottom and top linens on the bed. A drawsheet can aid moving the patient in bed.
16. Raise side rail. Assist the patient to roll over the folded linen in the middle of the bed toward you. Reposition pillow and bath blanket or top sheet. Move to the other side of the bed and lower the side rail.	This ensures patient safety. The movement allows the bed to be made on the other side. The bath blanket provides warmth and privacy.
17. Loosen and remove all bottom linen. Discard soiled linen in laundry bag or hamper. **Do not place on floor or furniture. Do not hold soiled linens against your uniform.**	Placing linens directly into the hamper helps prevent the spread of microorganisms. The floor is heavily contaminated; soiled linen will further contaminate furniture. Soiled linen contaminates the

ACTION	RATIONALE
	nurse's uniform, and this may spread organisms to another patient.
18. Ease clean linen from under the patient. Pull the bottom sheet taut and secure it at the corners of the head and foot of the mattress. Pull the drawsheet tight and smooth. Tuck the drawsheet securely under the mattress.	This removes wrinkles and creases in the linens, which are uncomfortable to lie on.
19. Assist the patient to turn back to the center of the bed. Remove pillow and change pillowcase. Open each pillowcase in the same manner as you opened other linens. Gather the pillowcase over one hand toward the closed end. Grasp the pillow with the hand inside the pillowcase. Keep a firm hold on the top of the pillow and pull the cover on to the pillow. Place the pillow under the patient's head.	Opening linens by shaking them causes organisms to be carried on air currents.
20. Apply top linen, sheet, and blanket, if desired, so that they are centered. Fold the top linens over at the patient's shoulders to make a cuff. Have the patient hold on to top linen and remove the bath blanket from underneath.	This allows bottom hems to be tucked securely under the mattress and provides for privacy.
21. Secure top linens under the foot of the mattress and miter corners (Refer to Skill Variation, Skill 11). Loosen top linens over the patient's feet by grasping them in the area of the feet and pulling gently toward foot of bed.	This provides for a neat appearance. Loosening linens over the patient's feet gives more room for movement.

ACTION	RATIONALE
22. Return the patient to a position of comfort. Remove your gloves. Raise side rail and lower bed. Reattach call bell.	Promotes patient comfort and safety. Removing gloves properly reduces the risk for infection transmission and contamination of other items.
23. Dispose of soiled linens according to agency policy.	Deters the spread of microorganisms.
24. Remove any other PPE, if used. Perform hand hygiene.	Removing PPE properly reduces the risk for infection transmission and contamination of other items. Hand hygiene prevents the spread of microorganisms.

EVALUATION
- The bed linens are changed without any injury to the patient or nurse.
- The patient verbalizes feelings of increased comfort after the bed is changed.

DOCUMENTATION
- Changing of bed linens does not need to be documented. The use of a specialty bed, or bed equipment, such as Balkan frame or foot cradle, should be documented. Document any significant observations and communication.

Skill · 11   **Making an Unoccupied Bed**

Usually bed linens are changed after the bath, but some agencies change linens only when soiled. If the patient can get out of bed, the bed should be made while it is unoccupied to decrease stress on the patient and the nurse. The following procedure explains how to make the bed using a fitted bottom sheet. Some facilities do not provide fitted bottom sheets, or sometimes a fitted bottom sheet may not be available. If this is the case, refer to the accompanying Skill Variation for using a flat bottom sheet, instead of a fitted sheet.

EQUIPMENT

- One large flat sheet
- One fitted sheet
- Drawsheet (optional)
- Blankets
- Bedspread
- Pillowcases
- Linen hamper or bag
- Bedside chair
- Waterproof protective pad (optional)
- Disposable gloves
- Additional PPE, as indicated

ASSESSMENT GUIDELINES

- Assess the patient's preferences regarding linen changes.
- Assess for any physical activity limitations.
- Check for any patient belongings that may have accidentally been placed in the bed linens, such as eyeglasses or prayer cloths.

NURSING DIAGNOSES

- Risk for Impaired Skin Integrity
- Risk for Activity Intolerance
- Impaired Physical Mobility

OUTCOME IDENTIFICATION AND PLANNING

Expected outcomes may include:
- The bed linens will be changed without injury to the nurse or patient.

IMPLEMENTATION

ACTION	RATIONALE
1. Assemble equipment and arrange on a bedside chair in the order in which items will be used.	Organization facilitates performance of task.
2. Perform hand hygiene. Put on PPE, as indicated.	Hand hygiene and PPE prevent the spread of microorganisms. PPE is required based on transmission precautions.
3. Adjust the bed to a comfortable working height, usually elbow height of the caregiver (VISN 8 Patient Safety Center, 2009). Drop the side rails.	Having the bed at the proper height prevents back and muscle strain. Having the side rails down reduces strain on the nurse while working.
4. Disconnect call bell or any tubes from bed linens.	Disconnecting devices prevents damage to the devices.

ACTION	RATIONALE
5. Put on gloves. Loosen all linen as you move around the bed, from the head of the bed on the far side to the head of the bed on the near side.	Gloves prevent the spread of microorganisms. Loosening the linen helps prevent tugging and tearing on linen. Loosening the linen and moving around the bed systematically reduce strain caused by reaching across the bed.
6. Fold reusable linens, such as sheets, blankets, or spread, in place on the bed in fourths and hang them over a clean chair.	Folding saves time and energy when reusable linen is replaced on the bed. Folding linens while they are on the bed reduces strain on the nurse's arms. Some agencies change linens only when soiled.
7. Snugly roll all the soiled linen inside the bottom sheet and place directly into the laundry hamper. **Do not place on the floor or furniture. Do not hold soiled linens against your uniform.**	Rolling soiled linens snugly and placing them directly into the hamper helps prevent the spread of microorganisms. The floor is heavily contaminated; soiled linen will further contaminate furniture. Soiled linen contaminates the nurse's uniform, and this may spread organisms to another patient.
8. If possible, shift mattress up to head of bed. If mattress is soiled, clean and dry according to facility policy before applying new sheets.	This allows more foot room for the patient.
9. Remove your gloves, unless indicated for transmission precautions. Place the bottom sheet with its center fold in the center of the bed. Open the sheet and fan-fold to the center.	Gloves are not necessary to handle clean linen. Removing gloves properly reduces the risk for infection transmission and contamination of other items. Opening linens on the bed reduces strain on the nurse's arms and diminishes the spread of microorganisms. Centering the sheet ensures sufficient coverage for both sides of the mattress.
10. If using, place the drawsheet with its center fold in the center of the bed and positioned so it will be located under the patient's midsection. Open	If the patient soils the bed, drawsheet and pad can be changed without the bottom and top linens on the bed. Having all bottom linens in place before tucking

ACTION	RATIONALE
the drawsheet and fan-fold to the center of the mattress. If a protective pad is used, place it over the drawsheet in the proper area and open to the center fold. Not all agencies use drawsheets routinely. The nurse may decide to use one. In some institutions, the protective pad doubles as a drawsheet.	them under the mattress avoids unnecessary moving about the bed. A drawsheet can aid moving the patient in bed.
11. Pull the bottom sheet over the corners at the head and foot of the mattress. (See accompanying Skill Variation for using a flat bottom sheet, instead of a fitted sheet.) Tuck the drawsheet securely under the mattress.	Making the bed on one side and then completing the bed on the other side saves time. Having bottom linens free of wrinkles reduces patient discomfort.
12. Move to the other side of the bed to secure bottom linens. Pull the bottom sheet tightly and secure over the corners at the head and foot of the mattress. Pull the drawsheet tightly and tuck it securely under the mattress.	This removes wrinkles from the bottom linens, which can cause patient discomfort and promote skin breakdown.
13. Place the top sheet on the bed with its center fold in the center of the bed and with the hem even with the head of the mattress. Unfold the top sheet. Follow same procedure with top blanket or spread, placing the upper edge about 6 inches below the top of the sheet.	Opening linens by shaking them spreads organisms into the air. Holding linens overhead to open them causes strain on the nurse's arms.
14. Tuck the top sheet and blanket under the foot of the bed on the near side. Miter the corners. (See accompanying Skill Variation.)	This saves time and energy and keeps the top linen in place.
15. Fold the upper 6 inches of the top sheet down over the spread and make a cuff.	This makes it easier for the patient to get into bed and pull the covers up.

ACTION	RATIONALE
16. Move to the other side of the bed and follow the same procedure for securing top sheets under the foot of the bed and making a cuff.	Working on one side of the bed at a time saves energy and is more efficient.
17. Place the pillows on the bed. Open each pillowcase in the same manner as you opened other linens. Gather the pillowcase over one hand toward the closed end. Grasp the pillow with the hand inside the pillowcase. Keep a firm hold on the top of the pillow and pull the cover onto the pillow. Place the pillow at the head of the bed.	Opening linens by shaking them causes organisms to be carried on air currents. Covering the pillow while it rests on the bed reduces strain on the nurse's arms and back.
18. Fan-fold or pie-fold the top linens.	Having linens opened makes it more convenient for the patient to get into bed.
19. Secure the signal device on the bed, according to agency policy.	The patient will be able to call for assistance as necessary. Promotes patient comfort and safety.
20. Raise side rail and lower bed.	Promotes patient comfort and safety.
21. Dispose of soiled linen according to agency policy.	Deters the spread of microorganisms.
22. Remove any other PPE, if used. Perform hand hygiene.	Removing PPE properly reduces the risk for infection transmission and contamination of other items. Hand hygiene prevents the spread of microorganisms.

EVALUATION

• The bed linens are changed without any injury to the patient or nurse.

DOCUMENTATION

• Changing of bed linens does not need to be documented. The use of a specialty bed, or bed equipment, such as Balkan frame or foot cradle, should be documented.

Skill Variation | Making a Bed with a Flat Bottom Sheet

1. Assemble equipment and arrange on a bedside chair in the order in which the items will be used. Two large flat sheets are needed.
2. Perform hand hygiene. Put on gloves.
3. Adjust bed to high position and drop side rails.
4. Disconnect call bell or any tubes from bed linens.
5. Loosen all linen as you move around the bed, from the head of the bed on the far side to the head of the bed on the near side.
6. Fold reusable linens, such as sheets, blankets, or spread, in place on the bed in fourths and hang them over a clean chair.
7. Snugly roll all the soiled linen inside the bottom sheet and place directly into the laundry hamper. Do not place on floor or furniture. Do not hold soiled linens against your uniform.
8. If possible, shift mattress up to head of bed.
9. Remove your gloves. Place the bottom sheet with its center fold in the center of the bed and high enough to be able to tuck under the head of the mattress. Open the sheet and fan-fold to the center.
10. If using, place the drawsheet with its center fold in the center of the bed and positioned so it will be located under the patient's midsection. Open the drawsheet and fan-fold to the center of the mattress. If a protective pad is used, place it over the drawsheet in the proper area and open to the center fold.
11. Tuck the bottom sheet securely under the head of the mattress on one side of the bed, making a corner. Corners are usually mitered. Grasp the side edge of the sheet about 18 inches down from the mattress top (Figure A). Lay the sheet on top of the mattress to form a triangular, flat-fold (Figure B). Tuck the portion of the sheet that is hanging loose below

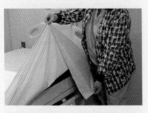

FIGURE A Grasping the side edge of the sheet and lifting up to form a triangle.

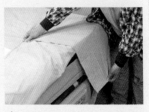

FIGURE B Laying sheet on top of the bed to make triangular flat-fold.

(continued on page 58)

Making a Bed with a Flat Bottom Sheet *continued*

the mattress under the mattress without pulling on the triangular fold (FIGURE C). Pick the top of the triangle fold and place it over the side of the mattress (FIGURE D). Tuck this loose portion of the sheet under the mattress. Continue tucking the remaining bottom sheet and drawsheet securely under the mattress (FIGURE E).

Move to the other side of the bed to secure bottom linens. Pull the sheets across the mattress from the center fold. Secure the bottom of the sheet under the head of the bed and miter the corners. Pull the remainder of the sheet and the drawsheet tightly and tuck under the mattress, starting at the head and moving toward the foot (FIGURE F).

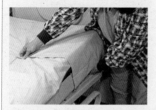

FIGURE C Tucking sheet under mattress.

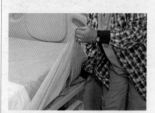

FIGURE D Placing top of triangular fold over mattress side.

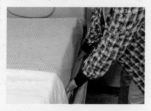

FIGURE E Tucking end of triangular linen fold under mattress to complete mitered corner.

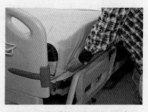

FIGURE F Tucking sheet snugly under mattress.

12. Place the top sheet on the bed with its center fold in the center of the bed and with the hem even with the head of the mattress. Unfold the top sheet. Follow same procedure with top blanket or spread, placing the upper edge about 6 inches below the top of the sheet.

13. Tuck the top sheet and blanket under the foot of the bed on the near side. Miter the corners.

(continued on page 59)

Making a Bed with a Flat Bottom Sheet *continued*

14. Fold the upper 6 inches of the top sheet down over the spread and make a cuff.
15. Move to the other side of the bed and follow the same procedure for securing top sheets under the foot of the bed and making a cuff.
16. Place the pillows on the bed. Open each pillowcase in the same manner as you opened other linens. Gather the pillowcase over one hand toward the closed end. Grasp the pillow with the hand inside the pillowcase. Keep a firm hold on the top of the pillow and pull the cover onto the pillow. Place the pillow at the head of the bed.
17. Fan-fold or pie-fold the top linens.
18. Secure the signal device on the bed, according to agency policy.
19. Adjust bed to low position.
20. Dispose of soiled linen, according to agency policy. Perform hand hygiene.

Skill · 12   **Assisting With the Use of a Bedpan**

Patients who cannot get out of bed because of physical limitations or physician's orders need to use a bedpan or urinal for voiding. Male patients confined to bed usually prefer to use the urinal for voiding and the bedpan for defecation; female patients usually prefer to use the bedpan for both. Many patients find it difficult and embarrassing to use the bedpan. When a patient uses a bedpan, promote comfort and normalcy and respect the patient's privacy as much as possible. Be sure to maintain a professional manner. In addition, provide skin care and perineal hygiene after bedpan use. Regular bedpans have a rounded, smooth upper end and a tapered, open lower end. The upper end fits under the patient's buttocks toward the sacrum, with the open end toward the foot of the bed. A special bedpan called a "fracture bedpan" is frequently used for patients with fractures of the femur or lower spine. Smaller and flatter than the ordinary bedpan, this type of bedpan is helpful for patients who cannot easily raise themselves onto the regular bedpan. Very thin or elderly patients often find it easier and more comfortable to use the fracture bedpan. The fracture pan has a shallow, narrow upper end with a flat wide rim, and a deeper, open lower end. The upper end fits under the patient's buttocks toward the sacrum, with the deeper, open lower end toward the foot of the bed.

EQUIPMENT
- Bedpan (regular or fracture)
- Toilet tissue
- Disposable clean gloves
- Additional PPE, as indicated
- Cover for bedpan or urinal (disposable waterproof pad or cover)

ASSESSMENT GUIDELINES

* Assess the patient's normal elimination habits. Determine why the patient needs to use a bedpan, (e.g., a medical order for strict bed rest or immobilization).
* Assess the patient's degree of limitation and ability to help with activity. Assess for activity limitations, such as hip surgery or spinal injury, which would contraindicate certain actions by the patient.
* Check for the presence of drains, dressings, intravenous fluid infusion sites/equipment, traction, or any other devices that could interfere with the patient's ability to help with the procedure or that could become dislodged.
* Assess the characteristics of the urine and the patient's skin.

NURSING DIAGNOSES

* Impaired Physical Mobility
* Deficient Knowledge
* Impaired Urinary Elimination
* Functional Urinary Incontinence
* Toileting Self-Care Deficit

OUTCOME IDENTIFICATION AND PLANNING

Expected outcomes may include:
* Patient is able to void with assistance.
* Patient maintains continence.
* Patient demonstrates how to use the bedpan with assistance.
* Patient maintains skin integrity.

IMPLEMENTATION

ACTION	RATIONALE
1. Review the patient's chart for any limitations in physical activity. (See Skill Variation: Assisting With Use of a Bedpan When the Patient Has Limited Movement.)	Activity limitations may contraindicate certain actions by the patient.
2. Bring bedpan and other necessary equipment to the bedside stand or overbed table.	Bringing everything to the bedside conserves time and energy. Arranging items nearby is convenient, saves time, and avoids unnecessary stretching and twisting of muscles on the part of the nurse.
3. Perform hand hygiene and put on PPE, if indicated.	Hand hygiene and PPE prevent the spread of microorganisms. PPE is required based on transmission precautions.

ACTION	RATIONALE
4. Identify the patient.	Identifying the patient ensures the right patient receives the intervention and helps prevent errors.
5. Close curtains around bed and close the door to the room, if possible. Discuss the procedure with the patient and assess the patient's ability to assist with the procedure, as well as personal hygiene preferences.	This ensures the patient's privacy. This discussion promotes reassurance and provides knowledge about the procedure. Dialogue encourages patient participation and allows for individualized nursing care.
6. Unless contraindicated, apply powder to the rim of the bedpan. Place bedpan and cover on chair next to bed. Put on gloves.	Powder helps keep the bedpan from sticking to the patient's skin and makes it easier to remove. Powder is not applied if the patient has respiratory problems or is allergic to powder or if a urine specimen is needed (could contaminate the specimen). The bedpan on the chair allows for easy access. Gloves prevent contact with blood and body fluids.
7. Adjust the bed to comfortable working height, usually elbow height of the caregiver (VISN 8 Patient Safety Center, 2009). Place the patient in a supine position, with the head of the bed elevated about 30 degrees, unless contraindicated.	Having the bed at the proper height prevents back and muscle strain. Supine position is necessary for correct placement of the patient on the bedpan.
8. Fold top linen back just enough to allow placement of the bedpan. If there is no waterproof pad on the bed and time allows, consider placing a waterproof pad under patient's buttocks before placing bedpan.	Folding back the linen in this manner minimizes unnecessary exposure while allowing the nurse to place the bedpan. The waterproof pad will protect the bed should there be a spill.
9. Ask the patient to bend the knees. Have the patient lift his or her hips upward. Assist the patient, if necessary, by	The nurse uses less energy when the patient can assist by placing some of his or her weight on the heels.

ACTION	RATIONALE
placing your hand that is closest to the patient palm up, under the lower back, and assist with lifting. Slip the bedpan into place with other hand.	
10. **Ensure that bedpan is in proper position and the patient's buttocks are resting on the rounded shelf of the regular bedpan or the shallow rim of the fracture bedpan.**	Having the bedpan in the proper position prevents spills onto the bed, ensures patient comfort, and prevents injury to the skin from a misplaced bedpan.
11. Raise the head of bed as near to sitting position as tolerated, unless contraindicated. Cover the patient with bed linens.	This position makes it easier for the patient to void or defecate, avoids strain on the patient's back, and allows gravity to aid in elimination. Covering promotes warmth and privacy.
12. **Place the call bell and toilet tissue within easy reach. Place the bed in the lowest position.** Leave patient if it is safe to do so. Use side rails appropriately.	Falls can be prevented if the patient does not have to reach for items he or she needs. Placing the bed in the lowest position promotes patient safety. Leaving the patient alone, if possible, promotes self-esteem and shows respect for privacy. Side rails assist the patient in repositioning.
13. Remove gloves and additional PPE, if used. Perform hand hygiene.	Proper removal of PPE prevents transmission of microorganisms. Hand hygiene deters the spread of microorganisms.

Removing the Bedpan

14. Perform hand hygiene and put on gloves and additional PPE, as indicated. Adjust bed to comfortable working height, usually elbow height of the caregiver (VISN 8 Patient Safety Center, 2009). Have a receptacle, such as plastic trash bag, handy for discarding tissue.	Hand hygiene deters the spread of microorganisms. Gloves prevent exposure to blood and body fluids. Having the bed at the proper height prevents back and muscle strain. Proper disposal of soiled tissue prevents transmission of microorganisms.

ACTION	RATIONALE
15. Lower the head of the bed, if necessary, to about 30 degrees. Remove bedpan in the same manner in which it was offered, being careful to hold it steady. Ask the patient to bend the knees and lift the buttocks up from the bedpan. Assist the patient, if necessary, by placing your hand that is closest to the patient palm up, under the lower back, and assist with lifting. Place the bedpan on the bedside chair and cover it.	Holding the bedpan steady prevents spills. The nurse uses less energy when the patient can assist by placing some of his or her weight on the heels. Covering the bedpan helps to prevent the spread of microorganisms.
16. If the patient needs assistance with hygiene, wrap tissue around the hand several times, and wipe patient clean, using one stroke from the pubic area toward the anal area. Discard tissue, and use more until patient is clean. Place patient on his or her side and spread buttocks to clean anal area.	Cleaning area from front to back minimizes fecal contamination of the vagina and urinary meatus. Cleaning the patient after he or she has used the bedpan prevents offensive odors and irritation to the skin.
17. Do not place toilet tissue in the bedpan if a specimen is required or if output is being recorded. Place toilet tissue in appropriate receptacle.	Mixing toilet tissue with a specimen makes laboratory examination more difficult and interferes with accurate output measurement.
18. Return the patient to a comfortable position. Make sure the linens under the patient are dry. Replace or remove pad under the patient, as necessary. Remove your gloves and ensure that the patient is covered.	Positioning helps to promote patient comfort. Removing contaminated gloves prevents spread of microorganisms.
19. Raise side rail. Lower bed height and adjust head of bed to a comfortable position. Reattach call bell.	These actions promote patient safety.

ACTION	RATIONALE
20. Offer the patient supplies to wash and dry his or her hands, assisting as necessary.	Washing hands after using the urinal helps prevent the spread of microorganisms.
21. Put on clean gloves. Empty and clean the bedpan, measuring urine in graduated container, as necessary. Discard trash receptacle with used toilet paper, per facility policy.	Gloves prevent exposure to blood and body fluids. Cleaning reusable equipment helps prevent the spread of microorganisms.
22. Remove additional PPE, if used. Perform hand hygiene.	Removing PPE properly reduces the risk for infection transmission and contamination of other items. Hand hygiene prevents the spread of microorganisms.

EVALUATION

* Patient voids using the bedpan.
* Patient remains dry.
* Patient does not experience episodes of incontinence.
* Patient demonstrates measures to assist with using the bedpan.
* Patient does not experience impaired skin integrity.

DOCUMENTATION

* Document the patient's tolerance of the activity. Record the amount of urine voided on the intake and output record, if appropriate. Document any other assessments, such as unusual urine characteristics or alterations in the patient's skin.

GENERAL CONSIDERATIONS

* A fracture bedpan is usually more comfortable for the patient, but it does not hold as large a volume as the regular bedpan.
* Bedpan should not be left in place for extended periods of time as this can result in excessive pressure and irritation to the patient's skin.

Skill Variation   Assisting With Use of a Bedpan When the Patient Has Limited Movement

Patients who are unable to lift themselves onto the bedpan or who have activity limitations that prohibit the required actions can be assisted onto the bedpan in an alternate manner using these actions:

(continued on page 65)

Assisting With Use of a Bedpan When the Patient Has Limited Movement *continued*

1. Discuss the procedure with the patient and assess his or her ability to assist with the procedure, as well as personal hygiene preferences. Review the patient's chart for any limitations in physical activity.

2. Bring bedpan and other necessary equipment to bedside. Put on PPE, as indicated, and perform hand hygiene. Check the patient's identification band.

3. Unless contraindicated, apply powder to the rim of the bedpan.

4. Place bedpan and cover on chair next to bed. Close curtains around bed and close the door to the room, if possible.

5. Adjust the bed to comfortable working height, usually elbow height of the caregiver (VISN 8 Patient Safety Center, 2009). Place the patient in a supine position, with the head of the bed elevated about 30 degrees, unless contraindicated. Put on disposable gloves.

6. Fold top linen just enough to turn the patient, while minimizing exposure. If there is no waterproof pad on the bed and time allows, consider placing a waterproof pad under patient's buttocks before placing the bedpan.

7. Assist the patient to roll to the opposite side or turn the patient into a side-lying position.

8. Hold the bedpan firmly against the patient's buttocks, with the upper end of the bedpan under the patient's buttocks toward the sacrum and down into the mattress.

9. Keep one hand against the bedpan. Apply gentle pressure to ensure the bedpan remains in place as you assist the patient to roll back onto the bedpan.

10. Ensure that bedpan is in proper position and the patient's buttocks are resting on the rounded shelf of the regular bedpan or the shallow rim of the fracture bedpan.

11. Raise the head of the bed as near to sitting position as tolerated, unless contraindicated. Cover the patient with bed linens.

12. Place call bell and toilet tissue within easy reach. Place the bed in the lowest position. Leave patient if it is safe to do so. Use side rails appropriately.

13. Remove gloves, and PPE, if used. Perform hand hygiene.

14. To remove the bedpan, perform hand hygiene and put on disposable gloves, and additional PPE, as indicated. Raise the bed to a comfortable working height. Have a receptacle handy for discarding tissue.

(continued on page 66)

Assisting With Use of a Bedpan When the Patient Has Limited Movement *continued*

15. Lower the head of the bed. Grasp the closest side of the bedpan. Apply gentle pressure to hold the bedpan flat and steady. Assist the patient to roll to the opposite side or turn the patient into a side-lying position with the assistance of a second caregiver. Remove the bedpan and set on chair. Cover the bedpan.

16. Wrap tissue around the hand several times, and wipe patient clean, using one stroke from the pubic area toward the anal area. Discard tissue in an appropriate receptacle, and use more until the patient is clean. Do not place toilet tissue in the bedpan if a specimen is required or if output is being recorded. Spread buttocks to clean anal area.

17. Return the patient to a comfortable position. Make sure the linens under the patient are dry and that the patient is covered.

18. Remove your gloves. Offer the patient supplies to wash and dry his or her hands, assisting as necessary.

19. Raise the side rail. Lower bed height and adjust the head of bed to a comfortable position. Reattach call bell.

20. Put on clean gloves. Empty and clean the bedpan, measuring urine in graduated container, as necessary. Remove gloves and additional PPE, if used. Perform hand hygiene.

Skill · 13   Using a Bed Scale

Obtaining a patient's weight is an important component of assessment. In addition to providing baseline information of the patient's overall status, weight is a valuable indicator of nutritional status and fluid balance. Changes in a patient's weight can provide clues to underlying problems, such as nutritional deficiencies or fluid excess or deficiency, or indicate the development of new problems, such as fluid overload. Weight also can be used to evaluate a patient's response to treatment. For example, if a patient was receiving nutritional supplementation, obtaining daily or biweekly weights would be used to determine achievement of the expected outcome (weight gain).

Typically, weight is measured by having the patient stand on an upright scale. However, doing so requires that the patient is mobile and can maintain his or her balance. For patients who are confined to the bed, have limited mobility, or cannot maintain a balanced standing position for a short period of time, a bed scale can be used. With a bed scale, the patient is placed in a sling and raised above the bed. To ensure safety, a second nurse should be on hand to assist with weighing the patient. Many facilities are providing beds for patient use with built-in scales. The following procedure explains how to weigh the patient with a portable bed scale.

EQUIPMENT
- Bed scale with sling
- Cover for sling
- Sheet or bath blanket
- PPE, as indicated

ASSESSMENT GUIDELINES
- Assess the patient's ability to stand for a weight measurement. If the patient cannot stand, assess the patient's ability to sit in a chair or to lie still for a weight measurement.
- Assess the patient for pain; medication may be given for pain or sedation before placing the patient on a bed scale.
- Assess for the presence of any material, such as tubes, drains, or IV tubing, which could become entangled in the scale or pulled during the weighing procedure.

NURSING DIAGNOSES
- Risk for Injury
- Impaired Physical Mobility
- Imbalanced Nutrition: Less Than Body Requirements
- Imbalanced Nutrition: More Than Body Requirements

OUTCOME IDENTIFICATION AND PLANNING
Expected outcomes may include:
- Patient's weight is assessed accurately, without injury, and the patient experiences minimal discomfort.

IMPLEMENTATION

ACTION	RATIONALE
1. Check medical order or nursing care plan for frequency of weight measurement. More frequent pulse measurement may be appropriate based on nursing judgment. Obtain the assistance of a second caregiver, based on patient's mobility and ability to cooperate with the procedure.	This provides for patient safety and appropriate care.

ACTION	RATIONALE

2. Perform hand hygiene and put on PPE, if indicated.

Hand hygiene and PPE prevent the spread of microorganisms. PPE is required based on transmission precautions.

3. Identify the patient.

Identifying the patient ensures the right patient receives the intervention and helps prevent errors.

4. Close curtains around bed and close the door to the room, if possible. Discuss the procedure with the patient and assess the patient's ability to assist with the procedure.

This ensures the patient's privacy. Explanation relieves anxiety and facilitates cooperation.

5. Place a cover over the sling of the bed scale.

Using a cover deters the spread of microorganisms.

6. Attach the sling to the bed scale. Lay the sheet or bath blanket in the sling. Turn on the scale. **Adjust the dial so that weight reads 0.0.**

Scale will add the sling into the weight unless it is zeroed with the sling, blanket, and cover.

7. Adjust bed to comfortable working position, usually elbow height of the caregiver (VISN 8 Patient Safety Center, 2009). Position one caregiver on each side of the bed, if two caregivers are present. Raise side rail on the opposite side of the bed from where the scale is located, if not already in place. Cover the patient with the sheet or bath blanket. Remove other covers and any pillows.

Having the bed at the proper height prevents back and muscle strain. Having one caregiver on each side of the bed provides for patient safety and appropriate care. Blanket maintains patient's dignity and provides warmth.

8. Turn the patient onto his or her side facing the side rail, keeping his or her body covered with the sheet or blanket. Remove the sling from the

Rolling the patient onto his or her side facilitates placing the patient onto the sling. Blanket maintains patient's dignity and provides warmth.

ACTION	RATIONALE
scale. Roll sling long ways. Place rolled sling under patient, making sure the patient is centered in the sling.	
9. Roll the patient back over the sling and onto the other side. Pull the sling through, as if placing a sheet under the patient, unrolling as it is pulled through.	This facilitates placing the patient onto the sling.
10. Roll scale over the bed so that the arms of the scale are directly over the patient. **Spread the base of the scale.** Lower arms of the scale and place arm hooks into holes on the sling.	By spreading the base, you are giving the scale a wider base, thus preventing the scale from toppling over with the patient. Hooking sling to scale provides secure attachment to the scale and prevents injury.
11. Once scale arms are hooked onto the sling, gradually elevate the sling so that the patient is lifted up off of the bed (FIGURE 1). Assess all tubes and drains, making sure that none have tension placed on them as the scale is lifted. Once the sling is no longer touching the bed, ensure that nothing else is hanging onto the sling (e.g., ventilator tubing, IV tubing). If any tubing is connected to the patient, raise it up so that it is not adding any weight to the patient.	Scale must be hanging free to obtain an accurate weight. Any tubing that is hanging off the scale will add weight to the patient.

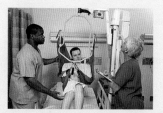

FIGURE 1 Using a bed scale.

ACTION	RATIONALE
12. Note weight reading on the scale. Slowly and gently, lower patient back onto the bed. Disconnect scale arms from the sling. Close base of scale and pull it away from the bed.	Lowering patient slowly does not alarm patient. Closing the base of the scale facilitates moving the scale.
13. Raise the side rail. Turn the patient to the side rail. Roll the sling up against the patient's backside.	Raising the side rail is a safety measure.
14. Raise the other side rail. Roll the patient back over the sling and up facing the other side rail. Remove sling from bed. Remove gloves, if used. Raise remaining side rail.	Patient needs to be removed from the sling before it can be removed from the bed.
15. Cover the patient and help him or her to a position of comfort. Place the bed in the lowest position.	Ensures patient comfort and safety.
16. Remove disposable cover from the sling and discard it in an appropriate receptacle.	Using a cover deters spread of microorganisms.
17. Remove additional PPE, if used. Perform hand hygiene.	Removing PPE properly reduces the risk for infection transmission and contamination of other items. Hand hygiene deters the spread of microorganisms.
18. Replace scale and sling in appropriate spot. Plug scale into electrical outlet.	Scale should be ready for use at any time.

EVALUATION

• Patient is weighed accurately without injury using the bed scale.

DOCUMENTATION

• Document weight, unit of measurement, and scale used.

Skill · 14 — Assessing Bladder Volume Using an Ultrasound Bladder Scanner

Portable bladder ultrasound devices are accurate, reliable, and noninvasive devices used to assess bladder volume. Bladder scanners do not pose a risk for the development of a urinary tract infection, unlike intermittent catheterization, which is also used to determine bladder volume. They are used when there is urinary frequency, absent or decreased urine output, bladder distention, or inability to void, and when establishing intermittent catheterization schedules. Protocols can be established to guide the decision to catheterize a patient. Some scanners offer the ability to print the scan results for documentation purposes.

Results are most accurate when the patient is in the supine position during the scanning. The device must be programmed for the gender of the patient by pushing the correct button on the device. If a female patient has had a hysterectomy, the male button is pushed (Altschuler & Diaz, 2006). A postvoid residual (PVR) volume less than 50 mL indicates adequate bladder emptying. A PVR of greater than 150 mL is often recommended as the guideline for catheterization, because residual urine volumes greater than 150 mL have been associated with the development of urinary tract infections (Stevens, 2005).

EQUIPMENT
- Bladder scanner
- Ultrasound gel or bladder scan gel pad
- Alcohol wipe or other sanitizer recommended by the scanner
- manufacturer and/or facility policy
- Clean gloves
- Additional PPE, as indicated
- Paper towel or washcloth

ASSESSMENT GUIDELINES
- Assess the patient for the need to check bladder volume, including signs of urinary retention, measurement of postvoid residual volume, verification that bladder is empty, identification of obstruction in an indwelling catheter, and evaluation of bladder distension to determine if catheterization is necessary.
- Verify medical order, if required by facility. Many facilities allow the use of a bladder scanner as a nursing judgment.

NURSING DIAGNOSES
- Impaired Urinary Elimination
- Urinary Retention

OUTCOME IDENTIFICATION AND PLANNING
Expected outcomes may include:
- Volume of urine in the patient's bladder will be accurately measured.
- Patient's urinary elimination will be maintained, with a urine output of at least 30 mL/hour.
- Patient's bladder will not be distended.

IMPLEMENTATION

ACTION	RATIONALE
1. Review the patient's chart for any limitations in physical activity.	Physical limitations may require adaptations in performing the skill.
2. Bring the bladder scanner and other necessary equipment to the bedside.	Bringing everything to the bedside conserves time and energy. Arranging items nearby is convenient, saves time, and avoids unnecessary stretching and twisting of muscles on the part of the nurse.
3. Perform hand hygiene and put on PPE, if indicated.	Hand hygiene and PPE prevent the spread of microorganisms. PPE is required based on transmission precautions.
4. Identify the patient.	Identifying the patient ensures the right patient receives the intervention and helps prevent errors.
5. Close curtains around bed and close the door to the room, if possible. Discuss the procedure with the patient and assess the patient's ability to assist with the procedure, as well as personal hygiene preferences.	This ensures the patient's privacy. Discussion promotes reassurance and provides knowledge about the procedure. Dialogue encourages patient participation and allows for individualized nursing care.
6. Adjust the bed to a comfortable working height; usually elbow height of the caregiver (VISN 8 Patient Safety Center, 2009). Place the patient in a supine position. Drape the patient. Stand on the patient's right side if you are right-handed, patient's left side if you are left-handed.	Having the bed at the proper height prevents back and muscle strain. Proper positioning allows accurate assessment of bladder volume. Keeping the patient covered as much as possible promotes patient comfort and privacy. Positioning allows for ease of use of dominant hand for the procedure.
7. Put on clean gloves.	Gloves prevent contact with blood and body fluids.

ACTION	RATIONALE
8. Press the ON button. Wait until the device warms up. Press the SCAN button to turn on the scanning screen.	Many devices require a few minutes to prepare the internal programs.
9. Press the appropriate gender button. The appropriate icon for male or female will appear on the screen.	The device must be programmed for the gender of the patient by pushing the correct button on the device. If a female patient has had a hysterectomy, push the male button (Altschuler & Diaz, 2006).
10. Clean the scanner head with the appropriate cleaner.	Cleaning the scanner head deters transmission of microorganisms.
11. **Gently palpate the patient's symphysis pubis. Place a generous amount of ultrasound gel or gel pad midline on the patient's abdomen, about 1 to 1.5 inches above the symphysis pubis (anterior midline junction of pubic bones).**	Palpation identifies the proper location and allows for correct placement of the scanner head over the patient's bladder.
12. **Place the scanner head on the gel or gel pad, with the directional icon on the scanner head toward the patient's head. Aim the scanner head toward the bladder (point the scanner head slightly downward toward the coccyx) (Patraca, 2005). Press and release the 'Scan' button (FIGURE 1).**	Proper placement allows for accurate reading of urine in the bladder.

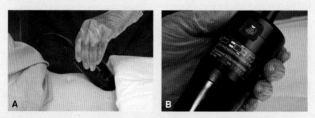

FIGURE 1 (**A**) Positioning the scanner head with directional icon toward the patient's head. (**B**) Pressing the scan button. (*Photos by B. Proud*)

ACTION	RATIONALE
13. Observe the image on the scanner screen. **Adjust the scanner head to center the bladder image on the cross-bars (FIGURE 2).**	This action allows for accurate reading of urine in bladder.

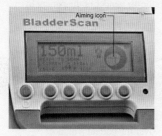

FIGURE 2 Centering the image on the crossbars. (From Patraca, K. (2005). Measure bladder volume without catheterization. *Nursing, 35*(4), 47, with permission.)

ACTION	RATIONALE
14. Press and hold the DONE button until it beeps. Read the volume measurement on the screen. Print the results, if required, by pressing PRINT.	This action provides for accurate documentation of reading.
15. Use a washcloth or paper towel to remove remaining gel from the patient's skin. Alternately, gently remove gel pad from the patient's skin. Return the patient to a comfortable position. Remove your gloves and ensure that the patient is covered.	Removal of the gel promotes patient comfort. Removing contaminated gloves prevents spread of microorganisms.
16. Lower bed height and adjust head of bed to a comfortable position. Reattach call bell, if necessary.	These actions promote patient safety.
17. Remove additional PPE, if used. Perform hand hygiene.	Removing PPE properly reduces the risk for infection transmission and contamination of other items. Hand hygiene prevents the spread of microorganisms.

EVALUATION

- Volume of urine in the bladder is accurately measured.
- Patient's urinary elimination is maintained, with a urine output of at least 30 mL/hour.
- Patient's bladder is not distended.

DOCUMENTATION

- Document the assessment data that led to the use of the bladder scanner, the urine volume measured, and the patient's response.

Skill · 15   **Obtaining a Capillary Blood Sample for Glucose Testing**

Blood glucose monitoring provides information about how the body is controlling glucose metabolism. Controlling the patient's blood glucose levels is an important part of medical care (ADA, 2008; Levetan, 2005). It is indicated in the care of patients with many conditions, including diabetes, seizures, enteral and parenteral feeding, liver disease, pancreatitis, head injury, stroke, alcohol and drug intoxication, and sepsis, and also with patients prescribed corticosteroids. Point-of-care testing (testing done at the bedside, where samples are not sent to the laboratory) provides a convenient, rapid, and accurate measurement of blood glucose (ADA, 2008; Ferguson, 2005). Blood samples are commonly obtained from the edges of the fingers for adults, but samples can be obtained from the palm of the hand, forearm, upper arm, and anterior thigh, depending on the time of testing and monitor used (Dale, 2006). Avoid fingertips, because they are more sensitive. Rotate sites to prevent skin damage. **It is important to be familiar with and follow the manufacturer's guidelines and facility policy and procedure to ensure accurate results.** Normal fasting glucose for adults is less than 110 mg/dL (Fischbach & Dunning, 2009).

EQUIPMENT

- Blood glucose meter
- Sterile lancet
- Cotton balls or gauze squares
- Testing strips for meter
- Nonsterile gloves
- Additional PPE, as indicated
- Soap and water or alcohol swab

ASSESSMENT GUIDELINES

- Assess the patient's understanding of the collection procedure, reason for testing, and ability to cooperate.
- Assess the patient's history for indications necessitating the monitoring of blood glucose levels, such as high-carbohydrate feedings, history of diabetes mellitus, or corticosteroid therapy.

• Assess the patient's knowledge about monitoring blood glucose.
• Inspect the area of the skin to be used for testing. Avoid bruised and open areas.

NURSING DIAGNOSES

• Risk for Unstable Blood Glucose Level
• Risk for Injury
• Deficient Knowledge
• Anxiety

OUTCOME IDENTIFICATION AND PLANNING

Expected outcomes may include:
• The blood glucose level is measured accurately without adverse effect.
• The patient demonstrates accurate understanding of testing instructions.
• The patient demonstrates a blood glucose level within acceptable parameters.
• The patient demonstrates ability to participate in monitoring.
• The patient verbalizes increased comfort with the procedure.

IMPLEMENTATION

ACTION	RATIONALE
1. Check the patient's medical record or nursing plan of care for monitoring schedule. The nurse may decide that additional testing is indicated based on nursing judgment and the patient's condition.	This confirms scheduled times for checking blood glucose. Independent nursing judgment may lead to the decision to test more frequently, based on the patient's condition.
2. Bring necessary equipment to the bedside stand or over-bed table.	Bringing everything to the bedside conserves time and energy. Arranging items nearby is convenient, saves time, and avoids unnecessary stretching and twisting of muscles on the part of the nurse. Organization facilitates performance of tasks.
3. Perform hand hygiene and put on PPE, if indicated.	Hand hygiene and PPE prevent the transmission of microorganisms. PPE is required based on transmission precautions.

ACTION	RATIONALE
4. Identify the patient. Explain the procedure to the patient and instruct the patient about the need for monitoring blood glucose.	Identifying the patient ensures the right patient receives the intervention and helps prevent errors. Explanation helps to alleviate anxiety and facilitates cooperation.
5. Close curtains around bed or close the door to the room, if possible.	Closing the door or curtain provides for patient privacy.
6. Turn on the monitor.	The monitor must be on for use.
7. Enter the patient's identification number, if required, according to facility policy.	Use of identification number allows for electronic storage and accurate identification of patient data.
8. Put on nonsterile gloves.	Gloves protect the nurse from exposure to blood or body fluids.
9. Prepare lancet using aseptic technique.	Aseptic technique maintains sterility.
10. Remove test strip from the vial. **Recap container immediately.** Test strips also come individually wrapped. **Check that the code number for the strip matches the code number on the monitor screen.**	Immediate recapping protects strips from exposure to humidity, light, and discoloration. Matching code numbers on the strip and glucose monitor ensures that the machine is calibrated correctly.
11. Insert strip into the meter according to directions for that specific device.	Correctly inserted strip allows meter to read blood glucose level accurately.
12. For adult, massage side of finger toward puncture site.	Massage encourages blood to flow to the area.
13. **Have patient wash hands with soap and warm water and dry thoroughly.** Alternately, **cleanse the skin with an alcohol swab. Allow skin to dry completely.**	Washing with soap and water or alcohol cleanses the puncture site. Warm water also helps to cause vasodilation. Alcohol can interfere with accuracy of results if not completely dried.
14. Hold lancet perpendicular to skin and pierce site with lancet (FIGURE 1).	Holding lancet in proper position facilitates proper skin penetration.
15. Wipe away first drop of blood with gauze square or	Manufacturers recommend discarding the first drop of blood,

ACTION	RATIONALE

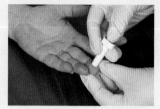

FIGURE 1 Piercing patient's finger with lancet.

cotton ball, if recommended by manufacturer of monitor.

16. Encourage bleeding by lowering the hand, making use of gravity. Lightly stroke the finger, if necessary, until a sufficient amount of blood has formed to cover the sample area on the strip, based on monitor requirements (check instructions for monitor). Take care not to squeeze the finger, not to squeeze at the puncture site, or not to touch the puncture site or blood.

17. Gently touch a drop of blood to pad to the test strip without smearing it (FIGURE 2).

which may be contaminated by serum or cleansing product, producing an inaccurate reading.

An appropriate-sized droplet facilitates accurate test results. Squeezing can cause injury to the patient and alter the test result (Ferguson, 2005).

Smearing blood on strip may result in inaccurate test results.

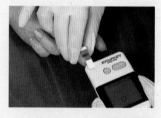

FIGURE 2 Applying blood to test strip.

18. Press time button if directed by manufacturer.

Correct timing produces accurate results.

ACTION	RATIONALE
19. Apply pressure to the puncture site with a cotton ball or dry gauze. **Do not use alcohol wipe.**	Pressure causes hemostasis. Alcohol stings and may prolong bleeding.
20. Read blood glucose results and document appropriately at bedside. Inform patient of test result.	Timing depends on type of meter.
21. Turn off meter, remove test strip, and dispose of supplies appropriately. Place lancet in sharps container.	Proper disposal prevents exposure to blood and accidental needlestick.
22. Remove gloves and any other PPE, if used. Perform hand hygiene.	Removing PPE properly reduces the risk for infection transmission and contamination of other items. Hand hygiene reduces the transmission of microorganisms.

EVALUATION

- The patient's blood glucose level is measured accurately without adverse effect.
- The patient demonstrates accurate understanding of testing instructions.
- The blood glucose level is within acceptable limits.
- The patient participates in monitoring.
- The patient verbalizes comfort with the procedure.

DOCUMENTATION

- Document blood glucose level on flow sheet in medical record, according to facility policy. Document pertinent patient assessments, any intervention related to glucose level, and any patient teaching. Report abnormal results and/or significant assessments to primary healthcare provider.

GENERAL CONSIDERATIONS

- Sampling of blood from an alternative site other than fingertips may have limitations. Blood in the fingertips show changes in glucose levels more quickly than blood in other parts of the body. This means that alternative site test results may be different from fingertip test results when glucose levels are changing rapidly (e.g., after a meal, taking insulin, or during or after exercise) because the actual glucose concentration is different. Patients should be cautioned to use a fingertip sample if it is less than 2 hours after eating; less than 2 hours after injecting rapid-acting insulin; during exercise or within 2 hours of exercise; when sick or under stress; when having symptoms of hypoglycemia; if patient is unable to recognize symptoms of hypoglycemia; or if site results do not agree with the way the patient feels (Dale, 2006).

- Meters require calibration at least monthly or according to the manufacturer's recommendation, and when a new bottle of test strips is opened. Manufacturer's directions for calibration should be followed. After calibration, the meter is checked for accuracy by testing a control solution containing a known amount of glucose.
- Inadequate sampling can cause errors in the results. It is very important to be aware of requirements for specific monitor used.
- Monitors that measure glucose collected from the skin have recently become available. One of these devices, which uses electrical stimulation to draw interstitial fluid through intact skin into a transdermal pad, is worn like a watch and provides a reading every 20 minutes. Another device is a monitor worn on a belt that uses a fine needle worn in the subcutaneous tissue to measure interstitial fluid glucose levels and transmit the results to a computer (Brown, 2008).

Skill · 16   Assessing Brachial Artery Blood Pressure

Blood pressure refers to the force of the blood against arterial walls. Systolic pressure is the highest point of pressure on arterial walls when the ventricles contract and push blood through the arteries at the beginning of systole. When the heart rests between beats during diastole, the pressure drops. The lowest pressure present on arterial walls during diastole is the diastolic pressure (Taylor et al., 2011). Blood pressure is measured in millimeters of mercury (mm Hg) and is recorded as a fraction. The numerator is the systolic pressure; the denominator is the diastolic pressure. The difference between the two is called the pulse pressure. For example, if the blood pressure is 120/80 mm Hg, 120 is the systolic pressure and 80 is the diastolic pressure. The pulse pressure, in this case, is 40.

To get an accurate assessment of blood pressure, you should know what equipment to use, which site to choose, and how to identify the sounds you hear. Take routine measurements after the patient has rested for a minimum of 5 minutes. In addition, make sure the patient does not have any caffeine or nicotine 30 minutes before measuring blood pressure.

The series of sounds for which to listen when assessing blood pressure are called Korotkoff sounds. Blood pressure may be assessed with different types of devices. Commonly, it is assessed by using a stethoscope and sphygmomanometer. Blood pressure may also be estimated with a Doppler ultrasound and by palpation, and assessed with electronic or automated devices. It is very important to use correct technique and properly functioning equipment when assessing blood pressure to avoid errors in measurement. It is necessary to use a cuff of the correct size for the patient, correct limb placement, recommended deflation rate, and correct interpretation of the sounds heard to ensure accurate blood pressure measurement (Smeltzer et al., 2010; Pickering, 2005; Pickering, et al., 2004).

Various sites may be used to assess blood pressure. The brachial artery and the popliteal artery are used most commonly. This skill discusses using the brachial artery site to obtain a blood pressure measurement. The skill begins with the procedure for estimating systolic pressure. Estimation of systolic pressure prevents inaccurate readings in the presence of an auscultatory gap (a pause in the auscultated sounds). To identify the first Korotkoff sound accurately, the cuff must be inflated to a pressure above the point at which the pulse can no longer be felt.

EQUIPMENT

- Stethoscope
- Sphygmomanometer
- Blood pressure cuff of appropriate size
- Pencil or pen, paper or flow sheet
- Alcohol swab
- PPE, as indicated

ASSESSMENT GUIDELINES

- Assess the brachial pulse, or the pulse appropriate for the site being used.
- Assess for an intravenous infusion or breast or axilla surgery on the side of the body corresponding to the arm used. Assess for the presence of a cast, arteriovenous shunt, or injured or diseased limb. If any of these conditions are present, do not use the affected arm to monitor blood pressure.
- Assess the size of the limb so that the appropriate-sized blood pressure cuff can be used. The correct cuff should have a bladder length that is 80% of the arm circumference and a width that is at least 40% of the arm circumference: a length to width ratio of 2:1.
- Assess for factors that could affect blood pressure reading, such as the patient's age, exercise, position, weight, fluid balance, smoking, and medications. Note baseline or previous blood pressure measurements. Assess the patient for pain.
- If the patient reports pain, give pain medication, as ordered, before assessing blood pressure. If the blood pressure is taken while the patient is in pain, make a notation concerning the pain if the blood pressure is elevated.

NURSING DIAGNOSES

- Decreased Cardiac Output
- Ineffective Health Maintenance
- Effective Therapeutic Regimen Management
- Risk for Falls

OUTCOME IDENTIFICATION AND PLANNING

Expected outcomes may include:
• Patient's blood pressure is measured accurately without injury.

IMPLEMENTATION

ACTION	RATIONALE
1. Check medical order or nursing care plan for frequency of blood pressure measurement. More frequent measurement may be appropriate based on nursing judgment.	Provides for patient safety.
2. Perform hand hygiene and put on PPE, if indicated.	Hand hygiene and PPE prevent the spread of microorganisms. PPE is required based on transmission precautions.
3. Identify the patient.	Identifying the patient ensures the right patient receives the intervention and helps prevent errors.
4. Close curtains around bed and close the door to the room, if possible. Discuss the procedure with the patient and assess the patient's ability to assist with the procedure. Validate that the patient has relaxed for several minutes.	This ensures the patient's privacy. Explanation relieves anxiety and facilitates cooperation. Activity immediately before measurement can result in inaccurate results.
5. Put on gloves, if appropriate or indicated.	Gloves prevent contact with blood and body fluids. Gloves are usually not required for measurement of blood pressure, unless contact with blood or body fluids is anticipated.
6. Select the appropriate arm for application of the cuff.	Measurement of blood pressure may temporarily impede circulation to the extremity.
7. Have the patient assume a comfortable lying or sitting position with the forearm supported at the level of the heart and the palm of the	The position of the arm can have a major influence when the blood pressure is measured; if the upper arm is below the level of the right atrium, the readings will

hand upward. If the measurement is taken in the supine position, support the arm with a pillow. In the sitting position, support the arm yourself or by using the bedside table. If the patient is sitting, have the patient sit back in the chair so that the chair supports his or her back. In addition, make sure the patient keeps the legs uncrossed.

be too high. If the arm is above the level of the heart, the readings will be too low (Pickering, et al., 2004). If the back is not supported, the diastolic pressure may be elevated falsely; if the legs are crossed, the systolic pressure may be elevated falsely (Pickering, et al., 2004). This position places the brachial artery on the inner aspect of the elbow so that the bell or diaphragm of the stethoscope can rest on it easily. This sitting position ensures accuracy.

8. Expose the brachial artery by removing garments, or move a sleeve, if it is not too tight, above the area where the cuff will be placed.

Clothing over the artery interferes with the ability to hear sounds and may cause inaccurate blood pressure readings. A tight sleeve would cause congestion of blood and possibly inaccurate readings.

9. Palpate the location of the brachial artery. **Center the bladder of the cuff over the brachial artery, about midway on the arm, so that the lower edge of the cuff is about 2.5 to 5 cm (1 to 2 inches) above the inner aspect of the elbow. Line the artery marking on the cuff up with the patient's brachial artery. The tubing should extend from the edge of the cuff nearer the patient's elbow (FIGURE 1).**

Pressure in the cuff applied directly to the artery provides the most accurate readings. If the cuff gets in the way of the stethoscope, readings are likely to be inaccurate. A cuff placed upside down with the tubing toward the patient's head may give a false reading.

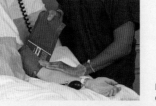

FIGURE 1 Placing blood pressure cuff. (*Photo by B. Proud.*)

ACTION	RATIONALE
10. Wrap the cuff around the arm smoothly and snugly, and fasten it. Do not allow any clothing to interfere with the proper placement of the cuff.	A smooth cuff and snug wrapping produce equal pressure and help promote an accurate measurement. A cuff wrapped too loosely results in an inaccurate reading.
11. Check that the needle on the aneroid gauge is within the zero mark. If using a mercury manometer, check to see that the manometer is in the vertical position and that the mercury is within the zero level with the gauge at eye level.	If the needle is not in the zero area, the blood pressure measurement may not be accurate. Tilting a mercury manometer, inaccurate calibration, or improper height for reading the gauge can lead to errors in determining the pressure measurements.

Estimating Systolic Pressure

12. Palpate the pulse at the brachial or radial artery by pressing gently with the fingertips.	Palpation allows for measurement of the approximate systolic reading.
13. Tighten the screw valve on the air pump.	The bladder within the cuff will not inflate with the valve open.
14. **Inflate the cuff while continuing to palpate the artery. Note the point on the gauge where the pulse disappears.**	The point where the pulse disappears provides an estimate of the systolic pressure. To identify the first Korotkoff sound accurately, the cuff must be inflated to a pressure above the point at which the pulse can no longer be felt.
15. Deflate the cuff and wait 1 minute.	Allowing a brief pause before continuing permits the blood to refill and circulate through the arm.

Obtaining Blood Pressure Measurement

16. Assume a position that is no more than 3 feet away from the gauge.	A distance of more than about 3 feet can interfere with accurate readings of the numbers on the gauge.
17. Place the stethoscope earpieces in your ears. Direct the earpieces forward into the canal and not against the ear itself.	Proper placement blocks extraneous noise and allows sound to travel more clearly.

ACTION	RATIONALE
18. Place the bell or diaphragm of the stethoscope firmly but with as little pressure as possible over the brachial artery. Do not allow the stethoscope to touch clothing or the cuff.	Having the bell or diaphragm directly over the artery allows more accurate readings. Heavy pressure on the brachial artery distorts the shape of the artery and the sound. Placing the bell or diaphragm away from clothing and the cuff prevents noise, which would distract from the sounds made by blood flowing through the artery.
19. Pump the pressure 30 mm Hg above the point at which the systolic pressure was palpated and estimated. Open the valve on the manometer and allow air to escape slowly (allowing the gauge to drop 2 to 3 mm per second).	Increasing the pressure above the point where the pulse disappeared ensures a period before hearing the first sound that corresponds with the systolic pressure. It prevents misinterpreting phase II sounds as phase I sounds.
20. **Note the point on the gauge at which the first faint, but clear, sound appears that slowly increases in intensity. Note this number as the systolic pressure. Read the pressure to the closest 2 mm Hg.**	Systolic pressure is the point at which the blood in the artery is first able to force its way through the vessel at a similar pressure exerted by the air bladder in the cuff. The first sound is phase I of Korotkoff sounds.
21. Do not reinflate the cuff once the air is being released to recheck the systolic pressure reading.	Reinflating the cuff while obtaining the blood pressure is uncomfortable for the patient and may cause an inaccurate reading. Reinflating the cuff causes congestion of blood in the lower arm, which lessens the loudness of Korotkoff sounds.
22. **Note the point at which the sound completely disappears.**	The point at which the sound disappears corresponds to the beginning of phase V Korotkoff sounds and is generally considered the diastolic pressure reading (Pickering, et al., 2004).
23. Allow the remaining air to escape quickly. Repeat any	False readings are likely to occur if there is congestion of blood in

ACTION	RATIONALE
suspicious reading, but wait at least 1 minute. Deflate the cuff completely between attempts to check the blood pressure.	the limb while obtaining repeated readings.
24. When measurement is completed, remove the cuff. Remove gloves, if worn. Cover the patient and help him or her to a position of comfort.	Removing PPE properly reduces the risk for infection transmission and contamination of other items and ensures patient comfort.
25. Remove additional PPE, if used. Perform hand hygiene.	Removing PPE properly reduces the risk for infection transmission and contamination of other items. Hand hygiene deters the spread of microorganisms.
26. Clean the diaphragm of the stethoscope with the alcohol wipe. Clean and store the sphygmomanometer, according to facility policy.	Appropriate cleaning deters the spread of microorganisms. Equipment should be left ready for use.

EVALUATION
• Patient's blood pressure is measured accurately without injury.

DOCUMENTATION
• Record the findings on paper, flow sheet, or computerized record. Report abnormal findings to the appropriate person. Identify arm used and site of assessment if other than brachial.

GENERAL CONSIDERATIONS
• If this is the initial nursing assessment of a patient, take the blood pressure on both arms. It is normal to have a 5- to 10-mm Hg difference in the systolic reading between arms. Use the arm with the higher reading for subsequent blood pressure measurements.
• If you have difficulty hearing the blood pressure sounds, raise the patient's arm, with cuff in place, over his or her head for 30 seconds before rechecking the blood pressure. Inflate the cuff while the arm is elevated, and then gently lower the arm while continuing to support it. Position the stethoscope and deflate the cuff at the usual rate while listening for Korotkoff sounds. Raising the arm over the head reduces vascular volume in the limb and improves blood flow to enhance the Korotkoff sounds (Pickering, et al., 2004).

- Blood pressure may be assessed using an electronic device or Doppler ultrasound (see Skill 17).
- Many electronic devices are not recommended for patients with irregular heart rates, tremors, or the inability to hold the extremity still. The machine will continue to inflate, causing pain for the patient.
- Monitors that measure blood pressure at the wrist are available. It is important for the wrist to be at heart level when readings are taken to avoid error due to hydrostatic effect of differences in the position of the wrist relative to the heart. Some wrist monitors will only record a measurement when the monitor is held at heart level (Pickering, et al., 2004).
- Diastolic pressure measured while the patient is sitting is approximately 5 mm Hg higher than when measured while the patient is supine; systolic pressure measured while the patient is supine is approximately 8 mm Hg higher than when measured in the patient who is sitting (Pickering, et al., 2004).

Skill · 17   **Assessing Blood Pressure Using a Doppler Ultrasound**

Blood pressure may be measured with an ultrasound or Doppler device, which amplifies sound. It is especially useful if the sounds are indistinct or inaudible with a regular stethoscope. This method provides only an estimate of systolic blood pressure.

EQUIPMENT

- Sphygmomanometer
- Blood pressure cuff of appropriate size
- Portable Doppler ultrasound
- Conducting gel
- Pencil or pen, paper or flow sheet
- Alcohol swab
- PPE, as indicated

ASSESSMENT GUIDELINES

- Assess the brachial pulse, or the pulse appropriate for the site being used.
- Assess for an intravenous infusion or breast or axilla surgery on the side of the body corresponding to the arm used. Assess for the presence of a cast, arteriovenous shunt, or injured or diseased limb. If any of these conditions are present, do not use the affected arm to monitor blood pressure.
- Assess the size of the limb so that the appropriate-sized blood pressure cuff can be used. The correct cuff should have a bladder length that is 80% of the arm circumference and a width that is at least 40% of the arm circumference; a length-to-width ratio of 2:1.

• Assess for factors that could affect blood pressure reading, such as the patient's age, exercise, position, weight, fluid balance, smoking, and medications. Note baseline or previous blood pressure measurements. Assess the patient for pain.

NURSING DIAGNOSES

• Decreased Cardiac Output
• Ineffective Health Maintenance
• Risk for Falls
• Effective Therapeutic Regimen Management

OUTCOME IDENTIFICATION AND PLANNING

Expected outcomes may include:
• Patient's systolic blood pressure is measured accurately without injury.

IMPLEMENTATION

ACTION	RATIONALE
1. Check medical order or nursing plan of care for frequency of blood pressure measurement. More frequent measurement may be appropriate based on nursing judgment. Assess the situation to determine the appropriateness and necessity for using a Doppler device to obtain systolic blood pressure measurement.	Provides for patient safety. Using a Doppler device provides measurement of only the systolic blood pressure and is often used only in an emergency situation.
2. Perform hand hygiene and put on PPE, if indicated.	Hand hygiene and PPE prevent the spread of microorganisms. PPE is required based on transmission precautions.
3. Identify the patient.	Identifying the patient ensures the right patient receives the intervention and helps prevent errors.
4. Close curtains around bed and close the door to the room, if possible. Discuss the procedure with the patient and assess the patient's	This ensures the patient's privacy. Explanation relieves anxiety and facilitates cooperation. Activity immediately before measurement can result in inaccurate results.

ACTION	RATIONALE
ability to assist with the procedure. Validate that the patient has relaxed for several minutes, as appropriate.	
5. Put on gloves, if appropriate or indicated.	Gloves prevent contact with blood and body fluids. Gloves are usually not required for measurement of blood pressure, unless contact with blood or body fluids is anticipated.
6. Select the appropriate arm for application of the cuff.	Measurement of blood pressure may temporarily impede circulation to the extremity.
7. Have the patient assume a comfortable lying or sitting position with the forearm supported at the level of the heart and the palm of the hand upward. If the measurement is taken in the supine position, support the arm with a pillow. In the sitting position, support the arm yourself or by using the bedside table. If the patient is sitting, have the patient sit back in the chair so that the chair supports his or her back. In addition, make sure the patient keeps the legs uncrossed.	The position of the arm can have a major influence when the blood pressure is measured; if the upper arm is below the level of the right atrium, the readings will be too high. If the arm is above the level of the heart, the readings will be too low (Pickering, et al., 2004). If the back is not supported, the diastolic pressure may be elevated falsely; if the legs are crossed, the systolic pressure may be elevated falsely (Pickering, et al., 2004.). This position places the brachial artery on the inner aspect of the elbow so that the bell or diaphragm of the stethoscope can rest on it easily. This sitting position ensures accuracy.
8. Expose the brachial artery by removing garments, or move a sleeve, if it is not too tight, above the area where the cuff will be placed.	Clothing over the artery interferes with the ability to hear sounds and may cause inaccurate blood pressure readings. A tight sleeve would cause congestion of blood and possibly inaccurate readings.
9. Palpate the location of the brachial artery. **Center the bladder of the cuff over the brachial artery, about**	Pressure in the cuff applied directly to the artery provides the most accurate readings. If the cuff gets in the way of the

ACTION	RATIONALE
midway on the arm, so that the lower edge of the cuff is about 2.5 to 5 cm (1 to 2 inches) above the inner aspect of the elbow. Line up the artery marking on the cuff with the patient's brachial artery. The tubing should extend from the edge of the cuff nearer the patient's elbow.	stethoscope, readings are likely to be inaccurate. A cuff placed upside down with the tubing toward the patient's head may give a false reading.
10. Wrap the cuff around the arm smoothly and snugly, and fasten it. Do not allow any clothing to interfere with the proper placement of the cuff.	A smooth cuff and snug wrapping produce equal pressure and help promote an accurate measurement. A cuff wrapped too loosely results in an inaccurate reading.
11. Check that the needle on the aneroid gauge is within the zero mark. If using a mercury manometer, check to see that the manometer is in the vertical position and that the mercury is within the zero level with the gauge at eye level.	If the needle is not in the zero area, the blood pressure may not be accurate. Tilting a mercury manometer, inaccurate calibration, or improper height for reading the gauge can lead to errors in determining the pressure measurements.
12. Place a small amount of conducting gel over the artery.	Conduction gel is necessary to provide conduction of sound from artery to Doppler.
13. Hold the Doppler device in your nondominant hand. Using your dominant hand, place the Doppler tip in the gel. Adjust the volume, as needed. Move the Doppler tip around until you hear the pulse.	Locates arterial pulse for reading.
14. Once the pulse is located using the Doppler, close the valve to the sphygmomanometer. Tighten the screw valve on the air pump. Inflate the cuff while continuing to use the Doppler on the artery (FIGURE 1).	The point where the pulse disappears provides a measurement of the systolic pressure.

ACTION	RATIONALE

Note the point on the gauge where the pulse disappears.

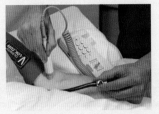

FIGURE 1 Inflating cuff while listening to artery pulsations. (*Photo by B. Proud.*)

15. Open the valve on the manometer and allow air to escape quickly. Repeat any suspicious reading, but wait at least 1 minute between readings to allow normal circulation to return in the limb. Deflate the cuff completely between attempts to check the blood pressure.	False readings are likely to occur if there is congestion of blood in the limb while obtaining repeated readings.
16. Remove the Doppler tip and turn off the Doppler device. Wipe excess gel off of the patient's skin with tissue. Remove the cuff. Wipe off any gel remaining on the Doppler probe with a tissue. Clean the Doppler device according to facility policy or manufacturer's recommendations.	Removing gel from the patient's skin promotes patient comfort. Appropriate cleaning deters the spread of microorganisms. Equipment should be left ready for use.
17. Remove gloves, if worn. Cover the patient and help him or her to a position of comfort.	Removing PPE properly reduces the risk for infection transmission and contamination of other items. Ensures patient comfort.
18. Remove additional PPE, if used. Perform hand hygiene.	Removing PPE properly reduces the risk for infection transmission and contamination of other items. Hand hygiene deters the spread of microorganisms.
19. Return the Doppler device to the charge base and store according to facility policy.	Equipment should be left ready for use.

EVALUATION

• Patient's blood pressure is measured accurately without injury.

DOCUMENTATION

• Record the findings on paper, flow sheet, or computerized record. Report abnormal findings to the appropriate person. Identify arm used and site of assessment if other than brachial.

Skill · 18 | **Assessing Blood Pressure Using an Electronic Device**

Automatic, electronic equipment is often used to monitor blood pressure in acute care settings, during anesthesia, postoperatively, or any time frequent assessments are necessary. This unit determines blood pressure by analyzing the sounds of blood flow or measuring oscillations. The machine can be set to take and record blood pressure readings at preset intervals. Irregular heart rates, excessive patient movement, and environmental noise can interfere with the readings. Because electronic equipment is more sensitive to outside interference, these readings are susceptible to error. The cuff is applied in the same manner as the auscultatory method, with the microphone or pressure sensor positioned directly over the artery. When using an automatic blood pressure device for serial readings, check the cuffed limb frequently. Incomplete deflation of the cuff between measurements can lead to inadequate arterial perfusion and venous drainage, compromising the circulation in the limb.

EQUIPMENT

• Electronic automated blood pressure device
• Blood pressure cuff of appropriate size
• Pencil or pen, paper or flow sheet
• Alcohol swab
• PPE, as indicated

ASSESSMENT GUIDELINES

• Assess the brachial pulse, or the pulse appropriate for the site being used.
• Assess for an intravenous infusion or breast or axilla surgery on the side of the body corresponding to the arm used. Assess for the presence of a cast, arteriovenous shunt, or injured or diseased limb. If any of these conditions are present, do not use the affected arm to monitor blood pressure.
• Assess the size of the limb so that the appropriate-sized blood pressure cuff can be used. The correct cuff should have a bladder length that is 80% of the arm circumference and a width that is at least 40% of the arm circumference; a length-to-width ratio of 2:1.

- Assess for factors that could affect blood pressure reading, such as the patient's age, exercise, position, weight, fluid balance, smoking, and medications. Note baseline or previous blood pressure measurements. Assess the patient for pain.
- If the patient reports pain, give pain medication, as ordered, before assessing blood pressure. If the blood pressure is taken while the patient is in pain, make a notation concerning the pain if the blood pressure is elevated.

NURSING DIAGNOSES
- Decreased Cardiac Output
- Ineffective Health Maintenance
- Risk for Falls

OUTCOME IDENTIFICATION AND PLANNING
Expected outcomes may include:
- Patient's blood pressure is measured accurately without injury.

IMPLEMENTATION

ACTION	RATIONALE
1. Check medical order or nursing care plan for frequency of blood pressure measurement. More frequent measurement may be appropriate based on nursing judgment.	Provides for patient safety.
2. Perform hand hygiene and put on PPE, if indicated.	Hand hygiene and PPE prevent the spread of microorganisms. PPE is required based on transmission precautions.
3. Identify the patient.	Identifying the patient ensures the right patient receives the intervention and helps prevent errors.
4. Close curtains around bed and close the door to the room, if possible. Discuss the procedure with the patient and assess the patient's ability to assist with the procedure. Validate that the patient	This ensures the patient's privacy. Explanation relieves anxiety and facilitates cooperation. Activity immediately before measurement can result in inaccurate results.

ACTION	RATIONALE
has relaxed for several minutes.	
5. Put on gloves, if appropriate or indicated.	Gloves prevent contact with blood and body fluids. Gloves are usually not required for measurement of blood pressure, unless contact with blood or body fluids is anticipated.
6. Select the appropriate arm for application of the cuff.	Measurement of blood pressure may temporarily impede circulation to the extremity.
7. Have the patient assume a comfortable lying or sitting position with the forearm supported at the level of the heart and the palm of the hand upward. If the measurement is taken in the supine position support the arm with a pillow. In the sitting position, support the arm yourself or by using the bedside table. If the patient is sitting, have the patient sit back in the chair so that the chair supports his or her back. In addition, make sure the patient keeps the legs uncrossed.	The position of the arm can have a major influence when the blood pressure is measured; if the upper arm is below the level of the right atrium, the readings will be too high. If the arm is above the level of the heart, the readings will be too low (Pickering, et al., 2004). If the back is not supported, the diastolic pressure may be elevated falsely; if the legs are crossed, the systolic pressure may be elevated falsely (Pickering, et al., 2004). This position places the brachial artery on the inner aspect of the elbow so that the bell or diaphragm of the stethoscope can rest on it easily. This sitting position ensures accuracy.
8. Expose the brachial artery by removing garments, or move a sleeve, if it is not too tight, above the area where the cuff will be placed.	Clothing over the artery interferes with the ability to hear sounds and may cause inaccurate blood pressure readings. A tight sleeve would cause congestion of blood and possibly inaccurate readings.
9. Palpate the location of the brachial artery. **Center the bladder of the cuff over the brachial artery, about midway on the arm, so that the lower edge of the cuff is about 2.5 to 5 cm (1 to**	Pressure in the cuff applied directly to the artery provides the most accurate readings. If the cuff gets in the way of the stethoscope, readings are likely to be inaccurate. A cuff placed upside down with the tubing toward the

ACTION	RATIONALE

2 inches) above the inner aspect of the elbow. Line the artery marking on the cuff up with the patient's brachial artery. The tubing should extend from the edge of the cuff nearer the patient's elbow.

patient's head may give a false reading.

10. Wrap the cuff around the arm smoothly and snugly, and fasten it. Do not allow any clothing to interfere with the proper placement of the cuff (FIGURE 1).

A smooth cuff and snug wrapping produce equal pressure and help promote an accurate measurement. A cuff wrapped too loosely results in an inaccurate reading.

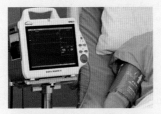

FIGURE 1 Electronic blood pressure device. (*Photo by B. Proud.*)

11. Turn on the machine. If the machine has different settings for infants, children, and adults, select the appropriate setting. Push the 'start' button. Instruct the patient to hold the limb still.

Turning on the device allows for blood pressure measurement. Improper setting on device and movement of limb can lead to errors in determining the pressure measurements.

12. Wait until the machine beeps and the blood pressure reading appears. Remove the cuff from the patient's limb and clean and store the equipment.

Machine signals when measurement is completed. Proper cleaning prevents the transmission of microorganisms.

13. Remove gloves, if worn. Cover the patient and help him or her to a position of comfort.

Removing PPE properly reduces the risk for infection transmission and contamination of other items. Ensures patient comfort.

14. Remove additional PPE, if used. Perform hand hygiene.

Removing PPE properly reduces the risk for infection transmission and contamination of other items. Hand hygiene deters the spread of microorganisms.

EVALUATION

• Patient's blood pressure is measured accurately without injury.

DOCUMENTATION

• Record the findings on paper, flow sheet, or computerized record. Report abnormal findings to the appropriate person. Identify arm used and assessment site, if other than brachial.

GENERAL CONSIDERATIONS

• If this is the initial nursing assessment of a patient, take the blood pressure on both arms. It is normal to have a 5- to 10-mm Hg difference in the systolic reading between arms. Use the arm with the higher reading for subsequent blood pressure measurements.
• Many electronic devices are not recommended for patients with irregular heart rates, tremors, or the inability to hold the extremity still. The machine will continue to inflate, causing the patient pain.
• Monitors that measure blood pressure at the wrist are available. It is important for the wrist to be at heart level when readings are taken to avoid error due to hydrostatic effect of differences in the position of the wrist relative to the heart. Some wrist monitors will only record a measurement when the monitor is held at heart level (Pickering, et al., 2004).
• Diastolic pressure measured while the patient is sitting is approximately 5 mm Hg higher than when measured while the patient is supine; systolic pressure measured while the patient is supine is approximately 8 mm Hg higher than when measured in the patient who is sitting (Pickering, et al., 2004).

> **Skill · 19** **Obtaining an Arterial Blood Specimen for Blood Gas Analysis**

The most common site for sampling arterial blood is the radial artery; other arteries may be used, but most institutions require a physician's order to obtain the sample from another artery. Arterial blood gas (ABG) analysis evaluates ventilation by measuring blood pH and the partial pressures of arterial oxygen (Pao_2) and partial pressure of arterial carbon dioxide ($Paco_2$). Blood pH measurement reveals the blood's acid–base balance. Pao_2 indicates the amount of oxygen that the lungs deliver to the blood, and $Paco_2$ indicates the lungs' capacity to eliminate carbon dioxide. ABG samples can also be analyzed for oxygen content and saturation, and for bicarbonate values. A respiratory technician or specially trained nurse can collect most ABG samples, but a physician usually performs collection from the femoral artery, depending on facility policy. An Allen's test should always be performed before using the radial artery to determine whether the ulnar artery delivers sufficient blood to the hand and fingers, in case of damage to the radial artery during the blood sampling. Refer to the guidelines in this skill for performing an Allen's test.

EQUIPMENT

- ABG kit, *or* heparinized, self-filling 10-mL syringe with 22-G, 1-inch needle attached
- Airtight cap for hub of syringe
- 2 × 2 gauze pad
- Band-Aid
- Antimicrobial swab, such as chlorhexidine
- Biohazard bag
- Appropriate label for specimen, based on facility policy and procedure
- Cup or bag of ice
- Nonsterile gloves
- Additional PPE, as indicated
- Rolled towel

ASSESSMENT GUIDELINES

- Review the patient's medical record and plan of care for information about the need for an ABG specimen. Ensure that the appropriate computer laboratory request has been completed.
- Assess the patient's cardiac status, including heart rate, blood pressure, and auscultation of heart sounds.
- Assess the patient's respiratory status, including respiratory rate, excursion, lung sounds, and use of oxygen, including the amount being used, if ordered.
- Determine the adequacy of peripheral blood flow to the extremity to be used by performing the Allen's test (detailed below). If Allen's test reveals no or little collateral circulation to the hand, do not perform an arterial stick to that artery. Assess the patient's radial pulse. If you are unable to palpate the radial pulse, consider using the other wrist.
- Assess the patient's understanding about the need for specimen collection. Ask the patient if he or she has ever felt faint, sweaty, or nauseated when having blood drawn.

NURSING DIAGNOSES

- Acute Pain
- Risk for Injury
- Anxiety
- Impaired Gas Exchange
- Decreased Cardiac Output
- Fear
- Ineffective Airway Clearance

OUTCOME IDENTIFICATION AND PLANNING

Expected outcomes may include:
- An uncontaminated specimen will be obtained from the artery without damage to the artery and sent to the laboratory promptly.
- The patient experiences minimal pain and anxiety during the procedure.
- The patient verbalizes an understanding of the reason for the testing.

IMPLEMENTATION

ACTION	RATIONALE
1. Gather the necessary supplies. Check product expiration dates. Identify ordered arterial blood gas analysis. Check the chart to make sure the patient has not been suctioned within the past 15 minutes. Check facility policy and/or procedure for guidelines on administering local anesthesia for arterial punctures. Administer anesthetic and allow sufficient time for full effect before beginning the procedure (AACN, 2005; Hudson, et al., 2006).	Organization facilitates efficient performance of the procedure. Ensures proper functioning of equipment. Suctioning may change the oxygen saturation and is a temporary change not to be confused with baseline for the patient. Arterial puncture is a source of pain and discomfort. Intradermal injection of lidocaine around the puncture site has been shown to decrease the incidence and severity of localized pain when used before arterial puncture (AACN, 2005; Hudson, et al., 2006).
2. Bring necessary equipment to the bedside stand or overbed table.	Bringing everything to the bedside conserves time and energy. Arranging items nearby is convenient, saves time, and avoids unnecessary stretching and twisting of muscles on the part of the nurse. Organization facilitates performance of tasks.
3. Perform hand hygiene and put on PPE, if indicated.	Hand hygiene and PPE prevent the transmission of microorganisms. PPE is required based on transmission precautions.
4. Check the patient's identification and confirm the patient's identity. Tell the patient you need to collect an arterial blood sample, and explain the procedure. Tell the patient that the needlestick will cause some discomfort but that he or she must remain still during the procedure.	Identifying the patient ensures the right patient receives the intervention and helps prevent errors. Explanation facilitates cooperation and provides reassurance for patient.

ACTION	RATIONALE
5. Close curtains around bed and close the door to the room, if possible.	Closing the door or curtain provides for patient privacy.
6. Check specimen label with patient identification bracelet. Label should include patient's name and identification number, time specimen was collected, route of collection, identification of person obtaining the sample, amount of oxygen the patient is receiving, and any other information required by agency policy.	Confirmation of patient identification information ensures specimen is labeled correctly for the right patient.
7. Provide for good light. Artificial light is recommended. Place a trash receptacle within easy reach.	Good lighting is necessary to perform the procedure properly. Having the trash receptacle in easy reach allows for safe disposal of contaminated materials.
8. If the patient is on bed rest, ask him or her to lie in a supine position, with the head slightly elevated and the arms at the sides. Ask the ambulatory patient to sit in a chair and support the arm securely on an armrest or a table. Place a waterproof pad under the site and a rolled towel under the wrist.	Positioning the patient comfortably helps minimize anxiety. Using a rolled towel under the wrist provides for easy access to the insertion site.
9. **Perform Allen's test (FIGURE 1) before obtaining a specimen from the radial artery:**	Allen's testing assesses patency of the ulnar and radial arteries.
a. Have the patient clench the wrist to minimize blood flow into the hand.	
b. Using your index and middle fingers, press on the radial and ulnar arteries (FIGURE 1A). Hold this position for a few seconds.	

ACTION	RATIONALE

c. Without removing your fingers from the arteries, ask the patient to unclench the fist and hold the hand in a relaxed position (FIGURE 1B). The palm will be blanched because pressure from your fingers has impaired the normal blood flow.

d. Release pressure on the ulnar artery (FIGURE 1C). If the hand becomes flushed, which indicates that blood is filling the vessels, it is safe to proceed with the radial artery puncture. This is considered a positive test. If the hand does not flush, perform the test on the other arm.

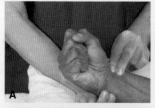

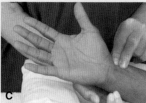

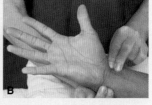

FIGURE 1 Performing Allen's test. (**A**) Compressing the arteries with patient's fist closed. (**B**) Maintaining compression as patient unclenches fist. (**C**) Compressing only the radial artery.

10. Put on nonsterile gloves. Locate the radial artery and lightly palpate it for a strong pulse.

Gloves reduce transmission of microorganisms. If you push too hard during palpation, the radial artery will be obliterated and hard to palpate.

ACTION	RATIONALE
11. Clean the site with the anti-microbial swab. If using chlorhexidine, use a back-and-forth motion, applying friction to the site for 30 seconds, or use procedure recommended by the manufacturer. Allow the site to dry. **After disinfection, do not palpate the site unless sterile gloves are worn.**	Site cleansing prevents potentially infectious skin flora from being introduced into the vessel during the procedure. Palpation after cleansing contaminates the area.
12. Stabilize the hand with the wrist extended over the rolled towel, palm up. Palpate the artery above the puncture site with the index and middle fingers of your nondominant hand while holding the syringe over the puncture site with your dominant hand. **Do not directly touch the area to be stuck.**	Stabilizing the hand and palpating the artery with one hand while holding the syringe in the other provides better access to the artery. Palpating the area to be stuck would contaminate the clean area.
13. Hold the needle bevel up at a 45-degree angle at the site of maximal pulse impulse, with the shaft parallel to the path of the artery. (When puncturing the brachial artery, hold the needle at a 60-degree angle.)	The proper angle of insertion ensures correct access to the artery. The artery is shallow and does not require a deeper angle to penetrate.
14. Puncture the skin and arterial wall in one motion. Watch for blood backflow in the syringe. The pulsating blood will flow into the syringe. Do not pull back on the plunger. Fill the syringe to the 5-mL mark.	The blood should enter the syringe automatically due to arterial pressure.
15. After collecting the sample, withdraw the syringe while your nondominant hand is beginning to place pressure proximal to the insertion site with the 2 × 2 gauze. Press a	If insufficient pressure is applied, a large, painful hematoma may form, hindering future arterial puncture at the site.

ACTION	RATIONALE
gauze pad firmly over the puncture site until the bleeding stops—at least 5 minutes. **If the patient is receiving anti-coagulant therapy or has a blood dyscrasia, apply pressure for 10 to 15 minutes; if necessary, ask a coworker to hold the gauze pad in place while you prepare the sample for transport to the laboratory, but do not ask the patient to hold the pad.**	
16. When the bleeding stops and the appropriate time has lapsed, apply a small adhesive bandage or small pressure dressing (fold a 2×2 gauze into fourths and firmly apply tape, stretching the skin tight).	Applying a dressing also prevents arterial hemorrhage and extravasation into the surrounding tissue, which can cause a hematoma.
17. Once the sample is obtained, check the syringe for air bubbles. If any appear, remove them by holding the syringe upright and slowly ejecting some of the blood onto a 2×2 gauze pad.	Air bubbles can affect the laboratory values.
18. Engage the needle guard and remove the needle. Place the airtight cap on the syringe. Gently rotate the syringe to ensure that heparin is well distributed. Do not shake. Insert the syringe into a cup or bag of ice.	This prevents the sample from leaking and keeps air out of the syringe, because blood will continue to absorb oxygen and will give a false reading if allowed to have contact with air. Heparin prevents blood from clotting. Ice prevents the blood from degrading. Vigorous shaking may cause hemolysis.
19. Place label on the syringe per facility policy. Place iced syringe in plastic sealable biohazard bag.	Labeling ensures the specimen is the correct one for the right patient. Packaging the specimen in a biohazard bag prevents the person transporting the samples from coming in contact with blood.

ACTION	RATIONALE

20. Discard needle in sharps container. Remove gloves and perform hand hygiene.

Proper disposal of equipment prevents accidental injury and reduces transmission of microorganisms. Removing gloves properly reduces the risk for infection transmission and contamination of other items. Hand hygiene reduces transmission of microorganisms.

21. Remove other PPE, if used. Perform hand hygiene.

Removing PPE properly reduces the risk for infection transmission and contamination of other items. Hand hygiene reduces the transmission of microorganisms.

22. Transport specimen to laboratory immediately.

Timely transport ensures accurate results.

EVALUATION

- An uncontaminated specimen is obtained from the artery without damage to the artery and sent to the laboratory promptly.
- The patient experiences minimal pain and anxiety during the procedure.
- The patient verbalizes an understanding of the reason for the testing.

DOCUMENTATION

- Document results of Allen's test, time the sample was drawn, arterial puncture site, amount of time pressure was applied to the site to control bleeding, type and amount of oxygen therapy that the patient was receiving, pulse oximetry values, respiratory rate, respiratory effort, and any other significant assessments.

GENERAL CONSIDERATIONS

- Be aware that use of a particular arterial site is contraindicated for the following reasons: absence of a palpable radial artery pulse; Allen's test showing only one artery supplying blood to the hand; Allen's test showing obstruction in the ulnar artery; cellulitis or infection at the site; presence of arteriovenous fistula or shunt; severe thrombocytopenia (platelet count 20,000/mm^3 or less, or based on facility policy), and a prolonged prothrombin time or partial thromboplastin time.

- Use a Doppler probe or finger pulse transducer to assess circulation and perfusion in patients with dark skin tones or uncooperative patients (Fischbach & Dunning, 2006).
- If the patient is receiving oxygen, make sure that this therapy has been underway for at least 15 minutes before collecting an arterial blood sample. Also be sure to indicate on the laboratory request and the specimen label the amount and type of oxygen therapy the patient is receiving. If the patient is receiving mechanical ventilation, note the fraction of inspired oxygen and tidal volume.
- If the patient is not receiving oxygen, indicate that he or she is breathing room air.
- If the patient has just received a nebulizer treatment, wait about 20 minutes before collecting the sample.
- Consider obtaining an order for the use of a local anesthetic (1% lidocaine solution) to minimize discomfort and pain for the patient, based on facility policy. The use of 1% lidocaine without epinephrine injected intradermally around the artery puncture site has been shown to decrease the incidence of localized pain (Hudson, et al., 2006; AACN, 2005). Be familiar with requirements and specifications for particular products available for use. Application needs to occur sufficiently in advance to allow enough time to become effective, which may be contraindicated by the patient's condition. Consider such use of lidocaine carefully because it can delay the procedure. The patient may be allergic to the drug, or the resulting vasoconstriction may prevent successful puncture.
- If the femoral site is used for the procedure, apply pressure for a minimum of 10 minutes.
- Arterial lines may be used to obtain blood samples. Refer to Skill 20. When sampling from arterial lines, record amount of blood drawn for each sampling. Frequent sampling can result in significant amount of blood being removed.

| **Skill · 20** | **Obtaining an Arterial Blood Specimen From an Arterial Line–Stopcock System** |

Obtaining an arterial blood sample requires percutaneous puncture of the brachial, radial, or femoral artery. However, an arterial blood sample can also be obtained from an arterial line. When collected, the sample can be analyzed to determine arterial blood gas (ABG), laboratory specimens, or other values.

The procedure below describes obtaining a sample from an open system. For information on obtaining an arterial blood sample from a closed reservoir system, please see the Skill Variation at the end of the skill.

EQUIPMENT

* Arterial blood gas (ABG) syringe with needleless cannula, if ABG is ordered
* Gloves
* Goggles
* Additional PPE, as indicated
* Two 5-mL syringes
* Vacutainer with needleless adapter and appropriate blood collection tubes for ordered tests
* Alcohol swabs or chlorhexidine, per facility policy
* Rubber cap for ABG syringe hub
* Ice-filled plastic bag or cup
* Label with patient identification information and test order number
* Laboratory request form, if necessary
* Biohazard bag

ASSESSMENT GUIDELINES

* Review the patient's medical record and plan of care for information about the patient's need for an arterial blood sample.
* Assess the patient's cardiac status, including heart rate, blood pressure, and auscultation of heart sounds.
* Assess the patient's respiratory status, including respiratory rate, excursion, lung sounds, and use of oxygen, if ordered.
* Check the patency and functioning of the arterial line. Determine the dead-space volume of the arterial line system immediately before withdrawing the laboratory sample (see Step 10). The dead space is the volume of the space from the tip of the catheter to the sampling port of the stopcock. The dead-space volume will depend on the gauge and length of the catheter, the length of the connecting tubing, and the number of stopcocks in the system. A sufficient amount of discard volume needs to be withdrawn before obtaining the blood sample to be tested in the laboratory. If an insufficient amount of discard volume is withdrawn, the specimen may be diluted and contaminated with flush solution. If an excessive amount of discard volume is withdrawn, the patient may experience an iatrogenic (treatment-induced) blood loss.
* Assess the patient's understanding about the need for specimen collection.

NURSING DIAGNOSES

* Impaired Gas Exchange
* Risk for Infection
* Decreased Cardiac Output
* Risk for Injury
* Anxiety

OUTCOME IDENTIFICATION AND PLANNING

Expected outcomes may include:
* Specimen is obtained without compromise to the patency of the arterial line.

• Patient experiences minimal discomfort and anxiety, remains free from infection, and demonstrates an understanding about the need for the specimen collection.

IMPLEMENTATION

ACTION	RATIONALE
1. Verify the order for laboratory testing on the patient's medical record.	This ensures that the correct intervention is performed on the correct patient.
2. Gather all equipment and bring to bedside.	Having equipment available saves time and facilitates accomplishment of procedure.
3. Perform hand hygiene and put on PPE, if indicated.	Hand hygiene and PPE prevent the spread of microorganisms. PPE is required based on transmission precautions.
4. Identify the patient.	Identifying the patient ensures the right patient receives the intervention and helps prevent errors.
5. Close curtains around bed and close the door to the room, if possible. Explain the procedure to the patient.	This ensures the patient's privacy. Explanation relieves anxiety and facilitates cooperation.
6. Compare specimen label with patient identification bracelet. Label should include patient's name and identification number, time specimen was collected, route of collection, identification of person obtaining sample, and any other information required by agency policy.	Verification of the patient's identity validates that the correct procedure is being done on the correct patient, and the specimen is accurately labeled.
7. Put on gloves and goggles or face shield.	Gloves and goggles (or face shield) prevent contact with blood and body fluids.
8. Turn off or temporarily silence the arterial pressure alarms, depending on facility policy.	The integrity of the system is being altered, which will cause the system to sound an alarm. Facility policy may require the alarm be left on.

ACTION	RATIONALE
9. Locate the stopcock nearest the arterial line insertion site. Use the alcohol swab or chlorhexidine to scrub the sampling port on the stopcock. Allow to air dry.	Cleansing prevents contamination from microorganisms on the sampling port.
10. Attach a 5-mL syringe into the sampling port on the stopcock to obtain the discard volume. Turn the stopcock off to the flush solution. Aspirate slowly until blood enters the syringe. Stop aspirating. Note the volume in the syringe, which is the dead-space volume. Continue to aspirate until the dead-space volume has been withdrawn a total of three times. For example, if the dead-space volume is 0.8 mL, aspirate 2.4 mL of blood.	A sufficient amount of discard volume needs to be withdrawn before obtaining the blood sample to be tested in the laboratory. This sample is discarded because it is diluted with flush solution, possibly leading to inaccurate test results. The dead space is the volume of the space from the tip of the catheter to the sampling port of the stopcock. The dead-space volume will depend on the gauge and length of the catheter, the length of the connecting tubing, and the number of stopcocks in the system. If an insufficient amount of discard volume is withdrawn, the specimen may be diluted and contaminated with flush solution. If an excessive amount of discard volume is withdrawn, the patient may experience an iatrogenic (treatment-induced) blood loss.
11. Turn the stopcock to the halfway position between the flush solution and the sampling port to close the system in all directions.	Turning off the stopcock maintains the integrity of the system.
12. Remove the discard syringe and dispose of it appropriately.	Observe Standard Precautions. Diluted blood still poses a risk for infection transmission.
13. Place the syringe for the laboratory sample or the Vacutainer in the sampling port of the stopcock. Turn off the stopcock to the flush solution, and slowly withdraw the	Turning off the stopcock to the flush solution prevents dilution from the flush device.

required amount of blood. For each additional sample required, repeat this procedure. If coagulation tests are included in the required tests, obtain blood for this sample from the final sample.

14. Turn the stopcock to the halfway position between the flush solution and the sampling port to close the system in all directions. Remove the syringe or Vacutainer. Apply the rubber cap to the ABG syringe hub, if necessary.

Turning off the stopcock maintains the integrity of the system.

15. Insert a 5-mL syringe into the sampling port of the stopcock. Turn off the stopcock to the patient. Activate the in-line flushing device. **Flush through the sampling port into the syringe to clear the stopcock and sampling port of any residual blood.**

Turning off the stopcock and in-line flushing maintains the integrity of the system, preventing clotting and infection.

16. Turn off the stopcock to the sampling port; remove the syringe. Remove sampling port cap and replace with new sterile one. **Intermittently flush the arterial catheter with the in-line flushing device until the tubing is clear of blood.**

Turning off the stopcock and in-line flushing maintains the integrity of the system, preventing clotting and infection.

17. Remove gloves. Reactivate the monitor alarms. Record date and time the samples were obtained on the labels, as well as the required information to identify the person obtaining the samples. If ABG was collected, record oxygen flow rate (or room air) on label. Apply labels to the specimens, according to

Removing gloves properly reduces the risk for infection transmission and contamination of other items. Reactivating the system ensures proper functioning. Proper labeling prevents error. Recording oxygen flow rate ensures accurate interpretation of results of ABG. Use of biohazard bag prevents contact with blood and body fluids. Ice maintains integrity of the sample.

ACTION	RATIONALE
facility policy. Place in bio-hazard bags; place ABG sample in bag with ice.	
18. Check the monitor for return of the arterial waveform and pressure reading.	This ensures proper functioning and integrity of the system.
19. Return the patient to a comfortable position. Lower bed height, if necessary, and adjust head of bed to a comfortable position.	Repositioning promotes patient comfort. Lowering the bed promotes patient safety.
20. Remove goggles and additional PPE, if used. Perform hand hygiene. Send specimens to the laboratory immediately.	Removing PPE properly reduces the risk for infection transmission and contamination of other items. Hand hygiene prevents transmission of microorganisms. Specimens must be processed in a timely manner to ensure accuracy.

EVALUATION

- Specimen is obtained without compromise to the patency of the arterial line.
- Patient experiences minimal discomfort and anxiety, remains free from infection, and demonstrates an understanding about the need for the specimen collection.

DOCUMENTATION

- Document any pertinent assessments, the laboratory specimens obtained, date and time specimens were obtained, and disposition of specimens.

GENERAL CONSIDERATIONS

- If the patient is receiving oxygen, make sure that this therapy has been underway for at least 15 minutes before collecting an arterial blood sample for ABG analysis. Indicate on the laboratory request slip the amount and type of oxygen therapy the patient is receiving. Also note the patient's current temperature, most recent hemoglobin level, and current respiratory rate. If the patient is receiving mechanical ventilation, note the fraction of inspired oxygen and tidal volume.
- If the patient is not receiving oxygen, indicate that he or she is breathing room air.
- If the patient has just received a nebulizer treatment, wait about 20 minutes before collecting the sample for ABG analysis.

| Skill Variation | Obtaining an Arterial Blood Sample From a Closed Reservoir System |

1. Gather all equipment and bring it to the bedside.

2. Perform hand hygiene. Put on PPE, as indicated.

3. Check the patient's identification. Compare the specimen label with the patient's identification.

4. Explain the procedure to the patient. Close curtains around bed and close the door to the room, if possible.

5. If bed is adjustable, raise it to a comfortable working height.

6. Put on gloves and goggles.

7. Locate the closed-system reservoir and blood-sampling site. Deactivate or temporarily silence monitor alarms (some facilities require that alarms be left on).

8. Clean the sampling site with an alcohol swab or chlorhexidine.

9. Holding the reservoir upright, grasp the flexures, and slowly fill the reservoir with blood over a 3- to 5-second period. If you feel resistance, reposition the extremity and check the catheter site for obvious problems (e.g., kinking of the tubing). Then, continue with blood withdrawal.

10. Turn off the one-way valve to the reservoir by turning the handle perpendicular to the tubing. Using a syringe with attached cannula, insert the cannula into the sampling site. Slowly fill the syringe. Then, grasp the cannula near the sampling site and remove the syringe and cannula as one unit. Repeat the procedure, as needed, to fill the required number of syringes. If coagulation tests have been ordered, obtain blood for those tests from the final syringe.

11. After filling the syringes, turn the one-way valve to its original position, parallel to the tubing. Push down evenly on the plunger until the flexures lock in place in the fully closed position and all fluid has been re-infused. The fluid should be re-infused over a 3- to 5-second period. Activate the fast-flush release.

12. Clean the sampling site with an alcohol swab or chlorhexidine. Reactivate the monitor alarms. Transfer blood samples to the appropriate specimen tubes, if necessary. Record on the labels the date and time the samples were obtained, as well as the required information to identify the person obtaining the samples. Apply labels to the specimens, according to facility policy. Place in biohazard bags; place ABG sample in bag with ice. Remove gloves.

(continued on page 111)

Obtaining an Arterial Blood Sample From a Closed Reservoir System *continued*

13. Check the monitor for return of the arterial waveform and pressure reading.

14. Remove any remaining equipment. Remove goggles and additional PPE, if used. Perform hand hygiene. Send specimens to the laboratory immediately.

Skill · 21 **Using Venipuncture to Collect a Venous Blood Sample for Routine Testing**

Venipuncture involves piercing a vein with a needle to obtain a venous blood sample, which is collected in a syringe or tube. The superficial veins of the arm are typically used for venipuncture; specifically, the vessels in the antecubital fossa (Fischbach & Dunning, 2009), which include the basilic, median cubital, and cephalic veins (FIGURE 1).

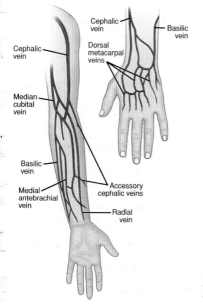

Cephalic vein

Cephalic vein

Median cubital vein

Basilic vein

Medial antebrachial vein

Cephalic vein

Basilic vein

Dorsal metacarpal veins

Accessory cephalic veins

Radial vein

FIGURE 1 Blood vessels in the arm typically used for venipuncture.

However, venipuncture can be performed on a vein in the dorsal fore-arm, the dorsum of the hand, or another accessible location. When performing a venipuncture, remember the following:

- Do not use the inner wrist because of the high risk for damage to underlying structures.
- Avoid areas that are edematous, paralyzed, or are on the same side as a mastectomy, arteriovenous shunt, or graft.
- Avoid areas of infection or with abnormal skin conditions (Fischbach & Dunning, 2006).
- Do not draw blood from the same extremity being used for administration of intravenous medications, fluids, or blood transfusions. Some facilities will allow use of such sites as a 'last resort,' after the infusion has been held for a period of time. If necessary, choose a site distal to the intravenous access site. Check facility policy and procedure (Infusion Nurses Society [INS], 2006; Fischbach & Dunning, 2009).
- Avoid venipuncture on a stroke patient's flaccid arm because the normal venous pump mechanism is lost, increasing the risk of vein thrombosis (Armed, 2008).

Explanation and communication with patients about the need for venipuncture can reduce anxiety. Information on the need for blood tests should be carefully explained to ensure patient understanding.

Measures to reduce the risk of infection are an important part of venipuncture. Hand hygiene, aseptic technique, the use of personal protective equipment, and safe disposal of sharps are key to providing safe venipuncture (Lavery & Ingram, 2005).

EQUIPMENT

- Tourniquet
- Nonsterile gloves
- Additional PPE, as indicated
- Antimicrobial swab, such as chlorhexidine or alcohol
- Sterile needle, gauge appropriate to the vein and sampling needs, using the smallest possible
- Vacutainer needle adaptor
- Blood-collection tubes appropriate for ordered tests
- Appropriate label for specimen, based on facility policy and procedure
- Biohazard bag
- Gauze pads (2×2)
- Adhesive bandage

ASSESSMENT GUIDELINES

- Review the patient's medical record and physician order for the blood specimens to be obtained. Ensure that the necessary computerized laboratory request has been completed.
- Assess the patient for any allergies, especially to the topical antimicrobial to be used for skin cleansing.
- Investigate for the presence of any conditions or use of medications that may prolong bleeding time, necessitating additional application of pressure to the puncture site. Ask the patient about any previous laboratory testing that he or she may have had, including any

problems, such as difficulty with venipuncture, fainting, or complaints of dizziness, light-headedness, or nausea.
- Assess the patient's anxiety level and understanding about the reasons for the blood test.
- Assess the patency of the veins in both upper limbs. Palpate the veins to assess condition of vessel; vein should be straight, feel soft, cylindrical, and bounce when lightly pressed. Appropriate vessels will compress without rolling, and have rapid rebound filling after compression (Scales, 2008). Avoid veins that are tender, sclerosed, thrombosed, fibrosed, or hard (Weinstein, 2006).

NURSING DIAGNOSES
- Deficient Knowledge
- Anxiety
- Risk for Injury
- Risk for Infection

OUTCOME IDENTIFICATION AND PLANNING
Expected outcomes may include:
- An uncontaminated specimen will be obtained and sent to the laboratory promptly.
- The patient does not experience undue anxiety, injury, or infection.
- The patient verbalizes an understanding of the reason for the testing.

IMPLEMENTATION

ACTION	RATIONALE
1. Gather the necessary supplies. Check product expiration dates. Identify ordered tests and select the appropriate blood-collection tubes.	Organization facilitates efficient performance of the procedure. Ensures proper functioning of equipment. Using correct tubes ensures accurate blood sampling.
2. Bring necessary equipment to the bedside stand or over-bed table.	Bringing everything to the bedside conserves time and energy. Arranging items nearby is convenient, saves time, and avoids unnecessary stretching and twisting of muscles on the part of the nurse. Organization facilitates performance of tasks.
3. Perform hand hygiene and put on PPE, if indicated.	Hand hygiene and PPE prevent the transmission of microorganisms. PPE is required based on transmission precautions.

ACTION	RATIONALE
4. Identify the patient. Explain the procedure. Allow the patient time to ask questions and verbalize concerns about the venipuncture procedure.	Identifying the patient ensures the right patient receives the intervention and helps prevent errors. Explanation provides reassurance and promotes cooperation.
5. Close curtains around bed and close the door to the room, if possible.	Closing the door or curtain provides for patient privacy.
6. Check specimen label with patient identification bracelet. Label should include patient's name and identification number, time specimen was collected, route of collection, identification of person obtaining sample, and any other information required by agency policy.	Confirmation of patient identification information ensures specimen is labeled correctly for the right patient.
7. Provide for good light. Artificial light is recommended. Place a trash receptacle within easy reach.	Good lighting is necessary to perform the procedure properly. Having the trash receptacle in easy reach allows for safe disposal of contaminated materials.
8. Assist the patient to a comfortable position, either sitting or lying. If the patient is lying in bed, raise the bed to a comfortable working height, usually elbow height of the caregiver (VISN 8 Patient Safety Center, 2009).	Proper positioning allows easy access to the site and promotes patient comfort and safety. Proper bed height helps reduce back strain while performing the procedure.
9. Determine the patient's preferred site for the procedure based on his or her previous experience. Expose the arm, supporting it in an extended position on a firm surface, such as a tabletop. Stand on the same side of the patient as the site selected. Apply a tourniquet to the upper arm on the chosen side approximately 3 to 4 inches above	Patient preference allows the patient to be involved in treatment and gives the nurse information that may aid in site selection (Lavery & Ingram, 2005). Positioning close to the chosen site reduces back strain. Tourniquet use increases venous pressure and distention to aid in vein identification. Tourniquet should remain in place no more than 60 seconds to prevent

ACTION	RATIONALE

the potential puncture site. Apply sufficient pressure to impede venous circulation but not arterial blood flow.

injury, stasis, and hemoconcentration, which may alter results (Fischbach & Dunning, 2009).

10. Put on gloves. Assess the veins using inspection and palpation to determine the best puncture site. Refer to the Assessment information above.

Gloves reduce transmission of microorganisms. Using the best site reduces the risk of injury to the patient. Palpation allows for making a distinction between other structures, such as tendons and arteries, in the area to avoid injury.

11. **Release the tourniquet. Check that the vein has decompressed (Lavery & Ingram, 2005).**

Releasing the tourniquet reduces the length of time the tourniquet is applied. Tourniquet should remain in place no more than 60 seconds to prevent injury, stasis, and hemoconcentration, which may alter results (Fischbach & Dunning, 2009). Thrombosed veins will remain firm and palpable and should not be used for venipuncture (Lavery & Ingram, 2005).

12. Attach the needle to the Vacutainer device. Place first blood-collection tube into the Vacutainer, but not engaged in the puncture device in the Vacutainer.

Device is prepared for use to ensure efficiency with the task.

13. Clean the patient's skin at the selected puncture site with the antimicrobial swab. If using chlorhexidine, use a back-and-forth motion, applying friction to the site for 30 seconds, or use procedure recommended by the manufacturer. If using alcohol, wipe in a circular motion spiraling outward. Allow the skin to dry before performing the venipuncture. Alternately, the skin can be dried with a sterile gauze (Fischbach & Dunning, 2009). Check facility policy.

Cleaning the patient's skin reduces the risk for transmission of microorganisms. Allowing the skin to dry maximizes antimicrobial action and prevents contact of the substance with the needle on insertion, thereby reducing the sting associated with insertion.

ACTION

RATIONALE

14. Reapply the tourniquet approximately 3 to 4 inches above the identified puncture site. **Apply sufficient pressure to impede venous circulation, but not arterial blood flow.**

Use of tourniquet increases venous pressure to aid in vein identification. Tourniquet should remain in place no more than 60 seconds to prevent injury, stasis, and hemoconcentration, which may alter results (Fischbach & Dunning, 2009).

15. Hold the patient's arm in a downward position with your nondominant hand. Align the needle and Vacutainer device with the chosen vein, holding the Vacutainer and needle in your dominant hand. Use the thumb or first finger of you nondominant hand to apply pressure and traction to the skin just below the identified puncture site.

Applying pressure helps immobilize and anchor the vein. Taut skin at the entry site aids smooth needle entry.

16. **Inform the patient that he or she is going to feel a pinch.** With the bevel of the needle up, insert the needle into the vein at a 15-degree angle to the skin (Fischbach & Dunning, 2009) (FIGURE 2).

Warning the patient prevents reaction related to surprise. Positioning the needle at the proper angle reduces the risk of puncturing through the vein.

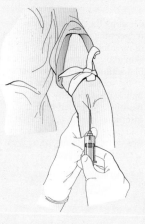

FIGURE 2 Inserting the needle at a 15-degree angle, with the bevel up.

ACTION	RATIONALE
17. Grasp the Vacutainer securely to stabilize it in the vein with your nondominant hand, and push the first collection tube into the puncture device in the Vacutainer, until the rubber stopper on the collection tube is punctured. You will feel the tube push into place on the puncture device. Blood will flow into the tube automatically.	The collection tube is a vacuum; negative pressure within the tube pulls blood into the tube.
18. **Remove the tourniquet as soon as blood flows adequately into the tube.**	Tourniquet removal reduces venous pressure and restores venous return to help prevent bleeding and bruising (Scales, 2008).
19. Continue to hold the Vacutainer in place in the vein and continue to fill the required tubes, removing one and inserting another. Gently rotate each tube as you remove it.	Filling the required tubes ensures that the sample is accurate. Gentle rotation helps to mix any additive in the tube with the blood sample.
20. After you have drawn all required blood samples, remove the last collection tube from the Vacutainer. **Place a gauze pad over the puncture site and slowly and gently remove the needle from the vein. Engage needle guard. Do not apply pressure to the site until the needle has been fully removed.**	Slow, gentle needle removal prevents injury to the vein. Releasing the vacuum before withdrawing the needle prevents vein injury and hematoma formation. Use of a needle guard prevents accidental needlestick injuries.
21. Apply gentle pressure to the puncture site for 2 to 3 minutes or until bleeding stops.	Applying pressure to the site after needle removal prevents injury, bleeding, and extravasation into the surrounding tissue, which can cause a hematoma.
22. After bleeding stops, apply an adhesive bandage.	The bandage protects the site and aids in applying pressure.

ACTION	**RATIONALE**
23. Remove equipment and return patient to a position of comfort. Raise side rail and lower bed.	Repositioning promotes patient comfort. Raising rails promotes safety.
24. Discard Vacutainer and needle in sharps container.	Proper disposal of equipment reduces transmission of microorganisms.
25. Remove gloves and perform hand hygiene.	Removing gloves properly reduces the risk for infection transmission and contamination of other items.
26. Place label on the container per facility policy. Place container in plastic sealable biohazard bag.	Proper labeling ensures accurate reporting of results. Packaging the specimen in a biohazard bag prevents the person transporting the container from coming in contact with blood and body fluids.
27. Check the venipuncture site to see if a hematoma has developed.	Development of a hematoma requires further intervention.
28. Remove other PPE, if used. Perform hand hygiene.	Removing PPE properly reduces the risk for infection transmission and contamination of other items. Hand hygiene reduces the transmission of microorganisms.
29. Transport the specimen to the laboratory immediately. If immediate transport is not possible, check with laboratory personnel or policy manual whether refrigeration is contraindicated.	Timely transport ensures accurate results.

EVALUATION

• An adequate uncontaminated blood specimen is obtained without adverse event and sent to the laboratory promptly.
• The patient states reason for blood test.
• The patient exhibits minimal anxiety during specimen collection.
• The patient verbalizes minor if any complaint of pain at venipuncture site.
• The patient exhibits no signs and symptoms of injury at venipuncture site.

DOCUMENTATION

- Record the date, time, and site of the venipuncture; the name of the test(s); the time the sample was sent to the laboratory; the amount of blood collected, if required; and any significant assessments or patient reactions.

GENERAL CONSIDERATIONS

- Be aware of the facility's policy regarding order of collection of multiple tubes of blood to ensure accurate results.
- If the flow of blood into the collection tube or syringe is sluggish, leave the tourniquet in place longer, but always remove it before withdrawing the needle. Do not leave the tourniquet on for more than 60 seconds.
- A blood pressure cuff inflated to a point between systolic and diastolic pressure values can be used as an alternative to a tourniquet (Fischbach & Dunning, 2009).
- Avoid collecting blood from edematous areas, arteriovenous shunts, an upper extremity on the same side as a previous lymph node dissection or mastectomy, infected sites, same extremity as an intravenous infusion, and sites of previous hematomas or vascular injury.
- Veins in the lower extremities should not be used for venipuncture, because of an increased risk of thrombophlebitis. Some facilities allow collection from lower extremities with a physician's order to collect blood from a leg or foot vein. Check your facility's policies.
- Warm compresses applied to the selected site 15 to 20 minutes before venipuncture can aid in distending veins that are difficult to locate.
- Consider the use of topical anesthetic creams to minimize discomfort and pain for the patient, based on facility policy. Be familiar with requirements and specifications for particular products available for use. Application needs to occur sufficiently in advance to allow enough time to become effective.
- Distraction has been shown to be of benefit in reducing anxiety related to venipuncture, especially with children. Asking the patient to concentrate on relaxing and performing deep breathing may help. Asking the patient to cough at the time of venipuncture is another technique that has been shown to be effective in reducing pain with venipuncture (Usichenko, et al., 2004).

Blood cultures are performed to detect bacterial invasion (bacteremia) and the systemic spread of such an infection (septicemia) through the bloodstream. In this procedure, a venous blood sample is collected by venipuncture into two bottles (one set), one containing an anaerobic medium and the other an aerobic medium. The bottles are incubated, encouraging any organisms that are present in the sample to grow in the media. Ideally, two to three sets of cultures, 1 hour apart or from separate sites, should be obtained.

The main problem encountered with blood-culture testing is that the specimen is easily contaminated with bacteria from the environment. Care must be taken to clean the skin at the venipuncture site properly to prevent contamination with skin flora, and aseptic technique must be used during the procedure. In addition, the access ports on the blood-culture bottles must be properly cleaned before access.

EQUIPMENT

- Tourniquet
- Nonsterile gloves
- Additional PPE, as indicated
- Antimicrobial swabs, such as chlorhexidine, per facility policy, for cleaning skin and culture bottle tops
- Vacutainer needle adaptor
- Sterile butterfly needle, gauge appropriate to the vein and sampling needs, using the smallest possible, with extension tubing
- Two blood-culture collection bottles for each set being obtained; one anaerobic bottle and one aerobic bottle
- Appropriate label for specimen, based on facility policy and procedure
- Biohazard bag
- Nonsterile 2 × 2 gauze pads
- Sterile 2 × 2 gauze pads
- Adhesive bandage

ASSESSMENT GUIDELINES

- Review the patient's medical record and the medical record for the number and type of blood cultures to be obtained. Ensure that the appropriate computer laboratory request has been completed.
- Assess the patient for signs and symptoms of infection, including vital signs, and note any antibiotic therapy being administered. Inspect any invasive monitoring insertion sites or incisions for indications of infection.
- Assess the patient for any allergies, especially related to the topical antimicrobial used for skin cleansing. Assess for the presence of any conditions or use of medications that may prolong bleeding time, necessitating additional application of pressure to the puncture site. Ask the patient about any previous laboratory testing that he or she

may have had, including any problems, such as difficulty with venipuncture, fainting, or complaints of dizziness, lightheadedness, or
nausea.
• Assess the patient's anxiety level and understanding about the
reasons for the blood test. Assess the patency of the veins in both
upper limbs. Palpate the veins to assess condition of vessel; vein
should be straight, feel soft, be cylindrical, and bounce when lightly
pressed. Appropriate vessels will compress without rolling, and have
rapid rebound filling after compression (Scales, 2008). Avoid veins
that are tender, sclerosed, thrombosed, fibrosed, or hard (Weinstein,
2006).

NURSING DIAGNOSES
• Hyperthermia
• Deficient Knowledge
• Anxiety
• Risk for Injury
• Risk for Infection

OUTCOME IDENTIFICATION AND PLANNING
Expected outcomes may include:
• An uncontaminated specimen will be obtained and sent to the labora-
tory promptly.
• The patient does not experience undue anxiety, injury, or infection.
• The patient verbalizes an understanding of the reason for the testing.

IMPLEMENTATION

ACTION	RATIONALE
1. Gather the necessary supplies. Check product expiration dates. Identify ordered number of blood culture sets and select the appropriate blood-collection bottles (at least one anaerobic and one aerobic bottle). If tests are ordered in addition to the blood cultures, collect the blood-culture specimens before other specimens.	Organization facilitates efficient performance of the procedure. Ensure proper functioning of equipment. Using correct bottles ensures accurate blood sampling.
2. Bring necessary equipment to the bedside stand or overbed table.	Bringing everything to the bedside conserves time and energy. Arranging items nearby is convenient, saves time, and avoids unnecessary stretching and

ACTION	RATIONALE
	twisting of muscles on the part of the nurse. Organization facilitates performance of tasks.
3. Perform hand hygiene and put on PPE, if indicated.	Hand hygiene and PPE prevent the transmission of microorganisms. PPE is required based on transmission precautions.
4. Identify the patient. Explain the procedure. Allow the patient time to ask questions and verbalize concerns about the venipuncture procedure.	Identifying the patient ensures the right patient receives the intervention and helps prevent errors. Explanation provides reassurance and promotes cooperation.
5. Close curtains around bed and close the door to the room, if possible.	Closing the door or curtain provides for patient privacy.
6. Check specimen label with patient identification bracelet. Label should include patient's name and identification number, time specimen was collected, route of collection, identification of the person obtaining the sample, and any other information required by agency policy.	Confirmation of patient identification information ensures specimen is labeled correctly for the right patient.
7. Provide for good light. Artificial light is recommended. Place a trash receptacle within easy reach.	Good lighting is necessary to perform the procedure properly. Having the trash receptacle in easy reach allows for safe disposal of contaminated materials.
8. Assist the patient to a comfortable position, either sitting or lying. If the patient is lying in bed, raise the bed to a comfortable working height, usually elbow height of the caregiver (VISN 8 Patient Safety Center, 2009).	Proper positioning allows easy access to the site and promotes patient comfort and safety. Proper bed height helps reduce back strain while performing the procedure.
9. Determine the patient's preferred site for the procedure based on his or her previous experience. Expose the arm,	Patient preference promotes patient participation in treatment and gives the nurse information

ACTION	RATIONALE
supporting it in an extended position on a firm surface, such as a tabletop. Position self on the same side of the patient as the site selected. Apply a tourniquet to the upper arm on the chosen side approximately 3 to 4 inches above the potential puncture site. Apply sufficient pressure to impede venous circulation but not arterial blood flow.	that may aid in site selection (Lavery & Ingram, 2005). Positioning close to the chosen site reduces back strain. Use of a tourniquet increases venous pressure to aid in vein identification. Tourniquet should remain in place no more than 90 seconds to prevent injury (Lavery & Ingram, 2005).
10. Put on nonsterile gloves. Assess the veins using inspection and palpation to determine the best puncture site. Refer to the Assessment information above.	Gloves reduce transmission of microorganisms. Using the best site reduces the risk of injury to the patient. Observation and palpation allow for making distinction between other structures, such as tendons and arteries, in area to avoid injury.
11. **Release the tourniquet. Check that the vein has decompressed (Lavery & Ingram, 2005).**	Releasing the tourniquet reduces the length of time the tourniquet is applied. Tourniquet should remain in place no more than 60 seconds to prevent injury, stasis, and hemoconcentration, which may alter results (Fischbach & Dunning, 2009). Thrombosed veins will remain firm and palpable and should not be used for venipuncture (Lavery & Ingram, 2005).
12. Attach the butterfly-needle extension tubing to the Vacutainer device.	Connection prepares device for use.
13. Move collection bottles to a location close to arm, with bottles sitting upright on tabletop.	Bottles must be close enough to reach with extension tubing on the butterfly needle to fill after venipuncture is completed. Bottles should remain upright to prevent backflow of contents to the patient.
14. Clean the patient's skin at the selected puncture site with the antimicrobial swab, according to facility policy.	Cleaning the patient's skin reduces the risk for transmission of microorganisms. Allowing the skin to dry maximizes

ACTION	RATIONALE
If using chlorhexidine, use a back-and-forth motion, applying friction for 30 seconds to the site, or use procedure recommended by the manufacturer. Allow the site to dry.	antimicrobial action and prevents contact of the substance with the needle on insertion, thereby reducing the sting associated with insertion.
15. Using a new antimicrobial swab, clean the stoppers of the culture bottles with the appropriate antimicrobial, per facility policy. Cover bottle top with sterile gauze square, based on facility policy.	Cleaning the bottle top reduces the risk for transmission of microorganisms into bottle. Covering top reduces risk of contamination.
16. Reapply the tourniquet approximately 3 to 4 inches above the identified puncture site. Apply sufficient pressure to impede venous circulation but not arterial blood flow. **After disinfection, not palpate the venipuncture site unless sterile gloves are worn.**	Use of a tourniquet increases venous pressure to aid in vein identification. Tourniquet should remain in place no more than 60 seconds to prevent injury, stasis, and hemoconcentration, which may alter results. Palpation is the greatest potential cause of blood culture contamination (Fischbach & Dunning, 2009).

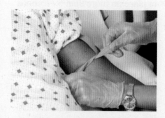

FIGURE 1 Applying the tourniquet. (*Photo by B. Proud.*)

17. Hold the patient's arm in a downward position with your nondominant hand. Align the butterfly needle with the chosen vein, holding the needle in your dominant hand. Use the thumb or first finger of nondominant hand to apply pressure and traction to the skin just below the identified puncture site. **Do not touch the insertion site.**	Applying pressure helps immobilize and anchor the vein. Taut skin at the entry site aids smooth needle entry. Not touching the insertion site helps to prevent contamination. Palpation is the greatest potential cause of blood culture contamination (Fischbach & Dunning, 2009).

ACTION	RATIONALE
18. **Inform the patient that he or she is going to feel a pinch.** With the bevel of the needle up, insert the needle into the vein at a 15-degree angle to the skin (Fischbach & Dunning, 2006). You should see a flash of blood in the extension tubing close to the needle when the vein is entered.	Warning the patient prevents reaction related to surprise. Positioning the needle at the proper angle reduces the risk of puncturing through the vein. Flash of blood indicates entrance into the vein.
19. Grasp the butterfly needle securely to stabilize it in the vein with your nondominant hand, and push Vacutainer onto the first collection bottle (anaerobic bottle), until the rubber stopper on the collection bottle is punctured. You will feel the bottle push into place on the puncture device. Blood will flow into the bottle automatically.	The collection bottle is a vacuum; negative pressure within the bottle pulls blood into the bottle.
20. **Remove the tourniquet as soon as blood flows adequately into the bottle.**	Tourniquet removal reduces venous pressure and restores venous return to help prevent bleeding and bruising (Scales, 2008).
21. Continue to hold butterfly needle in place in the vein. Once the first bottle is filled, remove it from the Vacutainer and insert the second bottle. After the blood culture specimens are obtained, continue to fill any additional required tubes, removing one and inserting another. Gently rotate each bottle and tube as you remove it.	Filling the required bottles ensures that the sample is accurate. Gentle rotation helps to mix any additive in the tube with the blood sample.
22. **After you have drawn all required blood samples, remove the last collection tube from the Vacutainer. Place a gauze pad over the puncture site and slowly and gently remove the needle from the vein. Engage the**	Slow, gentle needle removal prevents injury to the vein. Releasing vacuum before withdrawing the needle prevents injury to the vein and hematoma formation. Use of a needle guard prevents accidental needlestick injuries.

ACTION	RATIONALE
needle guard. Do not apply pressure to the site until the needle has been fully removed.	
23. Apply gentle pressure to the puncture site for 2 to 3 minutes or until bleeding stops.	Applying pressure to site after needle removal prevents injury, bleeding, and extravasation into the surrounding tissue, which can cause a hematoma.
24. After bleeding stops, apply an adhesive bandage.	The bandage protects the site and aids in applying pressure.
25. Remove equipment and return the patient to a position of comfort. Raise side rail and lower bed.	Repositioning promotes patient comfort. Raising rails promotes safety.
26. Discard Vacutainer and butterfly needle in sharps container.	Proper disposal of equipment reduces transmission of microorganisms.
27. Remove gloves and perform hand hygiene.	Removing gloves properly reduces the risk for infection transmission and contamination of other items. Hand hygiene reduces the transmission of microorganisms.
28. Place label on the container per facility policy. Place containers in plastic sealable biohazard bag. Refer to facility policy regarding the need for separate biohazard bags for blood culture specimens and other blood specimens.	Proper labeling ensures accurate reporting of results. Packaging the specimen in a biohazard bag prevents the person transporting the container from coming in contact with blood or body fluids. Some facility policies call for individual bagging.
29. Check the venipuncture site to see if a hematoma has developed.	Hematoma development requires further intervention.
30. Remove other PPE, if used. Perform hand hygiene.	Removing PPE properly reduces the risk for infection transmission and contamination of other items. Hand hygiene reduces the transmission of microorganisms.
31. Transport specimen to laboratory immediately. If immediate transport is not possible, check with laboratory personnel or policy manual as to appropriate handling.	Timely transport ensures accurate results.

EVALUATION

- An adequate and uncontaminated blood specimen is obtained without adverse event and sent to the laboratory promptly.
- The patient states reason for blood test.
- The patient exhibits minimal anxiety during specimen collection.
- The patient verbalizes minor if any complaint of pain at the venipuncture site.
- The patient exhibits no signs and symptoms of injury at venipuncture site.

DOCUMENTATION

- Record the date, time, and site of the venipuncture; the name of the test(s); the time the sample was sent to the laboratory; the amount of blood collected, if required; and any significant assessments or patient reactions.

GENERAL CONSIDERATIONS

- Be aware that the size of the culture bottles may vary according to facility policy, but the sample dilution should always be 1:10.
- Avoid using existing blood lines for cultures unless the sample is drawn when the line is inserted or catheter sepsis is suspected.
- Avoid collecting blood from edematous areas, arteriovenous shunts, an upper extremity on the same side as a previous lymph node dissection or mastectomy, infected sites, same extremity as an intravenous infusion, and sites of previous hematomas or vascular injury.
- Do not use veins in the lower extremities for venipuncture, because of an increased risk of thrombophlebitis. However, some facilities do allow collection from lower extremities with a physician's order to collect blood from a leg or foot vein. Check your facility's policies.
- Apply warm compresses to the selected site 15 to 20 minutes before venipuncture to aid in distending veins that are difficult to locate.
- Consider the use of topical anesthetic creams to minimize discomfort and pain for the patient, based on facility policy. Be familiar with requirements and specifications for particular product available for use. Application needs to occur far enough in advance to allow sufficient time to become effective.
- Use distraction, which has been shown to be of benefit in reducing anxiety related to venipuncture, especially with children. Asking the patient to concentrate on relaxing, and performing deep breathing may help. Asking the patient to cough at the time of venipuncture is another technique that has shown to be effective in reducing pain with venipuncture (Usichenko et al., 2004).

Skill · 23   Administering a Blood Transfusion

A blood transfusion is the infusion of whole blood or a blood component, such as plasma, red blood cells, or platelets into a patient's venous circulation. Before a patient can receive a blood product, his or her blood must be typed to ensure that he or she receives compatible blood. Otherwise, a serious and life-threatening transfusion reaction may occur involving clumping and hemolysis of the red blood cells and, possibly, death. The nurse must also verify the infusion rate, based on facility policy or medical order. Follow the facility's policies and guidelines to determine if the transfusion should be administered by electronic pump or by gravity.

EQUIPMENT

- Blood product
- Blood administration set (tubing with in-line filter and Y for saline administration)
- 0.9% normal saline for IV infusion
- IV pole
- Venous access; if peripheral site, preferably initiated

- with a 20-gauge catheter or larger
- Clean gloves
- Additional PPE, as indicated
- Tape (hypoallergenic)
- Second nurse for verification of blood product and patient information

ASSESSMENT GUIDELINES

- Obtain a baseline assessment of the patient, including vital signs, heart and lung sounds, and urinary output.
- Review the most recent laboratory values, in particular, the complete blood count (CBC).
- Ask the patient about any previous transfusions, including the number he or she has had and any reactions experienced during a transfusion.
- Assess the IV insertion site, noting that the size of the IV catheter is a 20 gauge or larger.

NURSING DIAGNOSES

- Risk for Injury
- Excess Fluid Volume
- Deficient Fluid Volume
- Ineffective Peripheral Tissue Perfusion
- Decreased Cardiac Output

OUTCOME IDENTIFICATION AND PLANNING

Expected outcomes may include:
- Patient will remain free of injury and any signs and symptoms of IV complications.
- Capped venous access device will remain patent.

IMPLEMENTATION

ACTION	RATIONALE
1. Verify the medical order for transfusion of blood product. Verify the completion of informed consent documentation in the medical record. Verify any medical order for pretransfusion medication. If ordered, administer medication at least 30 minutes before initiating transfusion.	Verification of order ensures patient receives correct intervention. Premedication is sometimes administered to decrease risk for allergic and febrile reactions for patients who have received multiple previous transfusions.
2. Gather all equipment and bring to bedside.	Having equipment available saves time and facilitates accomplishment of procedure.
3. Perform hand hygiene and put on PPE, if indicated.	Hand hygiene and PPE prevent the spread of microorganisms. PPE is required based on transmission precautions.
4. Identify the patient.	Identifying the patient ensures the right patient receives the intervention and helps prevent errors.
5. Close curtains around bed and close the door to the room, if possible. Explain what you are going to do and why you are going to do it to the patient. Ask the patient about previous experience with transfusion and any reactions. Advise patient to report any chills, itching, rash, or unusual symptoms.	This ensures the patient's privacy. Explanation relieves anxiety and facilitates cooperation. Previous reactions may increase the risk for reaction to this transfusion. Any reaction to the transfusion necessitates stopping the transfusion immediately and evaluating the situation.
6. Prime blood administration set with the normal saline IV fluid.	Normal saline is the solution of choice for blood product administration. Solutions with dextrose may lead to clumping of red blood cells and hemolysis.
7. Put on gloves. If patient does not have a venous access in place, initiate peripheral	Gloves prevent contact with blood and body fluids. Infusion of fluid via venous access

ACTION	RATIONALE
venous access. Connect the administration set to the venous access device via the extension tubing. Infuse the normal saline per facility policy.	maintains patency until the blood product is administered. Start an IV before obtaining the blood product in case the initiation takes longer than 30 minutes. Blood must be stored at a carefully controlled temperature (4°C) and transfusion must begin within 30 minutes of release from blood bank.
8. Obtain blood product from the blood bank according to agency policy. Scan for bar codes on blood products, if required.	Bar codes on blood products are currently being implemented in some agencies to identify, track, and assign data to transfusions as an additional safety measure.
9. Two nurses compare and validate the following information with the medical record, patient identification band, and the label of the blood product: • Medical order for transfusion of blood product • Informed consent • Patient identification number • Patient name • Blood group and type • Expiration date • Inspection of blood product for clots	Most states/agencies require two registered nurses to verify the following information: unit numbers match; ABO group and Rh type are the same; expiration date (after 35 days, red blood cells begin to deteriorate). Blood is never administered to a patient without an identification band. If clots are present, return blood to the blood bank.
10. Obtain baseline set of vital signs before beginning transfusion.	Any change in vital signs during the transfusion may indicate a reaction.
11. Put on gloves. If using an electronic infusion device, put the device on 'hold'. Close the roller clamp closest to the drip chamber on the saline side of the administration set. Close the roller clamp on administration set below the infusion device. Alternately, if using infusing via gravity,	Gloves prevent contact with blood and body fluids. Stopping the infusion prevents blood from infusing to the patient before completing preparations. Closing the clamp to saline allows blood product to be infused via an electronic infusion device.

ACTION	RATIONALE

close the roller clamp on the administration set.

12. Close the roller clamp closest to the drip chamber on the blood product side of the administration set. Remove the protective cap from the access port on the blood container. Remove the cap from the access spike on the administration set. Using a pushing and twisting motion, insert the spike into the access port on the blood container, taking care not to contaminate the spike. Hang blood container on the IV pole. Open the roller clamp on the blood side of the administration set. Squeeze drip chamber until the in-line filter is saturated. Remove gloves.

Filling the drip chamber prevents air from entering the administration set. The filter in the blood administration set removes particulate material formed during storage of blood. If the administration set is contaminated, the entire set would have to be discarded and replaced.

13. **Start administration slowly (no more than 25 to 50 mL for the first 15 minutes). Stay with the patient for the first 5 to 15 minutes of transfusion.** Open the roller clamp on the administration set below the infusion device. Set the flow rate and begin the transfusion. Alternately, start the flow of solution by releasing the clamp on the tubing and counting the drops. Adjust until the correct drop rate is achieved. Assess the blood flow and function of the infusion device. Inspect the insertion site for signs of infiltration.

Transfusion reactions typically occur during this period, and a slow rate will minimize the volume of red blood cells infused.

Verifying the rate and device settings ensures the patient receives the correct volume of solution. If the catheter or needle slips out of the vein, the blood will accumulate (infiltrate) into the surrounding tissue.

14. Observe patient for flushing, dyspnea, itching, hives or rash, and whether the patient makes any unusual comments.

These signs and symptoms may be an early indication of a transfusion reaction.

ACTION	RATIONALE
15. After the observation period (5 to 15 minutes), increase the infusion rate to the calculated rate to complete the infusion within the prescribed time frame, no more than 4 hours.	If there have been no adverse effects during this time, the infusion rate is increased. If complications occur, they can be observed and the transfusion can be stopped immediately. Verifying the rate and device settings ensures patient receives the correct volume of solution. Transfusion must be completed within 4 hours due to potential for bacterial growth in blood product at room temperature.
16. Reassess vital signs after 15 minutes. Obtain vital signs thereafter according to facility policy and nursing assessment.	Vital signs must be assessed as part of monitoring for possible adverse reaction. Facility policy and nursing judgment will dictate frequency.
17. Maintain the prescribed flow rate as ordered or as deemed appropriate based on the patient's overall condition, keeping in mind the outer limits for safe administration. Ongoing monitoring is crucial throughout the entire duration of the blood transfusion for early identification of any adverse reactions.	Rate must be carefully controlled, and the patient's reaction must be monitored frequently.
18. **During transfusion, assess frequently for transfusion reaction. Stop the blood transfusion if you suspect a reaction. Quickly replace the blood tubing with a new administration set primed with normal saline for IV infusion. Initiate an infusion of normal saline for IV at an open rate, usually 40 mL/hour. Obtain vital signs. Notify physician and blood bank.**	If a transfusion reaction is suspected, the blood must be stopped. Do not infuse the normal saline through the blood tubing because you would be allowing more of the blood into the patient's body, which could complicate a reaction. Besides a serious life-threatening blood transfusion reaction, the potential for fluid-volume overload exists in elderly patients and patients with decreased cardiac function.

ACTION	RATIONALE
19. When the transfusion is complete, close the roller clamp on blood side of the administration set and open the roller clamp on the normal saline side of the administration set. Initiate infusion of normal saline. When all of the blood has infused into the patient, clamp the administration set. Obtain vital signs. Put on gloves. Cap access site or resume previous IV infusion. Dispose of blood transfusion equipment or return to blood bank, according to facility policy.	Saline prevents hemolysis of red blood cells and clears the remainder of blood in IV line. Proper disposal of equipment reduces transmission of microorganisms and potential contact with blood and body fluids.
20. Remove equipment. Ensure patient's comfort. Remove gloves. Lower bed, if not in lowest position.	Promotes patient comfort and safety. Removing gloves properly reduces the risk for infection transmission and contamination of other items.
21. Remove additional PPE, if used. Perform hand hygiene.	Removing PPE properly reduces the risk for infection transmission and contamination of other items. Hand hygiene prevents transmission of microorganisms.

EVALUATION

• Patient receives the blood transfusion without any evidence of a transfusion reaction or complication.
• Patient exhibits signs and symptoms of fluid balance, improved cardiac output, and enhanced peripheral tissue perfusion.

DOCUMENTATION

• Document that the patient received the blood transfusion; include the type of blood product. Record the patient's condition throughout the transfusion, including pertinent data, such as vital signs, lung sounds, and the subjective response of the patient to transfusion. Document any complications or reactions or whether the patient received the transfusion without any complications or reactions. Document the assessment of the IV site, and any other fluids infused during the procedure.

Document transfusion volume and other IV fluid intake on the patient's intake and output record.

GENERAL CONSIDERATIONS

• If an electronic infusion device is used to maintain the prescribed rate, ensure it is designed for use with blood transfusions before initiation of transfusion.

• Never warm blood in a microwave. Use a blood-warming device, if indicated or ordered, especially with rapid transfusions through a CVAD. Rapid administration of cold blood can result in cardiac arrhythmias.

Skill · 24 Applying a Cardiac Monitor

Bedside cardiac monitoring provides continuous observation of the heart's electrical activity. It focuses on the detection of clinically significant dysrhythmias (Larson & Brady, 2008). Cardiac monitoring is used for patients with conduction disturbances and for those at risk for life-threatening arrhythmias, such as postoperative patients and patients who are sedated. As with other forms of electrocardiography (ECG), cardiac monitoring uses electrodes placed on the patient's chest to transmit electrical signals that are converted into a tracing of cardiac rhythm on an oscilloscope. Three-lead or five-lead systems may be used (FIGURE 1). The three-lead–wire monitoring system facilitates monitoring of the patient in any of the limb leads. The five-lead–wire monitoring system facilitates monitoring of the patient in any one of the standard 12 leads.

Two types of monitoring may be performed: hardwire or telemetry. In hardwire monitoring, the patient is connected to a monitor at the bedside.

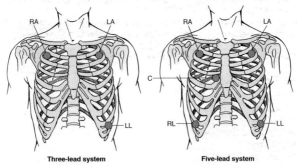

Three-lead system   **Five-lead system**
FIGURE 1 Three-lead or five-lead systems.

The rhythm display appears at the bedside, but may also be transmitted to a console at a remote location. Telemetry uses a small transmitter connected to the ambulatory patient to send electrical signals to another location, where they are displayed on a monitor screen. Battery-powered and portable, telemetry frees patients from cumbersome wires and cables and lets them be comfortably mobile. Telemetry is especially useful for monitoring arrhythmias that occur during sleep, rest, exercise, or stressful situations. Wireless telemetry devices are also being introduced, using microchips to record patient data, eliminating the need for new leads each time the patient is moved to a different location (Goulette, 2008).

Regardless of the type, cardiac monitors can display the patient's heart rate and rhythm, produce a printed record of cardiac rhythm, and sound an alarm if the heart rate exceeds or falls below specified limits. Monitors also recognize and count abnormal heartbeats as well as changes. Gel foam electrodes are commonly used. Electrodes should be changed every 24 hours, or according to facility policy, to prevent skin irritation. Hypoallergenic electrodes are available for patients with hypersensitivity to tape or adhesive. Any loose or nonadhering electrode should be replaced immediately to prevent inaccurate or missing data.

EQUIPMENT

- Lead wires
- Pregelled (gel foam) electrodes (number varies from 3 to 5)
- Alcohol pads
- Gauze pads
- Patient cable for hardwire cardiac monitor
- Transmitter, transmitter pouch, and telemetry battery pack for telemetry
- PPE, as indicated

ASSESSMENT GUIDELINES

- Review the patient's medical record and plan of care for information about the patient's need for cardiac monitoring.
- Assess the patient's cardiac status, including heart rate, blood pressure, and auscultation of heart sounds.
- Inspect the patient's chest for areas of irritation, breakdown, or excessive hair that might interfere with electrode placement. Electrode sites must be dry, with minimal hair.
- The patient may be sitting or supine, in a bed or chair.

NURSING DIAGNOSES

- Decreased Cardiac Output
- Excess Fluid Volume
- Impaired Gas Exchange
- Deficient Knowledge
- Acute Pain
- Activity Intolerance
- Anxiety

OUTCOME IDENTIFICATION AND PLANNING

Expected outcomes may include:
- A clear waveform, free from artifact, is displayed on the cardiac monitor.
- Patient displays understanding of the reason for monitoring.
- Patient experiences reduced anxiety.

IMPLEMENTATION

ACTION	RATIONALE
1. Verify the order for cardiac monitoring on the patient's medical record.	This ensures that the correct intervention is performed on the correct patient.
2. Gather all equipment and bring to bedside.	Having equipment available saves time and facilitates accomplishment of the procedure.
3. Perform hand hygiene and put on PPE, if indicated.	Hand hygiene and PPE prevent the spread of microorganisms. PPE is required based on transmission precautions.
4. Identify the patient.	Identifying the patient ensures the right patient receives the intervention and helps prevent errors.
5. Close curtains around bed and close the door to the room, if possible. Explain the procedure to the patient. Tell the patient that the monitoring records the heart's electrical activity. Emphasize that no electrical current will enter his or her body. Ask the patient about allergies to adhesive, as appropriate.	This ensures the patient's privacy. Explanation relieves anxiety and facilitates cooperation. Possible allergies may exist related to adhesive on ECG leads.
6. For hardwire monitoring, plug the cardiac monitor into an electrical outlet and turn it on to warm up the unit while preparing the equipment and the patient. For telemetry monitoring, insert a new battery	Proper setup ensures proper functioning. Not all models have a test button. Test according to manufacturer's directions.

ACTION	RATIONALE
into the transmitter. Match the poles on the battery with the polar markings on the transmitter case. Press the button at the top of the unit, test the battery's charge, and test the unit to ensure that the battery is operational.	
7. Insert the cable into the appropriate socket in the monitor.	Proper setup ensures proper functioning.
8. Connect the lead wires to the cable. In some systems, the lead wires are permanently secured to the cable. For telemetry, if the lead wires are not permanently affixed to the telemetry unit, attach them securely. If they must be attached individually, connect each one to the correct outlet.	Proper setup ensures proper functioning.
9. Connect an electrode to each of the lead wires, carefully checking that each lead wire is in its correct outlet.	Proper setup ensures proper functioning.
10. If the bed is adjustable, raise it to comfortable working height, usually elbow height of the caregiver (VISN 8 Patient Safety Center, 2009).	Having the bed at the proper height prevents back and muscle strain.
11. Expose the patient's chest and determine electrode positions, based on which system and leads are being used. If necessary, clip the hair from an area about 10 cm in diameter around each electrode site. Clean the area with soap and water and dry it completely to remove skin secretions that may interfere with electrode function.	These actions allow for better adhesion of the electrode and thus better conduction. Alcohol, benzoin, and antiperspirant are not recommended for use in preparing the skin.

ACTION	RATIONALE
12. Remove the backing from the pregelled electrode. Check the gel for moistness. If the gel is dry, discard it and replace it with a fresh electrode. **Apply the electrode to the site and press firmly to ensure a tight seal.** Repeat with the remaining electrodes to complete the three-lead or five-lead system.	Gel acts as a conduit and must be moist and secured tightly.
13. When all the electrodes are in place, connect the appropriate lead wire to each electrode. Check waveform for clarity, position, and size. **To verify that the monitor is detecting each beat, compare the digital heart rate display with an auscultated count of the patient's heart rate.** If necessary, use the gain control to adjust the size of the rhythm tracing, and use the position control to adjust the waveform position on the monitor.	This ensures accuracy of reading.
14. Set the upper and lower limits of the heart rate alarm, based on the patient's condition or unit policy.	Setting the alarm allows for audible notification if the heart rate is beyond limits. The default setting for the monitor automatically turns on all alarms; limits should be set for each patient.
15. For telemetry, place the transmitter in the pouch in the hospital gown. If not available in gown, use a portable pouch. Tie the pouch strings around the patient's neck and waist, making sure that the pouch fits snugly without causing discomfort. If no pouch is available, place the transmitter in the patient's bathrobe pocket.	Patient comfort leads to compliance.

ACTION	RATIONALE
16. To obtain a rhythm strip, press the RECORD key either at the bedside for monitoring or at the central station for telemetry. Label the strip with the patient's name and room number, date, time, and rhythm identification. Analyze the strip, as appropriate. Place the rhythm strip in the appropriate location in the patient's chart.	A rhythm strip provides a baseline.
17. Return the patient to a comfortable position. Lower bed height and adjust head of bed to a comfortable position.	Repositioning promotes patient comfort. Lowering the bed promotes patient safety.
18. Remove additional PPE, if used. Perform hand hygiene.	Removing PPE properly reduces the risk for infection transmission and contamination of other items. Hand hygiene prevents transmission of microorganisms.

EVALUATION

* Cardiac monitoring waveform displays the patient's cardiac rhythm, with a waveform that is detecting each beat, and is appropriate for clarity, position, and size.
* Patient demonstrates no undue anxiety and remains free of complications or injury.

DOCUMENTATION

* Record the date and time that monitoring began and the monitoring lead used in the medical record. Document a rhythm strip at least every 8 hours including any changes in the patient's condition (or as stated by facility's policy). Label the rhythm strip with the patient's name and room number, date, and time.

GENERAL CONSIDERATIONS

* Make sure all electrical equipment and outlets are grounded to avoid electric shock and interference (artifacts).
* Avoid opening the electrode packages until just before using to prevent the gel from drying out.

- Avoid placing the electrodes on bony prominences, hairy locations, areas where defibrillator pads will be placed, or areas for chest compression.
- If the patient's skin is very oily, scaly, or diaphoretic, rub the electrode site with a dry 4 × 4 gauze pad before applying the electrode to help reduce interference in the tracing.
- Assess skin integrity and examine the leads every 8 hours. Replace and reposition the electrodes, as necessary.
- If the patient is being monitored by telemetry, show him or her how the transmitter works. If applicable, identify the button that will produce a recording of the ECG at the central station. Instruct the patient to push the button whenever symptoms occur; this causes the central console to print a rhythm strip. Also, advise the patient to notify the nurse immediately if symptoms occur.
- If the medical order is in place, tell the patient to remove the transmitter during showering or bathing, if appropriate, but stress that he or she should let the nurse know the unit is being removed.

Skill · 25 **Performing Cardiopulmonary Resuscitation (CPR)**

Cardiopulmonary resuscitation (CPR), also known as basic life support, is used in the absence of spontaneous respirations and heartbeat to preserve heart and brain function while waiting for defibrillation and advanced cardiac life-support care. It is a combination of chest compressions, which manually pump the heart to circulate blood to the body systems, and "mouth-to-mouth" or rescue breathing, which supplies oxygen to the lungs.

Assess the patient, activate the emergency response system, and perform the ABCDs of CPR. Remember the ABCDs of CPR—airway, breathing, and circulation—followed by the 'D' of defibrillation to manage sudden cardiac death (American Heart Association [AHA], 2006).

In the hospital setting, it is imperative that personnel be aware of the patient's stated instructions regarding a wish not to be resuscitated. This should be clearly expressed and documented in the patient's medical record.

In 2008, the American Heart Association (AHA) instituted changes in their suggestions regarding emergency interventions outside of healthcare facilities. Learning conventional CPR is still recommended. However, the AHA alternately recommends when an adult suddenly collapses, persons near the victim should call 911 (activate the emergency response system), and push hard and fast in the center of the victim's chest. Studies of real emergencies that have occurred in homes, at work, or in public locations show that these two steps, called 'Hands-Only CPR,' can be as effective as conventional CPR. Providing Hands-Only CPR to an adult who has collapsed from a sudden cardiac arrest can more than double that person's chance of survival (AHA, 2008).

EQUIPMENT

- PPE, such as a face shield or one-way valve mask, and gloves, if available
- Ambu-bag and oxygen, if available

ASSESSMENT GUIDELINES

- Assess the patient's vital parameters and determine the patient's level of responsiveness.
- Check for partial or complete airway obstruction.
- Assess for the absence or ineffectiveness of respirations.
- Assess for the absence of signs of circulation and pulses.

NURSING DIAGNOSES

- Decreased Cardiac Output
- Ineffective Airway Clearance
- Risk for Ineffective Cerebral Tissue Perfusion
- Risk for Aspiration
- Impaired Gas Exchange
- Risk for Injury
- Impaired Spontaneous Ventilation

OUTCOME IDENTIFICATION AND PLANNING

Expected outcomes may include:
- CPR is performed effectively without adverse effect to the patient.
- Patient regains a pulse and respirations.
- Patient's heart and lungs maintain adequate function to sustain life.
- Advanced cardiac life support is initiated.

IMPLEMENTATION

ACTION	RATIONALE
1. Assess responsiveness. If the patient is not responsive, call for help, pull call bell, and call the facility emergency response number. Call for the automated external defibrillator (AED).	Assessing responsiveness prevents starting CPR on a conscious victim. Activating the emergency response system initiates a rapid response.
2. Put on gloves, if available. Position the patient supine on	Gloves prevent contact with blood and body fluids. The

ACTION

his or her back on a firm, flat surface, with arms alongside the body. If the patient is in bed, place a backboard or other rigid surface under the patient (often the footboard of the patient's bed).

3. Use the head tilt–chin lift maneuver to open the airway. Place one hand on the victim's forehead and apply firm, backward pressure with the palm to tilt the head back. Place the fingers of the other hand under the bony part of the lower jaw near the chin and lift the jaw upward to bring the chin forward and the teeth almost to occlusion. If trauma to the head or neck is present or suspected, use the jaw-thrust maneuver to open the airway. Place one hand on each side of the patient's head. Rest elbows on the flat surface under the patient, grasp the angle of the patient's lower jaw, and lift with both hands.

4. Look, listen, and feel for air exchange. Take at least 5 seconds and no more than 10 seconds (AHA, 2006).

5. If the patient resumes breathing or adequate respirations and signs of circulation are noted, place the patient in the recovery position.

6. If no spontaneous breathing is noted, seal the patient's mouth and nose with the face shield, one-way valve mask,

RATIONALE

supine position is required for resuscitative efforts and evaluation to be effective. Backboard provides a firm surface on which to apply compressions. If the patient must be rolled, move as a unit so the head, shoulders, and torso move simultaneously without twisting.

This maneuver may be sufficient to open the airway and promote spontaneous respirations.

These techniques provide information about the patient's breathing and the need for rescue breathing.

The recovery position maintains alignment of the back and spine while allowing for continued observation and also maintains access to the patient.

Sealing the patient's mouth and nose prevents air from escaping. Devices, such as masks, reduce the risk for transmission of infections.

ACTION	RATIONALE
or Ambu-bag (handheld resuscitation bag), if available. If not available, seal patient's mouth with rescuer's mouth.	
7. Instill two breaths, each lasting 1 second, making the chest rise.	Breathing into the patient provides oxygen to the patient's lungs. Hyperventilation results in increased positive chest pressure and decreased venous return. Blood flow to the lungs during CPR is only about 25% to 33% normal; patient requires less ventilation to provide oxygen and remove carbon dioxide. Longer breaths reduce the amount of blood that refills the heart, reducing blood flow generated by compressions. Delivery of large, forceful breaths may cause gastric inflation and distension.
8. If you are unable to ventilate the patient or the chest does not rise during ventilation, reposition the patient's head and reattempt to ventilate. If still unable to ventilate, begin CPR. Each subsequent time the airway is opened to administer breaths, look for an object. If an object is visible in the mouth, remove it. If no object is visible, continue with CPR.	Inability to ventilate indicates that the airway may be obstructed. Repositioning maneuvers may be sufficient to open the airway and promote spontaneous respirations. It is critical to minimize interruptions in chest compressions, to maintain circulatory perfusion.
9. Check the carotid pulse, simultaneously evaluating for breathing, coughing, or movement. This assessment should take at least 5 seconds and no more than 10 seconds. Place the patient in the recovery position if breathing resumes.	Pulse and other assessments evaluate cardiac function. The femoral pulse may be used for the pulse check.

ACTION	RATIONALE
10. If the patient has a pulse, but remains without spontaneous breathing, continue rescue breathing at a rate of one breath every 5 to 6 seconds, for a rate of 10 to 12 breaths per minute.	Rescue breathing maintains adequate oxygenation.
11. If the patient is without signs of circulation, position the heel of one hand in the center of the chest between the nipples, directly over the lower half of the sternum. Place the other hand directly on top of the first hand. Extend or interlace fingers to keep fingers above the chest. Straighten arms and position shoulders directly over hands.	Proper hand positioning ensures that the force of compressions is on the sternum, thereby reducing the risk of rib fracture, lung puncture, or liver laceration.
12. Perform 30 chest compressions at a rate of 100 per minute, counting "one, two, etc." up to 30, keeping elbows locked, arms straight, and shoulders directly over the hands. Chest compressions should depress the sternum 1½ to 2 inches. Push straight down on the patient's sternum. Allow full chest recoil (re-expand) after each compression.	Direct cardiac compression and manipulation of intrathoracic pressure supply blood flow during CPR. Compressing the chest 1½ to 2 inches ensures that compressions are not too shallow and provides adequate blood flow. Full chest recoil allows adequate venous return to the heart.
13. Give two rescue breaths after each set of 30 compressions. Do five complete cycles of 30 compressions and two ventilations.	Breathing and compressions simulate lung and heart function, providing oxygen and circulation.
14. **Defibrillation should be provided at the earliest possible moment, as soon as AED becomes available.** Refer to Skill 47: Manual External Defibrillation and	The interval from collapse to defibrillation is the most important determinant of survival from cardiac arrest (AHA, 2005).

ACTION	RATIONALE
Skill 48: Automated External Defibrillation.	
15. Continue CPR until advanced care providers take over, the patient starts to move, you are too exhausted to continue, or a physician discontinues CPR. Advanced care providers will indicate when a pulse check or other therapies are appropriate (AHA, 2006).	Once started, CPR must continue until one of these conditions is met. In a hospital setting, help should arrive within a few minutes.
16. Remove gloves, if used. Perform hand hygiene.	Removing PPE properly reduces the risk for infection transmission and contamination of other items. Hand hygiene prevents transmission of microorganisms.

EVALUATION
- CPR is performed effectively without adverse effect to the patient.
- Patient regains a pulse and respirations.
- Patient's heart and lungs maintain adequate function to sustain life.
- Advanced cardiac life support is initiated.
- Patient does not experience serious injury.

DOCUMENTATION
- Document the time you discovered the patient unresponsive and started CPR. Continued intervention, such as by the code team, is typically documented on a code form, which identifies the actions and drugs provided during the code. Provide a summary of these events in the patient's medical record.

GENERAL CONSIDERATIONS
- If the arrest is out-of-hospital and not witnessed, approximately 2 minutes of CPR (five cycles) should be given before applying the AED, checking the ECG rhythm, and attempting defibrillation (Brunetti, 2008; AHA, 2006).
- If the nurse is unsure whether the patient has a pulse, CPR should be initiated. Unnecessary CPR is less harmful than not performing CPR when it is truly needed (AHA, 2006).
- **Every effort to minimize interruptions in chest compressions should be taken. Causes for not providing compressions may include prolonged pulse checks, taking too long to give breaths, moving the patient, and using the AED. Try to limit interruptions**

to less than 10 seconds, except for intubation, defibrillation, or moving the patient from danger (AHA, 2006).

- Perform CPR in the same manner if the patient is obese.
- Perform CPR for pregnant patients using the same guidelines, with a few additional measures. Before initiating chest compressions, the patient must be placed in a 30-degree left lateral tilt position, which reduces vena cava compression and resulting decreased cardiac output (Castle, 2007). The left lateral tilt position is accomplished by using a foam wedge or other firm device behind the patient's back. The rescuer's hands are placed in the center of the patient's chest and compressions to move the sternum directed toward the spine, not vertically downward. Use additional pressure with chest compressions. Pregnancy-related decreased chest-wall compliance decreases the efficiency of chest compressions. Anterior-posterior placement of electrode pads can avoid difficulties associated with increased breast size (Castle, 2007).
- If it is not possible to seal the patient's mouth completely for reasons such as oral trauma, perform mouth-to-nose breathing. If the patient has a tracheostomy, provide ventilations through the tracheostomy instead of the mouth.
- Be aware that in 2008, the AHA instituted changes in their suggestions regarding emergency interventions outside of healthcare facilities. Learning conventional CPR is still recommended. However, the AHA alternately recommends when an adult suddenly collapses, persons near the victim should call 911 (activate the emergency response system), and push hard and fast in the center of the victim's chest. Studies of real emergencies that have occurred in homes, at work, or in public locations, show that these two steps, called Hands-Only CPR, can be as effective as conventional CPR. Providing Hands-Only CPR to an adult who has collapsed from a sudden cardiac arrest can more than double that person's chance of survival (AHA, 2008).
- Know that Hands-Only CPR is not recommended for victims of drowning, trauma, airway obstruction, and acute respiratory distress (AHA, 2008).

Skill · 26   Assisting with Cast Application

A cast is a rigid external immobilizing device that encases a body part. Casts are used to immobilize a body part in a specific position and to apply uniform pressure on the encased soft tissue. Casts generally allow the patient mobility while restricting movement of the affected body part. Nonplaster casts set in 15 minutes and can sustain weight-bearing or pressure in 15 to 30 minutes. Plaster casts can take 24 to 72 hours to dry, and weight-bearing or pressure is contraindicated during this period. Patient safety is of utmost importance during the application of a cast.

Typically, a physician or other advanced practice professional applies the cast. Nursing responsibilities include preparing the patient and equipment and assisting during the application. The nurse provides skin care to the affected area before, during, and after the cast is applied. In some settings, nurses with special preparation may apply or change casts.

EQUIPMENT

- Casting materials, such as plaster rolls or fiberglass, depending on the type of cast being applied
- Padding material, such as stockinette, sheet wadding, or Webri®, depending on the type of cast being applied
- Plastic bucket or basin filled with warm water
- Disposable nonsterile gloves and aprons
- Scissors
- Waterproof disposable pads
- PPE, as indicated

ASSESSMENT GUIDELINES

- Assess the skin condition in the affected area, noting redness, contusions, or open wounds.
- Assess the neurovascular status of the affected extremity, including distal pulses, color, temperature, presence of edema, capillary refill to fingers or toes, and sensation and motion.
- Perform a pain assessment. If the patient reports pain, administer the prescribed analgesic in sufficient time to allow for the full effect of the medication.
- Assess for muscle spasms and administer the prescribed muscle relaxant in sufficient time to allow for the full effect of the medication.
- Assess for the presence of disease processes that may contraindicate the use of a cast or interfere with wound healing, including skin diseases, peripheral vascular disease, diabetes mellitus, and open or draining wounds.

NURSING DIAGNOSES

- Risk for Impaired Skin Integrity
- Anxiety
- Acute Pain
- Disturbed Body Image
- Impaired Physical Mobility
- Ineffective Peripheral Tissue Perfusion
- Risk for Injury
- Deficient Knowledge
- Risk for Peripheral Neurovascular Dysfunction

OUTCOME IDENTIFICATION AND PLANNING

Expected outcomes may include:
- The cast is applied without interfering with neurovascular function and healing occurs.
- The patient is free from complications.
- The patient has knowledge of the treatment regimen.
- The patient experiences increased comfort.

IMPLEMENTATION

ACTION	RATIONALE
1. Review the medical record and medical orders to determine the need for the cast.	Reviewing the medical record and order validates the correct patient and correct procedure.
2. Perform hand hygiene. Put on gloves and/or other PPE, as indicated.	Hand hygiene and PPE prevent the spread of microorganisms. PPE is required based on transmission precautions.
3. Identify the patient. Explain the procedure to the patient and verify the area to be casted.	Patient identification validates the correct patient and correct procedure. Discussion and explanation help allay anxiety and prepare the patient for what to expect.
4. Perform a pain assessment and assess for muscle spasm. Administer prescribed medications in sufficient time to allow for the full effect of the analgesic and/or muscle relaxant.	Assessment of pain and analgesic administration ensure patient comfort and enhance cooperation.
5. Close curtains around bed and close the door to the room, if possible. Place the bed at an appropriate and comfortable working height, if necessary.	Closing the door or curtains provides privacy. Proper bed height helps reduce back strain while you are performing the procedure.
6. Position the patient, as needed, depending on the type of cast being applied and the location of the injury. Support the extremity or body part to be casted.	Proper positioning minimizes movement, maintains alignment, and increases patient comfort.
7. Drape the patient with the waterproof pads.	Draping provides warmth and privacy and helps protect other body parts from contact with casting materials.
8. Cleanse and dry the affected body part.	Skin care before cast application helps prevent skin breakdown.
9. Position and maintain the affected body part in the position indicated by the	Stockinette and other materials protect skin from casting materials and create a smooth, padded

ACTION

RATIONALE

physician as the stockinette, sheet wadding, and padding are applied (FIGURE 1). The stockinette should extend beyond the ends of the cast. As the wadding is applied, check for wrinkles.

edge, protecting the skin from abrasion. Padding protects the skin, tissues, and nerves from the pressure of the cast.

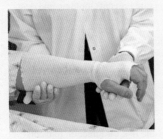

FIGURE 1 Stockinette in place.

10. Continue to position and maintain the affected body part in the position indicated by the physician or advanced practice professional as the casting material is applied. Assist with finishing by folding the stockinette or other padding down over the outer edge of the cast.

Smooth edges lessen the risk for skin irritation and abrasion.

11. **Support the cast during hardening.** Handle hardening plaster casts with the palms of hands, not fingers (FIGURE 2).

Proper handling avoids denting of the cast and development of pressure areas.

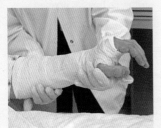

FIGURE 2 Using palms to move the casted limb.

ACTION	RATIONALE
Support the cast on a firm, smooth surface. Do not rest it on a hard surface or sharp edges. Avoid placing pressure on the cast.	
12. **Elevate the injured limb above heart level with pillow or bath blankets, as ordered, making sure pressure is evenly distributed under the cast.**	Elevation promotes venous return. Evenly distributed pressure prevents molding and denting of the cast and development of pressure areas.
13. Place the bed in the lowest position, with the side rails up. Make sure the call bell and other necessary items are within easy reach.	Having the bed at proper height and leaving the call bell and other items within reach ensure patient safety.
14. Remove gloves and any other PPE, if used. Perform hand hygiene.	Removing PPE properly reduces the risk for infection transmission and contamination of other items. Hand hygiene prevents the spread of microorganisms.
15. Instruct the patient to report pain, odor, drainage, changes in sensation, abnormal sensation, or the inability to move the fingers or toes of the affected extremity.	Pressure within a cast may increase with edema and lead to compartment syndrome. Patient complaints allow for early detection of and prompt intervention for complications such as skin irritation or impaired tissue perfusion.
16. Leave the cast uncovered and exposed to the air. Reposition the patient every 2 hours. Depending on facility policy, a fan may be used to dry the cast.	Keeping the cast uncovered promotes drying. Repositioning prevents development of pressure areas. Using a fan helps increase airflow and speeds drying.

EVALUATION

• Neurovascular function is maintained and healing occurs.
• The patient is free from complications.
• The patient has knowledge of the treatment regimen.
• The patient experiences increased comfort.

DOCUMENTATION

- Document the time, date, and site that the cast was applied. Include the skin assessment and care provided before application. Document the patient's response to the cast and the neurovascular status of the extremity.

GENERAL CONSIDERATIONS

- Perform frequent, regular assessment of neurovascular status. Early recognition of diminished circulation and nerve function is essential to prevent loss of function. Be alert for the presence of compartment syndrome.
- Fiberglass casts dry quickly, usually within 5 to 15 minutes.
- If a fiberglass cast was applied, remove any fiberglass resin residue on the skin with alcohol or acetone.
- Synthetic casts are lightweight, easy to clean, and somewhat water resistant. If a Gore-Tex liner is used when the cast is applied, the cast may be immersed in water without affecting the cast integrity.

Skin · 27 **Caring for a Cast**

A cast is a rigid external immobilizing device that encases a body part. Casts, made of plaster or synthetic materials, such as fiberglass, are used to immobilize a body part in a specific position and to apply uniform pressure on the encased soft tissue. They may be used to treat injuries, correct a deformity, stabilize weakened joints, or to promote healing after surgery. Casts generally allow the patient mobility while restricting movement of the affected body part. Nursing responsibilities after the cast is in place include maintaining the cast, preventing complications, and providing patient teaching related to cast care.

EQUIPMENT

- Washcloth
- Towel
- Skin cleanser
- Basin of warm water
- Waterproof pads
- Tape
- Pillows
- Nonsterile gloves and/or other PPE, as indicated

ASSESSMENT GUIDELINES

- Review the patient's medical record and nursing plan of care to determine the need for cast care and care of the affected area.
- Perform a pain assessment. If the patient reports pain, administer the prescribed analgesic in sufficient time to allow for the full effect of the medication.
- Assess the neurovascular status of the affected extremity, including distal pulses, color, temperature, presence of edema, capillary refill

to fingers or toes, and sensation and motion. Assess the skin distal to
the cast. Note any indications of infection, including any foul odor
from the cast, pain, fever, edema, and extreme warmth over an area
of the cast. Assess for complications of immobility, including alterations in skin integrity, reduced joint movement, decreased peristalsis,
constipation, alterations in respiratory function, and signs of
thrombophlebitis.
- Inspect the condition of the cast. Be alert for cracks, dents, or the
  presence of drainage from the cast.
- Assess the patient's knowledge of cast care.

NURSING DIAGNOSES
- Disturbed Body Image
- Acute Pain
- Risk for Injury
- Risk for Falls
- Risk for Disuse Syndrome
- Impaired Tissue Perfusion
- Deficient Knowledge
- Risk for Impaired Skin Integrity
- Impaired Physical Mobility
- Risk for Peripheral Neurovascular Dysfunction
- Self-Care Deficit (bathing, feeding, dressing, or toileting)

OUTCOME IDENTIFICATION AND PLANNING
Expected outcomes may include:
- The cast remains intact.
- The patient does not experience neurovascular compromise.
- The patient is free from infection.
- The patient experiences only mild pain and slight edema or
  soreness.
- The patient experiences only slight limitations of range of joint
  motion.
- The skin around the cast edges remains intact.
- The patient participates in activities of daily living.
- The patient demonstrates appropriate cast-care techniques.

IMPLEMENTATION

ACTION	RATIONALE
1. Review the medical record and the nursing plan of care to determine the need for cast care and care for the affected body part.	Reviewing the medical record and plan of care validates the correct patient and correct procedure.

ACTION	RATIONALE

2. Perform hand hygiene. Put on PPE, as indicated.

Hand hygiene and PPE prevent the spread of microorganisms. PPE is required based on transmission precautions.

3. Identify the patient. Explain the procedure to the patient.

Patient identification validates the correct patient and correct procedure. Discussion and explanation help allay anxiety and prepare the patient for what to expect.

4. Close curtains around bed and close the door to the room, if possible. Place the bed at an appropriate and comfortable working height, if necessary.

Closing the door or curtains provides privacy. Proper bed height helps reduce back strain while you are performing the procedure.

5. If a plaster cast was applied, handle the casted extremity or body area with the palms of your hands for the first 24 to 36 hours, until the cast is fully dry.

Proper handling of a plaster cast prevents dents in the cast, which may create pressure areas on the inside of the cast.

6. If the cast is on an extremity, elevate the affected area on pillows covered with waterproof pads. **Maintain the normal curvatures and angles of the cast.**

Elevation helps reduce edema and enhances venous return. Use of a waterproof pad prevents soiling of linen. Maintaining curvatures and angles maintains proper joint alignment, helps prevent flattened areas on the cast as it dries, and prevents pressure areas.

7. Keep cast (plaster) uncovered until fully dry.

Keeping the cast uncovered allows heat and moisture to dissipate and air to circulate to speed drying.

8. Assess the condition of the cast (FIGURE 1). Be alert for cracks, dents, or the presence of drainage from the cast. Perform skin and neurovascular assessment according to facility policy, as often as every 1 to 2 hours. **Check for pain, edema, inability to**

Assessment helps detect abnormal neurovascular function or infection and allows for prompt intervention. Assessing the neurovascular status determines the circulation and oxygenation of tissues. Pressure within a cast may increase with edema and lead to compartment syndrome.

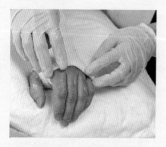

FIGURE 1 Assessing condition of cast.

move body parts distal to
the cast, pallor, pulses, and
abnormal sensations. If the
cast is on an extremity,
compare it with the
uncasted extremity.

9. If breakthrough bleeding or
drainage is noted on the cast,
mark the area on the cast,
according to facility policy
(FIGURE 2). Indicate the date
and time next to the area.
Follow physician orders or
facility policy regarding the
amount of drainage that
needs to be reported to the
physician.

Marking the area provides a
baseline for monitoring the
amount of bleeding or drainage.

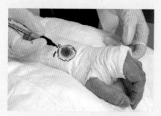

FIGURE 2 Marking any breakthrough bleeding on the cast,
indicating the date and time.

10. Assess for signs of infection.
Monitor the patient's temperature. Assess for a foul odor
from the cast, increased pain,
or extreme warmth over an
area of the cast.

Infection deters healing. Assessment allows for early detection
and prompt intervention.

ACTION	RATIONALE
11. Reposition the patient every 2 hours. Provide back and skin care frequently. Encourage range-of-motion exercises for unaffected joints. Encourage the patient to cough and deep breathe.	Repositioning promotes even drying of the cast and reduces the risk for the development of pressure areas under the cast. Frequent skin and back care prevents patient discomfort and skin breakdown. Range-of-motion exercises maintain joint function of unaffected areas. Coughing and deep breathing reduce the risk for respiratory complications associated with immobility.
12. Instruct the patient to report pain, odor, drainage, changes in sensation, abnormal sensation, or the inability to move the fingers or toes of the affected extremity.	Pressure within a cast may increase with edema and lead to compartment syndrome. Patient understanding of signs and symptoms allows for early detection and prompt intervention.

EVALUATION

- The patient exhibits a cast that is intact without evidence of neurovascular compromise to the affected body part.
- The patient is free from complications.
- The patient verbalizes only mild pain and slight edema or soreness.
- The patient demonstrates intact skin at cast edges.
- The patient is able to perform activities of daily living.
- The patient demonstrates appropriate cast-care techniques.

DOCUMENTATION

- Document all assessments and care provided. Document the patient's response to the cast, repositioning, and any teaching.

GENERAL CONSIDERATIONS

- Explain that itching under the cast is normal, but the patient should not stick objects down or into the cast to scratch.
- Begin patient teaching immediately after the cast is applied and continue until the patient or a significant other can provide care.
- If a cast is applied after surgery or trauma, monitor vital signs (the most accurate way to assess for bleeding).
- Synthetic casts are lightweight, easy to clean, and somewhat water resistant. If a Gore-Tex liner is used when the cast is applied, the cast may be immersed in water without affecting the cast integrity.

Skill · 28   Central Venous Access Device (CVAD): Accessing an Implanted Port

An implanted port consists of a subcutaneous injection port attached to a catheter. The distal catheter tip dwells in the lower one-third of the superior vena cava to the junction of the superior vena cava and the right atrium (INS, 2006), and the proximal end or port is usually implanted in a subcutaneous pocket of the upper chest wall. Implanted ports placed in the antecubital area of the arm are referred to as peripheral access system ports. When not in use, no external parts of the system are visible. When venous access is desired, the location of the injection port must be palpated. A special angled, noncoring needle is inserted through the skin and septum and into the port reservoir to access the system. Once accessed, patency is maintained by periodic flushing. The length and gauge of the needle used to access the port should be selected based on the patient's anatomy, amount of subcutaneous tissue at the site, and anticipated infusion requirements. In general, a ¾-inch 20-gauge needle is frequently used. If the patient has a significant amount of subcutaneous tissue, a longer length (1 or 1.5 inches) may be selected. A larger gauge (19-gauge) is preferred for administration of blood products.

EQUIPMENT

- Sterile tape or Steri-Strips
- Sterile semipermeable transparent dressing
- Several 2 × 2 gauzes
- Sterile towel or drape
- 2% chlorhexidine solution
- NSS vial and 10-mL syringe or prefilled 10-mL NSS syringe
- Heparin 100 U/mL in 10-mL syringe
- Noncoring needle (Huber needle) of appropriate length and gauge
- Masks (2)
- Clean gloves
- Sterile gloves
- Additional PPE, as indicated
- Skin protectant wipe
- Alcohol wipes
- Positive pressure end cap
- IV securement/stabilization device, as appropriate
- Bath blanket

ASSESSMENT GUIDELINES

- Inspect the skin over port, looking for any swelling, redness, or drainage. Also assess the site over the port for any pain or tenderness.
- Review the patient's history for the length of time the port has been in place. If the port has been placed recently, assess the surgical incision. Note presence of steri-strips, approximation, ecchymosis, redness, edema, and/or drainage.

NURSING DIAGNOSES

- Risk for Infection
- Acute Pain

• Deficient Knowledge
• Risk for Injury

OUTCOME IDENTIFICATION AND PLANNING

Expected outcomes may include:
• Port is accessed with minimal to no discomfort to the patient.
• Patient experiences no trauma to the site or infection.
• Patient verbalized an understanding of care associated with the port.

IMPLEMENTATION

ACTION	RATIONALE
1. Verify medical order and/or facility policy and procedure. Often, the procedure for accessing an implanted port and dressing changes will be a standing protocol. Gather equipment and bring to bedside.	Checking the order and/or policy ensures that the proper procedure is initiated. Having equipment available saves time and facilitates the task.
2. Perform hand hygiene and put on PPE, if indicated.	Hand hygiene and PPE prevent the spread of microorganisms. Unclean hands and improper technique are potential sources for infecting a CVAD. PPE is required based on transmission precautions.
3. Identify the patient.	Identifying the patient ensures the right patient receives the intervention and helps prevent errors.
4. Close curtains around bed and close the door to the room, if possible. Explain what you are going to do, and why you are going to do it, to the patient. Ask the patient about allergies to tape and skin antiseptics.	This ensures the patient's privacy. Explanation relieves anxiety and facilitates cooperation. Possible allergies may exist related to tape or antiseptics.
5. Place a waste receptacle or bag at a convenient location for use during the procedure.	Having a waste container handy means the soiled dressing may be discarded easily, without the spread of microorganisms.

ACTION	RATIONALE
6. Adjust bed to comfortable working height, usually elbow height of the caregiver (VISN 8 Patient Safety Center, 2009).	Having the bed at the proper height prevents back and muscle strain.
7. Assist the patient to a comfortable position that provides easy access to the port site. Use the bath blanket to cover any exposed area other than the site.	Patient positioning and use of a bath blanket provide for comfort and warmth.
8. Put a mask on. Ask the patient to turn his or her head away from the access site. Alternately, have the patient put on a mask. Move the overbed table to a convenient location within easy reach. Set up a sterile field on the table. Open dressing supplies and add to sterile field.	Masks help to deter the spread of microorganisms. Masks should be used when catheters have extended dwell times, when the catheter tip is centrally located, or when the patient is immunocompromised (INS, 2006, p. S57). Patient should wear a mask if unable to turn the head away from the site, or based on facility policy. Many facilities have all sterile dressing supplies gathered in a single package.
9. Put on clean gloves. Palpate the location of the port. Assess the site. Note the status of any surgical incisions that may be present. Remove gloves and discard.	Knowledge of location and boundaries of port is necessary to safely access the site.
10. Put on sterile gloves. Connect the end cap to the extension tubing on the noncoring needle. Clean end cap with alcohol wipe. Insert syringe with normal saline into end cap. Fill extension tubing with normal saline and apply clamp. Place on sterile field.	Priming the extension tubing removes air from the tubing and prevents administration of air when connected to the port.
11. Using the chlorhexidine swab, cleanse the port site. Press the applicator against the skin. **Apply chlorhexidine using a back and forth**	Site care and replacement of dressing are accomplished using sterile technique. Organisms on the skin can be introduced into the tissues or the bloodstream

ACTION	RATIONALE
friction scrub for at least 30 seconds. Moving outward from the site, use a circular, scrubbing motion to continue to clean, covering at least a 2- to 3-inch area. **Do not wipe or blot. Allow to dry completely.**	with the needle. Chlorhexidine is recommended for CVAD site care. It is effective against the most common causes of catheter-associated central line infections (CDC, 2002; INS, 2006). Scrubbing motion and length of time (minimum 30 seconds) are necessary for chlorhexidine to be effective (ICT, 2005).
12. Using the nondominant hand, locate the port. Hold the port stable, keeping the skin taut.	The edges of the port must be palpated so that the needle can be inserted into the center of the port. Hold the port with your nondominant hand so that the needle is inserted into the port with the dominant hand.
13. Visualize the center of the port. Pick up the needle. Coil extension tubing into the palm of the hand. Holding needle at a 90-degree angle to the skin, insert **through the skin into the port septum** (FIGURE 1) **until the needle hits the back of the port** (FIGURE 2).	To function properly, the needle must be located in the middle of the port and inserted to the back of the port.

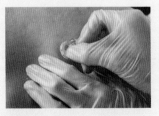

FIGURE 1 Inserting needle through skin into the port. (*Photo by B. Proud.*)

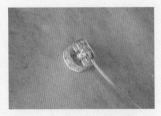

FIGURE 2 Huber (noncoring) needle in place. (*Photo by B. Proud.*)

| 14. Cleanse the end cap on the extension tubing with an antimicrobial swab and insert the syringe with normal | If the needle is not inserted correctly, fluid will leak into tissue, causing the tissue to swell and producing signs of infiltration. |

ACTION	RATIONALE
saline. Open the clamp on the extension tubing and flush with 3 to 5 mL of saline, while observing the site for fluid leak or infiltration. It should flush easily, without resistance.	Flushing without resistance is also a sign that the needle is inserted correctly.
15. Pull back on the syringe plunger to aspirate for blood return. Aspirate only a few milliliters of blood; do not allow blood to enter the syringe. If positive, instill the solution over 1 minute or flush the line according to facility policy. Remove the syringe. Insert heparin syringe and instill the solution over 1 minute or according to facility policy. Remove syringe and clamp the extension tubing. Alternately, if IV fluid infusion is to be started, do not flush with heparin.	Positive blood return indicates the port is patent. Positive blood return confirms patency before administration of medications and solutions (INS, 2006). Not allowing blood to enter the syringe ensures that the needle will be flushed with pure saline. Flushing maintains IV line patency. **Amount of saline and heparin flushes varies depending on specific CVAD and facility policy.** Action of the positive-pressure end cap is maintained with removal of syringe before clamp is engaged. Clamping prevents air from entering the CVAD. Indwelling heparin is recommended to prevent clotting of the CVAD (Hadaway, 2006; INS, 2006).
16. If using a 'Gripper' needle, remove the gripper portion from the needle by squeezing the sides together and lifting off the needle while holding the needle securely to the port with the other hand.	Gripper facilitates needle insertion and needs to be removed before application of dressing.
17. Apply the skin protectant to the site, avoiding direct application to the needle insertion site. Allow to dry.	Skin protectant improves adhesion of dressing and protects skin from damage and irritation when the dressing is removed.
18. Apply tape or Steri-Strips in a starlike pattern over the needle to secure it.	Secures needle to help prevent the needle from accidentally pulling out.
19. Apply transparent site dressing or securement/stabilization	Dressing prevents contamination of the IV catheter and protects

ACTION	RATIONALE
device, centering over insertion site.	the insertion site. Securement/stabilization device prevents accidental dislodgement and/or removal of the needle.
20. Label dressing with date, time of change, and initials. If IV fluid infusion is ordered, attach the administration set to extension tubing and begin administration. Refer to Skill 30.	Labeling helps ensure communication about venous access site dressing change.
21. Remove equipment. Ensure patient's comfort. Lower bed, if not in lowest position.	Promotes patient comfort and safety.
22. Remove additional PPE, if used. Perform hand hygiene.	Removing PPE properly reduces the risk for infection transmission and contamination of other items. Hand hygiene prevents transmission of microorganisms.

EVALUATION

- Port is accessed without difficulty or pain.
- Patient remains free of signs and symptoms of infection or trauma.
- Patient verbalizes an understanding of care related to port.

DOCUMENTATION

- Document the location of the port and the needle size used to access the port. Document the presence of a blood return and the ease of ability to flush the port. Record the patient's reaction to the procedure and if the patient is experiencing any pain or discomfort related to the port. Document the assessment of the site. Record any appropriate patient teaching.

GENERAL CONSIDERATIONS

- Implanted ports require larger flush volumes due to volume required to fill device.
- Groshong devices do not require the use of heparin for flushing.
- Some institutions call for a power flush (rapidly pushing the flush in small amounts).
- Heparin-induced thrombocytopenia (HIT) has been reported with the use of heparin flush solutions. Monitor all patients closely for signs

and symptoms of HIT. If present or suspected, discontinue heparin (INS, 2006).
- Monitor platelet counts for patient receiving heparin flush solution when there is an increased risk of HIT (INS, 2006).
- Patients often are discharged with a CVAD. The patient and family or significant other requires teaching to care for CVAD in the home.
- Implanted ports need to be accessed every 4 to 6 weeks (according to facility policy) to be flushed.

| Skill · 29 | **Central Venous Access Device (CVAD): Changing Site Dressing and Flushing Central Venous Access Devices** |

Central venous access devices (CVADs) are devices where the tip of the catheter terminates in the central venous circulation, usually in the superior vena cava just above the right atrium. Types of CVADs include peripherally inserted central catheters (PICCs), nontunneled percutaneous central venous catheters, tunneled central venous catheters, and implanted ports. They provide access for a variety of IV fluids, medications, blood products, and TPN solutions and allow a means for hemodynamic monitoring and blood sampling. The patient's diagnosis, the type of care that is required, and other factors (e.g., limited venous access, irritating drugs, patient request, or the need for long-term intermittent infusions) determine the type of CVAD used. Dressings are placed at the insertion site to occlude the site and prevent the introduction of microorganisms into the bloodstream. Scrupulous care of the site is required to control contamination. Facility policy generally determines the type of dressing used and the intervals for dressing change, but any dressing that is damp, loosened, or soiled should be changed immediately.

EQUIPMENT
- Sterile tape or Steri-Strips
- Sterile semipermeable transparent dressing
- Several 2 × 2 gauzes
- Sterile towel or drape
- 2% chlorhexidine solution
- NSS vial and 10-mL syringe or prefilled 10-mL NSS syringe; one for each lumen of the CVAD
- Heparin 100 U/mL in 10-mL syringe, one for each lumen of the CVAD
- Masks (2)
- Clean gloves
- Sterile gloves
- Additional PPE, as indicated
- Skin protectant wipe
- Alcohol wipes
- Positive pressure end caps; one for each lumen of the CVAD
- IV securement/stabilization device, as appropriate
- Bath blanket

ASSESSMENT GUIDELINES

- Inspect the insertion site closely for any color change, drainage, swelling, or pain. Palpate for tenderness.
- Assess the catheter condition.
- Ask the patient about any complaints at the insertion site.

NURSING DIAGNOSES

- Risk for Infection
- Deficient Knowledge
- Risk for Injury

OUTCOME IDENTIFICATION AND PLANNING

Expected outcomes may include:
- Patient will remain free of any signs and symptoms of infection.
- CVAD site will be clean and dry, with an intact dressing, and will show no signs or symptoms of IV complications, such as redness, drainage, swelling, or pain.
- CVAD will remain patent.

IMPLEMENTATION

ACTION	RATIONALE
1. Verify the medical order and/or facility policy and procedure. Often the procedure for CVAD flushing and dressing changes will be a standing protocol. Gather equipment and bring to bedside.	Checking the order and/or policy ensures that the proper procedure is initiated. Having equipment available saves time and facilitates the task.
2. Perform hand hygiene and put on PPE, if indicated.	Hand hygiene and PPE prevent the spread of microorganisms. Unclean hands and improper technique are potential sources for infecting a CVAD. PPE is required based on transmission precautions.
3. Identify the patient.	Identifying the patient ensures the right patient receives the intervention and helps prevent errors.
4. Close curtains around bed and close the door to the room, if possible. Explain	This ensures the patient's privacy. Explanation relieves anxiety and facilitates cooperation.

ACTION	RATIONALE
what you are going to do and why you are going to do it to the patient. Ask the patient about allergies to tape and skin antiseptics.	Possible allergies may exist related to tape or antiseptics.
5. Place a waste receptacle or bag at a convenient location for use during the procedure.	Having a waste container handy means the soiled dressing may be discarded easily, without the spread of microorganisms.
6. Adjust the bed to a comfortable working height, usually elbow height of the caregiver (VISN 8 Patient Safety Center, 2009).	Having the bed at the proper height prevents back and muscle strain.
7. Assist the patient to a comfortable position that provides easy access to the CVAD insertion site and dressing. If the patient has a PICC, position the patient with the arm extended from the body below heart level. Use the bath blanket to cover any exposed area other than the site.	Patient positioning and use of a bath blanket provide for comfort and warmth. This position is recommended to reduce the risk of air embolism.
8. Apply a mask. Ask the patient to turn his or her head away from access site. Alternately, have the patient put on a mask. Move the overbed table to a convenient location within easy reach. Set up a sterile field on the table. Open dressing supplies and add to the sterile field. If an IV solution is infusing via CVAD, interrupt and place on hold during dressing change. Apply slide clamp on each lumen of the CVAD.	Masks help to deter the spread of microorganisms. Masks should be used when catheters have extended dwell times, when the catheter tip is centrally located, or when the patient is immunocompromised (INS, 2006). Patient should wear a mask if unable to turn head away from the site, or based on facility policy. Many facilities have all sterile dressing supplies gathered in a single package. Stopping infusion and clamping each lumen prevents air from entering the CVAD.
9. Put on clean gloves. Assess CVAD insertion site (for inflammation, redness, and so on) through old dressing.	If the CVAD is a PICC line, note how the PICC is secured. A PICC line may not be sutured in place; it may be held in place

ACTION	RATIONALE
Note the status of any sutures that may be present. Remove old dressing by lifting it distally and then working proximally, making sure to stabilize the catheter. Discard dressing in trash receptacle. Remove gloves and discard.	only by the dressing. Care should be taken to avoid dislodgment when changing dressings.
10. Put on sterile gloves. Starting at insertion site and continuing in a circle, wipe off any old blood or drainage with a sterile antimicrobial wipe. Using the chlorhexidine swab, cleanse the site. Cleanse directly over the insertion site by pressing the applicator against the skin. **Apply chlorhexidine using a back-and-forth friction scrub for at least 30 seconds.** Moving outward from the site, use scrubbing motion to continue to clean, covering at least a 2- to 3-inch area. **Do not wipe or blot. Allow to dry completely.** Apply the skin protectant to the same area, avoiding direct application to the insertion site and allow to dry.	Site care and replacement of dressing are accomplished using sterile technique. Organisms on the skin can be introduced into the tissues or the bloodstream with the needle. Chlorhexidine is recommended for CVAD site care. It is effective against the most common causes of catheter-associated central line infections (CDC, 2002; INS, 2006). Scrubbing motion and length of time (minimum 30 seconds) is necessary for chlorhexidine to be effective (ICT, 2005). Skin protectant improves adhesion of dressing and protects skin from damage and irritation when the dressing is removed.
11. Stabilize catheter hub by holding it in place with your nondominant hand. Use an alcohol wipe to clean each lumen of the catheter, starting at the insertion site and moving outward.	Organisms on the skin can be introduced into the tissues or the bloodstream with the needle.
12. Apply transparent site dressing or securement/stabilization device, centering it over the insertion site (FIGURE 1). If the patient has PICC in place, measure the length of	Dressing prevents contamination of the IV catheter and protects the insertion site. Securement/stabilization device prevents accidental dislodgment and/or removal of the needle. Measurement of the

ACTION	RATIONALE

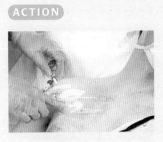

FIGURE 1 Applying site dressing and stabilization device.

the catheter that extends out from the insertion site.

extending catheter can be compared with the documented length at time of insertion to assess if the catheter has migrated inward or moved outward.

13. Working with one lumen at a time, remove end cap. Cleanse the end of the lumen with an alcohol swab and apply new end cap. Repeat for each lumen. Secure catheter lumens and/or tubing that extend outside dressing with tape.
If required, flush each lumen of the CVAD. Amount of saline and heparin flushes varies depending on specific CVAD and facility policy.

The catheter ends should be cleansed and injection caps changed to prevent infection. Weight of tubing and/or tugging on tubing could cause catheter dislodgment.

14. Cleanse end cap with an antimicrobial swab.

Cleaning the cap reduces the risk for contamination.

15. Insert the saline flush syringe into the cap on the extension tubing. Pull back on the syringe to aspirate the catheter for positive blood return. If positive, instill the solution over 1 minute or flush the line according to facility policy. Remove syringe. Insert heparin syringe and instill the volume of solution designated by facility policy over

Positive blood return confirms patency before administration of medications and solutions (INS, 2006). Flushing maintains patency of the IV line. Action of positive pressure end cap is maintained with removal of syringe before the clamp is engaged. Clamping prevents air from entering the CVAD. Indwelling heparin is recommended to prevent clotting of

ACTION	RATIONALE
1 minute or according to facility policy. Remove syringe and reclamp the lumen. Remove gloves.	CVAD (Hadaway, 2006; INS, 2006). Removing gloves properly reduces the risk for infection transmission and contamination of other items.
16. Label dressing with date, time of change, and initials. Resume fluid infusion, if indicated. Check that IV flow is accurate and the system is patent.	Labeling helps ensure communication about venous access site dressing change.
17. Remove equipment. Ensure patient's comfort. Lower bed, if not in lowest position.	Promotes patient comfort and safety.
18. Remove additional PPE, if used. Perform hand hygiene.	Removing PPE properly reduces the risk for infection transmission and contamination of other items. Hand hygiene prevents transmission of microorganisms.

EVALUATION

- CVAD dressing is changed without any complications, including dislodgement of the CVAD.
- Patient exhibits an insertion site that is clean and dry without redness or swelling.
- CVAD dressing is clean, dry, and intact.
- CVAD remains patent.

DOCUMENTATION

- Document the location and appearance of the CVAD site. The site should be free of redness, drainage, or swelling. Record if the patient is experiencing any pain or discomfort related to the CVAD. The CVAD lumens should flush without difficulty. Document and report abnormal findings, such as dislodgement of the CVAD, abnormal insertion assessment findings, or inability to flush the CVAD.

GENERAL CONSIDERATIONS

- Flushing of PICC devices requires the use of syringes no smaller than 10-mL volume to avoid excessive pressure. Syringes smaller than 10 mL may provide pressures great enough to damage the PICC catheter.

- Implanted ports require larger flush volumes due to volume required to fill device.
- Groshong devices do not require the use of heparin for flushing.
- Some institutions call for a power flush (rapidly pushing the flush in small amounts).
- Heparin-induced thrombocytopenia (HIT) has been reported with the use of heparin flush solutions. Monitor all patients closely for signs and symptoms of HIT. If present or suspected, discontinue heparin (INS, 2006).
- Monitor platelet counts for patient receiving heparin flush solution when there is an increased risk of HIT (INS, 2006).

Skill · 30   **Central Venous Access Device (CVAD): Deaccessing an Implanted Port**

When an implanted port will not be used for a period of time, such as when a patient is being discharged, the port can be deaccessed. Deaccessing a port involves removing the needle from the port.

EQUIPMENT

- Clean gloves
- Additional PPE, as indicated
- Syringe filled with 10 mL saline
- Syringe filled with 5 mL heparin (100 U/mL or institution's recommendations)
- Sterile gauze sponge
- Alcohol wipe
- Band-Aid

ASSESSMENT GUIDELINES

- Inspect the insertion site, looking for any swelling, redness, or drainage.
- Assess site over port for any pain or tenderness.
- Review the patient's history for the length of time the port and needle have been in place.

NURSING DIAGNOSES

- Risk for Infection
- Acute Pain
- Deficient Knowledge
- Risk for Injury

OUTCOME IDENTIFICATION AND PLANNING

Expected outcomes may include:
- Needle is removed with minimal to no discomfort to the patient.
- Patient experiences no trauma or infection.
- Patient verbalizes an understanding of port care.

IMPLEMENTATION

ACTION	RATIONALE
1. Verify medical order and/or facility policy and procedure. Often the procedure for accessing an implanted port and dressing changes will be a standing protocol. Gather equipment and bring to bedside.	Checking the order and/or policy ensures that the proper procedure is initiated. Having equipment available saves time and facilitates the task.
2. Perform hand hygiene and put on PPE, if indicated.	Hand hygiene and PPE prevent the spread of microorganisms. Unclean hands and improper technique are potential sources for infecting a CVAD. PPE is required based on transmission precautions.
3. Identify the patient.	Identifying the patient ensures the right patient receives the intervention and helps prevent errors.
4. Close curtains around bed and close the door to the room, if possible. Explain what you are going to do and why you are going to do it to the patient.	This ensures the patient's privacy. Explanation relieves anxiety and facilitates cooperation.
5. Adjust bed to comfortable working height, usually elbow height of the caregiver (VISN 8 Patient Safety Center, 2009).	Having the bed at the proper height prevents back and muscle strain.
6. Assist the patient to a comfortable position that provides easy access to the port site. Use the bath blanket to cover any exposed area other than the site.	Patient positioning and use of a bath blanket provide for comfort and warmth.
7. Put on gloves. Stabilize port needle with your nondominant hand. Gently pull back transparent dressing, beginning with edges and proceeding around the edge of the dressing.	Gloves prevent contact with blood and body fluids. Gently pulling the edges of the dressing is less traumatic to the patient.

ACTION	RATIONALE
Carefully remove all the tape that is securing the needle in place.	
8. Clean the end cap on the extension tubing and insert the saline-filled syringe. Unclamp the extension tubing and flush with a minimum of 10 mL normal saline.	It is important to flush all substances out of the well of the implanted port, because it may be inactive for an extended period. **Amount of saline and heparin flushes varies depending on specific CVAD and facility policy.**
9. Remove the syringe and insert the heparin-filled syringe, flushing with 5 mL heparin (100 U/mL, or per facility policy). Remove syringe and clamp the extension tubing.	**Amount of saline and heparin flushes varies depending on specific CVAD and facility policy.** Action of positive pressure end cap is maintained with removal of the syringe before the clamp is engaged. Clamping prevents air from entering the CVAD. Indwelling heparin is recommended to prevent clotting of CVAD (Hadaway, 2006; INS, 2006).
10. Secure the port on either side with the fingers of your nondominant hand. Grasp the needle/wings with the fingers of your dominant hand. Firmly and smoothly, pull the needle straight up at a 90-degree angle from the skin to remove it from the septum. Engage needle guard.	The port is held in place while the needle is removed.
11. Apply gentle pressure with the gauze to the insertion site. Apply a Band-Aid over the port if any oozing occurs. Otherwise, a dressing is not necessary. Remove gloves.	A small amount of blood may form from the needlestick. Intact skin provides a barrier to infection.
12. Ensure patient's comfort. Lower bed, if not in lowest position. Put on one glove to handle needle. Dispose of needle with extension tubing in sharps container.	Promotes patient comfort and safety. Proper needle disposal prevents accidental injury.

ACTION	RATIONALE
13. Remove gloves and additional PPE, if used. Perform hand hygiene.	Removing PPE properly reduces the risk for infection transmission and contamination of other items. Hand hygiene prevents transmission of microorganisms.

EVALUATION

- Port flushes easily and the needle is removed.
- Port site is clean, dry, without evidence of redness, irritation, or warmth.
- Patient verbalizes an understanding of port care.

DOCUMENTATION

- Document the location of the port and the ease or difficulty of flushing the port. Document removal of the access needle. Record the appearance of the site, including any drainage, swelling, or redness. Record any appropriate patient teaching.

GENERAL CONSIDERATIONS

- Groshong devices do not require heparin.
- Some institutions call for a power flush (rapidly pushing the flush in small amounts).
- Heparin-induced thrombocytopenia (HIT) has been reported with the use of heparin flush solutions. Monitor all patients closely for signs and symptoms of HIT. If present or suspected, discontinue heparin (INS, 2006).
- Monitor platelet counts for patient receiving heparin flush solution when there is an increased risk of HIT (INS, 2006).
- Patients often are discharged with a CVAD. The patient and family or significant other requires teaching to care for CVAD in the home.
- Implanted ports need to be accessed every 4 to 6 weeks (according to agency policy) to be flushed.

| **Skill · 31** | **Central Venous Access Device (CVAD): Removing a Peripherally Inserted Central Catheter (PICC)** |

When PICC is no longer required or when the insertion site shows signs of local complications, it will be discontinued. Nurses or specialized IV team nurses may be responsible for removing a PICC line. Specific protocols must be followed to prevent breakage or fracture of the catheter.

EQUIPMENT
- Clean gloves
- Additional PPE, as indicated
- Sterile gauze sponges
- Tape
- Disposable measuring tape

ASSESSMENT GUIDELINES
- Inspect the insertion site, looking for any swelling, redness, or drainage.
- Check pertinent laboratory values, particularly coagulation times and platelet counts. Patients with alterations in coagulation will require that pressure is applied for a longer period of time after catheter removal.
- Measure the length of the PICC after removal.

NURSING DIAGNOSES
- Risk for Infection
- Deficient Knowledge
- Risk for Injury

OUTCOME IDENTIFICATION AND PLANNING
Expected outcomes may include:
- PICC is removed with minimal to no discomfort to the patient.
- Patient experiences no trauma or infection.

IMPLEMENTATION

ACTION	RATIONALE
1. Verify medical order for PICC removal and facility policy and procedure. Gather equipment and bring to bedside.	Checking the order and/or policy ensures that the proper procedure is initiated. Having equipment available saves time and facilitates the task.

ACTION	**RATIONALE**

2. Perform hand hygiene and put on PPE, if indicated.

Hand hygiene and PPE prevent the spread of microorganisms. Unclean hands and improper technique are potential sources for infecting a CVAD. PPE is required based on transmission precautions.

3. Identify the patient.

Identifying the patient ensures the right patient receives the intervention and helps prevent errors.

4. Close curtains around bed and close the door to the room, if possible. Explain what you are going to do and why you are going to do it to the patient.

This ensures the patient's privacy. Explanation relieves anxiety and facilitates cooperation.

5. Adjust bed to comfortable working height, usually elbow height of the caregiver (VISN 8 Patient Safety Center, 2009).

Having the bed at the proper height prevents back and muscle strain.

6. Assist the patient to a supine position with the arm straight and the catheter insertion site below heart level. Use the bath blanket to cover any exposed area other than the site.

This position is recommended to reduce the risk of air embolism. Use of a bath blanket provides for comfort and warmth.

7. Put on gloves. Stabilize catheter hub with your nondominant hand. Gently pull back the transparent dressing, beginning with edges and proceeding around the edge of the dressing. Carefully remove all the tape that is securing the catheter in place.

Gloves prevent contact with blood and body fluids. Gently pulling the edges of the dressing is less traumatic to the patient.

8. Using your dominant hand, remove the catheter slowly. Grasp the catheter close to

Gentle pressure reduces risk of breakage. Catheter should come out easily.

ACTION	RATIONALE
the insertion site and slowly ease the catheter out, keeping it parallel to the skin. Continue removing in small increments, using a smooth and gentle motion (*Best Practices*, 2007).	
9. After removal, apply pressure to the site with a sterile gauze until hemostasis is achieved (minimum 1 minute). Then apply a small sterile dressing to the site.	Adequate pressure prevents hematoma formation.
10. Measure the catheter and compare it with the length listed in the chart when it was inserted. Inspect the catheter for patency. Dispose of the PICC according to facility policy.	Measurement and inspection ensures the entire catheter was removed. Proper disposal reduces transmission of microorganisms and prevents contact with blood and body fluids.
11. Remove gloves. Ensure patient's comfort. Lower bed, if not in lowest position.	Promotes patient comfort and safety.
12. Remove additional PPE, if used. Perform hand hygiene.	Removing PPE properly reduces the risk for infection transmission and contamination of other items. Hand hygiene prevents transmission of microorganisms.

EVALUATION
• PICC is removed with minimal to no discomfort to the patient.
• Patient experiences no trauma or infection.

DOCUMENTATION
• Document the location of the PICC and its removal. Record the catheter length and patency. Record the appearance of the site, including any drainage, swelling, or redness. Record any appropriate patient teaching.

Patients suspected of having injuries to the cervical spine must be immobilized with a cervical collar to prevent further damage to the spinal cord. A cervical collar maintains the neck in a straight line, with the chin slightly elevated and tucked inward. Care must be taken when applying the collar not to hyperflex or hyperextend the patient's neck.

EQUIPMENT

- Nonsterile gloves
- Additional PPE, as indicated
- Tape measure
- Cervical collar of appropriate size
- Washcloth
- Soap and water or skin cleanser
- Towel

ASSESSMENT GUIDELINES

- Assess for a patent airway. If airway is occluded, try repositioning using the jaw thrust–chin lift method, which helps open the airway without moving the patient's neck.
- Inspect and palpate the cervical spine area for tenderness, swelling, deformities, or crepitus. Do not ask the patient to move the neck if a cervical spinal cord injury is suspected.
- Assess the patient's level of consciousness and ability to follow commands to determine any neurologic dysfunction. If the patient is able to follow commands, instruct him or her not to move the head or neck.
- Have a second person stabilize the cervical spine by holding the patient's head firmly on either side directly above the ears.

NURSING DIAGNOSES

- Risk for Injury
- Risk for Aspiration
- Acute Pain
- Ineffective Breathing Pattern

OUTCOME IDENTIFICATION AND PLANNING

Expected outcomes may include:
- Patient's cervical spine is immobilized, preventing further injury to the spinal cord.
- Patient maintains head and neck without movement.
- Patient experiences minimal to no pain.
- Patient demonstrates an understanding about the need for immobilization.

IMPLEMENTATION

ACTION	RATIONALE
1. Review the medical record and nursing plan of care to determine the need for placement of a cervical collar. Identify any movement limitations.	Reviewing the record and plan of care validates the correct patient and correct procedure. Identification of limitations prevents injury.
2. Gather the necessary supplies and bring to the bedside stand or overbed table.	Preparation promotes efficient time management and organized approach to the task. Bringing everything to the bedside conserves time and energy. Arranging items nearby is convenient, saves time, and avoids unnecessary stretching and twisting of muscles on the part of the nurse.
3. Perform hand hygiene and put on PPE, if indicated.	Hand hygiene and PPE prevent the spread of microorganisms. PPE is required based on transmission precautions.
4. Identify the patient.	Identifying the patient ensures the right patient receives the intervention and helps prevent errors.
5. Close curtains around bed and close the door to the room, if possible. Explain what you are going to do and why you are going to do it to the patient.	This ensures the patient's privacy. Explanation relieves anxiety and facilitates cooperation.
6. Assess the patient for any changes in neurologic status.	Patients with cervical spine injuries are at risk for problems with the neurologic system.
7. Place the bed at an appropriate and comfortable working height, usually elbow height of the caregiver (VISN 8 Patient Safety Center, 2009). Lower the side rails, as necessary.	Having the bed at the proper height and lowering the rails prevents back and muscle strain.
8. Gently clean the face and neck with a mild soap and water. If the patient has	Blood, glass, leaves, and twigs may be present on the patient's neck. The area should be clean

ACTION	RATIONALE

experienced trauma, inspect the area for broken glass or other material that could cut the patient or the nurse. Pat the area dry.

before applying the cervical collar to prevent skin breakdown.

9. Have a second caregiver in position to hold the patient's head firmly on either side above the ears. Measure from the bottom of the chin to the top of the sternum, and measure around the neck. Match these height and circumference measurements to the manufacturer's recommended size chart.

Stabilize the cervical spine by holding the head firmly on either side above the ears. To immobilize the cervical spine and to prevent skin breakdown under the collar, the correct size of collar must be used.

10. Slide the flattened back portion of the collar under the patient's head. **The center of the collar should line up with the center of the patient's neck. Do not allow the patient's head to move when passing the collar under the head.**

Stabilizing the cervical spine is crucial to prevent the head from moving, which could cause further damage to the cervical spine. Placing the collar in the center ensures that the neck is aligned properly.

11. Center the front of the collar over the chin, while ensuring that the chin area fits snugly in the recess. Be sure that the front half of the collar overlaps the back half. Secure Velcro straps on both sides. Check to see that at least one finger can be inserted between collar and patient's neck.

The collar should fit snugly to prevent the patient from moving the neck and causing further damage to the cervical spine. Velcro will help hold the collar securely in place. Collar should not be too tight to cause discomfort.

12. Raise the side rails. Place the bed in lowest position. Make sure the call bell is in reach.

Bed in lowest position and access to call bell contribute to patient safety.

13. Reassess the patient's neurologic status and comfort level.

Reassessment helps to evaluate the effects of movement on the patient.

ACTION	RATIONALE
14. Remove PPE, if used. Perform hand hygiene.	Removing PPE properly reduces the risk for infection transmission and contamination of other items. Hand hygiene prevents transmission of microorganisms.
15. **Check the skin under the cervical collar at least every 4 hours for any signs of skin breakdown. Remove** the top half of the collar daily and cleanse the skin under the collar. **When the collar is removed, have a second person immobilize the cervical spine.**	Skin breakdown may occur under the cervical collar if the skin is not inspected and cleansed.

EVALUATION
- Patient's cervical spine is immobilized without further injury.
- Patient verbalizes minimal to no pain.
- Patient demonstrates an understanding of the rationale for cervical spine immobilization.

DOCUMENTATION
- Document the application of the collar, including size and any skin care necessary before the application; condition of skin under the cervical collar; and patient's pain level, neurologic assessments, and any other assessment findings.

GENERAL CONSIDERATIONS
- Cervical collar-related pressure ulcers may develop on the occiput, chin, ears, mandible, suprascapular area, and over the larynx. The occipital area has very little subcutaneous tissue overlying the bone, making it a particularly vulnerable area (Jacobson, et al., 2008). Proper sizing and skin care are an integral part of managing care for these patients.

Skill · 33	Chest Tube: Providing Care of a Chest Drainage System

Chest tubes may be inserted to drain fluid (pleural effusion), blood (hemothorax), or air (pneumothorax) from the pleural space. A chest tube is a firm, plastic tube with drainage holes in the proximal end that is inserted in the pleural space. Once inserted, the tube is secured with a suture and tape, covered with an airtight dressing, and attached to a drainage system that may or may not be attached to suction. Other components of the system may include a closed water-seal drainage system that prevents air from reentering the chest once it has escaped and a suction control chamber that prevents excess suction pressure from being applied to the pleural cavity. The suction chamber may be a water-filled or a dry chamber. A water-filled suction chamber is regulated by the amount of water in the chamber, whereas dry suction is automatically regulated to changes in the patient's pleural pressure. Many healthcare agencies use a molded plastic, three-compartment disposable chest drainage unit for management of chest tubes. There are also portable drainage systems that use gravity for drainage. The following procedure is based on the use of a traditional water-seal, three-compartment chest drainage system. The Skill Variation following the procedure describes a technique for caring for a chest drainage system using dry seal or suction.

EQUIPMENT

- Bottle of sterile normal saline or water
- Two pairs of padded or rubber-tipped Kelly clamps
- Pair of clean scissors
- Disposable gloves
- Additional PPE, as indicated
- Foam tape or bands
- Prescribed drainage system, if changing is required

ASSESSMENT GUIDELINES

- Assess the patient's vital signs. Significant changes from baseline may indicate complications.
- Assess the patient's respiratory status, including oxygen saturation level. If chest tube is not functioning appropriately, the patient may become tachypneic and hypoxic.
- Assess the patient's lung sounds. The lung sounds over the chest tube site may be diminished due to the presence of fluid, blood, or air.
- Assess the patient for pain. Sudden pressure or increased pain indicates potential complications. In addition, many patients report pain at the chest tube insertion site and request medication for the pain.
- Assess the patient's knowledge of the chest tube to ensure that he or she understands the rationale for the chest tube.

NURSING DIAGNOSES
- Risk for Activity Intolerance
- Deficient Knowledge
- Acute Pain
- Anxiety

OUTCOME IDENTIFICATION AND PLANNING
Expected outcomes may include:
- Patient will not experience any complications related to the chest drainage system or respiratory distress.
- Patient understands need for the chest tube.
- Patient will have adequate pain control at chest tube insertion site.
- Patient's lung sounds will be clear and equal bilaterally.
- Patient will be able to increase activity tolerance gradually.

IMPLEMENTATION

ACTION	RATIONALE
1. Bring necessary equipment to the bedside stand or over-bed table.	Bringing everything to the bedside conserves time and energy. Arranging items nearby is convenient, saves time, and avoids unnecessary stretching and twisting of muscles on the part of the nurse.
2. Perform hand hygiene and put on PPE, if indicated.	Hand hygiene and PPE prevent the spread of microorganisms. PPE is required based on transmission precautions.
3. Identify the patient.	Identifying the patient ensures the right patient receives the intervention and helps prevent errors.
4. Close curtains around bed and close the door to the room, if possible.	This ensures the patient's privacy.
5. Explain what you are going to do and the reason for doing it to the patient.	Explanation relieves anxiety and facilitates cooperation.

ACTION	RATIONALE
6. Assess the patient's level of pain. Administer prescribed medication, as needed.	Regular pain assessments are required to maintain adequate analgesic relief from the discomfort and pain caused by chest drains (Sullivan, 2008).
7. Put on clean gloves.	Gloves prevent contact with contaminants and body fluids.

Assessing the Drainage System

8. Move the patient's gown to expose the chest tube insertion site. Keep the patient covered as much as possible, using a bath blanket to drape the patient, if necessary. **Observe the dressing around the chest tube insertion site and ensure that it is dry, intact, and occlusive.**	Keeping the patient as covered as possible maintains the patient's privacy and limits unnecessary exposure of the patient. If the dressing is not intact and occlusive, air can leak into the space, causing displacement of the lung tissue, and the site could be contaminated. Some patients experience significant drainage or bleeding at the insertion site, and the dressing needs to be replaced to maintain occlusion of the site.
9. Check that all connections are securely taped. Gently palpate around the insertion site, feeling for subcutaneous emphysema, a collection of air or gas under the skin. This may feel crunchy or spongy, or like "popping" under your fingers.	Small amounts of subcutaneous emphysema will be absorbed by the body after the chest tube is removed. If larger amounts or increasing amounts are present, it could indicate improper placement of the tube or an air leak and can cause discomfort to the patient.
10. Check drainage tubing to ensure that there are no dependent loops or kinks. Position the drainage collection device below the tube insertion site.	Dependent loops or kinks in the tubing can prevent the tube from draining appropriately (Sullivan, 2008; Halm, 2007). The drainage collection device must be positioned below the tube insertion site so that drainage can move out of the tubing and into the collection device.
11. If the chest tube is ordered to be suctioned, note the fluid level in the suction chamber and check it with the amount	Some fluid is lost due to evaporation. If suction is set too low, the amount needs to be increased to ensure that sufficient negative

of ordered suction. Look for bubbling in the suction chamber. Temporarily disconnect the suction to check the level of water in the chamber. Add sterile water or saline, if necessary, to maintain correct amount of suction.

12. Observe the water-seal chamber for fluctuations of the water level with the patient's inspiration and expiration (tidaling). If suction is used, temporarily disconnect the suction to observe for fluctuation. **Assess for the presence of bubbling in the water-seal chamber.** Add water, if necessary, to maintain the level at the 2-cm mark, or the mark recommended by the manufacturer.

13. Assess the amount and type of fluid drainage. Measure drainage output at the end of each shift by marking the level on the container or placing a small piece of tape at the drainage level to indicate date and time. The amount should be a running total, because the drainage system is never emptied. If the drainage system fills, it is removed and replaced.

14. Remove gloves. Assist the patient to a comfortable position. Raise the bed rail and place the bed in the lowest position, as necessary.

pressure is placed in the pleural space to drain the pleural space sufficiently. If suction is set too high, the amount needs to be decreased to prevent any damage to the fragile lung tissue. Gentle bubbling in the suction chamber indicates that suction is being applied to assist drainage.

Fluctuations of the water level in the water-seal chamber with inspiration and expiration is an expected and normal finding. Bubbles in the water-seal chamber after the initial insertion of the tube or when air is being removed are a normal finding. Constant bubbles in the water-seal chamber after initial insertion period indicate an air leak in the system. Leaks can occur within the drainage unit at the insertion site.

Measurement allows for accurate intake and output measurement, assessment of therapy effectiveness, and contributes to the decision to remove the tube. The drainage system would lose its negative pressure if it were opened.

Removing PPE properly reduces the risk for infection transmission and contamination of other items. Ensures patient comfort. Proper positioning with raised side rails and proper bed height provides for patient comfort and safety.

ACTION	RATIONALE

15. Remove additional PPE, if used. Perform hand hygiene.

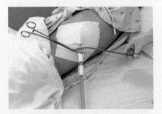

Removing PPE properly reduces the risk for infection transmission and contamination of other items. Hand hygiene prevents the spread of microorganisms.

Changing the Drainage System

16. Obtain two padded Kelly clamps, a new drainage system, and bottle of sterile water. Add water to the water-seal chamber in the new system until it reaches the 2-cm mark or the mark recommended by the manufacturer. Follow manufacturer's directions to add water to the suction system if suction is ordered.

Gathering equipment provides for an organized approach. Appropriate level of water in the water-seal chamber is necessary to prevent air from entering the chest. Appropriate level of water in the suction chamber provides the ordered suction.

17. Put on clean gloves and additional PPE, as indicated.

Gloves prevent contact with contaminants and body fluids.

18. **Apply Kelly clamps 1½ to 2½ inches from insertion site and 1 inch apart, going in opposite directions (FIGURE 1).**

Clamp provides a more complete seal and prevents air from entering the pleural space through the chest tube.

FIGURE 1 Using padded clamps on chest tube.

19. Remove the suction from the current drainage system. Unroll or use scissors to carefully cut away any foam tape on connection of chest tube and drainage system. Using a slight twisting motion, remove the drainage system. **Do not pull on the chest tube.**

Removing suction permits application to a new system. In many institutions, bands or foam tape are placed where the chest tube meets the drainage system to ensure that the chest tube and the drainage system remain connected. Due to the negative pressure, a slight twisting motion may be needed to separate the

ACTION	RATIONALE

tubes. The chest tube is sutured in place; do not tug on the chest tube and dislodge it.

20. **Keeping the end of the chest tube sterile, insert the end of the new drainage system into the chest tube (FIGURE 2). Remove Kelly clamps. Reconnect suction if ordered. Apply plastic bands or foam tape to chest tube/drainage system connection site.**

Chest tube is sterile. Tube must be reconnected to suction to form a negative pressure and allow for re-expansion of lung or drainage of fluid. Prolonged clamping can result in a pneumothorax. Bands or foam tape help prevent the separation of the chest tube from the drainage system.

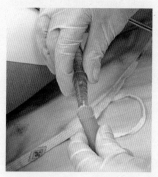

FIGURE 2 Attaching new drainage tube.

21. Assess the patient and the drainage system as outlined (Steps 5–15).

Assess for changes related to the manipulation of the system and placement of new drainage system.

22. Remove additional PPE, if used. Perform hand hygiene.

Removing PPE properly reduces the risk for infection transmission and contamination of other items. Hand hygiene prevents the spread of microorganisms.

EVALUATION

• The patient's chest drainage system is patent and functioning.
• Patient remains free of signs and symptoms of respiratory distress and complications related to the chest drainage system.
• Patient verbalizes adequate pain relief; gradually increases activity tolerance; and demonstrates an understanding of the need for the chest tube.

DOCUMENTATION

- Document the site of the chest tube, amount and type of drainage, amount of suction applied, and any bubbling, tidaling, or subcutaneous emphysema noted. Document the type of dressing in place and the patient's pain level, as well as any measures performed to relieve the patient's pain.

GENERAL CONSIDERATIONS

- Ensure that a bottle of sterile water or normal saline is at the bedside at all times. Never clamp chest tubes except to change the drainage system. If the chest tube becomes accidentally disconnected from the drainage system, place the end of the chest tube into the sterile solution. This prevents more air from entering the pleural space through the chest tube but allows for any air that does enter the pleural space, through respirations, to escape once pressure builds up.
- Keep two rubber-tipped clamps and additional dressing material at the bedside for quick access, if needed.
- If the patient has a small pneumothorax with little or no drainage and suction is not used, the tube may be connected to a Heimlich valve. A Heimlich valve is a water-seal chamber that allows air to exit from, but not enter, the chest tube. Check to assure that the valve is pointing in the correct direction. The blue end should be connected to the chest tube and the clear end is open as the vent. The arrow on the casing points away from the patient.
- Maintain the chest drainage system in an upright position and lower than the level of the tube insertion site. This is necessary for proper function of the system and to aid drainage.
- Encourage the use of an incentive spirometer if ordered and/or frequent deep breathing and coughing by the patient. This helps drain the lungs, promotes lung expansion, and prevents atelectasis.

Skill Variation | Caring for a Chest Drainage System Using Dry Seal or Suction

1. Bring necessary equipment to the bedside stand or overbed table.

2. Perform hand hygiene and put on PPE, if indicated.

3. Identify the patient.

4. Close curtains around bed and close the door to the room, if possible.

5. Explain what you are going to do and the reason for doing it to the patient.

6. Put on clean gloves.

7. Move the patient's gown to expose chest-tube insertion site. Keep the patient covered as much as possible, using a bath blanket to

Caring for a Chest Drainage System Using Dry Seal or Suction *continued*

drape the patient, if necessary. Observe the dressing around the chest tube insertion site and ensure that it is dry, intact, and occlusive.

8. Check that all connections are taped securely. Gently palpate around the insertion site, feeling for subcutaneous emphysema, a collection of air or gas under the skin. This may feel crunchy or spongy, or like 'popping' under your fingers.

9. Check drainage tubing to ensure that there are no dependent loops or kinks. The drainage collection device must be positioned below the tube insertion site.

10. If the chest tube is ordered to be to suctioned, assess the amount of suction set on the chest tube against the amount of suction ordered. Assess for the presence of the suction control indicator, which is a bellows or float device, when adjusting the regulator to the desired level of suction, if prescribed.

11. Assess for fluctuations in the diagnostic indicator with the patient's inspiration and expiration.

12. Check the air-leak indicator for leaks in dry systems with a one-way valve.

13. Assess the amount and type of fluid drainage. Measure drainage output at the end of each shift by marking the level on the container or placing a small piece of tape at the drainage level to indicate date and time. The amount should be a running total, because the drainage system is never emptied. If the drainage system fills, it is removed and replaced.

14. Some portable chest drainage systems require manual emptying of the collection chamber. Follow the manufacturer's recommendations for timing of emptying. Typically, the unit should not be allowed to fill completely as drainage could spill out. Wear gloves, clean the syringe port with an alcohol wipe, use a 60-mL Luer-Lok syringe, screw the syringe into the port, and aspirate to withdraw fluid. Repeat, as necessary, to empty the chamber. Dispose of the fluid according to facility policy.

15. Remove gloves, and additional PPE, if used. Perform hand hygiene.

Skill · 34   Assisting With Removal of a Chest Tube

Chest tubes are removed after the lung is re-expanded and drainage is minimal. Chest tube removal is usually performed by the physician, advance practice nurse, or physician's assistant. The practitioner will determine when the chest tube is ready for removal by evaluating the chest x-ray and assessing the patient and the amount of drainage from the tube.

EQUIPMENT

- Disposable gloves
- Additional PPE, as indicated
- Suture removal kit (tweezers and scissors)
- Sterile Vaseline-impregnated gauze and 4 × 4 gauze dressings
- Occlusive tape, such as foam tape

ASSESSMENT GUIDELINES

- Assess the patient's respiratory status, including respiratory rate and oxygen saturation level. This provides a baseline for comparison after the tube is removed. If the patient begins to have respiratory distress, he or she will usually become tachypneic and hypoxic.
- Assess the patient's lung sounds. The lung sounds over the chest tube site may be diminished due to the tube.
- Assess the patient for pain. Many patients report pain at the chest tube insertion site and request medication for the pain. If the patient has not recently received pain medication, it may be given before the chest tube removal to decrease the pain felt with the procedure.

NURSING DIAGNOSES

- Deficient Knowledge
- Acute Pain
- Impaired Skin Integrity

OUTCOME IDENTIFICATION AND PLANNING

Expected outcomes may include:
- Patient will remain free of respiratory distress.
- Patient's tube insertion site will remain clean and dry without evidence of infection.
- Patient will experience adequate pain control during the chest tube removal.
- Patient's lung sounds will be clear and equal bilaterally.
- Patient will be able to increase activity tolerance gradually.

IMPLEMENTATION

ACTION

RATIONALE

1. Bring necessary equipment to the bedside stand or over-bed table.

   Bringing everything to the bed-side conserves time and energy. Arranging items nearby is convenient, saves time, and avoids unnecessary stretching and twisting of muscles on the part of the nurse.

2. Perform hand hygiene and put on PPE, if indicated.

   Hand hygiene and PPE prevent the spread of microorganisms. PPE is required based on transmission precautions.

3. Identify the patient.

   Identifying the patient ensures the right patient receives the intervention and helps prevent errors.

4. Administer pain medication as prescribed. **Premedicate the patient before removing the chest tube, at a sufficient interval to allow for the medication to take effect, based on the medication prescribed.**

   Most patients report discomfort during chest tube removal.

5. Close curtains around bed and close the door to the room, if possible.

   This ensures the patient's privacy.

6. Explain what you are going to do and the reason for doing it to the patient. Explain any nonpharmacologic pain interventions the patient may use to decrease discomfort during tube removal.

   Explanation relieves anxiety and facilitates cooperation. Nonpharmacologic pain management interventions, such as relaxation exercises, have been shown to help decrease pain during chest tube removal (Friesner, et al., 2006).

7. Put on clean gloves.

   Gloves prevent contact with contaminants and body fluids.

8. Provide reassurance to the patient while the physician removes the dressing and then the tube.

   Removal of the dressing and the tube can increase the patient's anxiety level. Offering reassurance will help the patient feel more secure and help decrease anxiety.

ACTION	RATIONALE
9. After the primary care provider has removed the chest tube and secured the occlusive dressing, assess the patient's lung sounds, respiratory rate, oxygen saturation, and pain level.	In most institutions, physicians remove chest tubes, but some institutions train nurses to remove them. Once the tube is removed, the patient's respiratory status will need to be assessed to ensure that no distress is noted.
10. Anticipate the physician ordering a chest x-ray.	The physician may want a chest x-ray taken to evaluate the status of the lungs after chest tube removal.
11. Dispose of equipment appropriately.	This reduces the risk for transmission of microorganisms and contamination of other items.
12. Remove gloves and additional PPE, if used. Perform hand hygiene.	Removing PPE properly reduces the risk for infection transmission and contamination of other items. Hand hygiene prevents the spread of microorganisms.

EVALUATION

• Patient exhibits no signs and symptoms of respiratory distress after the chest tube is removed.
• Patient verbalizes adequate pain control.
• Patient's lung sounds are clear and equal.
• Patient's activity level gradually increases.

DOCUMENTATION

• Document the patient's respiratory rate, oxygen saturation, lung sounds, total chest tube output, and status of insertion site and dressing.

Skill · 35   Applying Cold Therapy

Cold constricts the peripheral blood vessels, reducing blood flow to the tissues and decreasing the local release of pain-producing substances. Cold reduces the formation of edema and inflammation, reduces muscle spasm, and promotes comfort by slowing the transmission of pain stimuli. The application of cold therapy reduces bleeding and hematoma formation. The application of cold, using ice, is appropriate after direct trauma, for dental pain, for muscle spasms, after muscle sprains, and for the treatment of chronic pain. Ice can be used to apply cold therapy, usually in the form of an ice bag or ice collar, or in a glove. Commercially prepared cold packs are also available. For electronically controlled cooling devices, see the accompanying Skill Variation.

EQUIPMENT

- Ice
- Ice bag, ice collar, glove
- Commercially prepared cold packs
- Small towel or washcloth
- PPE, as indicated
- Disposable waterproof pad
- Gauze wrap or tape
- Bath blanket

ASSESSMENT GUIDELINES

- Assess the situation to determine the appropriateness for the application of cold therapy.
- Assess the patient's physical and mental status and the condition of the body area to be treated with the cold therapy.
- Confirm the medical order, including frequency, type of therapy, body area to be treated, and length of time for the application.
- Assess the equipment to be used to make sure it will function properly.

NURSING DIAGNOSES

- Impaired Skin Integrity
- Ineffective Tissue Perfusion
- Delayed Surgical Recovery
- Chronic Pain

OUTCOME IDENTIFICATION AND PLANNING

Expected outcomes may include:
- Patient experiences increased comfort.
- Patient experiences decreased muscle spasms.
- Patient experiences decreased inflammation.
- Patient does not show signs of bleeding or hematoma at the treatment site.

IMPLEMENTATION

ACTION	RATIONALE
1. Review the medical order or nursing plan of care for the application of cold therapy, including frequency, type of therapy, body area to be	Reviewing the order validates the correct patient and correct procedure.

ACTION	RATIONALE

    treated, and length of time
for the application.

2. Gather the necessary supplies
and bring to the bedside
stand or overbed table.

Preparation promotes efficient
time management and organized
approach to the task. Bringing
everything to the bedside conserves time and energy. Arranging items nearby is convenient,
saves time, and avoids unnecessary stretching and twisting of
muscles on the part of the nurse.

3. Perform hand hygiene and

    put on PPE, if
indicated.

Hand hygiene and PPE prevent
the spread of microorganisms.
PPE is required based on transmission precautions.

4. Identify the patient. Determine if the patient has
had any previous
adverse reaction to
hypothermia therapy.

Identifying the patient ensures
the right patient receives the
intervention and helps prevent
errors. Individual differences
exist in tolerating specific
therapies.

5. Close curtains around bed and
close the door to the room, if
possible. Explain what you are
going to do and why you are
going to do it to the patient.

This ensures the patient's privacy. Explanation relieves anxiety and facilitates cooperation.

6. Assess the condition of the
skin where the ice is to be
applied.

Assessment supplies baseline data
for post-treatment comparison and
identifies any conditions that may
contraindicate the application.

7. Assist the patient to a comfortable position that provides easy access to the area
to be treated. Expose the area
and drape the patient with a
bath blanket, if needed. Put
the waterproof pad under the
wound area, if necessary.

Patient positioning and use of a
bath blanket provide for comfort
and warmth. Waterproof pad protects the patient and the bed
linens.

8. Prepare device:
Fill the bag, collar, or glove
about three-fourths full with
ice. **Remove any excess air**

Ice provides a cold surface. Excess
air interferes with cold conduction.
Fastening the end prevents leaks.

ACTION	RATIONALE
from the device. Securely fasten the end of the bag or collar; tie the glove closed, checking for holes and leakage of water. Prepare commercially prepared ice pack, if appropriate.	
9. **Cover the device with a towel or washcloth.** (If the device has a cloth exterior, this is not necessary.)	The cover protects the skin and absorbs condensation.
10. Position cooling device on top of designated area and lightly secure in place, as needed.	Proper positioning ensures the cold therapy is applied to the specific area of the body.
11. **Remove the ice and assess the site for redness after 30 seconds. Ask the patient about the presence of burning sensations.**	These actions prevent burn injury.
12. Replace the device snugly against the site if no problems are evident. Secure it in place with gauze wrap, ties, or tape.	Wrapping or taping stabilizes the device in the proper location.
13. Reassess the treatment area every 5 minutes or according to facility policy.	Assessment of the patient's skin is necessary for early detection of adverse effects, thereby allowing prompt intervention to avoid complications.
14. **After 20 minutes or the prescribed amount of time, remove the ice and dry the skin.**	Limiting the time of application prevents injury due to overexposure to cold. Prolonged application of cold may result in decreased blood flow, with resulting tissue ischemia. A compensatory vasodilation or rebound phenomenon may occur as a means to provide warmth to the area.
15. Remove PPE, if used. Perform hand hygiene.	Removing PPE properly reduces the risk for infection transmission and contamination of other items. Hand hygiene prevents the spread of microorganisms.

EVALUATION

- Patient reports a relief of pain and increased comfort.
- Patient verbalizes a decrease in muscle spasms.
- Patient exhibits a reduction in inflammation.
- Patient remains free of any injury, including signs of bleeding or hematoma at the treatment site.

DOCUMENTATION

- Document the location of the application, time of placement, and time of removal. Record the assessment of the area where the cold therapy was applied, including the patient's mobility, sensation, color, temperature, and any presence of numbness, tingling, or pain. Document the patient's response, such as any decrease in pain or change in sensation. Include any pertinent patient and family education.

GENERAL CONSIDERATIONS

- The patient may experience a secondary defense reaction, vasodilation, that causes body temperature to rebound, defeating the purpose of the therapy.
- Older adults are more at risk for skin and tissue damage because of their thin skin, loss of cold sensation, decreased subcutaneous tissue, and changes in the body's ability to regulate temperature. Check these patients more frequently during therapy.

Skill Variation — Applying an Electronically Controlled Cooling Device

Electronically controlled cooling devices are used in situations to deliver a constant cooling effect. Postoperative orthopedic patients as well as other patients with acute musculoskeletal injuries may benefit from this therapy. A medical order is required for use of this device. Initial assessment of the extremity is involved, as well as ongoing assessment throughout the period of use. As with the application of any electronic device, ongoing monitoring for proper functioning and temperature regulation is necessary.

1. Gather equipment and verify the medical order.

2. Perform hand hygiene. Put on PPE, as indicated.

3. Identify the patient and explain the procedure to the patient.

4. Assess the involved extremity or body part.

5. Set the correct temperature on the device.

(continued on page 194)

Applying an Electronically Controlled Cooling Device *continued*

6. Wrap the cooling water-flow pad around the involved body part.

7. Wrap Ace bandage or gauze pads around the water-flow pads.

8. Assess to ensure that the cooling pads are functioning properly.

9. Remove PPE, if used. Perform hand hygiene.

10. Recheck frequently to ensure proper functioning of equipment.

11. Unwrap at intervals to assess skin integrity of the body part.

Skill · 36   Irrigating a Colostomy

Irrigations are infrequently used to promote regular evacuation of some colostomies. Various factors, such as the site of the colostomy in the colon (sigmoid colostomy) and the patient's and physician's preferences, determine whether a colostomy is to be irrigated. Ileostomies are not irrigated because the fecal content of the ileum is liquid and cannot be controlled.

When successful, colostomy irrigation can offer a regular, predictable elimination pattern for the patient, allowing for the use of a small covering over the colostomy between irrigations instead of a regular appliance (Karadag, Mentes & Ayaz, 2005).

EQUIPMENT

- Disposable irrigation system and irrigation sleeve
- Waterproof pad
- Bedpan or toilet
- Water-soluble lubricant
- IV pole
- Disposable gloves
- Additional PPE, as indicated
- Lukewarm solution at a temperature of 105°F to 110°F (40°C to 43°C) (as ordered by physician; normally tap water)
- Washcloth, soap, and towels
- Paper towel
- New ostomy appliance, if needed, or stoma cover

ASSESSMENT GUIDELINES

- Ask patient if he or she has been experiencing any abdominal discomfort.
- Ask patient about date of last irrigation and whether there have been any changes in stool pattern or consistency. If the patient irrigates his or her colostomy at home, ask if he or she has any special routines

during irrigation, such as reading the newspaper or listening to music. Also determine how much solution the patient typically uses for irrigation. The normal amount of irrigation fluid varies, but is usually around 750 to 1,000 mL for an adult.

- If this is a first irrigation, the normal irrigation volume is around 250 to 500 mL.
- Assess the ostomy, ensuring that the diversion is a colostomy. Note placement of colostomy on abdomen, color and size of ostomy, color and condition of stoma, and amount and consistency of stool.

NURSING DIAGNOSES

- Deficient Knowledge
- Anxiety
- Constipation
- Ineffective Coping
- Risk for Injury
- Disturbed Body Image

OUTCOME IDENTIFICATION AND PLANNING

Expected outcomes may include:
- Patient expels soft, formed stool.
- Patient remains free of any evidence of trauma to the stoma and intestinal mucosa.
- Patient demonstrates the ability to participate in care.
- Patient voices increased confidence with ostomy care.
- Patient demonstrates positive coping mechanisms.

IMPLEMENTATION

ACTION	RATIONALE
1. Verify the order for the irrigation. Bring necessary equipment to the bedside stand or overbed table.	Verifying the medical order is crucial to ensuring that the proper treatment is administered to the right patient. Bringing everything to the bedside conserves time and energy. Arranging items nearby is convenient, saves time, and avoids unnecessary stretching and twisting of muscles on the part of the nurse.
2. Perform hand hygiene and put on PPE, if indicated.	Hand hygiene and PPE prevent the spread of microorganisms. PPE is required based on transmission precautions.

ACTION	RATIONALE
3. Identify the patient. 	Identifying the patient ensures the right patient receives the intervention and helps prevent errors.
4. Close curtains around bed and close the door to the room, if possible. Explain what you are going to do and why you are going to do it to the patient. Plan where he or she will receive irrigation. Assist the patient onto bedside commode or into nearby bathroom.	This ensures the patient's privacy. Explanation relieves anxiety and facilitates cooperation. Discussion promotes cooperation and helps to minimize anxiety. The patient cannot hold the irrigation solution. A large immediate return of irrigation solution and stool usually occurs.
5. Warm solution in amount ordered, and check temperature with a bath thermometer, if available. If bath thermometer is not available, warm to room temperature or slightly higher, and test on inner wrist. If tap water is used, adjust temperature as it flows from faucet.	If the solution is too cool, patient may experience cramps or nausea. Solution that is too warm or hot can cause irritation and trauma to intestinal mucosa.
6. Add irrigation solution to container. Release clamp and allow fluid to progress through tube before reclamping.	This causes any air to be expelled from the tubing. Although allowing air to enter the intestine is not harmful, it may further distend the intestine.
7. Hang container so that bottom of bag will be at patient's shoulder level when seated.	Gravity forces the solution to enter the intestine. The amount of pressure determines the rate of flow and pressure exerted on the intestinal wall.
8. Put on nonsterile gloves.	Gloves prevent contact with blood, body fluids, and microorganisms.
9. Remove ostomy appliance and attach irrigation sleeve. Place drainage end into toilet bowl or commode.	The irrigation sleeve directs all irrigation fluid and stool into the toilet or bedpan for easy disposal.

ACTION	RATIONALE
10. Lubricate end of cone with water-soluble lubricant.	This facilitates passage of the cone into the stoma opening.
11. Insert the cone into the stoma. Introduce solution slowly over a period of 5 to 6 minutes. Hold cone and tubing (or if patient is able, allow patient to hold) all the time that solution is being instilled. Control rate of flow by closing or opening the clamp.	If the irrigation solution is administered too quickly, the patient may experience nausea and cramps due to rapid distention and increased pressure in the intestine.
12. **Hold cone in place for an additional 10 seconds after the fluid is infused.**	This will allow a small amount of dwell time for the irrigation solution.
13. Remove cone. Patient should remain seated on toilet or bedside commode.	An immediate return of solution and stool will usually occur, followed by a return in spurts for up to 45 more minutes.
14. After most of the solution has returned, allow the patient to clip (close) the bottom of the irrigating sleeve and continue with daily activities.	An immediate return of solution and stool will usually occur, followed by a return in spurts for up to 45 more minutes.
15. After the solution has stopped flowing from the stoma, put on clean gloves. Remove irrigating sleeve and cleanse skin around stoma opening with mild soap and water. Gently pat peristomal skin dry.	Gloves prevent contact with blood and body fluids. Peristomal skin must be clean and free of any liquid or stool before application of new appliance.
16. Attach new appliance to stoma or stoma cover, as needed.	Some patients will not require an appliance, but may use a stoma cover. Protects stoma.
17. Remove gloves. Return the patient to a comfortable position. Make sure the linens under the patient are dry, if appropriate. Ensure that the patient is covered.	Promotes patient comfort. Removing contaminated gloves prevents spread of microorganisms.

ACTION	RATIONALE
18. Raise side rail. Lower bed height and adjust head of bed to a comfortable position, as necessary.	Promotes patient safety.
19. Remove gloves and additional PPE, if used. Perform hand hygiene.	Removing PPE properly reduces the risk for infection transmission and contamination of other items. Hand hygiene prevents the spread of microorganisms.

EVALUATION

- Irrigation solution flows easily into the stoma opening and the patient expels soft formed stool.
- Patient remains free of any evidence of trauma to the stoma and intestinal mucosa.
- Patient participates in irrigation with increasing confidence.
- Patient demonstrates positive coping mechanisms.

DOCUMENTATION

- Document the procedure, including the amount of irrigating solution used; color, amount, and consistency of stool returned. Document the condition of the stoma, degree of patient participation, and patient's reaction to irrigation.

GENERAL CONSIDERATIONS

- In myelosuppressed patients, irrigation is contraindicated. Do not manipulate the stoma of a neutropenic patient (NCI, 2008).

Skill · 37   Promoting Patient Comfort

Patient discomfort and pain can be relieved through various pain management therapies. Interventions may include the administration of analgesics, emotional support, comfort measures, and nonpharmacologic interventions. Nonpharmacologic methods of pain management can diminish the emotional components of pain, strengthen coping abilities, give patients a sense of control, contribute to pain relief, decrease fatigue, and promote sleep (McCaffery & Pasero, 1999; Tracy et al., 2006). The following skill identifies potential interventions related to discomfort and pain. The interventions are listed sequentially for teaching purposes; the order is not sequential and should be adjusted based on patient assessment and nursing judgment. Not every intervention discussed will be appropriate for every patient. Additional interventions for discomfort and pain are discussed in other skills, such as the application of heat or cold therapy, and the administration of medications for pain relief.

EQUIPMENT

- Pain assessment tool and/or scale
- Oral hygiene supplies ,
- Nonsterile gloves, if necessary
- Additional PPE, as indicated

ASSESSMENT GUIDELINES

- Review the patient's medical record and plan of care for information about the patient's status and contraindications to any of the potential interventions.
- Inquire about any allergies.
- Assess the patient's level of discomfort.
- Assess the patient's pain using an appropriate assessment tool. Assess the characteristics of any pain.
- Assess for other symptoms that often occur with the pain, such as headache or restlessness.
- Ask the patient what interventions have and have not been successful in the past to promote comfort and relieve pain.
- Assess the patient's vital signs.
- Check the patient's medication administration record for the time an analgesic was last administered.
- Assess cultural beliefs related to pain.
- Assess the patient's response to a particular intervention to evaluate effectiveness and presence of adverse effect.

NURSING DIAGNOSES

- Acute Pain
- Disturbed Sleep Pattern
- Chronic Pain
- Fatigue
- Anxiety
- Ineffective Coping
- Activity Intolerance
- Deficient Knowledge
- Self-Care Deficit

OUTCOME IDENTIFICATION AND PLANNING

Expected outcomes may include:
- Patient experiences relief from discomfort and/or pain without adverse effect.
- Patient experiences decreased anxiety and improved relaxation.
- Patient is able to participate in activities of daily living.
- Patient verbalizes an understanding of and satisfaction with the pain management plan.

IMPLEMENTATION

ACTION	RATIONALE
1. Perform hand hygiene and put on PPE, if indicated.	Hand hygiene and PPE prevent the spread of microorganisms. PPE is required based on transmission precautions.
2. Identify the patient.	Identifying the patient ensures the right patient receives the intervention and helps prevent errors.
3. Discuss pain with the patient, acknowledging that the patient's pain exists. Explain how pain medications and other pain management therapies work together to provide pain relief. Allow the patient to help choose interventions for pain relief.	Pain discussion and patient involvement strengthen the nurse–patient relationship and promote pain relief (Taylor et al., 2011). Explanation encourages patient understanding and cooperation and reduces apprehension.
4. Assess the patient's pain, using an appropriate assessment tool and measurement scale.	Accurate assessment is necessary to guide treatment/relief interventions and evaluate the effectiveness of pain control measures.
5. Provide pharmacologic interventions, if indicated and ordered.	Analgesics and adjuvant drugs reduce perception of pain and alter responses to discomfort.
6. Adjust the patient's environment to promote comfort.	The environment can improve or detract from the patient's sense of well-being and can be a source of stimulation that aggravates pain and reduces comfort.
a. Adjust and maintain the room temperature per the patient's preference.	A too warm or too cool environment can be a source of stimulation that aggravates pain and reduces comfort.
b. Reduce harsh lighting, but provide adequate lighting per the patient's preference.	Harsh lighting can be a source of stimulation that aggravates pain and reduces comfort.
c. Reduce harsh and unnecessary noise. Avoid carrying out conversations	Noise, including talking, can be a source of stimuli that aggravates pain and reduces comfort.

ACTION	RATIONALE
immediately outside the patient's room.	
d. Close room door and/or curtain whenever possible.	Closing the door or curtain provides privacy and reduces noise and other extraneous stimuli that may aggravate pain and reduce comfort.
e. Provide good ventilation in the patient's room. Reduce unpleasant odors by promptly emptying bedpans, urinals, and emesis basins after use. Remove trash and laundry promptly.	Odors can be a source of stimuli that aggravates pain and reduces comfort.
7. Prevent unnecessary interruptions and coordinate patient activities to group activities together. Allow for and plan rest periods without disturbance.	Frequent interruptions and disturbances for assessment or treatment can be a source of stimuli that aggravate pain and reduce comfort. Fatigue reduces tolerance for pain and can increase the pain experience (Taylor et al., 2011).
8. Assist the patient to change position frequently. Assist the patient to a comfortable position, maintaining good alignment and supporting extremities, as needed. Raise the head of the bed as appropriate.	Positioning in proper alignment with supports ensures that the patient will be able to maintain the desired position and reduces pressure.
9. Provide oral hygiene as often as necessary to keep the mouth and mucous membranes clean and moist, as often as every 1 or 2 hours, if necessary. This is especially important for patients who cannot drink or are not permitted fluids by mouth.	Moisture helps maintain the integrity of mucous membranes. Dry mucous membranes can be a source of stimuli that aggravate pain and reduce comfort.
10. Ensure the availability of appropriate fluids for drinking, unless contraindicated. Make sure the patient's water	Thirst and dry mucous membranes can be sources of stimuli that reduce comfort and aggravate pain.

ACTION	RATIONALE
pitcher is filled and within reach. Make other fluids of the patient's choice available.	
11. Remove physical situations that may cause discomfort.	
a. Change soiled and/or wet dressings; replace soiled and/or wet bed linens.	Moisture can cause discomfort and irritation to skin.
b. Smooth wrinkles in bed linens.	Wrinkled bed linens apply pressure to skin and can cause discomfort and irritation to skin.
c. Ensure patient is not lying or sitting on tubes, tubing, wires, or other equipment.	Tubing and equipment apply pressure to skin and can cause discomfort and irritation to skin.
12. Assist the patient, as necessary, with ambulation, active range-of-motion exercises, and/or passive ROM exercises, as appropriate.	Activity prevents stiffness and loss of mobility, which can reduce comfort and aggravate pain.
13. Assess the patient's spirituality needs related to the pain experience. Ask the patient if he/she would like a spiritual counselor to visit.	Some individuals' spiritual beliefs facilitate positive coping with the effects of illness, including pain.
14. Consider the use of distraction. Distraction requires the patient to focus on something other than the pain.	Conscious attention often appears to be necessary to experience pain. Preoccupation with other things has been observed to distract the patient from pain. Distraction is thought to raise the threshold of pain and/or increase pain tolerance (Taylor et al., 2011).
a. Have the patient recall a pleasant experience or focus attention on an enjoyable experience.	
b. Offer age/developmentally appropriate games, toys, books, audiobooks, access to television and/or videos, or other items of interest to the patient.	

ACTION	RATIONALE

   c. Encourage the patient to hold or stroke a loved person, pet, or toy.

   d. Offer access to music the patient prefers. Turn on the music when pain begins, or before anticipated painful stimuli. The patient can close his or her eyes and concentrate on listening. Raising or lowering the volume as pain increases or decreases can be helpful.

15. Consider the use of guided imagery.

Guided imagery helps the patient gradually become less aware of the discomfort or pain. Positive emotions evoked by the image help reduce the pain experience.

   a. Help the patient to identify a scene or experience that the patient describes as happy, pleasant, or peaceful.

   b. Encourage the patient to begin with several minutes of focused breathing, relaxation, or meditation.

   c. Help the patient concentrate on the peaceful, pleasant image.

   d. If indicated, read a description of the identified scene or experience, using a soothing, soft voice.

   e. Encourage the patient to concentrate on the details of the image, such as its sight, sounds, smells, tastes, and touch.

16. Consider the use of relaxation activities, such as deep breathing.

Relaxation techniques reduce skeletal muscle tension and lessen anxiety, which can reduce comfort and aggravate pain. Relaxation can also be a distraction, providing help in reducing the

ACTION	RATIONALE
	pain experience (Kwekkeboom et al., 2008; Schaffer & Yucha, 2004; Taylor et al., 2011).
a. Have the patient sit or recline comfortably and place hands on stomach. Close the eyes.	
b. Ask the patient to mentally count to maintain a comfortable rate and rhythm. Have the patient inhale slowly and deeply while letting the abdomen expand as much as possible. Have the patient hold his or her breath for a few seconds.	
c. Tell the patient to exhale slowly through mouth, blowing through puckered lips. Have the patient continue to count to maintain a comfortable rate and rhythm, concentrating on the rise and fall of the abdomen.	
d. When the patient's abdomen feels empty, have the patient begin again with a deep inhalation.	
e. Encourage the patient to practice at least twice a day, for 10 minutes, and then use, as needed, to assist with pain management (Schaffer & Yucha, 2004).	
17. Consider the use of relaxation activities, such as progressive muscle relaxation.	Relaxation techniques reduce skeletal muscle tension and lessen anxiety, which can reduce comfort and aggravate pain. Relaxation can also be a distraction, providing help in reducing the pain experience (Kwekkeboom et al., 2008; Schaffer & Yucha, 2004; Taylor et al., 2011).

ACTION	RATIONALE

ACTION

a. Assist the patient to a comfortable position.

b. Direct the patient to focus on a particular muscle group. Start with the muscles of the jaw, then repeat with the neck muscles, shoulder muscles, upper and lower arm, hand, abdomin, buttocks, thigh, lower leg, and foot muscles.

c. Ask the patient to tighten the muscle group and note the sensation that the tightened muscles produced. After 5 to 7 seconds, tell the patient to relax the muscles all at once and concentrate on the sensation of the relaxed state, noting the difference in feeling in the muscles when contracted and relaxed.

d. Have the patient continue to tighten–hold–relax each muscle group until the entire body has been covered.

e. Encourage the patient to practice at least twice a day, for 10 minutes, and then use, as needed, to assist with pain management (Schaffer & Yucha, 2004).

18. Consider the use of cutaneous stimulation, such as the intermittent application of heat or cold, or both.

RATIONALE

Heat helps relieve pain by stimulating specific nerve fibers, closing the gate that allows the transmission of pain stimuli to centers in the brain. Heat accelerates the inflammatory response to promote healing, and reduces muscle tension to promote relaxation and to help to relieve

ACTION

RATIONALE

muscle spasms and joint stiffness. Cold reduces blood flow to tissues and decreases the local release of pain-producing substances, such as histamine, serotonin, and bradykinin, and reduces the formation of edema and inflammation.

Cold reduces muscle spasm, alters tissue sensitivity (producing numbness), and promotes comfort by slowing the transmission of pain stimuli (Taylor et al., 2011).

19. Consider the use of cutaneous stimulation, such as massage. See Skill 8, Giving a Back Massage.

Cutaneous stimulation techniques stimulate the skin's surface, closing the gating mechanism in the spinal cord, decreasing the number of pain impulses that reach the brain for perception.

20. Discuss the potential for use of cutaneous stimulation, such as TENS, with the patient and primary care provider. See Skill 4, Applying and Caring for a Patient Using a TENS Unit.

Cutaneous stimulation techniques stimulate the skin's surface, closing the gating mechanism in the spinal cord, decreasing the number of pain impulses that reach the brain for perception.

21. Remove equipment and return the patient to a position of comfort. Remove gloves, if used. Raise side rail and lower bed.

Equipment removal and repositioning promote patient comfort. Removing gloves properly reduces the risk for infection transmission and contamination of other items. Lowering bed promotes patient safety.

22. Remove additional PPE, if used. Perform hand hygiene.

Removing PPE properly reduces the risk for infection transmission and contamination of other items. Hand hygiene prevents transmission of microorganisms.

23. Evaluate the patient's response to interventions. Reassess level of discomfort or pain using original assessment tools. Reassess and alter plan of care as appropriate.

Evaluation allows for individualization of plan of care and promotes optimal patient comfort.

EVALUATION

• Patient experiences relief from discomfort and/or pain without adverse effect.
• Patient experiences decreased anxiety and improved relaxation.
• Patient is able to participate in activities of daily living.
• Patient verbalizes an understanding of and satisfaction with the pain management plan.

DOCUMENTATION

• Document pain assessment and other significant assessments. Document pain relief therapies used and patient responses. Record alternative treatments to consider, if appropriate.

GENERAL CONSIDERATIONS

• The use of alternate and adjunct therapies is often a 'try and see process.' Many interventions may be tried to achieve the best combination for a particular patient. Individuals respond to pain differently; what works for one person may not help another.

Skill · 38 **Assisting With the Use of a Bedside Commode**

Patients who experience difficulty getting to the bathroom may benefit from the use of a bedside commode. Bedside commodes are portable toilet substitutes that can be used for voiding and defecation. A bedside commode can be placed close to the bed for easy use. Many have armrests attached to the legs that may interfere with ease of transfer. The legs usually have some type of end cap on the bottom to reduce movement, but care must be taken to prevent the commode from moving during transfer, resulting in patient injury or falls.

EQUIPMENT

• Commode with cover (usually attached)
• Toilet tissue
• Nonsterile gloves
• Additional PPE, as indicated

ASSESSMENT GUIDELINES

• Assess the patient's normal elimination habits. Determine why the patient needs to use a commode, such as weakness or unsteady gait.
• Assess the patient's degree of limitation and ability to help with activity.
• Check for the presence of drains, dressings, intravenous fluid infusion sites/equipment, or other devices that could interfere with the

patient's ability to help with the procedure or that could become dislodged.
• Assess the characteristics of the urine and the patient's skin.

NURSING DIAGNOSES
• Impaired Physical Mobility
• Deficient Knowledge
• Risk for Falls
• Functional Urinary Incontinence
• Impaired Urinary Elimination
• Toileting Self-Care Deficit

OUTCOME IDENTIFICATION AND PLANNING
Expected outcomes may include:
• Patient is able to void with assistance.
• Patient maintains continence.
• Patient demonstrates how to use the commode.
• Patient maintains skin integrity.
• Patient remains free from injury.

IMPLEMENTATION

ACTION	RATIONALE
1. Review the patient's chart for any limitations in physical activity.	Physical limitations may require adaptations in performing the skill.
2. Bring the commode and other necessary equipment to the bedside. Obtain assistance for patient transfer from another staff member, if necessary.	Bringing everything to the bedside conserves time and energy. Arranging items nearby is convenient, saves time, and avoids unnecessary stretching and twisting of muscles on the part of the nurse. Assistance from another person may be required to transfer patient safely to the commode.
3. Perform hand hygiene and put on PPE, if indicated.	Hand hygiene and PPE prevent the spread of microorganisms. PPE is required based on transmission precautions.
4. Identify the patient.	Identifying the patient ensures the right patient receives the intervention and helps prevent errors.

ACTION	RATIONALE
5. Close the curtains around the bed and close the door to the room, if possible. Discuss the procedure with patient and assess the patient's ability to assist with the procedure, as well as personal hygiene preferences.	This ensures the patient's privacy. Discussion promotes reassurance and provides knowledge about the procedure. Dialogue encourages patient participation and allows for individualized nursing care.
6. Place the commode close to, and parallel with, the bed. Raise or remove the seat cover.	Allows for easy access.
7. Assist the patient to a standing position and then help the patient pivot to the commode. **While bracing one commode leg with your foot, ask the patient to place his or her hands one at a time on the armrests. Assist the patient to lower himself or herself slowly onto the commode seat.**	Standing and then pivoting ensures safe patient transfer. Bracing the commode leg with a foot prevents the commode from shifting while the patient is sitting down.
8. Cover the patient with a blanket. Place call bell and toilet tissue within easy reach. Leave patient if it is safe to do so.	Covering patient promotes warmth. Falls can be prevented if the patient does not have to reach for items he or she needs. Leaving the patient alone, if possible, promotes self-esteem and shows respect for privacy.

Assisting Patient Off Commode

9. Perform hand hygiene. Put on gloves and additional PPE, as indicated.	Hand hygiene deters the spread of microorganisms. Gloves prevent exposure to blood and body fluids.
10. Assist the patient to a standing position. If patient needs assistance with hygiene, wrap toilet tissue around your hand several times, and wipe patient clean, using one stroke from	Cleaning area from front to back minimizes fecal contamination of the vagina and urinary meatus. Cleaning the patient after he or she has used the commode

ACTION	RATIONALE
the pubic area toward the anal area. Discard tissue in an appropriate receptacle, according to facility policy, and continue with additional tissue until the patient is clean.	prevents offensive odors and irritation to the skin.
11. Do not place toilet tissue in the commode if a specimen is required or if output is being recorded. Replace or lower the seat cover.	Mixing toilet tissue with a specimen makes laboratory examination more difficult and interferes with accurate output measurement. Covering the commode helps to prevent the spread of microorganisms.
12. Remove your gloves. Return the patient to the bed or chair. If the patient returns to the bed, raise side rails, as appropriate. Ensure that the patient is covered and call bell is readily within reach.	Removing contaminated gloves prevents the spread of microorganisms. Returning the patient to the bed or chair promotes patient comfort. Side rails assist with patient movement in the bed. Having the call device readily available promotes patient safety.
13. Offer patient supplies to wash and dry his or her hands, assisting as necessary.	Washing hands after using the commode helps prevent the spread of microorganisms.
14. Put on clean gloves. Empty and clean the commode, measuring urine in graduated container, as necessary.	Gloves prevent exposure to blood and body fluids. Accurate measurement of urine is necessary for accurate intake and output records.
15. Remove gloves and additional PPE, if used. Perform hand hygiene.	Removing PPE properly reduces the risk for infection transmission and contamination of other items. Hand hygiene prevents the spread of microorganisms.

EVALUATION

• Patient successfully uses the bedside commode.
• Patient remains dry.
• Patient does not experience episodes of incontinence.
• Patient demonstrates measures to assist with using the commode.
• Patient does not experience impaired skin integrity or falls.

DOCUMENTATION

• Document the patient's tolerance of the activity, including his or her ability to use the commode. Record the amount of urine voided and/or stool passed on the intake and output record, if appropriate. Document any other assessments, such as unusual urine or stool characteristics or alterations in the patient's skin.

GENERAL CONSIDERATIONS

• Commode can be left within the patient's reach, to be used without assistance, if appropriate and safe to do so, based on the patient's activity limitations and mobility. Adjust room door or curtain to provide privacy for the patient in the event the commode is used.

Skill · 39   **Applying a Warm Compress**

Warm moist compresses are used to help promote circulation, encourage healing, decrease edema, promote consolidation of exudate, and decrease pain and discomfort. Moist heat softens crusted material and is less drying to the skin. Moist heat also penetrates tissues more deeply than dry heat.

The heat of a warm compress dissipates quickly, so the compresses must be changed frequently. If a constant warm temperature is required, a heating device such as an Aquathermia pad (refer to Skill 83) is applied over the compress. However, because moisture conducts heat, a low temperature setting is needed on the heating device. Many facilities have warming devices to heat the dressing package to an appropriate temperature for the compress. These devices help reduce the risk of burning or skin damage.

EQUIPMENT

• Prescribed solution to moisten the compress material, warmed to 105°F to 110°F
• Container for solution
• Gauze dressings or compresses
• Alternately, obtain the appropriate number of commercially packaged, prewarmed dressings from the warming device
• Clean disposable gloves
• Additional PPE, as indicated
• Waterproof pad and bath blanket
• Dry bath towel
• Tape or ties
• Aquathermia or other external heating device, if ordered or required to maintain the temperature of the compress

ASSESSMENT GUIDELINES

- Assess for circulatory compromise in the area where the compress will be applied, including skin color, pulses distal to the site, evidence of edema, and the presence of sensation.
- Assess the situation to determine the appropriateness for the application of heat.
- Confirm the medical order for the compresses, including the solution to be used, frequency, body area to be treated, and length of time for the application.
- Assess the equipment to be used, if necessary, including the condition of cords, plugs, and heating elements. Look for fluid leaks. Once the equipment is turned on, make sure there is a consistent distribution of heat and the temperature is within safe limits.
- Assess the application site frequently during the treatment, because tissue damage can occur.

NURSING DIAGNOSES

- Anxiety
- Disturbed Body Image
- Acute Pain
- Chronic Pain
- Impaired Skin Integrity
- Risk for Impaired Skin Integrity
- Impaired Tissue Integrity
- Deficient Knowledge

OUTCOME IDENTIFICATION AND PLANNING

Expected outcomes may include:
- Patient shows signs, such as decreased inflammation, decreased muscle spasms, or decreased pain, which indicate problems have been relieved.
- Patient experiences improved wound healing.
- Patient remains free from injury.

IMPLEMENTATION

ACTION	RATIONALE
1. Review the medical order for the application of a moist warm compress, including frequency, and length of time for the application.	Reviewing the order and plan of care validates the correct patient and correct procedure.
2. Gather the necessary supplies and bring to the bedside stand or overbed table.	Preparation promotes efficient time management and organized approach to the task. Bringing

ACTION	RATIONALE

everything to the bedside conserves time and energy. Arranging items nearby is convenient, saves time, and avoids unnecessary stretching and twisting of muscles on the part of the nurse.

3. Perform hand hygiene and put on PPE, if indicated.

Hand hygiene and PPE prevent the spread of microorganisms. PPE is required based on transmission precautions.

4. Identify the patient.

Identifying the patient ensures the right patient receives the intervention and helps prevent errors.

5. Assess the patient for possible need for nonpharmacologic pain-reducing interventions or analgesic medication before beginning the procedure. Administer appropriate analgesic, consulting physician's orders, and allow enough time for analgesic to achieve its effectiveness before beginning procedure.

Pain is a subjective experience influenced by past experience. Depending on the site of application, manipulation of the area may cause pain for some patients.

6. Close curtains around bed and close door to room if possible. Explain what you are going to do and why you are going to do it to the patient.

This ensures the patient's privacy. Explanation relieves anxiety and facilitates cooperation.

7. If using an electronic heating device, check that the water in the unit is at the appropriate level. Fill the unit two-thirds full with distilled water, or to the fill mark, if necessary. Check the temperature setting on the unit to ensure it is within the safe range.

Sufficient water in the unit is necessary to ensure proper function of the unit. Tap water leaves mineral deposits in the unit. Checking the temperature setting helps to prevent skin or tissue damage.

ACTION	RATIONALE
8. Assist the patient to a comfortable position that provides easy access to the area. Use a bath blanket to cover any exposed area other than the intended site. Place a waterproof pad under the site.	Patient positioning and use of a bath blanket provide for comfort and warmth. Waterproof pad protects underlying surfaces.
9. Place a waste receptacle at a convenient location for use during the procedure.	Having a waste container handy means that the used materials may be discarded easily, without the spread of microorganisms.
10. Pour the warmed solution into the container and drop the gauze for the compress into the solution. Alternately, if commercially packaged pre-warmed gauze is used, open packaging.	Prepares compress for application.
11. Put on clean gloves. Assess the application site for inflammation, skin color, and ecchymosis.	Gloves protect the nurse from potential contact with microorganisms. Assessment provides information about the area, the healing process and about the presence of infection and allows for documentation of the condition of the area before the compress is applied.
12. Retrieve the compress from the warmed solution, squeezing out any excess moisture (FIGURE 1). Alter-	Excess moisture may contaminate the surrounding area and is uncomfortable for the patient. Molding the compress to the skin

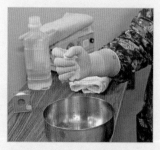

FIGURE 1 Squeezing excess solution out of a dressing.

ACTION

RATIONALE

nately, remove pre-warmed gauze from open package. Apply the compress by gently and carefully molding it to the intended area. Ask patient if the application feels too hot.

promotes retention of warmth around the site.

13. Cover the site with a single layer of gauze (FIGURE 2) and with a clean dry bath towel (FIGURE 3); secure in place if necessary.

Towel provides extra insulation.

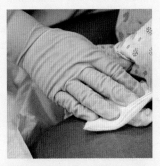

FIGURE 2 Applying single layer of gauze.

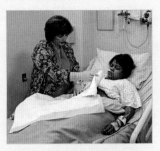

FIGURE 3 Applying clean bath towel.

14. Place the Aquathermia or heating device, if used, over the towel.

Use of heating device maintains the temperature of the compress and extends the therapeutic effect.

15. Remove gloves and discard them appropriately. Perform hand hygiene.

Hand hygiene prevents the spread of microorganisms.

16. Remove additional PPE, if 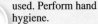 used. Perform hand hygiene.

Removing PPE properly reduces the risk for infection transmission and contamination of other items. Hand hygiene prevents the spread of microorganisms.

ACTION	RATIONALE
17. **Monitor the time the compress is in place to prevent burns and skin/tissue damage. Monitor the condition of the patient's skin and the patient's response at frequent intervals.**	Extended use of heat results in an increased risk for burns from the heat. Impaired circulation may affect the patient's sensitivity to heat.
18. After the prescribed time for the treatment (up to 30 minutes), remove the external heating device (if used) and put on gloves.	Gloves protect the nurse from potential contact with microorganisms.
19. Carefully remove the compress while assessing the skin condition around the site and observing the patient's response to the heat application. Note any changes in the application area.	Assessment provides information about the healing process; the presence of irritation or infection should be documented.
20. Remove gloves. Place the patient in a comfortable position. Lower the bed. Dispose of any other supplies appropriately.	Repositioning promotes patient comfort and safety.
21. Remove additional PPE, if used. Perform hand hygiene.	Removing PPE properly reduces the risk for infection transmission and contamination of other items. Hand hygiene prevents the spread of microorganisms.

EVALUATION

• Patient reports relief of symptoms, such as decreased inflammation, pain, or muscle spasms.
• Patient remains free of signs and symptoms of injury.

DOCUMENTATION

• Document the procedure, the length of time the compress was applied, including use of an Aquathermia pad. Record the temperature of the Aquathermia pad and length of application time. Include a description of the application area noting any edema, redness, or ecchymosis. Document the patient's reaction to the procedure, including pain assessment. Record any patient and family education that was provided.

GENERAL CONSIDERATIONS

• Patients with diabetes, stroke, spinal cord injury, and peripheral neuropathy are at risk for thermal injury, as are patients with very thin or damaged skin.
• Be extremely careful when applying to heat-sensitive areas, such as scar tissue and stomas.

Skill · 40   Applying an External Condom Catheter

When voluntary control of urination is not possible for male patients, an alternative to an indwelling catheter is the external condom catheter. This soft, pliable sheath made of silicone material is applied externally to the penis. Most devices are self-adhesive. The condom catheter is connected to drainage tubing and a collection bag. The collection bag may be a leg bag. The risk for urinary tract infection with a condom catheter is lower than the risk associated with an indwelling urinary catheter. Nursing care of a patient with a condom catheter includes vigilant skin care to prevent excoriation. This includes removing the condom catheter daily, washing the penis with soap and water and drying carefully, and inspecting the skin for irritation. In hot and humid weather, more frequent changing may be required. Always follow the manufacturer's instructions for applying the condom catheter because there are several variations. In all cases, care must be taken to fasten the condom sufficiently secure to prevent leakage, yet not so tight as to constrict the blood vessels in the area. In addition, the tip of the tubing should be kept 1 to 2 inches (2.5 to 5 cm) beyond the tip of the penis to prevent irritation to the sensitive glans area.

Maintaining free urinary drainage is another nursing priority. Institute measures to prevent the tubing from becoming kinked and urine from backing up in the tubing. Urine can lead to excoriation of the glans, so position the tubing that collects the urine from the condom so that it draws urine away from the penis.

Always use a measuring or sizing guide supplied by the manufacturer to ensure the correct size of sheath is applied. Skin barriers, such as 3M or Skin Prep can be applied to the penis to protect penile skin from irritation and changes in integrity.

EQUIPMENT

- Condom sheath in appropriate size
- Skin protectant, such as 3M or Skin Prep
- Bath blanket
- Reusable leg bag with tubing or urinary drainage setup

- Basin of warm water and soap
- Disposable gloves
- Additional PPE, as indicated
- Washcloth and towel
- Scissors

ASSESSMENT GUIDELINES

- Assess the patient's knowledge of the need for the use of a condom catheter.
- Ask the patient about any allergies, especially to latex or tape.
- Assess the size of the patient's penis to ensure that the appropriate-sized condom catheter is used.
- Inspect the skin in the groin and scrotal area, noting any areas of redness, irritation, or breakdown.

NURSING DIAGNOSES

- Impaired Urinary Elimination
- Risk for Impaired Skin Integrity
- Functional Urinary Incontinence

OUTCOME IDENTIFICATION AND PLANNING

Expected outcomes may include:
- Patient's urinary elimination will be maintained, with a urine output of at least 30 mL/hour, and the bladder is not distended.
- Patient's skin remains clean, dry, and intact, without evidence of irritation or breakdown.

IMPLEMENTATION

ACTION	RATIONALE
1. Bring necessary equipment to the bedside.	Bringing everything to the bedside conserves time and energy. Arranging items nearby is convenient, saves time, and avoids unnecessary stretching and twisting of muscles on the part of the nurse.
2. Perform hand hygiene and put on PPE, if indicated.	Hand hygiene and PPE prevent the spread of microorganisms. PPE is required based on transmission precautions.

ACTION	RATIONALE

3. Identify the patient.

Identifying the patient ensures the right patient receives the intervention and helps prevent errors.

4. Close curtains around bed and close the door to the room, if possible. Discuss the procedure with the patient. Ask the patient if he has any allergies, especially to latex.

This ensures the patient's privacy. Discussion promotes reassurance and provides knowledge about the procedure. Dialogue encourages patient participation and allows for individualized nursing care. Some condom catheters are made of latex.

5. Adjust bed to comfortable working height, usually elbow height of the caregiver (VISN 8 Patient Safety Center, 2009). Stand on the patient's right side if you are right-handed, or on patient's left side if you are left-handed.

Having the bed at the proper height prevents back and muscle strain. Positioning on one side allows for ease of use of dominant hand for catheter application.

6. Prepare urinary drainage setup or reusable leg bag for attachment to the condom sheath.

Provides for an organized approach to the task.

7. Position patient on his back with thighs slightly apart. Drape patient so that only the area around the penis is exposed. Slide waterproof pad under the patient.

Positioning allows access to site. Draping prevents unnecessary exposure and promotes warmth. The waterproof pad will protect bed linens from moisture.

8. Put on disposable gloves. Trim any long pubic hair that is in contact with the penis.

Gloves prevent contact with blood and body fluids. Trimming pubic hair prevents pulling of hair by adhesive without the risk of infection associated with shaving.

9. Clean the genital area with washcloth, skin cleanser, and warm water. If patient is uncircumcised, retract

Washing removes urine, secretions, and microorganisms. The penis must be clean and dry to minimize skin irritation. If the

ACTION	RATIONALE
foreskin and clean glans of penis. Replace foreskin. Clean the tip of the penis first, moving the washcloth in a circular motion from the meatus outward. Wash the shaft of the penis using downward strokes toward the pubic area. Rinse and dry. Remove gloves. Perform hand hygiene again.	foreskin is left retracted, it may cause venous congestion in the glans of the penis, leading to edema.
10. Apply skin protectant to the penis and allow to dry.	Skin protectant minimizes the risk of skin irritation from adhesive and moisture and increases adhesive's ability to adhere to skin.
11. Roll condom sheath outward onto itself. Grasp penis firmly with nondominant hand. **Apply condom sheath by rolling it onto penis with dominant hand (FIGURE 1). Leave 1 to 2 inches (2.5 to 5 cm) of space between the tip of the penis and the end of the condom sheath.**	Rolling the condom sheath outward allows for easier application. The space prevents irritation to the tip of the penis and allows free drainage of urine.

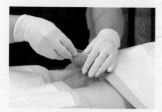

FIGURE 1 Unroll sheath onto penis.

ACTION	RATIONALE
12. **Apply pressure to the sheath at the base of the penis for 10 to 15 seconds.**	Application of pressure ensures good adherence of adhesive with skin.
13. Connect condom sheath to drainage setup. Avoid kinking or twisting drainage tubing.	The collection device keeps the patient dry. Kinked tubing encourages backflow of urine.

ACTION	RATIONALE
14. Remove gloves. Secure drainage tubing to the patient's inner thigh with Velcro leg strap or tape. Leave some slack in tubing for leg movement.	Proper attachment prevents tension on the sheath and potential inadvertent removal.
15. Assist the patient to a comfortable position. Cover the patient with bed linens. Place the bed in the lowest position.	Positioning and covering provide warmth and promote comfort. Bed in the lowest position promotes patient safety.
16. Secure drainage bag below the level of the bladder. Check that drainage tubing is not kinked and that movement of side rails does not interfere with the drainage bag.	This facilitates drainage of urine and prevents the backflow of urine.
17. Remove equipment. Remove gloves and additional PPE, if used. Perform hand hygiene.	Proper disposal of equipment prevents transmission of microorganisms. Removing PPE properly reduces the risk for infection transmission and contamination of other items. Hand hygiene prevents the spread of microorganisms.

EVALUATION

- Condom catheter is applied without adverse effect.
- Patient's urinary elimination is maintained, with a urine output of at least 30 mL/hour.
- Patient's skin remains clean, dry, and intact, without evidence of irritation or breakdown.

DOCUMENTATION

- Document the application of the condom catheter and the condition of the patient's skin. Record urine output on the intake and output record.

Skill · 41   Removing Contact Lenses

If a patient wears contact lenses but cannot remove them, the nurse may be responsible for removing them. This may occur, for example, when the nurse is caring for an unconscious patient. Whenever an unconscious patient is admitted without any family present, always assess the patient to determine whether he or she wears contact lenses. Leaving contact lenses in place for long periods could result in permanent eye damage. Before removing hard or gas-permeable lenses, use gentle pressure to center the lens on the cornea. Once removed, be sure to identify the lenses as being for the right or left eye, because the two lenses are not necessarily identical. If an eye injury is present, do not try to remove lenses because of the danger of causing an additional injury.

EQUIPMENT

- Disposable gloves
- Additional PPE, if indicated
- Container for contact lenses (if unavailable, two small sterile containers marked 'L' and 'R' will suffice)
- Sterile normal saline solution
- Rubber pincer, if available (for removal of soft lenses)
- Suction-cup remover, if available (for removal of hard lenses)

ASSESSMENT GUIDELINES

- Assess both eyes for contact lenses; some people wear them in only one eye.
- Assess eyes for any redness or drainage, which may indicate an infection of the eye or an allergic response.
- Assess for any eye injury. If an injury is present, notify the physician about the presence of the contact lens. Do not try to remove the contact lens in this situation due to the risk for additional eye injury.

NURSING DIAGNOSES

- Risk for Injury

OUTCOME IDENTIFICATION AND PLANNING

Expected outcomes may include:
- The lenses are removed without trauma to the eye and stored safely.

IMPLEMENTATION

ACTION	RATIONALE

1. Perform hand hygiene and put on PPE, if indicated.

Hand hygiene and PPE prevent the spread of microorganisms. PPE is required based on transmission precautions.

2. Identify the patient. Explain the procedure to the patient.

Patient identification validates the correct patient and correct procedure. Discussion and explanation help allay anxiety and prepare the patient for what to expect.

3. Assemble equipment on overbed table within reach.

Organization facilitates performance of the task.

4. Close curtains around bed and close the door to the room, if possible.

This ensures the patient's privacy.

5. Assist patient to a supine position. Elevate bed. Lower side rail closest to you.

Supine position with the bed raised and the side rail down is the least stressful position for the nurse to remove the contact lens.

6. If containers are not already labeled, do so now. Place 5 mL of normal saline in each container.

Many patients have different prescription strengths for each eye. The saline will prevent the contact from drying out.

7. Put on gloves. Remove soft contact lens:

Gloves prevent the spread of microorganisms.

   a. Have the patient look forward. Retract the lower lid with one hand. Using the pad of the index finger of the other hand, move the lens down to the sclera (FIGURE 1).

   b. Using the pads of the thumb and index finger, grasp the lens with a gentle pinching motion and remove (FIGURE 2).

ACTION

RATIONALE

See accompanying Skill Variation display for other techniques for removing both hard and soft lenses.

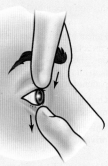

FIGURE 1 Retracting the lower lid with one hand and using the pad of the index finger of the other hand to move the lens down to the sclera.

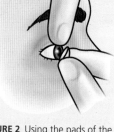

FIGURE 2 Using the pads of the thumb and index finger to grasp the lens with a gentle pinching motion and remove.

8. Place the first lens in its designated cup in the storage case before removing the second lens.

Lenses may be different for each eye. Avoids mixing them up.

9. Repeat actions to remove other contact lens.

10. If patient is awake and has glasses at bedside, offer patient glasses.

Not being able to see clearly creates anxiety.

11. Remove equipment and return patient to a position of comfort. Remove your gloves. Raise side rail and lower bed.

Promotes patient comfort and safety. Removing gloves properly reduces the risk for infection transmission and contamination of other items.

12. Remove additional PPE, if used. Perform hand hygiene.

Removing PPE properly reduces the risk for infection transmission and contamination of other items. Hand hygiene prevents transmission of microorganisms.

EVALUATION

- The patient remains free of injury.
- The patient's eye exhibits no signs and symptoms of trauma, irritation, or redness.

DOCUMENTATION

- Record your assessment, significant observations, and unusual findings, such as drainage or pain. Document any teaching done. Document the removal of the contact lenses, storage, and patient response.

Skill Variation | Removing Different Types of Contact Lenses

1. Perform hand hygiene.

2. Check the patient's identification.

3. Explain what you are going to do.
4. Close curtains around bed and close the door to the room, if possible.
5. Assist patient to supine position. Elevate bed. Lower side rail closest to you.
6. If containers are not already labeled, do so now. Place 5 mL of normal saline in each container.
7. Put on clean gloves.

To Remove Hard Contact Lenses—Patient is Able to Blink:
a. If the lens is not centered over the cornea, apply gentle pressure on the lower eyelid to center the lens.
b. Gently pull the outer corner of the eye toward the ear.
c. Position the other hand below the lens to catch it and ask the patient to blink.

To Remove Hard Contact Lenses—Patient is Unable to Blink:
a. Gently spread the eyelids beyond the top and bottom edges of the lens.
b. Gently press the lower eyelid up against the bottom of the lens.
c. After the lens is tipped slightly, move the eyelids toward one another to cause the lens to slide out between the eyelids.

To Remove Hard Contact Lenses With a Suction Cup—Patient is Unable to Blink:
a. Ensure that contact lens is centered on cornea. Place a drop of sterile saline on the suction cup.
b. Place the suction cup in the center of the contact lens and gently pull the contact lens off the eye.
c. To remove the suction cup from the lens, slide the lens off sideways.

(continued on page 226)

Removing Different Types of Contact Lenses *continued*

To Remove Soft Contact Lenses With a Rubber Pincer:

 a. Locate the contact lens and place the rubber pincers in the center of the lens.

 b. Gently squeeze the pincers and remove the lens from the eye.

8. Place the first lens in its designated cup in the stor-

age case before removing the second lens.

9. Repeat actions to remove the other contact lens.

10. If patient is awake and has glasses at bedside, offer patient glasses.

11. Remove gloves. Perform hand hygiene.

Skill · 42   **Administering a Continuous Closed Bladder Irrigation**

Indwelling catheters sometimes require continuous irrigation, or flushing, with solution to restore or maintain the patency of the drainage system. Sediment or debris, as well as blood clots, might block the catheter, preventing the flow of urine out of the catheter. Irrigations might also be used to instill medications that will act directly on the bladder wall. Irrigating a catheter through a closed system is preferred to opening the catheter because opening the catheter could lead to contamination and infection. If the irrigation is to be continuous, a triple-lumen or three-way catheter is placed to maintain a closed system.

EQUIPMENT

- Sterile irrigating solution (at room temperature or warmed to body temperature)
- Sterile tubing with drip chamber and clamp for connection to irrigating solution
- IV pole
- IV pump (if bladder is being irrigated with a solution containing medication)
- Three-way indwelling catheter in place in patient's bladder
- Indwelling catheter drainage setup (tubing and collection bag)
- Alcohol swabs
- Bath blanket
- Disposable gloves
- Additional PPE, as indicated

ASSESSMENT GUIDELINES

- Verify the order in the medical record for continuous bladder irrigation, including type and amount of irrigant.

- Assess the catheter to ensure that it has an irrigation port (if the patient has an indwelling catheter already in place).
- Assess the characteristics of urine present in the tubing and drainage bag.
- Review the patient's medical record for and ask the patient about any allergies to medications.
- Assess the bladder for fullness, either by palpation or with a handheld bladder ultrasound device.
- Assess for signs of adverse effects, which may include pain, bladder spasm, bladder distension/fullness, or lack of drainage from the catheter.

NURSING DIAGNOSES
- Impaired Urinary Elimination
- Risk for Infection

OUTCOME IDENTIFICATION AND PLANNING
Expected outcomes may include:
- Patient exhibits free-flowing urine through the catheter. Initially, clots or debris may be noted. These should decrease over time, with the patient ultimately exhibiting urine that is free of clots or debris.
- Bladder irrigation continues without adverse effect.
- Drainage is greater than the hourly amount of irrigation solution being placed in the bladder.
- Patient exhibits no signs and symptoms of infection.

IMPLEMENTATION

ACTION	RATIONALE
1. Confirm the order for catheter irrigation in the medical record. Calculate the drip rate via gravity infusion for the prescribed infusion rate.	Verifying the medical order ensures that the correct intervention is administered to the right patient. Solution must be administered via gravity at the appropriate rate as prescribed.
2. Bring necessary equipment to the bedside.	Bringing everything to the bedside conserves time and energy. Arranging items nearby is convenient, saves time, and avoids unnecessary stretching and twisting of muscles on the part of the nurse.
3. Perform hand hygiene and put on PPE, if indicated.	Hand hygiene and PPE prevent the spread of microorganisms. PPE is required based on transmission precautions.

ACTION	RATIONALE
4. Identify the patient.	Identifying the patient ensures the right patient receives the intervention and helps prevent errors.
5. Close curtains around the bed and close the door to the room, if possible. Discuss the procedure with the patient.	This ensures the patient's privacy. Discussion promotes reassurance and provides knowledge about the procedure. Dialogue encourages patient participation and allows for individualized nursing care.
6. Adjust bed to comfortable working height, usually elbow height of the caregiver (VISN 8 Patient Safety Center, 2009).	Having the bed at the proper height prevents back and muscle strain.
7. Empty the catheter drainage bag and measure the amount of urine, noting the amount and characteristics of the urine.	Emptying the drainage bag allows for accurate assessment of drainage after the irrigation solution is instilled. Assessment of urine provides baseline for future comparison.
8. Assist patient to a comfortable position and expose the irrigation port on the catheter setup. Place waterproof pad under catheter and aspiration port.	This provides adequate visualization. Waterproof pad protects the patient and bed from leakage.
9. Prepare sterile irrigation bag for use as directed by manufacturer. Clearly label the solution as 'Bladder Irrigant.' Include the date and time on the label. Hang bag on IV pole 2½ to 3 feet above level of patient's bladder. Secure tubing clamp and insert sterile tubing with drip chamber to container using aseptic technique. Release clamp and remove protective cover on end of tubing without contaminating it. Allow solution	Proper labeling provides accurate information for caregivers. Sterile solution not used within 24 hours of opening should be discarded. Aseptic technique prevents contamination of solution irrigation system. Priming the tubing before attaching irrigation bag clears air from the tubing that might cause bladder distention.

ACTION	RATIONALE
to flush tubing and remove air. Clamp tubing and replace end cover.	
10. Put on gloves. **Cleanse the irrigation port on the catheter with an alcohol swab. Using aseptic technique, attach irrigation tubing to irrigation port of three-way indwelling catheter.**	Aseptic technique prevents the spread of microorganisms into the bladder.
11. Check the drainage tubing to make sure the clamp, if present, is open.	An open clamp prevents accumulation of solution in the bladder.
12. **Release clamp on irrigation tubing and regulate flow at determined drip rate, according to the ordered rate.** If the bladder irrigation is to be done with a medicated solution, use an electronic infusion device to regulate the flow.	This allows for continual gentle irrigation without causing discomfort to the patient. An electronic infusion device regulates the flow of the medication.
13. Remove gloves. Assist the patient to a comfortable position. Cover the patient with bed linens. Place the bed in the lowest position.	Positioning and covering provide warmth and promote comfort and safety.
14. Assess patient's response to the procedure, and quality and amount of drainage.	Assessment is necessary to determine effectiveness of intervention and detection of adverse effects.
15. Remove equipment. Remove gloves and additional PPE, if used. Perform hand hygiene	Proper disposal of equipment prevents transmission of microorganisms. Removing PPE properly reduces the risk for infection transmission and contamination of other items. Hand hygiene prevents the spread of microorganisms.
16. As irrigation fluid container nears empty, clamp the administration tubing. Do not allow drip chamber to empty. Disconnect empty bag and	This eliminates the need to separate tubing from the catheter and clear air from the tubing. Opening the drainage system provides access for microorganisms.

ACTION	RATIONALE
attach a new full irrigation solution bag.	
17. Put on gloves and empty drainage collection bag as each new container is hung and recorded.	Gloves protect against exposure to blood, body fluids, and microorganisms.

EVALUATION

• Patient exhibits the free flow of urine through the catheter, and the irrigant and urine are returned into the drainage bag.
• Effectiveness of therapy is determined by the urine characteristics. On completion of the therapy with a continuous bladder irrigation, the patient should exhibit urine that is clear, without evidence of clots or debris.
• Continuous bladder irrigation is administered without adverse effect.
• Drainage is greater than the hourly amount of irrigation solution being instilled in bladder.
• Patient exhibits no signs and symptoms of infection.

DOCUMENTATION

• Document baseline assessment of patient. Document the amount and type of irrigation solution used and the patient's tolerance of the procedure. Record urine amount emptied from the drainage bag before the procedure and the amount of irrigant used on intake and output record. Record the amount of urine and irrigant emptied from the drainage bag. **Subtract the amount of irrigant instilled from the total volume of drainage to obtain the volume of urine output.**

Skill • 43   Applying a Continuous Passive Motion Device

A continuous passive motion (CPM) device promotes range of motion, circulation, and healing of a joint. It is frequently used after total knee arthroplasty as well as after surgery on other joints, such as shoulders (Lynch et al., 2005). The amount of flexion and extension of the joint and the cycle rate (the number of revolutions per minute) are determined by the physician, but nurses place the patient in and out of the device and monitor the patient's response to the therapy.

EQUIPMENT

- CPM device
- Single-patient-use soft-goods kit
- Tape measure
- Goniometer
- Nonsterile gloves and/or other PPE, if indicated

ASSESSMENT GUIDELINES

- Review the medical record and nursing plan of care for orders for degrees of flexion and extension.
- Assess the neurovascular status of the involved extremity.
- Perform a pain assessment. Administer the prescribed medication in sufficient time to allow for the full effect of the analgesic before starting the device.
- Assess for proper alignment of the joint in the CPM device. Assess the patient's ability to tolerate the prescribed treatment.

NURSING DIAGNOSES

- Impaired Physical Mobility
- Acute Pain
- Activity Intolerance
- Risk for Impaired Skin Integrity
- Anxiety
- Delayed Surgical Recovery
- Risk for Injury
- Fatigue
- Risk for Peripheral Neurovascular Dysfunction

OUTCOME IDENTIFICATION AND PLANNING

Expected outcomes may include:
- The patient experiences increased joint mobility.
- The patient displays improved or maintained muscle strength.
- Muscle atrophy and contractures are prevented.
- Circulation is promoted in the affected extremity.

IMPLEMENTATION

ACTION	RATIONALE
1. Review the medical record and nursing plan of care for the appropriate degrees of flexion and extension, the cycle rate, and the length of time the CPM is to be used.	Reviewing the medical record and plan of care validates the correct patient and correct procedure and reduces the risk for injury.
2. Obtain equipment. Apply the soft goods to the CPM device.	Equipment preparation promotes efficient time management and provides an organized approach to the task. The soft goods help

ACTION	RATIONALE
	to prevent friction to the extremity during motion.
3. Perform hand hygiene. Put on PPE, as indicated.	Hand hygiene and PPE prevent the spread of microorganisms. PPE is required based on transmission precautions.
4. Identify the patient. Explain the procedure to the patient.	Patient identification validates the correct patient and correct procedure. Discussion and explanation help allay anxiety and prepare the patient for what to expect.
5. Close curtains around the bed and close the door to the room, if possible. Place the bed at an appropriate and comfortable working height, usually elbow height of the caregiver (VISN 8 Patient Safety Center, 2009).	Closing the door or curtains provides privacy. Proper bed height helps reduce back strain.
6. Using the tape measure, determine the distance between the gluteal crease and the popliteal space.	The thigh length on the CPM device is adjusted based on this measurement.
7. Measure the leg from the knee to 14 inches beyond the bottom of the foot.	The position of the footplate is adjusted based on this measurement.
8. Position the patient in the middle of the bed. The affected extremity should be in a slightly abducted position.	Proper positioning promotes correct body alignment and prevents pressure on the unaffected extremity.
9. Support the affected extremity and elevate it, placing it in the padded CPM device.	Support and elevation assist in movement of the affected extremity without injury.
10. **Make sure the knee is at the hinged joint of the CPM device.**	Proper positioning in the device prevents injury.
11. **Adjust the footplate to maintain the patient's foot in a neutral position. Assess the patient's position to**	Adjustment helps ensure proper positioning and prevents injury.

ACTION	RATIONALE

make sure the leg is not internally or externally rotated.

12. Apply the restraining straps under the CPM device and around the leg. **Check that two fingers fit between the strap and the leg (FIGURE 1).**

Restraining straps maintain the leg in position. Leaving a space between the strap and leg prevents injury from excessive pressure from the strap.

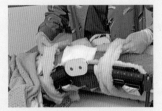

FIGURE 1 Using two fingers to check the fit between the straps and the leg.

13. Explain the use of the STOP/GO button to the patient. Set the controls to the prescribed levels of flexion and extension and cycles per minute. Turn on the power to the CPM.

Explanation decreases anxiety by allowing the patient to participate in care.

14. Set the device to ON and start the therapy by pressing the GO button. Observe the patient and the device during the first cycle. Determine the angle of flexion when the device reaches its greatest height using the goniometer (FIGURE 2). Compare with prescribed degree.

Observation ensures that the device is working properly, thereby ensuring patient safety. Measuring with a goniometer ensures the device is set to the prescribed parameters.

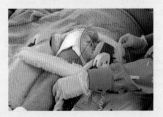

FIGURE 2 Using the goniometer, determining the angle of joint flexion when the device reaches its greatest height.

ACTION	RATIONALE
15. Check the patient's level of comfort and perform skin and neurovascular assessment at least every 8 hours or per facility policy.	Frequent assessments provide for early detection and prompt intervention should problems arise.
16. Place the bed in the lowest position, with the side rails up. Make sure the call bell and other necessary items are within easy reach.	Having the bed at the proper height and having the call bell and other items handy ensure patient safety.
17. Remove PPE, if used. Perform hand hygiene.	Removing PPE properly reduces the risk for infection transmission and contamination of other items. Hand hygiene prevents the spread of microorganisms.

EVALUATION

- The patient demonstrates increased joint mobility.
- The patient exhibits improved muscle strength without evidence of atrophy or contractures.

DOCUMENTATION

- Document the time and date of CPM application, the extension and flexion settings, the device speed, the patient's response to the therapy, and your assessment of the extremity.

Skill · 44 Caring for a Patient Receiving Continuous Wound Perfusion Pain Management

Continuous wound perfusion pain management systems deliver a continuous infusion of local analgesia to surgical wound beds. These systems are used as an adjuvant in the management of postoperative pain in a wide range of surgical procedures, such as cardiothoracic and orthopedic procedures. The system consists of a balloon-type pump filled with local anesthetic and a catheter placed near an incision, nerve close to a surgical site, or in a wound bed (FIGURE 1). The catheter delivers a consistent flow rate and uniform distribution to the surgical site. The local anesthetic directly blocks transmission of pain and inhibits local inflammatory response, which contributes to pain and hyperalgesia (Liu et al.,

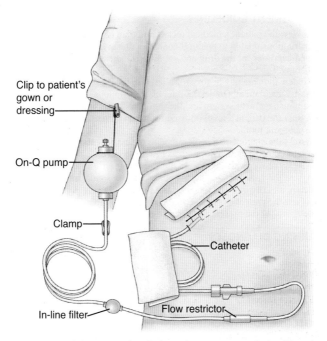

FIGURE 1 Continuous wound perfusion pain management device. Wound perfusion pain management system, which consists of a balloon (pump), filter, and catheter, delivers a specific amount of prescribed local anesthetic at the rate determined by the prescriber. (Redrawn from I-Flow Corporation, Lake Forest, CA, with permission.)

2006). Continuous wound perfusion catheters decrease postoperative pain and opioid use and side effects, and have been associated with decreased postoperative nausea and vomiting (Charous, 2008; Liu et al., 2006; D'Arcy, 2007b). The catheter is placed during surgery and is not sutured into place; it is held in place by the dressing.

EQUIPMENT

- CMAR, MAR, or patient record, based on facility policy
- Gauze and tape, or other dressing, based on facility policy
- Nonsterile gloves
- Additional PPE, as indicated

ASSESSMENT GUIDELINES

- Review the patient's medical record and plan of care for specific instructions related to epidural analgesia therapy, including the medical order for the drug and conditions indicating the need for therapy.
- Review the patient's history for allergy to the prescribed medication.
- Assess the patient's understanding of a continuous wound perfusion pain management system and the rationale for its use.
- Assess the patient's level of discomfort and pain using an appropriate assessment tool.
- Assess the characteristics of any pain. Assess for other symptoms that often occur with the pain, such as headache or restlessness.
- Assess the surgical site. Assess the catheter insertion site dressing.
- Assess the patient's vital signs and respiratory status, including rate, depth, and rhythm, and oxygen saturation level using pulse oximetry.
- Assess the patient's response to the intervention to evaluate effectiveness and for the presence of adverse effects.

NURSING DIAGNOSES

- Acute Pain
- Anxiety
- Deficient Knowledge
- Risk for Injury
- Risk for Infection

OUTCOME IDENTIFICATION AND PLANNING

- Patient reports increased comfort and/or decreased pain, without adverse effects.
- Patient displays decreased anxiety.
- Patient exhibits a dry, intact dressing with catheter in place.
- Patient remains free from infection.
- Patient verbalizes an understanding of the therapy and the reason for its use.

IMPLEMENTATION

ACTION	RATIONALE
1. Check the medication order against the original medical order according to agency policy. Clarify any inconsistencies. Check the patient's chart for allergies.	This comparison helps to identify errors that may have occurred when orders were transcribed. The medical order is the legal record of medication orders for each agency.

ACTION	RATIONALE

2. Know the actions, special nursing considerations, safe dose ranges, purpose of administration, and adverse effects of the medications to be administered. Consider the appropriateness of the medication for this patient.

This knowledge aids the nurse in evaluating the therapeutic effect of the medication in relation to the patient's disorder and can also be used to educate the patient about the medication.

3. Perform hand hygiene and put on PPE, if indicated.

Hand hygiene and PPE prevent the spread of microorganisms. PPE is required based on transmission precautions.

4. Identify the patient.

Identifying the patient ensures the right patient receives the intervention and helps prevent errors.

5. Close curtains around the bed and close the door to the room, if possible.

Closing the door or curtain provides patient privacy.

6. Assess the patient's pain. Administer postoperative analgesic, as ordered.

Continuous wound perfusion pain management is an adjuvant therapy; patients will likely require postoperative pain medication, with reduced frequency.

7. Check the medication label attached to the balloon. Compare with the medical order and MAR, per facility policy. Assess the patient for perioral numbness/tingling, numbness/tingling of fingers or toes, blurred vision, ringing in the ears, metallic taste in the mouth, confusion, seizures, drowsiness, nausea and/or vomiting. Assess the patient's vital signs.

Checking the medication label with the order and MAR ensures correct therapy for the patient. These symptoms may indicate local anesthetic toxicity (D'Arcy, 2007b). Changes in vital signs may indicate adverse effect. Cardiac dysrhythmias and hypertension are possible adverse effects (I-Flow, 2006; Layzell, 2008).

8. Put on gloves. Assess the wound perfusion system. Inspect tubing for kinks; check that the white tubing

Gloves prevent contact with blood and body fluids. Tubing must be unclamped and free of kinks and/or crimping to

ACTION	RATIONALE
clamps are open. If tubing appears crimped, massage area on tubing to facilitate flow. Check filter in tubing, which should be unrestricted and free from tape.	maintain consistent flow of analgesic. Tape over filter interferes with properly functioning system.
9. Check the flow restrictor to ensure it is in contact with the patient's skin. Tape in place, as necessary.	Checking the flow restrictor for adequate contact ensures accurate flow rate.
10. Check the insertion site dressing. Ensure that it is intact. Assess for leakage and dislodgement. Assess for redness, warmth, swelling, pain at site, and drainage.	Catheter is held in place by transparent dressing. Dressing must stay in place to prevent accidental dislodgement or removal. These symptoms may indicate infection.
11. Review the device with the patient. Review the function of the device and the reason for its use. Reinforce the purpose and action of the medication to the patient.	Explanation encourages patient understanding and cooperation and reduces apprehension.

To Remove the Catheter

12. Check to ensure that infusion is complete. Infusion is complete when the delivery time has passed and the balloon is no longer inflated.	Depending on the size and volume of the balloon, the infusion typically lasts 2 to 5 days. Infusion time should be recorded in the operative note or postoperative instructions. The balloon will no longer appear full; the outside bag will be flat, and a hard tube can be felt in the middle of the balloon (I-Flow, 2006).
13. Perform hand hygiene. Identify the patient. Put on gloves. Remove the catheter site dressing. Loosen adhesive skin closure strips at the catheter site.	Hand hygiene and use of gloves reduces the risk of infection transmission. Identifying the patient ensures the right patient receives the intervention and helps prevent errors. Loosening of materials allows the catheter to be free of constraints.

ACTION	RATIONALE
14. Grasp the catheter close to the patient's skin at the insertion site. Gently pull the catheter to remove it. Catheter should be easy to remove and not painful. Do not tug or quickly pull on the catheter during removal. Check the distal end of the catheter for the black marking.	Gentle removal prevents patient discomfort and accidental breakage of catheter. Checking for the black mark at the distal end ensures the entire catheter was removed.
15. Cover puncture site with a dry dressing, according to facility policy.	Covering the wound prevents contamination.
16. Dispose of the balloon, tubing, and catheter according to facility policy.	Proper disposal reduces the risk for infection transmission and contamination of other items.
17. Remove gloves and additional PPE, if used. Perform hand hygiene.	Removing PPE properly reduces the risk for infection transmission and contamination of other items. Hand hygiene prevents transmission of microorganisms.

EVALUATION

- Patient verbalizes pain relief.
- Patient exhibits a dry, intact dressing, and the catheter exit site is free of signs and symptoms of complications, injury, or infection.
- Patient reports a decrease in anxiety and an increased ability to cope with pain.
- Patient verbalizes information related to the functioning of the system and the reasons for its use.

DOCUMENTATION

- Document system patency, the condition of the insertion site and dressing, vital signs and assessment information, analgesics administered, and the patient's response.

GENERAL CONSIDERATIONS

- Be aware that a change in the appearance and size of the pump may not be evident for more than 24 hours after surgery due to the slow flow rate of the device.
- Do not expect to observe a fluid level line in the balloon and fluid moving through the system tubing.

- Over time, expect to see the outside bag on the balloon becoming looser with creases beginning to form in the bag.
- Know that as the medication is delivered, the balloon gradually becomes smaller.
- Do not forcefully remove the catheter.
- Do not reuse or refill the balloon. System is intended for one-time use.
- Protect the balloon and catheter site from water.
- Clip the balloon to the patient's clothing or dressing to prevent the application of tension on the system and site.
- Avoid placing cold therapy in the area of the flow restrictor. Contact with cold therapy will decrease the flow rate.

Skill · 45   Using a Cooling Blanket

A cooling blanket, or hypothermia pad, is a blanket-sized Aquathermia pad that conducts a cooled solution, usually distilled water, through coils in a plastic blanket or pad. Placing a patient on a hypothermia blanket or pad helps to lower body temperature. The nurse monitors the patient's body temperature and can reset the blanket setting accordingly. The blanket also may be preset to maintain a specific body temperature; the device continually monitors the patient's body temperature using a temperature probe (which is inserted rectally or in the esophagus, or placed on the skin) and adjusts the temperature of the circulating liquid accordingly.

EQUIPMENT

- Disposable cooling blanket or pad
- Electronic control panel
- Distilled water to fill the device, if necessary
- Thermometer, if needed, to monitor the patient's temperature
- Sphygmomanometer
- Stethoscope
- Temperature probe, if needed
- Thin blanket or sheet
- Towels
- Clean gloves
- Additional PPE, as indicated

ASSESSMENT GUIDELINES

- Assess the patient's condition, including current body temperature, to determine the need for the cooling blanket. Consider alternative measures to help lower the patient's body temperature before implementing the blanket.
- Verify the medical order for the application of a hypothermia blanket.
- Assess the patient's vital signs, neurologic status, peripheral circulation, and skin integrity.

- Assess the equipment to be used, including the condition of cords, plugs, and cooling elements. Look for fluid leaks. Once the equipment is turned on, make sure there is a consistent distribution of cooling.

NURSING DIAGNOSES
- Hyperthermia
- Risk for Impaired Skin Integrity
- Risk for Injury
- Ineffective Thermoregulation
- Acute Pain

OUTCOME IDENTIFICATION AND PLANNING
Expected outcomes may include:
- Patient maintains the desired body temperature.
- Patient does not experience shivering.
- Patient's vital signs are within normal limits.
- Patient does not experience alterations in skin integrity, neurologic status, peripheral circulation, fluid and electrolyte status, and edema.

IMPLEMENTATION

ACTION	RATIONALE
1. Review the medical order for the application of the hypothermia blanket. Obtain consent for the therapy per facility policy.	Reviewing the order validates the correct patient and correct procedure.
2. Gather the necessary supplies and bring to the bedside stand or overbed table.	Preparation promotes efficient time management and an organized approach to the task. Bringing everything to the bedside conserves time and energy. Arranging items nearby is convenient, saves time, and avoids unnecessary stretching and twisting of muscles on the part of the nurse.
3. Perform hand hygiene and put on PPE, if indicated.	Hand hygiene and PPE prevent the spread of microorganisms. PPE is required based on transmission precautions.

ACTION	RATIONALE
4. Identify the patient. Determine if the patient has had any previous adverse reaction to hypothermia therapy.	Identifying the patient ensures the right patient receives the intervention and helps prevent errors. Individual differences exist in tolerating specific therapies.
5. Close curtains around bed and close the door to the room, if possible. Explain what you are going to do and why you are going to do it to the patient.	This ensures the patient's privacy. Explanation relieves anxiety and facilitates cooperation.
6. Check that the water in the electronic unit is at the appropriate level. Fill the unit two-thirds full with distilled water, or to the fill mark, if necessary. Check the temperature setting on the unit to ensure it is within the safe range.	Sufficient water in the unit is necessary to ensure proper function of the unit. Tap water leaves mineral deposits in the unit. Checking the temperature setting helps to prevent skin or tissue damage.
7. Assess the patient's vital signs, neurologic status, peripheral circulation, and skin integrity.	Assessment supplies baseline data for comparison during therapy and identifies conditions that may contraindicate the application.
8. Adjust bed to comfortable working height, usually elbow height of the caregiver (VISN 8 Patient Safety Center, 2006).	Having the bed at the proper height prevents back and muscle strain.
9. Make sure the patient's gown has cloth ties, not snaps or pins.	Cloth ties minimize the risk of cold injury.
10. Apply lanolin or a mixture of lanolin and cold cream to the patient's skin where it will be in contact with the blanket.	These agents help protect the skin from cold.
11. Turn on the blanket and make sure the cooling light is on. Verify that the temperature limits are set within the desired safety range.	Turning on the blanket prepares it for use. Keeping temperature within the safety range prevents excessive cooling.

ACTION	RATIONALE
12. Cover the hypothermia blanket with a thin sheet or bath blanket.	A sheet or blanket protects the patient's skin from direct contact with the cooling surface, reducing the risk for injury.
13. Position the blanket under the patient so that the top edge of the pad is aligned with the patient's neck.	The blanket's rigid surface may be uncomfortable. The cold may lead to tissue breakdown.
14. Put on gloves. Lubricate the rectal probe and insert it into the patient's rectum, unless contraindicated. Or, tuck the skin probe deep into the patient's axilla and tape it in place. For patients who are comatose or anesthetized, use an esophageal probe. Remove gloves. Attach the probe to the control panel for the blanket.	The probe allows continuous monitoring of the patient's core body temperature. Rectal insertion may be contraindicated in patients with a low white blood cell count or platelet count.
15. Wrap the patient's hands and feet in gauze if ordered, or if the patient desires. For male patients, elevate the scrotum off the cooling blanket with towels.	These actions minimize chilling, promote comfort, and protect sensitive tissues from direct contact with cold.
16. Place the patient in a comfortable position. Lower the bed. Dispose of any other supplies appropriately.	Repositioning promotes patient comfort and safety.
17. Recheck the thermometer and settings on the control panel.	Rechecking verifies that the blanket temperature is maintained at a safe level.
18. Remove any additional PPE, if used. Perform hand hygiene.	Removing PPE properly reduces the risk for infection transmission and contamination of other items. Hand hygiene prevents the spread of microorganisms.
19. **Turn and position the patient regularly (every 30 minutes to 1 hour). Keep linens free from condensation. Reapply**	Turning and repositioning prevent alterations in skin integrity and provide for assessment of potential skin injuries.

ACTION	RATIONALE
cream, as needed. Observe the patient's skin for change in color, changes in lips and nail beds, edema, pain, and sensory impairment.	
20. **Monitor vital signs and perform a neurologic assessment, per facility policy, usually every 15 minutes, until the body temperature is stable.** In addition, monitor the patient's fluid and electrolyte status.	Continuous monitoring provides evaluation of the patient's response to the therapy and permits early identification and intervention if adverse effects occur.
21. Observe for signs of shivering, including verbalized sensations, facial muscle twitching, hyperventilation, or twitching of extremities.	Shivering increases heat production, and is often controlled with medications.
22. Assess the patient's level of comfort.	Hypothermia therapy can cause discomfort. Prompt assessment and action can prevent injuries.
23. Turn off blanket according to facility policy, usually when the patient's body temperature reaches 1 degree above the desired temperature. Continue to monitor the patient's temperature until it stabilizes.	Body temperature can continue to fall after this therapy.

EVALUATION

• Patient maintains the desired body temperature and other vital signs within acceptable parameters.
• Patient remains free from shivering; does not experience alterations in skin integrity, neurologic status, peripheral circulation, fluid and electrolyte status, and edema.

DOCUMENTATION

• Document assessments, such as vital signs, neurologic status, peripheral circulation, and skin integrity status before use of hypothermia blanket. Record verification of medical order and that the procedure was explained to the patient. Document the control settings, time of application and removal, and the route of the temperature monitoring. Include the application of lanolin cream to skin as well as the frequency of position changes. Document the patient's response to the therapy using facility flow sheet, especially noting decrease in temperature and discomfort assessment. Record the possible use of medication to reduce shivering or other discomforts. Include any pertinent patient and family teaching.

GENERAL CONSIDERATIONS

• The patient may experience a secondary defense reaction, vasodilation, that causes body temperature to rebound, defeating the purpose of the therapy.
• Older adults are more at risk for skin and tissue damage because of their thin skin, loss of cold sensation, decreased subcutaneous tissue, and changes in the body's ability to regulate temperature. Check these patients more frequently during therapy.

Skill · 46 — **Deep Breathing Exercises, Coughing, and Splinting**

During surgery, the cough reflex is suppressed, mucus accumulates in the tracheobronchial passages, and the lungs do not ventilate fully. After surgery, respirations are often less effective as a result of anesthesia, pain medication, and pain from the incision, particularly thoracic and high abdominal incisions. Alveoli do not inflate and may collapse. Along with retained secretions the risk for atelectasis and respiratory infection increases. Deep breathing exercises hyperventilate the alveoli and prevent them from collapsing again, improve lung expansion and volume, help to expel anesthetic gases and mucus, and facilitate oxygenation of tissues. Coughing helps to remove mucus from the respiratory tract and usually is taught in conjunction with deep breathing. Because coughing is often painful, the patient with a thoracic or abdominal incision should be taught how to splint the incision.

EQUIPMENT

• Small pillow or folded bath blanket
• PPE, as indicated

ASSESSMENT GUIDELINES

• Identify patients who are considered at greater risk, such as the very young and very old; obese or malnourished patients; patients with fluid and electrolyte imbalances; patients with chronic

disease; patients who have underlying lung or cardiac disease; patients who have decreased mobility; and patients who are at risk for decreased compliance with postoperative activities, such as those with alterations in cognitive function. Depending on the particular at-risk patient, specific assessments and interventions may be warranted.
• Assess the patient's current level of knowledge regarding deep breathing, coughing, and splinting.

NURSING DIAGNOSES
• Deficient Knowledge
• Impaired Physical Mobility
• Risk for Infection
• Readiness for Enhanced Knowledge

OUTCOME IDENTIFICATION AND PLANNING
Expected outcomes may include:
• Patient and/or significant other verbalizes an understanding of the instructions and is able to demonstrate the activities.

IMPLEMENTATION

ACTION	RATIONALE
1. Check the patient's chart for the type of surgery and review the medical orders.	This check ensures that the care will be provided for the right patient and any specific teaching based on the type of surgery will be addressed.
2. Gather the necessary supplies and bring to the bedside stand or overbed table.	Preparation promotes efficient time management and an organized approach to the task. Bringing everything to the bedside conserves time and energy. Arranging items nearby is convenient, saves time, and avoids unnecessary stretching and twisting of muscles on the part of the nurse.
3. Perform hand hygiene and put on PPE, if indicated.	Hand hygiene and PPE prevent the spread of microorganisms. PPE is required based on transmission precautions.

ACTION

RATIONALE

4. Identify the patient.

Identifying the patient ensures the right patient receives the intervention and helps prevent errors.

5. Close curtains around bed and close the door to the room, if possible. Explain what you are going to do and why you are going to do it to the patient.

This ensures the patient's privacy. Explanation relieves anxiety and facilitates cooperation.

6. Identify the patient's learning needs. Identify the patient's level of knowledge regarding deep breathing exercises, coughing, and splinting of the incision. If the patient has had surgery before, ask about this experience.

Identification of baseline knowledge contributes to individualized teaching. Previous surgical experience may have an impact on preoperative/postoperative care positively or negatively, depending on this past experience.

7. Explain the rationale for performing deep breathing exercises, coughing, and splinting of the incision.

Explanation facilitates patient cooperation. An understanding of the rationale may contribute to increased compliance.

8. Provide teaching about deep breathing exercises.

Deep breathing exercises improve lung expansion and volume, help expel anesthetic gases and mucus from the airway, and facilitate the oxygenation of body tissues.

a. Assist or ask the patient to sit up (semi-Fowler's position) (FIGURE 1) and instruct the patient to place the palms of both hands

The upright position promotes chest expansion and lessens exertion of the abdominal muscles. Positioning the hands on the rib cage allows the patient to feel

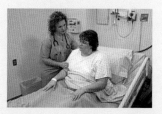

FIGURE 1 Assisting patient to semi- or high-Fowler's position.

ACTION	RATIONALE
along the lower anterior rib cage.	the chest rise and the lungs expand as the diaphragm descends.
b. Instruct the patient to exhale gently and completely.	Deep inhalation promotes lung expansion.
c. Instruct the patient to breathe in through the nose as deeply as possible and hold his or her breath for 3 seconds.	Return demonstration ensures that the patient is able to perform the exercises properly. Practice promotes effectiveness and compliance.
d. Instruct the patient to exhale through the mouth, pursing the lips like when whistling.	
e. Have the patient practice the breathing exercise three times. Instruct the patient that this exercise should be performed every 1 to 2 hours for the first 24 hours after surgery.	
9. Provide teaching regarding coughing and splinting (providing support to the incision).	Coughing helps remove retained mucus from the respiratory tract. Splinting minimizes pain while coughing or moving.
a. Ask the patient to sit up (semi-Fowler's position) and apply a folded bath blanket or pillow against the part of the body where the incision is located (e.g., abdomen or chest).	These interventions aim to decrease discomfort while coughing.
b. Instruct the patient to inhale and exhale through the nose three times.	
c. Ask the patient to take a deep breath and hold it for 3 seconds and then cough out three short breaths.	
d. Ask the patient to take a breath through his or her mouth and strongly cough again two times.	

ACTION	RATIONALE
e. Instruct the patient to perform these actions every 2 hours when awake after surgery.	
10. Validate the patient's understanding of information. Ask the patient to give a return demonstration. Ask the patient if he or she has any questions. Encourage the patient to practice the activities and ask questions, if necessary.	Validation facilitates the patient's understanding of information and performance of activities.
11. Remove PPE, if used. Perform hand hygiene.	Removing PPE properly reduces the risk for infection transmission and contamination of other items. Hand hygiene prevents the spread of microorganisms.

EVALUATION
• Patient and/or significant other verbalizes an understanding of the instructions related to deep breathing, coughing, and splinting, and is able to demonstrate the activities.

DOCUMENTATION
• Document the components of teaching related to deep breathing exercises, coughing, and splinting that were reviewed with the patient and family, if present. Record the patient's ability to demonstrate deep breathing exercises, coughing, and splinting and response to the teaching, and note if any follow-up instruction needs to be performed.

GENERAL CONSIDERATIONS
• Respiratory disorders, such as pneumonia and chronic obstructive pulmonary diseases, increase the risk for respiratory depression from anesthesia as well as postoperative pneumonia and atelectasis.
• Deep breathing and coughing can be accomplished through play to enhance a child's participation (Kyle, 2008).

Skill · 47 Performing Emergency Manual External Defibrillation (Asynchronous)

Electrical therapy is used to quickly terminate or control potentially lethal dysrhythmias. Electrical therapy can be administered by defibrillation, cardioversion, or a pacemaker. Defibrillation delivers large amounts of electric current to a patient over a brief period. It is the standard treatment for ventricular fibrillation (VF) and is also used to treat ventricular tachycardia (VT), in which the patient has no pulse. The goal is temporarily to depolarize the irregularly beating heart and allow more coordinated contractile activity to resume. It does so by completely depolarizing the myocardium, producing a momentary asystole. This provides an opportunity for the natural pacemaker centers of the heart to resume normal activity. The electrode paddles delivering the current may be placed on the patient's chest or, during cardiac surgery, directly on the myocardium. Because ventricular fibrillation leads to death if not corrected, the success of defibrillation depends on early recognition and quick treatment of this dysrhythmia.

Manual defibrillation depends on the operator for analysis of rhythm, charging, proper application of the paddles to the patient's thorax, and delivery of countershock. It requires the user to have immediate and accurate dysrhythmia recognition skills. The following guidelines are based on the American Heart Association 2005 guidelines. AHA guidelines state that these recommendations may be modified for the in-hospital setting, where continuous electrocardiographic or hemodynamic monitoring may be in place.

In the hospital setting, it is imperative that personnel be aware of the patient's stated instructions regarding a wish not to be resuscitated. This should be clearly expressed and documented in the patient's medical record.

EQUIPMENT

- Defibrillator (monophasic or biphasic)
- External paddles (or internal paddles sterilized for cardiac surgery)
- Conductive medium pads
- Electrocardiogram (ECG) monitor with recorder (often part of the defibrillator)
- Oxygen therapy equipment
- Handheld resuscitation bag
- Airway equipment
- Emergency pacing equipment
- Emergency cardiac medications

ASSESSMENT GUIDELINES

- Assess the patient for unresponsiveness, effective breathing, and signs of circulation.
- Assess the patient's vital parameters and determine the patient's level of responsiveness.

- Check for partial or complete airway obstruction.
- Assess for the absence or ineffectiveness of respirations.
- Assess for the absence of signs of circulation and pulses.
- Call for help and perform cardiopulmonary resuscitation (CPR) until the defibrillator and other emergency equipment arrive.

NURSING DIAGNOSES

- Decreased Cardiac Output
- Ineffective Airway Clearance
- Impaired Gas Exchange
- Risk for Injury
- Impaired Spontaneous Ventilation

OUTCOME IDENTIFICATION AND PLANNING

Expected outcomes may include:
- Manual external defibrillation is performed correctly without adverse effect to the patient.
- Patient regains signs of circulation.
- Patient regains respirations.
- Patient's heart and lungs maintain adequate function to sustain life.
- Patient does not experience serious injury.
- Advanced cardiac life support is initiated.

IMPLEMENTATION

ACTION	RATIONALE
1. Assess responsiveness. If the patient is not responsive, call for help and pull call bell, and call the facility emergency response number. Call for the AED. Put on gloves, if available. Perform cardiopulmonary resuscitation (CPR) until the defibrillator and other emergency equipment arrive.	Assessing responsiveness prevents starting CPR on a conscious victim. Activating the emergency response system initiates a rapid response. Gloves prevent contact with blood and body fluids. Initiating CPR preserves heart and brain function while awaiting defibrillation.
2. Turn on the defibrillator.	Charging and placement prepare for defibrillation.
3. If the defibrillator has 'quick-look' capability, place the paddles on the patient's chest. Otherwise, connect the monitoring leads of the defibrillator to the patient and assess the patient's cardiac rhythm.	Connecting the monitor leads to the patient allows for a quick view of the cardiac rhythm.

ACTION	RATIONALE
4. Expose the patient's chest, and apply conductive pads at the paddle placement positions. For anterolateral placement, place one pad to the right of the upper sternum, just below the right clavicle, and the other over the fifth or sixth intercostal space at the left anterior axillary line (FIGURE 1). 'Hands-free' defibrillator pads can be used with the same placement positions, if available. For anteroposterior placement, place the anterior paddle directly over the heart at the precordium, to the left of the lower sternal border. Place the flat posterior paddle under the patient's body beneath the heart and immediately below the scapulae (but not on the vertebral column) (FIGURE 2).	This placement ensures that the electrical stimulus needs to travel only a short distance to the heart.

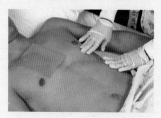

FIGURE 1 Anterolateral pad placement.

5. Set the energy level for 360 joules for an adult patient when using a monophasic defibrillator. Use clinically appropriate energy levels for biphasic defibrillators, beginning with 150 to 200 J (AHA, 2005b).	Proper setup ensures proper functioning.

ACTION   RATIONALE

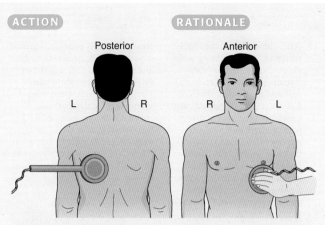

Posterior   Anterior

FIGURE 2 Anteroposterior placement of defibrillator pads. (From Smeltzer, S. C., Bare, B. G., et al. (2010). *Brunner and Suddarth's textbook of medical-surgical nursing.* 12th ed.). Philadelphia, PA: Lippincott Williams & Wilkins, with permission.)

ACTION	RATIONALE
6. Charge the paddles by pressing the charge buttons, which are located either on the machine or on the paddles themselves.	Proper setup ensures proper functioning.
7. **Place the paddles over the conductive pads and press firmly against the patient's chest, using 25 lb (11 kg) of pressure. If using hands-off pads, do not touch the paddles.**	Proper setup ensures proper functioning. Solid adhesion is necessary for conduction.
8. Reassess the cardiac rhythm.	The rhythm may have changed during preparation.
9. **If the patient remains in VF or pulseless VT, instruct all personnel to stand clear of the patient and the bed, including the operator.**	Standing clear of the bed and patient helps prevent electrical shocks to personnel.
10. Discharge the current by pressing both paddle charge buttons simultaneously. If using remote defibrillator pads, press the discharge or shock button on the machine.	Pressing the charge buttons discharges the electric current for defibrillation.

ACTION	RATIONALE
11. After the shock, immediately resume CPR, beginning with chest compressions. After five cycles (about 2 minutes), reassess the cardiac rhythm. Continue until advanced care providers take over, the patient starts to move, you are too exhausted to continue, or a physician discontinues CPR. Advanced care providers will indicate when a pulse check or other therapies are appropriate.	Resuming CPR provides optimal treatment. CPR preserves heart, and neurologic function (based on AHA 2006 recommended guidelines). Even when a shock eliminates the dysrhythmia, it may take several minutes for a heart rhythm to establish and even longer to achieve perfusion. Chest compressions can provide coronary and cerebral perfusion during this period (Zed et al., 2008).
12. If necessary, prepare to defibrillate a second time. Energy level on the monophasic defibrillator should remain at 360 J for subsequent shocks (AHA, 2005).	Additional shocking may be needed to stimulate the heart.
13. Announce that you are preparing to defibrillate and follow the procedure described above.	Additional shocking may be needed to stimulate the heart.
14. If defibrillation restores a normal rhythm:	
a. Check for signs of circulation; check the central and peripheral pulses, and obtain a blood pressure reading, heart rate, and respiratory rate.	The patient will need continuous monitoring to prevent further problems. Continuous monitoring helps provide for early detection and prompt intervention should additional problems arise.
b. If signs of circulation are present, check breathing. If breathing is inadequate, assist breathing. Start rescue breathing (one breath every 5 seconds).	
c. If breathing is adequate, place the patient in the recovery position. Continue to assess the patient.	Reassessment determines the need for continued intervention. Provides optimal treatment.

ACTION	RATIONALE
d. Assess the patient's level of consciousness, cardiac rhythm, breath sounds, and skin color and temperature.	
e. Obtain baseline ABG levels and a 12-lead ECG, if ordered.	
f. Provide supplemental oxygen, ventilation, and medications, as needed.	
15. Check the chest for electrical burns and treat them, as ordered, with corticosteroid or lanolin-based creams. If using 'hands-free' pads, keep pads on in case of recurrent ventricular tachycardia or ventricular fibrillation.	Skin inspection identifies injury. Keeping pads in place provides preparation for future use.
16. Remove gloves, if used. Perform hand hygiene.	Removing PPE properly reduces the risk for infection transmission and contamination of other items. Hand hygiene prevents transmission of microorganism.
17. Prepare the defibrillator for immediate reuse.	Patients may remain unstable and could require further intervention.

EVALUATION

• Manual external defibrillation is performed correctly without adverse effect to the patient and the patient regains signs of circulation.
• Patient regains respirations.
• Patient's heart and lungs maintain adequate function to sustain life.
• Patient does not experience serious injury.
• Advanced cardiac life support is initiated.

DOCUMENTATION

• Document the time you noted the patient to be unresponsive and initiated CPR. Document the procedure, including the patient's ECG rhythms both before and after defibrillation. Record the number of times defibrillation was performed and the voltage used during each attempt. Document the return of a pulse; the dosage, route, and time of drug administration; whether CPR was used; how the airway was maintained; and the patient's outcome. Continued intervention, such as by the code team, is typically documented on a code form, which identifies the actions and drugs provided during the code. Provide a summary of these events in the patient's medical record.

GENERAL CONSIDERATIONS

- Defibrillation can cause accidental electric shock to those providing care.
- Defibrillators vary among manufacturers. Be familiar with each particular facility's equipment.
- Defibrillator operation should be checked at least every 8 hours, or per facility policy, and after each use.
- Defibrillation can be affected by several factors, including paddle size and placement, condition of the patient's myocardium, duration of the arrhythmia, chest resistance, and the number of countershocks.

Skill · 48   **Performing Emergency Automated External Defibrillation**

The most frequent initial cardiac rhythm in witnessed sudden cardiac arrest is ventricular fibrillation (AHA, 2005b). Electrical defibrillation is the most effective treatment for ventricular fibrillation. Electrical therapy can be administered by defibrillation, cardioversion, or a pacemaker. Early defibrillation is critical to increase patient survival (AHA, 2006).

Defibrillation delivers large amounts of electric current to a patient over brief periods of time. It is the standard treatment for ventricular fibrillation (VF) and is also used to treat pulseless ventricular tachycardia (VT). The goal is temporarily to depolarize the irregularly beating heart and allow more coordinated contractile activity to resume. It does so by completely depolarizing the myocardium, producing a momentary asystole. This provides an opportunity for the natural pacemaker centers of the heart to resume normal activity.

The automated external defibrillator (AED) is a portable external defibrillator that automatically detects and interprets the heart's rhythm and informs the operator if a shock is indicated. AEDs are appropriate for use in situations where the patient is unresponsive, not breathing, and has no pulse (AHA, 2006). The defibrillator responds to the patient information by advising 'shock' or 'no shock.' Fully automatic models automatically perform rhythm analysis and shock, if indicated. These are usually found in out-of-hospital settings. Semiautomatic models require the operator to press an 'Analyze' button to initiate rhythm analysis and then press a

'Shock' button to deliver the shock, if indicated. Semiautomatic models are usually found in the hospital setting. AEDs will not deliver a shock unless the electrode pads are correctly attached and a shockable rhythm is detected. Some AEDs have motion-detection devices that ensure the defibrillator will not discharge if there is motion, such as motion from personnel in contact with the patient. The strength of the charge is preset. Once the pads are in place and the device is turned on, follow the prompts given by the device. The following guidelines are based on the American Heart Association (AHA, 2005a) guidelines. AHA guidelines state that these recommendations may be modified for the in-hospital setting, where continuous electrocardiographic or hemodynamic monitoring may be in place.

Current recommendations call for the application of the AED as soon as it is available, allowing for analysis of cardiac status and delivery of an initial shock, if indicated, for adults and children. After the initial shock, deliver five cycles of chest compressions/ventilations (30/2), and then reanalyze the cardiac rhythm. Provide sets of one shock alternating with 2 minutes of CPR until the AED indicates a 'no shock indicated' message or until ACLS is available (AHA, 2006).

In the hospital setting, it is imperative that personnel be aware of the patient's stated instructions regarding a wish not to be resuscitated. This should be clearly expressed and documented in the patient's medical record.

EQUIPMENT

- Automated external defibrillator (AED)
- Self-adhesive, pregelled monitor-defibrillator pads (6)
- Cables to connect the pads and AED
- Razor
- Towel
- Some models have the pads, cables, and AED preconnected.

ASSESSMENT GUIDELINES

- Assess the patient for unresponsiveness, effective breathing, and signs of circulation.
- Assess the patient's vital parameters and determine the patient's level of responsiveness.
- Check for partial or complete airway obstruction. Assess for the absence or ineffectiveness of respirations.
- Assess for the absence of signs of circulation and pulses. AEDs should be used only when a patient is unresponsive, not breathing, and without signs of circulation (pulseless, lack of effective respirations, coughing, moving).
- Determine the age of the patient; some AED systems are designed to deliver both adult and child shock doses. Choose correct electrode pad for size/age of patient. For children less than 8 years of age, use child pads or child system for children, if available.

NURSING DIAGNOSES

- Decreased Cardiac Output
- Impaired Gas Exchange
- Ineffective Airway Clearance
- Risk for Ineffective Cerebral Tissue Perfusion
- Impaired Spontaneous Ventilation
- Risk for Injury

OUTCOME IDENTIFICATION AND PLANNING

Expected outcomes may include:
- Automatic external defibrillation is performed correctly without adverse effect to the patient.
- Patient regains signs of circulation, with organized electrical rhythm and pulse.
- Patient regains respirations.
- Patient's heart and lungs maintain adequate function to sustain life.
- Patient does not experience serious injury.
- Advanced cardiac life support is initiated.

IMPLEMENTATION

ACTION	RATIONALE
1. Assess responsiveness. If the patient is not responsive, call for help and pull call bell, and call the facility emergency response number. Call for the AED. Put on gloves, if available. Perform cardiopulmonary resuscitation (CPR) until the defibrillator and other emergency equipment arrive.	Assessing responsiveness prevents starting CPR on a conscious victim. Activating the emergency response system initiates a rapid response. Gloves prevent contact with blood and body fluids. Initiating CPR preserves heart and brain function while awaiting defibrillation.
2. Prepare the AED. Power on the AED. Push the power button. Some devices will turn on automatically when the lid or case is opened.	Proper setup ensures proper functioning.
3. Attach AED connecting cables to the AED (may be preconnected). Attach AED cables to the adhesive electrode pads (may be preconnected).	Proper setup ensures proper functioning.

ACTION	RATIONALE
4. Stop chest compressions. Peel away the covering from the electrode pads to expose the adhesive surface. Attach the electrode pads to the patient's chest. Place one pad on the upper right sternal border, directly below the clavicle. Place the second pad lateral to the left nipple, with the top margin of the pad a few inches below the axilla (FIGURE 1).	Proper setup ensures proper functioning. The use of self-adhesive pads allows hands-free defibrillation and excellent skin–electrode contact, which provides lower impedance, less artifact, and greater user safety (Dwyer et al., 2004).

FIGURE 1 AED electrode pad placement.

5. Once the pads are in place and the device is turned on, follow the prompts given by the device. Clear the patient and analyze the rhythm. Ensure no one is touching the patient. Loudly state a 'Clear the patient' message. Press 'Analyze' button to initiate analysis, if necessary. Some devices automatically begin analysis when the pads are attached. Avoid all movement affecting the patient during analysis.	Movement and electrical impulses cause artifact during analysis. Avoidance of artifact ensures accurate rhythm analysis. Avoidance of contact with patient avoids accidental shock to personnel.
6. If ventricular tachycardia or ventricular fibrillation is present, the device will announce that a shock is indicated and	The shock message is delivered through a written or visual message on the AED screen, an auditory

ACTION	RATIONALE
begin charging. Once the AED is charged, a message will be delivered to shock the patient.	alarm, or a voice-synthesized statement.
7. Before pressing the 'Shock' button, loudly state a 'Clear the patient' message. Visually check that no one is in contact with the patient. Press the 'Shock' button. If the AED is fully automatic, a shock will be delivered automatically.	Ensuring a clear patient avoids accidental shocking of personnel.
8. Immediately resume CPR, beginning with chest compressions. After five cycles (about 2 minutes), allow the AED to analyze the heart rhythm. If a shock is not advised, resume CPR, beginning with chest compressions. Do not recheck to see if there is a pulse. Follow the AED voice prompts. Continue until advanced care providers take over, the patient starts to move, you are too exhausted to continue, or a physician discontinues CPR. Advanced care providers will indicate when a pulse check or other therapies are appropriate (AHA, 2006).	Resuming CPR provides optimal treatment. CPR preserves heart, and neurologic function (based on AHA 2006 recommended guidelines). Even when a shock eliminates the dysrhythmia, it may take several minutes for a heart rhythm to establish and even longer to achieve perfusion. Chest compressions can provide coronary and cerebral perfusion during this period (Zed et al., 2008). Some AEDs in the community for use by lay persons are automatically programmed to cycle through three analysis/shock cycles in one set. This would necessitate turning the AED off after the first shock and turning it back on for future analysis and defibrillation. Be familiar with the type of AED available for use.
9. Remove gloves, if used. Perform hand hygiene.	Removing PPE reduces the risk for infection transmission and contamination of other items. Hand hygiene prevents transmission of microorganisms.

EVALUATION

• Automatic external defibrillation is applied correctly, without adverse effect to the patient.

• Patient regains signs of circulation.

- Patient regains respirations.
- Patient's heart and lungs maintain adequate function to sustain life.
- Patient does not experience injury.
- Advanced cardiac life support is initiated.

DOCUMENTATION

- Document the time it was discovered that the patient was unresponsive and CPR was initiated. Document the time(s) AED shocks are initiated. Continued intervention, such as by the code team, is typically documented on a code form, which identifies the actions and drugs provided during the code. Provide a summary of these events in the patient's medical record.

GENERAL CONSIDERATIONS

- Appropriate maintenance of the AED is critical for proper operation. Check the AED for any visible signs of damage. Check the 'ready for use' indicator on the AED daily. Perform maintenance according to the manufacturer's recommendations and facility policy.
- Anterior-posterior placement of electrode pads can avoid difficulties associated with increased breast size in patients who are pregnant (Castle, 2007).

Skill · 49   **Providing Denture Care**

Plaque can accumulate on dentures and can promote oropharyngeal colonization of pathogens (Yoon & Steele, 2007). Diligent oral hygiene care can improve oral health and limit the growth of pathogens in the oropharyngeal secretions, decreasing the incidence of aspiration pneumonia and other systemic diseases (Yoon & Steele, 2007; AACN, 2006). Dentures should be cleaned at least daily, to prevent irritation and infection. They may be cleaned more often, based on need and the patient's personal preference. Dentures are often removed at night. Handle dentures with care to prevent breakage.

EQUIPMENT

- Soft toothbrush or denture brush
- Toothpaste
- Denture cleaner (optional)
- Denture adhesive (optional)
- Glass of cool water
- Emesis basin
- Denture cup (optional)
- Nonsterile gloves
- Additional PPE, as indicated
- Towel
- Mouthwash (optional)
- Washcloth or paper towel
- Lip lubricant (optional)
- Gauze

ASSESSMENT GUIDELINES
- Assess the patient's oral hygiene preferences: frequency, time of day, and type of hygiene products.
- Assess for any physical activity limitations.
- Assess patient's oral cavity and dentition. Look for any inflammation or bleeding of the gums. Look for ulcers, lesions, and yellow or white patches. The yellow or white patches may indicate a fungal infection called thrush. Look at the lips for dryness or cracking. Ask the patient if he or she is having pain, dryness, soreness, or difficulty chewing or swallowing.
- Assess patient's ability to perform own care.

NURSING DIAGNOSES
- Ineffective Health Maintenance
- Impaired Oral Mucous Membrane
- Disturbed Body Image
- Deficient Knowledge

OUTCOME IDENTIFICATION AND PLANNING
Expected outcomes may include:
- The patient's mouth and dentures will be clean.
- The patient verbalizes positive body image.
- The patient will verbalize the importance of oral care.

IMPLEMENTATION

ACTION	RATIONALE
1. Perform hand hygiene and put on PPE, if indicated.	Hand hygiene and PPE prevent the spread of microorganisms. PPE is required based on transmission precautions.
2. Identify patient. Explain the procedure to the patient.	Identifying the patient ensures the right patient receives the intervention and helps prevent errors. Explanation facilitates cooperation.
3. Assemble equipment on overbed table within reach.	Organization facilitates performance of task.
4. Provide privacy for patient.	Cleaning another person's mouth is invasive and may be embarrassing (Holman et al., 2005). Patient may be embarrassed by removal of dentures.

ACTION	RATIONALE
5. Lower side rail and assist patient to sitting position, if permitted, or turn patient onto side. Place towel across patient's chest. Raise bed to a comfortable working position, usually elbow height of the caregiver (VISN 8 Patient Safety Center, 2009). Put on gloves.	The sitting or side-lying position prevents aspiration of fluids into the lungs. The towel protects the patient from dampness. Proper bed height helps reduce back strain while performing the procedure. Gloves prevent the spread of microorganisms.
6. Apply gentle pressure with 4 × 4 gauze to grasp upper denture plate and remove (FIGURE 1). Place it immediately in denture cup. Lift lower dentures with gauze, using slight rocking motion. Remove, and place in denture cup.	Rocking motion breaks suction between denture and gum. Using 4 × 4 gauze prevents slippage and discourages spread of microorganisms.

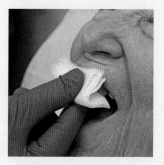

FIGURE 1 Removing dentures with a gauze sponge.

7. Place paper towels or washcloth in sink while brushing. Using the toothbrush and paste, brush all surfaces gently but thoroughly (FIGURE 2). If patient prefers, add denture cleaner to cup with water and follow directions on preparation.	Putting paper towels or a washcloth in the sink protects against breakage. Dentures collect food and microorganisms and require daily cleaning.

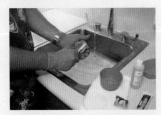

ACTION	RATIONALE

FIGURE 2 Cleaning dentures at the sink.

8. Rinse thoroughly with water. Apply denture adhesive if appropriate.

Water aids in removal of debris and acts as a cleaning agent.

9. Use a toothbrush and paste gently clean gums, mucous membranes, and tongue. Offer water and/or mouthwash so patient can rinse mouth before replacing dentures.

Cleaning removes food particles and plaque, permitting proper fit and preventing infection. Mouthwash leaves a pleasant taste in the mouth.

10. Insert upper denture in mouth and press firmly. Insert lower denture. Check that the dentures are securely in place and comfortable.

This ensures patient comfort.

11. If the patient desires, dentures can be stored in the denture cup in cold water, instead of returning to the mouth. Label the cup and place in the patient's bedside table.

Storing in water prevents warping of dentures. Proper storage prevents loss and damage.

12. Remove equipment and return patient to a position of comfort. Remove your gloves. Raise side rail and lower bed.

Promotes patient comfort and safety. Removing gloves properly reduces the risk for infection transmission and contamination of other items.

13. Remove additional PPE, if used. Perform hand hygiene.

Removing PPE properly reduces the risk for infection transmission and contamination of other items. Hand hygiene prevents transmission of microorganisms.

EVALUATION

- The patient received oral care and experienced little to no discomfort.
- The patient stated mouth feels refreshed.
- The patient verbalized an understanding of the reasons for proper oral care.

DOCUMENTATION

- Record oral assessment, significant observations and unusual findings, such as bleeding or inflammation. Document any teaching done. Document procedure and patient response.

GENERAL CONSIDERATIONS

- Encourage the patient to wear his or her dentures, if not contraindicated. Dentures enhance appearance, assist eating, facilitate speech, and maintain the gum line. Denture fit may be altered with long periods of nonuse.
- Encourage the patient to refrain from wrapping the denture in paper towels or napkins because they could be mistaken for trash.
- Encourage the patient to refrain from placing the dentures in the bed clothes because they can be lost in the laundry.
- Store dentures in cold water when not in the patient's mouth. Leaving dentures dry can cause warping, leading to discomfort when worn (Holman et al., 2005).

Skill · 50   Digital Removal of Stool

When a patient develops a fecal impaction (prolonged retention or an accumulation of fecal material that forms a hardened mass in the rectum), the stool must sometimes be broken up manually. Digital removal of feces is considered as a last resort after other methods of bowel evacuation have been unsuccessful (Kyle et al., 2004). Patient discomfort and irritation of the rectal mucosa may occur. Many patients find that a sitz bath or tub bath after this procedure soothes the irritated perineal area. An oil-retention enema may be ordered to be given before the procedure to soften stool.

EQUIPMENT

- Disposable gloves
- Additional PPE, as indicated
- Water-soluble lubricant
- Waterproof pad
- Bedpan
- Toilet paper, washcloth, and towel
- Sitz bath (optional)

ASSESSMENT GUIDELINES
- Verify the time of the patient's last bowel movement by asking the patient and checking the patient's medical record.
- Assess the abdomen, including auscultating for bowel sounds, percussing, and palpating.
- Inspect the rectal area for any fissures, hemorrhoids, sores, or rectal tears. If any of these are noted, consult the prescriber for the appropriateness of the intervention.
- Assess the results of the patient's laboratory work, specifically the platelet count and white blood cell (WBC) count. Digital removal of stool is contraindicated for patients with a low platelet count or low WBC count. Digital removal of stool may irritate or traumatize the gastrointestinal mucosa, causing bleeding, bowel perforation, or infection. Do not perform any unnecessary procedures that would place the patient at risk for bleeding or infection.
- Assess for dizziness, light-headedness, diaphoresis, and clammy skin. Assess pulse rate and blood pressure before and after the procedure. The procedure may stimulate a vagal response, which increases parasympathetic stimulation, causing a decrease in heart rate and blood pressure.
- Do not perform digital removal of stool on patients who have bowel inflammation or bowel infection, or after rectal, prostate, and colon surgery.

NURSING DIAGNOSES
- Constipation
- Acute Pain
- Risk for Injury

OUTCOME IDENTIFICATION AND PLANNING
Expected outcomes may include:
- Patient will expel feces with assistance.
- Patient verbalizes decreased discomfort.
- Abdominal distention is absent.
- Patient remains free of any evidence of trauma to the rectal mucosa or other adverse effect.

IMPLEMENTATION

ACTION	RATIONALE
1. Verify the order. Bring necessary equipment to the bedside stand or overbed table.	Digital removal of stool is considered an invasive procedure and requires a physician's order. Verifying the medical order is crucial to ensuring that the

ACTION	RATIONALE

| | proper procedure is administered to the right patient. Bringing everything to the bedside conserves time and energy. Arranging items nearby is convenient, saves time, and avoids unnecessary stretching and twisting of muscles on the part of the nurse. |

2. Perform hand hygiene and put on PPE, if indicated.

Hand hygiene and PPE prevent the spread of microorganisms. PPE is required based on transmission precautions.

3. Identify the patient.

Identifying the patient ensures the right patient receives the intervention and helps prevent errors.

4. Close curtains around bed and close the door to the room, if possible. Explain what you are going to do and why you are going to do it to the patient. Discuss signs and symptoms of a slow heart rate. Instruct the patient to alert you if any of these symptoms are felt during the procedure. Have a bedpan ready for use.

This ensures the patient's privacy. Explanation relieves anxiety and facilitates cooperation. The patient is better able to relax and cooperate if he or she is familiar with the procedure.

5. Adjust bed to comfortable working height, usually elbow height of the caregiver (VISN 8 Patient Safety Center, 2009). Position the patient on the left side (Sims' position), as dictated by patient comfort and condition. Fold top linen back just enough to allow access to the patient's rectal area. Place a waterproof pad under the patient's hip.

Having the bed at the proper height prevents back and muscle strain. Sims' position facilitates access into the rectum and colon. Folding back the linen in this manner minimizes unnecessary exposure and promotes the patient's comfort and warmth. The waterproof pad will protect the bed.

6. Put on nonsterile gloves.

This protects the nurse from microorganisms in feces. The GI tract is not a sterile environment.

ACTION	RATIONALE

7. Generously lubricate index finger with water-soluble lubricant and insert finger gently into anal canal, pointing toward the umbilicus.

Lubrication reduces irritation of the rectum. The presence of the finger added to the mass tends to cause discomfort for the patient if the work is not done slowly and gently.

8. Gently work the finger around and into the hardened mass to break it up (FIGURE 1) and then remove pieces of it. Instruct the patient to bear down, if possible, while extracting feces to ease in removal.

Fecal mass may be large and may need to be removed in smaller pieces.

Place extracted stool in bedpan.

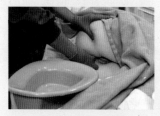

FIGURE 1 Gently work the finger around and into the hardened mass to break it up.

9. Remove impaction at intervals if it is severe. **Instruct patient to alert you if he or she begins to feel lightheaded or nauseated. If patient reports either symptom, stop removal and assess patient.**

This helps to prevent discomfort, irritation, and vagal nerve stimulation.

10. Put on clean gloves. Assist patient, if necessary, with cleaning of anal area. Offer washcloths, soap, and water for handwashing. If patient is able, offer sitz bath.

Cleaning deters the transmission of microorganisms and promotes hygiene. Sitz bath may relieve the irritated perianal area.

11. Remove gloves. Return the patient to a comfortable position. Make sure the linens under the patient are dry. Ensure that the patient is covered.

Removing contaminated gloves prevents spread of microorganisms. The other actions promote patient comfort.

ACTION	RATIONALE
12. Raise side rail. Lower bed height and adjust head of bed to a comfortable position.	These promote patient safety.
13. Remove additional PPE, if used. Perform hand hygiene.	Removing PPE properly reduces the risk for infection transmission and contamination of other items. Hand hygiene prevents the spread of microorganisms.

EVALUATION

• Fecal impaction is removed and the patient expels feces with assistance.
• Patient verbalizes decreased discomfort.
• Abdominal distention is absent.
• Patient remains free of any evidence of trauma to the rectal mucosa or other adverse effect.

DOCUMENTATION

• Document the following: color, consistency, and amount of stool removed; condition of perianal area after procedure; pain assessment; and patient's reaction to the procedure.

GENERAL CONSIDERATIONS

• In myelosuppressed patients and/or patients at risk for myelosuppression and mucositis, rectal agents and manipulation are discouraged because they can lead to development of bleeding, anal fissures, or abscesses, which are portals for infection (NCI, 2006).

Skill · 51   **Caring for a Hemovac Drain**

A Hemovac drain is placed into a vascular cavity where blood drainage is expected after surgery, such as with abdominal and orthopedic surgery. The drain consists of perforated tubing connected to a portable vacuum unit. Suction is maintained by compressing a spring-like device in the collection unit. After a surgical procedure, the surgeon places one end of the drain in or near the area to be drained. The other end passes through the skin via a separate incision. These drains are usually sutured in place. The site may be treated as an additional surgical wound, but often these sites are left open to air the first 24 hours after surgery.

As the drainage accumulates in the collection unit, it expands and suction is lost, requiring recompression. Typically, the drain is emptied every 4 or 8 hours and when it is half full of drainage or air. However, based on the medical orders and nursing assessment and judgment, it could be emptied and recompressed more frequently.

EQUIPMENT

- Graduated container for measuring drainage
- Clean disposable gloves
- Additional PPE, as indicated
- Cleansing solution, usually sterile normal saline
- Sterile gauze pads
- Skin-protectant wipes
- Dressing materials for site dressing, if used

ASSESSMENT GUIDELINES

- Confirm any medical orders relevant to drain care and any drain care included in the nursing plan of care.
- Assess the situation to determine the need for wound cleaning, a dressing change, or emptying of the drain.
- Assess the patient's level of comfort and the need for analgesics before wound care. Assess if the patient experienced any pain related to prior dressing changes and the effectiveness of interventions used to minimize the patient's pain.
- Assess the current dressing. Assess for the presence of excess drainage or bleeding or saturation of the dressing.
- Assess the patency of the drain and the drain site. Note the characteristics of the drainage in the collection bag.
- Inspect the wound and the surrounding tissue. Assess the appearance of the incision for the approximation of wound edges, the color of the wound and surrounding area, and signs of dehiscence. Note the stage of the healing process and characteristics of any drainage.
- Assess the surrounding skin for color, temperature, and edema, ecchymosis, or maceration.

NURSING DIAGNOSES

- Anxiety
- Acute Pain
- Disturbed Body Image
- Impaired Skin Integrity
- Deficient Knowledge
- Delayed Surgical Recovery
- Impaired Tissue Integrity

OUTCOME IDENTIFICATION AND PLANNING

Expected outcomes may include:
- Hemovac drain is patent and intact.
- Care is accomplished without contaminating the wound area, and without causing trauma to the wound or the patient to experience pain or discomfort.

- Patient's wound continues to show signs of healing progression.
- Drainage amounts are measured accurately at the frequency required by facility policy and recorded as part of the intake and output record.
- Patient demonstrates understanding about drain care.

IMPLEMENTATION

ACTION	RATIONALE
1. Review the medical orders for wound care or the nursing plan of care related to wound/drain care.	Reviewing the order and plan of care validates the correct patient and correct procedure.
2. Gather the necessary supplies and bring to the bedside stand or overbed table.	Preparation promotes efficient time management and an organized approach to the task. Bringing everything to the bedside conserves time and energy. Arranging items nearby is convenient, saves time, and avoids unnecessary stretching and twisting of muscles on the part of the nurse.
3. Perform hand hygiene and put on PPE, if indicated.	Hand hygiene and PPE prevent the spread of microorganisms. PPE is required based on transmission precautions.
4. Identify the patient.	Identifying the patient ensures the right patient receives the intervention and helps prevent errors.
5. Close curtains around bed and close the door to the room, if possible. Explain what you are going to do and why you are going to do it to the patient.	This ensures the patient's privacy. Explanation relieves anxiety and facilitates cooperation.
6. Assess the patient for possible need for nonpharmacologic pain-reducing interventions or analgesic medication before wound care dressing change.	Pain is a subjective experience influenced by past experience. Wound care and dressing changes may cause pain for some patients.

ACTION	RATIONALE
Administer appropriate pre-scribed analgesic. Allow sufficient time for the analgesic to achieve its effectiveness before beginning the procedure.	
7. Place a waste receptacle at a convenient location for use during the procedure.	Having a waste container handy means that the soiled dressing may be discarded easily, without the spread of microorganisms.
8. Adjust bed to comfortable working height, usually elbow height of the caregiver (VISN 8 Patient Safety Center, 2009).	Having the bed at the proper height prevents back and muscle strain.
9. Assist the patient to a comfortable position that provides easy access to the drain and/or wound area. Use a bath blanket to cover any exposed area other than the wound. Place a waterproof pad under the wound site.	Patient positioning and use of a bath blanket provide for comfort and warmth. Waterproof pad protects underlying surfaces.
10. Put on clean gloves; put on mask or face shield, if indicated.	Gloves prevent the spread of microorganisms; mask reduces the risk of transmission should splashing occur.
11. Place the graduated collection container under the outlet of the drain. Without contaminating the outlet, pull the cap off. The chamber will expand completely as it draws in air. **Empty the chamber's contents completely into the container. Use the gauze pad to clean the outlet. Fully compress the chamber by pushing the top and bottom together with your hands. Keep the device tightly compressed while you apply the cap** (FIGURE 1).	Emptying the drainage allows for accurate measurement. Cleaning the outlet reduces the risk of contamination and helps prevent the spread of microorganisms. Compressing the chamber reestablishes the suction.

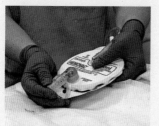

FIGURE 1 Compressing the Hemovac and securing the cap.

12. Check the patency of the equipment. Make sure the tubing is free from twists and kinks.

Patent, untwisted, or unkinked tubing promotes appropriate drainage from wound.

13. Secure the Hemovac drain to the patient's gown below the wound with a safety pin, making sure that there is no tension on the tubing.

Securing the drain prevents injury to the patient and accidental removal of the drain.

14. Carefully measure and record the character, color, and amount of the drainage. Discard the drainage according to facility policy.

Documentation promotes continuity of care and communication. Appropriate disposal of biohazard material reduces the risk for microorganism transmission.

15. Put on clean gloves. If the drain site has a dressing, redress the site as outlined in Skill 55. Also clean the sutures with the gauze pad moistened with normal saline. Dry sutures with gauze before applying new dressing.

Dressing protects the site. Cleaning and drying sutures deters the growth of microorganisms.

16. If the drain site is open to air, observe the sutures that secure the drain to the skin. Look for signs of pulling, tearing, swelling, or infection of the surrounding skin. Gently clean the sutures with the gauze pad moistened with normal saline. Dry with a

Early detection of problems leads to prompt intervention and prevents complications. Gentle cleaning and drying prevent the growth of microorganisms. Skin protectant prevents skin irritation and breakdown.

ACTION	RATIONALE
new gauze pad. Apply skin protectant to the surrounding skin, if needed.	
17. Remove and discard gloves. Remove all remaining equipment; place the patient in a comfortable position, with side rails up and bed in the lowest position.	Proper removal of gloves prevents spread of microorganisms. Proper patient and bed positioning promotes safety and comfort.
18. Remove additional PPE, if used. Perform hand hygiene.	Removing PPE properly reduces the risk for infection transmission and contamination of other items. Hand hygiene prevents the spread of microorganisms.
19. Check drain status at least every 4 hours. Check all wound dressings every shift. More frequent checks may be needed if the wound is more complex or dressings become saturated quickly.	Checking the drain ensures proper functioning and early detection of problems. Checking dressings ensures the assessment of changes in patient condition and timely intervention to prevent complications.

EVALUATION

- Patient exhibits a patent and intact Hemovac drain with a wound area that is free of contamination and trauma.
- Patient verbalizes minimal to no pain or discomfort.
- Patient exhibits signs and symptoms of progressive wound healing, with drainage being measured accurately at the frequency required by facility policy, and amounts recorded as part of the intake and output record.
- Patient verbalizes an understanding of the rationale for and/or the technique for drain care.

DOCUMENTATION

- Document the location of the wound and drain, the assessment of the wound and drain site, and patency of the drain. Note if sutures are intact. Document the presence of drainage and characteristics on the old dressing upon removal. Include the appearance of the surrounding skin. Document cleansing of the drain site. Record any skin care and the dressing applied. Note that the drain was emptied and recompressed. Note pertinent patient and family education and any patient reaction to this procedure, including patient's pain level and the effectiveness of nonpharmacologic interventions or analgesia, if administered. Document the amount and characteristics of drainage obtained on the appropriate intake and output record.

GENERAL CONSIDERATIONS

• When the patient with a drain is ready to ambulate, empty and compress the drain before activity. Secure the drain to the patient's gown below the wound, making sure there is no tension on the drainage tubing. This removes excess drainage, maintains maximal suction, and avoids strain on the drain's suture line.

Skill · 52   Caring for a Jackson-Pratt Drain

A Jackson-Pratt (J-P) or grenade drain collects wound drainage in a bulblike device that is compressed to create gentle suction. It consists of perforated tubing connected to a portable vacuum unit. After a surgical procedure, the surgeon places one end of the drain in or near the area to be drained. The other end passes through the skin via a separate incision. These drains are usually sutured in place. The site may be treated as an additional surgical wound, but often these sites are left open to air after the first 24 hours after surgery. They are typically used with breast and abdominal surgery.

As the drainage accumulates in the bulb, the bulb expands and suction is lost, requiring recompression. Typically, these drains are emptied every 4 to 8 hours, and when they are half full of drainage or air. However, based on nursing assessment and judgment, the drain could be emptied and recompressed more frequently.

EQUIPMENT

• Graduated container for measuring drainage
• Clean disposable gloves
• Additional PPE, as indicated
• Cleansing solution, usually sterile normal saline

• Sterile gauze pads
• Skin-protectant wipes
• Dressing materials for site dressing, if used

ASSESSMENT GUIDELINES

• Confirm any medical orders relevant to drain care and any drain care included in the nursing plan of care.
• Assess the situation to determine the need for wound cleaning, a dressing change, or emptying of the drain.

- Assess the patient's level of comfort and the need for analgesics before wound care. Assess if the patient experienced any pain related to prior dressing changes and the effectiveness of interventions used to minimize the patient's pain.
- Assess the current dressing. Assess for the presence of excess drainage or bleeding or saturation of the dressing.
- Assess the patency of the drain and the drain site. Note the characteristics of the drainage in the collection bag. Inspect the wound and the surrounding tissue.
- Assess the appearance of the incision for the approximation of wound edges, the color of the wound and surrounding area, and signs of dehiscence. Note the stage of the healing process and characteristics of any drainage.
- Assess the surrounding skin for color, temperature, and edema, ecchymosis, or maceration.

NURSING DIAGNOSES
- Anxiety
- Acute Pain
- Disturbed Body Image
- Impaired Skin Integrity
- Deficient Knowledge
- Delayed Surgical Recovery
- Impaired Tissue Integrity

OUTCOME IDENTIFICATION AND PLANNING

Expected outcomes may include:
- Jackson-Pratt drain is patent and intact.
- Care is accomplished without contaminating the wound area, without causing trauma to the wound or causing the patient to experience pain or discomfort.
- Patient's wound continues to show signs of healing progression.
- Drainage amounts are measured accurately at the frequency required by facility policy and recorded as part of the intake and output record.
- Patient demonstrates understanding about drain care.

IMPLEMENTATION

ACTION

RATIONALE

1. Review the medical orders for wound care or the nursing plan of care related to wound/drain care.

Reviewing the order and plan of care validates the correct patient and correct procedure.

2. Gather the necessary supplies and bring to the bedside stand or overbed table.

Preparation promotes efficient time management and an organized approach to the task.

ACTION	RATIONALE
	Bringing everything to the bedside conserves time and energy. Arranging items nearby is convenient, saves time, and avoids unnecessary stretching and twisting of muscles on the part of the nurse.
3. Perform hand hygiene and put on PPE, if indicated.	Hand hygiene and PPE prevent the spread of microorganisms. PPE is required based on transmission precautions.
4. Identify the patient.	Identifying the patient ensures the right patient receives the intervention and helps prevent errors.
5. Close curtains around bed and close the door to the room, if possible. Explain what you are going to do and why you are going to do it to the patient.	This ensures the patient's privacy. Explanation relieves anxiety and facilitates cooperation.
6. Assess the patient for possible need for nonpharmacologic pain-reducing interventions or analgesic medication before wound care dressing change. Administer appropriate prescribed analgesic. Allow sufficient time for the analgesic to achieve its effectiveness before beginning the procedure.	Pain is a subjective experience influenced by past experience. Wound care and dressing changes may cause pain for some patients.
7. Place a waste receptacle at a convenient location for use during the procedure.	Having a waste container handy means that the soiled dressing may be discarded easily, without the spread of microorganisms.
8. Adjust bed to comfortable working height, usually elbow height of the caregiver (VISN 8 Patient Safety Center, 2009).	Having the bed at the proper height prevents back and muscle strain.

ACTION	RATIONALE
9. Assist the patient to a comfortable position that provides easy access to the drain and/or wound area. Use a bath blanket to cover any exposed area other than the wound. Place a waterproof pad under the wound site.	Patient positioning and use of a bath blanket provide for comfort and warmth. Waterproof pad protects underlying surfaces.
10. Put on clean gloves; put on mask or face shield, if indicated.	Gloves prevent the spread of microorganisms; mask reduces the risk of transmission should splashing occur.
11. Place the graduated collection container under the outlet of the drain. Without contaminating the outlet valve, pull off the cap. The chamber will expand completely as it draws in air. **Empty the chamber's contents completely into the container. Use the gauze pad to clean the outlet. Fully compress the chamber with one hand and replace the cap with your other hand (FIGURE 1).**	Emptying the drainage allows for accurate measurement. Cleaning the outlet reduces the risk of contamination and helps prevent the spread of microorganisms. Compressing the chamber reestablishes the suction.

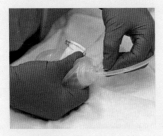

FIGURE 1 Compressing Jackson-Pratt drain and replacing cap.

| 12. Check the patency of the equipment. Make sure the tubing is free from twists and kinks. | Patent, untwisted, or unkinked tubing promotes appropriate drainage from the wound. |

ACTION	RATIONALE
13. Secure the Jackson-Pratt drain to the patient's gown below the wound with a safety pin, making sure that there is no tension on the tubing.	Securing the drain prevents injury to the patient and accidental removal of the drain.
14. Carefully measure and record the character, color, and amount of the drainage. Discard the drainage according to facility policy. Remove gloves.	Documentation promotes continuity of care and communication. Appropriate disposal of biohazard material reduces the risk for microorganism transmission. Proper disposal of gloves deters transmission of microorganisms.
15. Put on clean gloves. If the drain site has a dressing, redress the site as outlined in Skill 55. Also clean the sutures with the gauze pad moistened with normal saline. Dry sutures with gauze before applying a new dressing.	Dressing protects the site. Cleaning and drying sutures deters growth of microorganisms.
16. If the drain site is open to air, observe the sutures that secure the drain to the skin. Look for signs of pulling, tearing, swelling, or infection of the surrounding skin. Gently clean the sutures with the gauze pad moistened with normal saline. Dry with a new gauze pad. Apply skin protectant to the surrounding skin, if needed.	Early detection of problems leads to prompt intervention and prevents complications. Gentle cleaning and drying prevent the growth of microorganisms. Skin protectant prevents skin irritation and breakdown.
17. Remove and discard gloves. Remove all remaining equipment; place the patient in a comfortable position, with side rails up and bed in the lowest position.	Proper removal and disposal of gloves prevent the spread of microorganisms. Proper patient and bed positioning promotes safety and comfort.
18. Remove additional PPE, if used. Perform hand hygiene.	Removing PPE properly reduces the risk for infection transmission and contamination of other items. Hand hygiene prevents the spread of microorganisms.

ACTION	RATIONALE
19. Check drain status at least every 4 hours. Check all wound dressings every shift. More frequent checks may be needed if the wound is more complex or dressings become saturated quickly.	Checking the drain ensures proper functioning and early detection of problems. Checking dressings ensures the assessment of changes in patient condition and timely intervention to prevent complications

EVALUATION

• Patient exhibits a patent and intact Jackson-Pratt drain with a wound area that is free of contamination and trauma.
• Patient verbalizes minimal to no pain or discomfort.
• Patient exhibits signs and symptoms of progressive wound healing, with drainage being measured accurately at the frequency required by facility policy, and amounts recorded as part of the intake and output record.
• Patient verbalizes an understanding of the rationale for and/or the technique for drain care.

DOCUMENTATION

• Document the location of the wound and drain, the assessment of the wound and drain site, and patency of the drain. Note if sutures are intact. Document the presence of drainage and characteristics of the old dressing upon removal. Include the appearance of the surrounding skin. Document cleansing of the drain site. Record any skin care and the dressing applied. Note that the drain was emptied and recompressed. Note pertinent patient and family education and any patient reaction to this procedure, including patient's pain level and effectiveness of nonpharmacologic interventions or analgesia, if administered. Document the amount and characteristics of drainage obtained on the appropriate intake and output record.

GENERAL CONSIDERATIONS

• Often patients have more than one Jackson-Pratt drain. Number or letter the drains for easy identification. Record the drainage from each drain separately, identified by the number or letter, on the intake and output record.
• When the patient with a drain is ready to ambulate, empty and compress the drain before activity. Secure the drain to the patient's gown below the wound, making sure there is no tension on the drainage tubing. This removes excess drainage, maintains maximal suction, and avoids strain on the drain's suture line.

Skill · 53   Caring for a Penrose Drain

Drains are inserted into or near a wound when it is anticipated that a collection of fluid in a closed area would delay healing. A Penrose drain is a hollow, open-ended rubber tube. It allows fluid to drain via capillary action into absorbent dressings. Penrose drains are commonly used after a surgical procedure or for drainage of an abscess. After a surgical procedure, the surgeon places one end of the drain in or near the area to be drained. The other end passes through the skin, directly through the incision or through a separate opening referred to as a stab wound. A Penrose drain is not sutured. A large safety pin is usually placed in the part outside the wound to prevent the drain from slipping back into the incised area. This type of drain can be advanced or shortened to drain different areas. The patency and placement of the drain are included in the wound assessment.

EQUIPMENT

- Sterile gloves
- Gauze dressings
- Sterile cotton-tipped applicators, if appropriate
- Sterile drain sponges
- Surgical or abdominal pads
- Sterile dressing set or suture set (for the sterile scissors and forceps)
- Sterile cleaning solution, as ordered (commonly 0.9% normal saline solution)
- Sterile container to hold cleaning solution
- Clean safety pin
- Clean disposable gloves
- Plastic bag or other appropriate waste container for soiled dressings
- Waterproof pad and bath blanket
- Tape or ties
- Skin-protectant wipes, if needed
- Additional dressings and supplies needed or as required for ordered wound care

ASSESSMENT GUIDELINES

- Assess the situation to determine the necessity for wound cleaning and a dressing change. Confirm any medical orders relevant to drain care and any drain care included in the nursing plan of care.
- Assess the patient's level of comfort and the need for analgesics before wound care. Assess if the patient experienced any pain related to prior dressing changes and the effectiveness of interventions used to minimize the patient's pain.
- Assess the current dressing to determine if it is intact, and assess for the presence of excess drainage, bleeding, or saturation of the dressing.
- Assess the patency of the Penrose drain.

- Inspect the wound and the surrounding tissue. Assess the appearance of the wound for the approximation of wound edges, the color of the wound and surrounding area, and signs of dehiscence. Note the stage of the healing process and the characteristics of any drainage.
- Assess the surrounding skin for color, temperature, and the presence of edema, ecchymosis, or maceration.

NURSING DIAGNOSES

- Anxiety
- Acute Pain
- Disturbed Body Image
- Impaired Skin Integrity
- Deficient Knowledge
- Delayed Surgical Recovery
- Impaired Tissue Integrity

OUTCOME IDENTIFICATION AND PLANNING

Expected outcomes may include:
- Penrose drain remains patent and intact; the care is accomplished without contaminating the wound area, or causing trauma to the wound, and without causing the patient to experience pain or discomfort.
- Patient's wound shows signs of progressive healing without evidence of complications.
- Patient demonstrates understanding about drain care.

IMPLEMENTATION

ACTION	RATIONALE
1. Review the medical orders for wound care or the nursing plan of care related to wound/drain care.	Reviewing the order and plan of care validates the correct patient and correct procedure.
2. Gather the necessary supplies and bring to the bedside stand or overbed table.	Preparation promotes efficient time management and an organized approach to the task. Bringing everything to the bedside conserves time and energy. Arranging items nearby is convenient, saves time, and avoids unnecessary stretching and twisting of muscles on the part of the nurse.

ACTION	RATIONALE
3. Perform hand hygiene and put on PPE, if indicated.	Hand hygiene and PPE prevent the spread of microorganisms. PPE is required based on transmission precautions.
4. Identify the patient.	Identifying the patient ensures the right patient receives the intervention and helps prevent errors.
5. Close curtains around bed and close the door to the room, if possible. Explain what you are going to do and why you are going to do it to the patient.	This ensures the patient's privacy. Explanation relieves anxiety and facilitates cooperation.
6. Assess the patient for possible need for nonpharmacologic pain-reducing interventions or analgesic medication before wound care dressing change. Administer appropriate prescribed analgesic. Allow sufficient time for the analgesic to achieve its effectiveness before beginning the procedure.	Pain is a subjective experience influenced by past experience. Wound care and dressing changes may cause pain for some patients.
7. Place a waste receptacle at a convenient location for use during the procedure.	Having a waste container handy means that the soiled dressing may be discarded easily, without the spread of microorganisms.
8. Adjust bed to comfortable working height, usually elbow height of the caregiver (VISN 8 Patient Safety Center, 2009).	Having the bed at the proper height prevents back and muscle strain.
9. Assist the patient to a comfortable position that provides easy access to the drain and/or wound area. Use a bath blanket to cover any exposed area other than the wound. Place a waterproof pad under the wound site.	Patient positioning and use of a bath blanket provide for comfort and warmth. Waterproof pad protects underlying surfaces.

ACTION	RATIONALE
10. Put on clean gloves. Check the position of the drain or drains before removing the dressing. Carefully and gently remove the soiled dressings. If there is resistance, use a silicone-based adhesive remover to help remove the tape. If any part of the dressing sticks to the underlying skin, use small amounts of sterile saline to help loosen and remove it.	Gloves protect the nurse from handling contaminated dressings. Checking the position ensures that a drain is not removed accidentally if one is present. Cautious removal of the dressing is more comfortable for the patient and ensures that any drain present is not removed. A silicone-based adhesive remover allows for the easy, rapid, and painless removal without the associated problems of skin stripping (Rudoni, 2008; Stephen-Haynes, 2008). Sterile saline moistens the dressing for easier removal and minimizes damage and pain.
11. After removing the dressing, note the presence, amount, type, color, and odor of any drainage on the dressings. Place soiled dressings in the appropriate waste receptacle.	The presence of drainage should be documented. Discarding dressings appropriately prevents the spread of microorganisms.
12. Inspect the drain site for appearance and drainage. Assess if any pain is present.	The wound healing process and/or the presence of irritation or infection must be documented.
13. Using sterile technique, prepare a sterile work area and open the needed supplies.	Supplies are within easy reach and sterility is maintained.
14. Open the sterile cleansing solution. Pour the cleansing solution into the basin. Add the gauze sponges.	Sterility of dressings and solution is maintained.
15. Put on sterile gloves.	Sterile gloves help to maintain surgical asepsis and sterile technique and prevent the spread of microorganisms.
16. Cleanse the drain site with the cleansing solution. Use the forceps and the moistened gauze or cotton-tipped applicators. **Start at the drain insertion site, moving**	Using a circular motion ensures that cleaning occurs from the least to most contaminated area and a previously cleaned area is not contaminated again.

ACTION	RATIONALE

in a circular motion toward the periphery. Use each gauze sponge or applicator only once. Discard and use new gauze if additional cleansing is needed.

17. Dry the skin with a new gauze pad in the same manner. Apply skin protectant to the skin around the drain; extend out to include the area of skin that will be taped. Place a presplit drain sponge under the drain (FIGURE 1). Closely observe the safety pin in the drain. If the pin or drain is crusted, replace the pin with a new sterile pin. **Take care not to dislodge the drain.**

Drying prevents skin irritation. Skin protectant prevents skin irritation and breakdown. The gauze absorbs drainage and prevents the drainage from accumulating on the patient's skin.

Microorganisms grow more easily in a soiled environment. The safety pin ensures proper placement because the drain is not sutured in place.

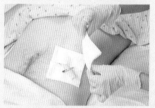

FIGURE 1 Presplit dressing around Penrose drain.

18. Apply gauze pads over the drain. Apply ABD pads over the gauze.

The gauze absorbs drainage. Pads provide extra absorption for excess drainage and a moisture barrier.

19. Remove and discard gloves. Apply tape, Montgomery straps, or roller gauze to secure the dressings.

Proper disposal of gloves prevents the spread of microorganisms. Tape or other securing products are easier to apply after gloves have been removed.

20. After securing the dressing, label it with date and time. Remove all remaining equipment; place the patient in a comfortable position, with side rails up and bed in the lowest position.

Recording date and time provides communication and demonstrates adherence to plan of care. Proper patient and bed positioning promotes safety and comfort.

ACTION	RATIONALE
21. Remove additional PPE, if used. Perform hand hygiene.	Removing PPE properly reduces the risk for infection transmission and contamination of other items. Hand hygiene prevents the spread of microorganisms.
22. Check all wound dressings every shift. More frequent checks may be needed if the wound is more complex or dressings become saturated quickly.	Checking dressings ensures the assessment of changes in patient condition and timely intervention to prevent complications.

EVALUATION

• Patient exhibits a wound that is clean, dry, and intact, with a patent, intact Penrose drain.
• Patient remains free of wound contamination and trauma.
• Patient reports minimal to no pain or discomfort.
• Patient exhibits signs and symptoms of progressive wound healing.
• Patient verbalizes an understanding of the rationale for and/or the technique for drain care.

DOCUMENTATION

• Document the location of the wound and drain, the assessment of the wound and drain site, and status of the Penrose drain. Document the presence of drainage and characteristics of the old dressing upon removal. Include the appearance of the surrounding skin. Document cleansing of the drain site. Record any skin care and the dressing applied. Note pertinent patient and family education and any patient reaction to this procedure, including patient's pain level and effectiveness of nonpharmacologic interventions or analgesia, if administered.

GENERAL CONSIDERATIONS

• Evaluate a sudden increase in the amount of drainage or bright red drainage and notify the primary care provider of these findings.
• Wound care is often uncomfortable, and patients may experience significant pain. Assess the patient's comfort level and past experiences with wound care. Offer analgesics, as ordered, to maintain the patient's level of comfort.

Skill · 54   Caring for a T-Tube Drain

A biliary drain or T-tube is sometimes placed in the common bile duct after removal of the gallbladder (cholecystectomy) or a portion of the bile duct (choledochostomy). The tube drains bile while the surgical site is healing. A portion of the tube is inserted into the common bile duct and the remaining portion is anchored to the abdominal wall, passed through the skin, and connected to a closed drainage system. Often, a three-way valve is inserted between the drain tube and the drainage system to allow for clamping and flushing of the tube, if necessary. The drainage amount is measured every shift, recorded, and included in output totals.

EQUIPMENT

- Sterile gloves
- Clean disposable gloves
- Additional PPE, as indicated
- Sterile gauze pads
- Sterile drain sponges
- Cleansing solution, usually sterile normal saline
- Sterile cotton-tipped applicators (if appropriate)
- Transparent dressing
- Graduated collection container
- Waste receptacle
- Sterile basin
- Sterile forceps
- Tape
- Skin-protectant wipes
- Waterproof pad and bath blanket, if needed

ASSESSMENT GUIDELINES

- Assess the situation to determine the need for wound cleaning, a dressing change, or emptying of the drain.
- Confirm any medical orders relevant to drain care and any drain care included in the nursing plan of care.
- Assess the patient's level of comfort and the need for analgesics before wound care. Assess if the patient experienced any pain related to prior dressing changes and the effectiveness of interventions used to minimize the patient's pain.
- Assess the current dressing to determine if it is intact, and assess for evidence of excessive drainage or bleeding or saturation of the dressing.
- Assess the patency of the T-tube and the drain site. Note the characteristics of the drainage in the collection bag.
- Inspect the wound and the surrounding tissue. Assess the appearance of the incision for the approximation of wound edges, the color of the wound and surrounding area, and signs of dehiscence. Note the stage of the healing process and characteristics of any drainage.
- Assess the surrounding skin for color, temperature, and edema, ecchymosis, or maceration.

NURSING DIAGNOSES

• Acute Pain
• Disturbed Body Image
• Anxiety
• Impaired Skin Integrity
• Deficient Knowledge
• Delayed Surgical Recovery
• Impaired Tissue Integrity

OUTCOME IDENTIFICATION AND PLANNING

Expected outcomes may include:
• Patient's T-tube drain remains patent and intact.
• Drain care is accomplished without contaminating the wound area and/or without causing trauma to the wound; and the patient does not experience pain or discomfort.
• Patient's wound continues to show signs of healing progression.
• Drainage amounts are measured accurately at the frequency required by facility policy and recorded as part of the intake and output record.
• Patient demonstrates understanding about drain care.

IMPLEMENTATION

ACTION	RATIONALE
1. Review the medical orders for wound care or the nursing plan of care related to wound/drain care.	Reviewing the order and plan of care validates the correct patient and correct procedure.
2. Gather the necessary supplies and bring to the bedside stand or overbed table.	Preparation promotes efficient time management and an organized approach to the task. Bringing everything to the bedside conserves time and energy. Arranging items nearby is convenient, saves time, and avoids unnecessary stretching and twisting of muscles on the part of the nurse.
3. Perform hand hygiene and put on PPE, if indicated.	Hand hygiene and PPE prevent the spread of microorganisms. PPE is required based on transmission precautions.

ACTION	RATIONALE

4. Identify the patient.

Identifying the patient ensures the right patient receives the intervention and helps prevent errors.

5. Close curtains around bed and close the door to the room, if possible. Explain what you are going to do and why you are going to do it to the patient.

This ensures the patient's privacy. Explanation relieves anxiety and facilitates cooperation.

6. Assess the patient for possible need for nonpharmacologic pain-reducing interventions or analgesic medication before wound care dressing change. Administer appropriate prescribed analgesic. Allow sufficient time for the analgesic to achieve its effectiveness before beginning the procedure.

Pain is a subjective experience influenced by past experience. Wound care and dressing changes may cause pain for some patients.

7. Place a waste receptacle at a convenient location for use during the procedure.

Having a waste container handy means that the soiled dressing may be discarded easily, without the spread of microorganisms.

8. Adjust bed to comfortable working height, usually elbow height of the caregiver (VISN 8 Patient Safety Center, 2009).

Having the bed at the proper height prevents back and muscle strain.

9. Assist the patient to a comfortable position that provides easy access to the drain and/or wound area. Use a bath blanket to cover any exposed area other than the wound. Place a waterproof pad under the wound site.

Patient positioning and use of a bath blanket provide for comfort and warmth. Waterproof pad protects underlying surfaces.

Emptying Drainage

10. Put on clean gloves; put on mask or face shield, if indicated.

Gloves prevent the spread of microorganisms; mask reduces the risk of transmission should splashing occur.

ACTION	RATIONALE
11. Using sterile technique, open a gauze pad, making a sterile field with the outer wrapper.	Using sterile technique deters the spread of microorganisms.
12. Place the graduated collection container under the outlet valve of the drainage bag. **Without touching the outlet, pull off the cap and empty the bag's contents completely into the container. Use the gauze to wipe the outlet, and replace the cap.**	Draining contents into a container allows for accurate measurement of the drainage. Touching the outlet with gloves or other surface contaminates the valve, potentially introducing pathogens. Wiping the outlet with gauze prevents contamination of the valve. Recapping prevents the spread of microorganisms.
13. Carefully measure and note the characteristics of the drainage. Discard the drainage according to facility policy.	Documentation promotes continuity of care and communication. Appropriate disposal of biohazard material reduces the risk for microorganism transmission.
14. Remove gloves and perform hand hygiene.	Proper glove removal and performing hand hygiene prevent spread of microorganisms.

Cleaning the Drain Site

15. Put on clean gloves. Check the position of the drain or drains before removing the dressing. Carefully and gently remove the soiled dressings. If there is resistance, use a silicone-based adhesive remover to help remove the tape. If any part of the dressing sticks to the underlying skin, use small amounts of sterile saline to help loosen and remove it. Do not reach over the drain site.	Gloves protect the nurse from handling contaminated dressings. Checking the position ensures that a drain is not removed accidentally if one is present. Cautious removal of the dressing is more comfortable for the patient and ensures that any drain present is not removed. A silicone-based adhesive remover allows for the easy, rapid, and painless removal without the associated problems of skin stripping (Rudoni, 2008; Stephen-Haynes, 2008). Sterile saline moistens the dressing for easier removal and minimizes damage and pain.

ACTION	RATIONALE
16. After removing the dressing, note the presence, amount, type, color, and odor of any drainage on the dressings. Place soiled dressings in the appropriate waste receptacle. Remove gloves and dispose of in appropriate waste receptacle.	The presence of drainage should be documented. Proper disposal of gloves prevents spread of microorganisms.
17. Inspect the drain site for appearance and drainage. Assess if any pain is present.	Wound healing process and/or the presence of irritation or infection should be documented.
18. Using sterile technique, prepare a sterile work area and open the needed supplies.	Preparing a sterile work area ensures that supplies are within easy reach and sterility is maintained.
19. Open the sterile cleansing solution. Pour the cleansing solution into the basin. Add the gauze sponges.	Sterility of dressings and solution is maintained.
20. Put on sterile gloves.	Use of sterile gloves maintains surgical asepsis and sterile technique and reduces the risk of microorganism transmission.
21. Cleanse the drain site with the cleansing solution. Use the forceps and the moistened gauze or cotton-tipped applicators. **Start at the drain insertion site, moving in a circular motion toward the periphery. Use each gauze sponge only once. Discard and use new gauze if additional cleansing is needed.**	Cleansing is done from the least to most contaminated area so that a previously cleaned area is not contaminated again.
22. Dry with new sterile gauze in the same manner. Apply skin protectant to the skin around the drain; extend out to include the area of skin that will be taped.	Drying prevents skin irritation. Skin protectant prevents skin irritation and breakdown.

ACTION	RATIONALE
23. Place a presplit drain sponge under the drain. Apply gauze pads over the drain. Remove and discard gloves.	The gauze absorbs drainage and prevents the drainage from accumulating on the patient's skin. Proper disposal of gloves prevents spread of microorganisms.
24. Secure the dressings with tape, as needed. Alternatively, before removing gloves, place a transparent dressing over the tube and insertion site. **Be careful not to kink the tubing.**	Kinked tubing could block drainage. Facility policy often determines type of dressing used.
25. After securing the dressing, label dressing with date and time. Remove all remaining equipment; place the patient in a comfortable position, with side rails up and bed in the lowest position.	Recording date and time provides communication and demonstrates adherence to plan of care. Proper patient and bed positioning promotes safety and comfort.
26. Remove additional PPE, if used. Perform hand hygiene.	Removing PPE properly reduces the risk for infection transmission and contamination of other items. Hand hygiene prevents the spread of microorganisms.
27. Check drain status at least every 4 hours. Check all wound dressings every shift. More frequent checks may be needed if the wound is more complex or dressings become saturated quickly.	Checking drain ensures proper functioning and early detection of problems. Checking dressings ensures the assessment of changes in patient condition and timely intervention to prevent complications.

EVALUATION

• Patient exhibits a patent and intact T-tube drain with a wound area that is free of contamination and trauma.
• Patient verbalizes minimal to no pain or discomfort.
• Patient exhibits signs and symptoms of progressive wound healing, with drainage being measured accurately at the frequency required by facility policy, and amounts recorded as part of the intake and output record.
• Patient verbalizes an understanding of the rationale for and/or the technique for drain care.

DOCUMENTATION

• Document the location of the wound and drain, the assessment of the wound and drain site, and patency of the drain. Note if sutures are intact. Document the presence of drainage and characteristics of the old dressing upon removal. Include the appearance of the surrounding skin. Document cleansing of the drain site. Record any skin care and the dressing applied. Note pertinent patient and family education and any patient reaction to this procedure, including patient's pain level and effectiveness of nonpharmacologic interventions or analgesia, if administered. Document the amount of bile drainage obtained from the drainage bag on the appropriate intake and output record.

GENERAL CONSIDERATIONS

• When the patient with a drain is ready to ambulate, empty the drain before activity. Secure the drain to the patient's gown below the wound, making sure there is no tension on the drainage tubing. This removes excess drainage, maintains maximal suction, and avoids strain on the drain's suture line.

• Evaluate a sudden increase in the amount of drainage or bright red drainage and notify the primary care provider of these findings.

• Wound care is often uncomfortable, and patients may experience significant pain. Assess the patient's comfort level and past experiences with wound care. Offer analgesics, as ordered, to maintain the patient's level of comfort.

Skill · 55 **Cleaning a Wound and Applying a Dry, Sterile Dressing**

Wound care may include cleaning of the wound and the use of a dressing as a protective covering over the wound. Wound cleansing is performed to remove debris, contaminants, and excess exudate. Sterile normal saline is the preferred cleansing solution.

There is no standard frequency for how often dressings should be changed. It depends on the amount of drainage, the primary practitioner's preference, the nature of the wound, and the particular wound care product being used. It is customary for the surgeon or other advanced practice professional to perform the first dressing change on a surgical wound, usually within 24 to 48 hours after surgery.

EQUIPMENT

- Sterile gloves
- Clean disposable gloves
- Additional PPE, as indicated
- Gauze dressings
- Surgical or abdominal pads
- Sterile dressing set or suture set (for the sterile scissors and forceps)
- Sterile cleaning solution as ordered (commonly 0.9% normal saline solution, or a commercially prepared wound cleanser)

- Sterile basin (may be optional)
- Sterile drape (may be optional)
- Plastic bag or other appropriate waste container for soiled dressings
- Waterproof pad and bath blanket
- Tape or ties
- Bath blanket or other linens for draping patient
- Additional dressings and supplies needed or required by the primary care provider's order

ASSESSMENT GUIDELINES

- Assess the situation to determine the need for wound cleaning and a dressing change. Confirm any medical orders relevant to wound care and any wound care included in the nursing plan of care.
- Assess the patient's level of comfort and the need for analgesics before wound care. Assess if the patient experienced any pain related to prior dressing changes and the effectiveness of interventions used to minimize the patient's pain.
- Assess the current dressing to determine if it is intact. Assess for excess drainage, bleeding, or saturation of the dressing.
- Inspect the wound and the surrounding tissue. Assess the appearance of the wound for the approximation of wound edges, the color of the wound and surrounding area, and signs of dehiscence. Assess for the presence of sutures, staples, or adhesive closure strips. Note the stage of the healing process and characteristics of any drainage. Also assess the surrounding skin for color, temperature, and edema, ecchymosis, or maceration.

NURSING DIAGNOSES

- Risk for Infection
- Acute Pain
- Anxiety
- Impaired Skin Integrity
- Disturbed Body Image
- Deficient Knowledge
- Impaired Tissue Integrity
- Delayed Surgical Recovery

OUTCOME IDENTIFICATION AND PLANNING

Expected outcomes may include:
- Patient's wound is cleaned and protected with a dressing without contaminating the wound area, without causing trauma to the wound, and without causing the patient to experience pain or discomfort.

• Patient's wound continues to show signs of healing progression.
• Patient demonstrates understanding of the need for wound care and dressing change.

IMPLEMENTATION

ACTION	RATIONALE
1. Review the medical orders for wound care or the nursing plan of care related to wound care.	Reviewing the order and plan of care validates the correct patient and correct procedure.
2. Gather the necessary supplies and bring to the bedside stand or overbed table.	Preparation promotes efficient time management and an organized approach to the task. Bringing everything to the bedside conserves time and energy. Arranging items nearby is convenient, saves time, and avoids unnecessary stretching and twisting of muscles on the part of the nurse.
3. Perform hand hygiene and put on PPE, if indicated.	Hand hygiene and PPE prevent the spread of microorganisms. PPE is required based on transmission precautions.
4. Identify the patient.	Identifying the patient ensures the right patient receives the intervention and helps prevent errors.
5. Close curtains around bed and close the door to the room, if possible. Explain what you are going to do and why you are going to do it to the patient.	This ensures the patient's privacy. Explanation relieves anxiety and facilitates cooperation.
6. Assess the patient for possible need for nonpharmacologic pain-reducing interventions or analgesic medication before wound care dressing change. Administer appropriate prescribed analgesic. Allow sufficient time for the analgesic to achieve its effectiveness.	Pain is a subjective experience influenced by past experience. Wound care and dressing changes may cause pain for some patients.

ACTION	RATIONALE
7. Place a waste receptacle or bag at a convenient location for use during the procedure.	Having a waste container handy means the soiled dressing may be discarded easily, without the spread of microorganisms.
8. Adjust bed to comfortable working height, usually elbow height of the caregiver (VISN 8 Patient Safety Center, 2009).	Having the bed at the proper height prevents back and muscle strain.
9. Assist the patient to a comfortable position that provides easy access to the wound area. Use the bath blanket to cover any exposed area other than the wound. Place a waterproof pad under the wound site.	Patient positioning and use of a bath blanket provide for comfort and warmth. Waterproof pad protects underlying surfaces.
10. Check the position of drains, tubes, or other adjuncts before removing the dressing. Put on clean, disposable gloves and loosen tape on the old dressings. If necessary, use an adhesive remover to help remove the tape.	Checking ensures that a drain is not removed accidentally if one is present. Gloves protect the nurse from contaminated dressings and prevent the spread of microorganisms. Adhesive-tape remover helps reduce patient discomfort during removal of the dressing.
11. Carefully remove the soiled dressings. If there is resistance, use a silicone-based adhesive remover to help remove the tape. If any part of the dressing sticks to the underlying skin, use small amounts of sterile saline to help loosen and remove it.	Cautious removal of the dressing is more comfortable for the patient and ensures that any drain present is not removed. A silicone-based adhesive remover allows for the easy, rapid, and painless removal without the associated problems of skin stripping (Rudoni, 2008; Stephen-Haynes, 2008). Sterile saline moistens the dressing for easier removal and minimizes damage and pain.
12. After removing the dressing, note the presence, amount, type, color, and odor of any drainage on the dressings. Place soiled dressings in the appropriate waste receptacle. Remove your gloves and dispose of them in an appropriate waste receptacle.	The presence of drainage should be documented. Proper disposal of soiled dressings and used gloves prevents spread of microorganisms.

ACTION	RATIONALE
13. Inspect the wound site for size, appearance, and drainage. Assess if any pain is present. Check the status of sutures, adhesive closure strips, staples, and drains or tubes, if present. Note any problems to include in your documentation.	Wound healing or the presence of irritation or infection should be documented.
14. **Using sterile technique, prepare a sterile work area and open the needed supplies.**	Supplies are within easy reach and sterility is maintained.
15. Open the sterile cleaning solution. Depending on the amount of cleaning needed, the solution might be poured directly over gauze sponges over a container for small cleaning jobs, or into a basin for more complex or larger cleaning.	Sterility of dressings and solution is maintained.
16. Put on sterile gloves.	Use of sterile gloves maintains surgical asepsis and sterile technique and reduces the risk for spreading microorganisms.
17. Clean the wound. **Clean the wound from top to bottom and from the center to the outside (FIGURE 1). Following this pattern, use new gauze for each wipe, placing the used gauze in the waste receptacle. Alternately, spray the wound from top to bottom with a commercially prepared wound cleanser.**	Cleaning from top to bottom and center to outside ensures that cleaning occurs from the least to most contaminated area and a previously cleaned area is not contaminated again. Using a single gauze for each wipe ensures that the previously cleaned area is not recontaminated.

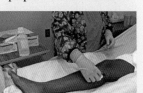

FIGURE 1 Cleaning wound with dampened gauze.

ACTION	RATIONALE
18. Once the wound is cleaned, dry the area using a gauze sponge in the same manner. Apply ointment or perform other treatments, as ordered.	Moisture provides a medium for growth of microorganisms. The growth of microorganisms may be inhibited and the healing process improved with the use of ordered ointments or other applications.
19. If a drain is in use at the wound location, clean around the drain. Refer to Skills 51–54.	Cleaning the insertion site helps prevent infection.
20. Apply a layer of dry, sterile dressing over the wound. Forceps may be used to apply the dressing.	Primary dressing serves as a wick for drainage. Use of forceps helps ensure that sterile technique is maintained.
21. Place a second layer of gauze over the wound site.	A second layer provides for increased absorption of drainage.
22. Apply a surgical or abdominal pad (ABD) over the gauze at the site as the outermost layer of the dressing.	The dressing acts as additional protection for the wound against microorganisms in the environment.
23. Remove and discard gloves. Apply tape, Montgomery straps, or roller gauze to secure the dressings. Alternately, many commercial wound products are self-adhesive and do not require additional tape.	Proper disposal of gloves prevents the spread of microorganisms. Tape or other securing products are easier to apply after gloves have been removed.
24. After securing the dressing, label it with date and time. Remove all remaining equipment; place the patient in a comfortable position, with side rails up and bed in the lowest position.	Recording date and time provides communication and demonstrates adherence to plan of care. Proper patient and bed positioning promotes safety and comfort.
25. Remove PPE, if used. Perform hand hygiene.	Removing PPE properly reduces the risk for infection transmission and contamination of other items. Hand hygiene prevents the spread of microorganisms.
26. Check all wound dressings every shift. More frequent checks may be needed if the wound is more complex or dressings become saturated quickly.	Checking dressings ensures the assessment of changes in patient condition and timely intervention to prevent complications.

EVALUATION

- Patient exhibits a clean, intact wound with a clean dressing in place.
- Patient's wound is free of contamination and trauma.
- Patient reports little to no pain or discomfort during care.
- Patient demonstrates signs and symptoms of progressive wound healing.

DOCUMENTATION

- Document the location of the wound and that the dressing was removed. Record assessment of the wound, including approximation of wound edges, presence of sutures, staples, or adhesive closure strips, and the condition of the surrounding skin. Note if redness, edema, or drainage is observed. Document cleansing of the incision with normal saline and any application of antibiotic ointment as ordered. Record the type of dressing that was reapplied. Note pertinent patient and family education and any patient reaction to this procedure, including patient's pain level and effectiveness of nonpharmacologic interventions or analgesia if administered.

GENERAL CONSIDERATIONS

- Instruct the patient, if appropriate, and ancillary staff members to observe for excessive drainage that may overwhelm the dressing. They should also report when dressings become soiled or loosened from the skin.
- The skin of older adults is less elastic and more sensitive; use paper tape, Montgomery straps (Refer to Skill 109), or roller gauze (on extremities) to prevent tearing of the skin.

Skill · 56 **Applying a Hydrocolloid Dressing**

Hydrocolloid dressings are wafer-shaped dressings that come in many shapes, sizes, and thicknesses. An adhesive backing provides adherence to the wound and surrounding skin. These dressings absorb drainage, maintain a moist wound surface, and decrease the risk for infection by covering the wound surface. Many commercially prepared dressing and wound care products are applied in a similar manner. It is very important for the nurse to be aware of the products available in a particular facility and be familiar with the indications for, and correct use of, each type of dressing and wound care product.

EQUIPMENT

- Hydrocolloid dressing
- Clean disposable gloves
- Sterile gloves, if indicated
- Additional PPE, as indicated
- Sterile dressing instrument set or suture set (for the scissors and forceps)
- Sterile cleaning solution as ordered (commonly 0.9% normal saline solution)

- Skin-protectant wipes
- Additional supplies needed for wound cleansing
- Sterile cotton-tipped applicators
- Waterproof pad
- Bath blanket
- Measuring tape or other supplies, such as sterile flexible applicator, for assessing wound measurements, as indicated

ASSESSMENT GUIDELINES

- Assess the situation to determine the need for a dressing change. Check the date when the current dressing (if present) was placed. Confirm any medical orders relevant to wound care and any wound care included in the nursing plan of care. Assess the current dressing to determine if it is intact.
- Assess the patient's level of comfort and the need for analgesics before wound care. Assess if the patient experienced any pain related to prior dressing changes and the effectiveness of interventions used to minimize the patient's pain.
- Assess the current dressing to determine if it is intact. Assess for excess drainage or bleeding or saturation of the dressing.
- Inspect the wound and the surrounding tissue. Assess the location, appearance of the wound, stage (if appropriate), drainage, and types of tissue present in the wound. Measure the wound. Note the stage of the healing process and characteristics of any drainage.
- Assess the surrounding skin for color, temperature, and edema, ecchymosis, or maceration.

NURSING DIAGNOSES

- Anxiety
- Disturbed Body Image
- Risk for Infection
- Chronic Pain
- Acute Pain
- Impaired Tissue Integrity

OUTCOME IDENTIFICATION AND PLANNING

Expected outcomes may include:
- Procedure is accomplished without contaminating the wound area, without causing trauma to the wound, and without causing the patient to experience pain or discomfort.
- Sterile technique is maintained (if appropriate).
- Wound healing is promoted.

• Patient's skin surrounding the wound is without signs of irritation, infection, and maceration; and the wound continues to show signs of healing progression.

IMPLEMENTATION

ACTION	RATIONALE
1. Review the medical orders for wound care or the nursing plan of care related to wound care.	Reviewing the order and plan of care validates the correct patient and correct procedure.
2. Gather the necessary supplies and bring to the bedside stand or overbed table.	Preparation promotes efficient time management and an organized approach to the task. Bringing everything to the bedside conserves time and energy. Arranging items nearby is convenient, saves time, and avoids unnecessary stretching and twisting of muscles on the part of the nurse.
3. Perform hand hygiene and put on PPE, if indicated.	Hand hygiene and PPE prevent the spread of microorganisms. PPE is required based on transmission precautions.
4. Identify the patient. 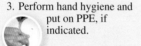	Identifying the patient ensures the right patient receives the intervention and helps prevent errors.
5. Close curtains around bed and close the door to the room, if possible. Explain what you are going to do and why you are going to do it to the patient.	This ensures the patient's privacy. Explanation relieves anxiety and facilitates cooperation.
6. Assess the patient for possible need for nonpharmacologic pain-reducing interventions or analgesic medication before wound care dressing change. Administer appropriate prescribed analgesic. Allow sufficient time for the analgesic to achieve its effectiveness before beginning the procedure.	Pain is a subjective experience influenced by past experience. Wound care and dressing changes may cause pain for some patients.

ACTION	RATIONALE
7. Place a waste receptacle or bag at a convenient location for use during the procedure.	Having a waste container handy means the soiled dressing may be discarded easily, without the spread of microorganisms.
8. Adjust bed to comfortable working height, usually elbow height of the caregiver (VISN 8 Patient Safety Center, 2009).	Having the bed at the proper height prevents back and muscle strain.
9. Assist the patient to a comfortable position that provides easy access to the wound area. Position the patient so the wound cleanser or irrigation solution will flow from the clean end of the wound toward the dirtier end, if being used (See Skill 55 for wound cleansing and Skill 183 for irrigation techniques). Use the bath blanket to cover any exposed area other than the wound. Place a waterproof pad under the wound site.	Patient positioning and use of a bath blanket provide for comfort and warmth. Gravity directs the flow of liquid from the least contaminated to the most contaminated area. Waterproof pad protects underlying surfaces.
10. Put on clean gloves. Carefully and gently remove the soiled dressings. If there is resistance, use a silicone-based adhesive remover to help remove the tape. If any part of the dressing sticks to the underlying skin, use small amounts of sterile saline to help loosen and remove it.	Gloves protect the nurse from handling contaminated dressings. Cautious removal of the dressing is more comfortable for the patient and ensures that any drain present is not removed. A silicone-based adhesive remover allows for the easy, rapid, and painless removal without the associated problems of skin stripping (Rudoni, 2008; Stephen-Haynes, 2008). Sterile saline moistens the dressing for easier removal and minimizes damage and pain.
11. After removing the dressing, note the presence, amount, type, color, and odor of any drainage on the dressings. Place soiled dressings in the appropriate waste receptacle.	The presence of drainage should be documented. Discarding dressings appropriately prevents the spread of microorganisms.

ACTION	RATIONALE
12. Assess the wound for appearance, stage, the presence of eschar, granulation tissue, epithelialization, undermining, tunneling, necrosis, sinus tract, and drainage. Assess the appearance of the surrounding tissue. Measure the wound.	This information provides evidence about the wound healing process and/or the presence of infection.
13. Remove your gloves and put them in the receptacle.	Discarding gloves prevents the spread of microorganisms.
14. Set up a sterile field, if indicated, and wound cleaning supplies. Put on sterile gloves. Alternately, clean gloves (clean technique) may be used when cleaning a chronic wound.	Sterile gloves maintain surgical asepsis. Clean technique is appropriate for cleaning chronic wounds.
15. Clean the wound (Refer to Skill 55). Alternately, irrigate the wound, as ordered or required (See Skill 183).	Cleaning the wound removes previous drainage and wound debris.
16. Dry the surrounding skin with gauze dressings.	Moisture provides a medium for growth of microorganisms. Excess moisture can contribute to skin irritation and breakdown.
17. Apply a skin protectant to the surrounding skin.	A skin protectant prevents skin irritation and breakdown.
18. Cut the dressing to size, if indicated, using sterile scissors. Size the dressing generously, allowing at least a 1-inch margin of healthy skin around the wound to be covered with the dressing.	These actions ensure proper adherence, coverage of the wound, and wear of the dressing.
19. Remove the release paper from the adherent side of the dressing. Apply the dressing to the wound without stretching the dressing. Smooth wrinkles as the dressing is applied (FIGURE 1).	Proper application prevents shearing force on the wound and minimizes irritation.

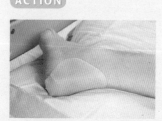

FIGURE 1 Hydrocolloid dressing in place.

20. If necessary, secure the dressing edges with tape. Apply additional skin barrier to the areas to be covered with tape, if necessary. Dressings that are near the anus need to have the edges taped. Apply additional skin barrier to the areas to be covered with tape, if necessary.

Taping helps keep the dressing intact. Skin protectant prevents surrounding skin irritation and breakdown. Taping the edges of dressings near the anus prevents wound contamination from fecal material.

21. After securing the dressing, label it with date and time. Remove all remaining equipment; place the patient in a comfortable position, with side rails up and bed in the lowest position.

Recording date and time provides communication and demonstrates adherence to plan of care. Proper patient and bed positioning promotes safety and comfort.

22. Remove PPE, if used. Perform hand hygiene.

Removing PPE properly reduces the risk for infection transmission and contamination of other items. Hand hygiene prevents the spread of microorganisms.

23. Check all wound dressings every shift. More frequent checks may be needed if the wound is more complex or dressings become saturated quickly.

Checking dressings ensures the assessment of changes in patient condition and timely intervention to prevent complications.

EVALUATION

- Procedure is accomplished without contaminating the wound area, without causing trauma to the wound, and without causing the patient to experience pain or discomfort.
- Sterile technique is maintained (if appropriate).
- Wound healing is promoted.
- Patient's skin surrounding the wound is without signs of irritation, infection, and maceration; and the wound continues to show signs of healing progression.

DOCUMENTATION

- Document the location of the wound and that the dressing was removed. Record assessment of the wound, including evidence of granulation tissue, presence of necrotic tissue, stage (if appropriate), and characteristics of drainage. Include the appearance of the surrounding skin. Document the cleansing or irrigation of the wound and solution used. Record the type of hydrocolloid dressing that was applied. Note pertinent patient and family education and any patient reaction to this procedure, including patient's pain level and effectiveness of nonpharmacologic interventions or analgesia if administered.

GENERAL CONSIDERATIONS

- Guidelines from the Wound, Ostomy, Continence Nurses Society (WOCN) and National Pressure Ulcer Advisory Panel (NPUAP) recommend that clean gloves may be used to treat chronic wounds and pressure ulcers as long as the infection-control procedures are followed. The *no-touch technique* may be used within these guidelines. Clean gloves are used to handle dressing material. Irrigants and dressings are sterile. The wound is re-dressed by picking up dressing materials by the corner and placing the untouched side over the wound (NPUAP, 2007b; Wooten & Hawkins, 2005).
- Many products are available to treat chronic and pressure ulcers. Treatment varies based on facility policy, nursing protocol, clinical specialist referrals, and primary care provider's orders.

Skill · 57   **Changing a Peripheral Venous Access Dressing**

The IV site is a potential entry point for microorganisms into the bloodstream. To prevent this, sealed IV dressings are used to occlude the site and prevent complications. Whenever these dressings need to be changed, it is important to observe meticulous aseptic technique to minimize the possibility of contamination. The particular facility's policies determine the type of dressing used and when these dressings are changed. Peripheral venous access site dressing changes often coincide with site rotations. However, dressing changes might be required more often, based on nursing assessment and judgment. Any access site dressing that is damp, loosened, or soiled should be changed immediately.

EQUIPMENT

- Transparent occlusive dressing
- 2% chlorhexidine, povidone-iodine, 70% alcohol
- Adhesive remover (optional)
- Alcohol swabs
- Tape
- Clean gloves
- Towel or disposable pad
- Masks for nurse and patient; sterile gloves (used for catheter with extended dwell time or if patient is immunocompromised [INS, 2006])
- Additional PPE, as indicated

ASSESSMENT GUIDELINES

- Assess IV site. Note any drainage, redness, leakage, or other indications that the dressing needs to be changed.
- Note the insertion date and date of last dressing change, if different from insertion date.
- Assess the patient's need to maintain venous access. If patient does not need the access, discuss the possibility of discontinuation with the primary care provider.
- Ask the patient about any allergies.

NURSING DIAGNOSES

- Risk for Infection
- Risk for Injury

OUTCOME IDENTIFICATION AND PLANNING

Expected outcomes may include:

- Patient will exhibit an access site that is clean, dry, and without any signs and symptoms of infection, infiltration, or phlebitis.
- Dressing will be clean, dry, and intact.
- Patient will not experience injury.

IMPLEMENTATION

ACTION	RATIONALE
1. Determine the need for a dressing change. Check facility policy. Gather all equipment and bring to bedside.	The particular facility's policies determine the type of dressing used and when these dressings are changed. Dressing changes might be required more often,

ACTION

RATIONALE

based on nursing assessment and judgment. Immediately change any access site dressing that is damp, loosened, or soiled.

Having equipment available saves time and facilitates accomplishment of procedure.

2. Perform hand hygiene and put on PPE, if indicated.

Hand hygiene and PPE prevent the spread of microorganisms. PPE is required based on transmission precautions.

3. Identify the patient.

Identifying the patient ensures the right patient receives the intervention and helps prevent errors.

4. Close curtains around bed and close the door to the room, if possible. Explain what you are going to do and why you are going to do it to the patient. Ask the patient about allergies to tape and skin antiseptics.

This ensures the patient's privacy. Explanation relieves anxiety and facilitates cooperation. Possible allergies may exist related to tape or antiseptics.

5. Put on mask and place on patient, if indicated. Put on gloves. Place towel or disposable pad under the arm with the venous access. If a solution is currently infusing, temporarily stop it. Hold the catheter in place with your nondominant hand and **carefully remove old dressing and/or stabilization/securing device.** Use adhesive remover as necessary. Discard dressing.

Masks should be used for catheter with extended dwell time or if the patient is immunocompromised (INS, 2006, p. S57). Gloves prevent contact with blood and body fluids. Pad protects underlying surface. Proper disposal of dressing prevents transmission of microorganisms.

6. **Inspect IV site for presence of phlebitis (inflammation), infection, or infiltration. Discontinue and relocate IV, if noted.**

Inflammation (phlebitis), infection, and infiltration cause trauma to tissues and necessitate removal of the venous access device.

ACTION	RATIONALE
7. **Cleanse site with an antiseptic solution, such as chlorhexidine, or according to facility policy. Press applicator against the skin and apply chlorhexidine using a back and forth friction scrub for at least 30 seconds. Do not wipe or blot. Allow to dry completely.**	Scrubbing motion and length of time (minimum 30 seconds) is necessary for chlorhexidine to be effective (Infusion Control Today [ICT], 2005). Organisms on the skin can be introduced into the tissues or the bloodstream with the needle. Chlorhexidine is the preferred antiseptic solution, but iodine, povidone-iodine, and 70% alcohol are considered acceptable alternatives (INS, 2006).
8. Open the skin protectant wipe. Apply the skin protectant to the site, making sure to cover at, minimum, the area to be covered with the dressing. Allow to dry. Place sterile transparent dressing or catheter securing/ stabilization device over the venipuncture site.	Skin protectant aids in adhesion of the dressing and decreases the risk for skin trauma when the dressing is removed. Transparent dressing allows easy visualization and protects the site. Stabilization/securing devices preserve the integrity of the access device and prevent catheter migration and loss of access (INS, 2006, p. S44). Some stabilization devices act as a site dressing also.
9. Label dressing with date, time of change, and initials. Loop the tubing near the entry site, and anchor it with tape (nonallergenic) close to the site. Resume fluid infusion, if indicated. Check that the IV flow is accurate and the system is patent.	Labeling helps ensure communication about venous access site dressing change. The weight of the tubing is sufficient to pull it out of the vein if it is not well anchored. Nonallergenic tape is less likely to tear fragile skin.
10. Remove equipment. Ensure patient's comfort. Remove gloves. Lower bed, if not in lowest position.	Promotes patient comfort and safety. Removing gloves properly reduces the risk for infection transmission and contamination of other items.
11. Remove additional PPE, if used. Perform hand hygiene.	Removing PPE properly reduces the risk for infection transmission and contamination of other items. Hand hygiene prevents transmission of microorganisms.

EVALUATION

- Patient remains free of any signs and symptoms of infection, phlebitis, or infiltration at the venous access site.
- Access site dressing is clean, dry, and intact.
- Patient has not experienced injury.

DOCUMENTATION

- Document the location of the venous access as well as the condition of the site. Include the presence or absence of signs of erythema, redness, swelling, or drainage. Document the clinical criteria for site complications. Record the subjective comments of the patient regarding the absence or presence of pain at the site. Record the patient's reaction to the procedure and pertinent patient teaching, such as alerting the nurse if the patient experiences any pain from the IV or notices any swelling at the site.

Skill · 58 **Applying a Saline-Moistened Dressing**

Gauze can be moistened with saline to keep the surface of open wounds moist. Many commercially prepared wound care products are also available to maintain a moist wound environment. This type of dressing promotes moist wound healing and protects the wound from contamination and trauma. A moist wound surface enhances the cellular migration necessary for tissue repair and healing. It is important that the dressing material be moist, not wet, when placed in open wounds. Dressing materials are soaked in normal saline solution and squeezed to remove excess saline so that the dressing is only slightly moist. The dressing can be loosely packed in the wound bed, if appropriate, and then covered with a secondary dressing to absorb drainage.

Many commercially prepared dressing and wound care products are applied in a similar manner. It is very important for the nurse to be aware of the products available in a particular facility and be familiar with the indications for, and correct use of, each type of dressing and wound care product.

EQUIPMENT

- Clean disposable gloves
- Sterile gloves, if indicated
- Additional PPE, as indicated
- Sterile dressing set or suture set (for the sterile scissors and forceps)
- Sterile thin-mesh gauze dressing for packing, if ordered
- Sterile gauze dressings
- Surgical or abdominal pads
- Skin-protectant wipes
- Sterile basin

- Sterile cleaning solution as ordered (commonly 0.9% normal saline solution)
- Sterile saline
- Tape or ties
- Plastic bag or other appropriate waste container for soiled dressings
- Sterile cotton-tipped applicators
- Supplies for wound cleansing or irrigation, as necessary
- Waterproof pad and bath blanket

ASSESSMENT GUIDELINES

- Assess the situation to determine the need for a dressing change. Confirm any medical orders relevant to wound care and any wound care included in the nursing plan of care.
- Assess the patient's level of comfort and the need for analgesics before wound care. Assess if the patient experienced any pain related to previous dressing changes and the effectiveness of interventions used to minimize the patient's pain.
- Assess the current dressing to determine if it is intact. Assess for excess drainage, bleeding, or saturation of the dressing.
- Inspect the wound and the surrounding tissue. Assess the location, appearance of the wound, wound stage (if appropriate), drainage, and types of tissue present in the wound.
- Measure the wound. Note the stage of the healing process and characteristics of any drainage. Also assess the surrounding skin for color, temperature, and edema, ecchymosis, or maceration.

NURSING DIAGNOSES

- Anxiety
- Disturbed Body Image
- Risk for Infection
- Impaired Skin Integrity
- Chronic Pain
- Acute Pain
- Deficient Knowledge
- Impaired Tissue Integrity

OUTCOME IDENTIFICATION AND PLANNING

Expected outcomes may include:
- Procedure is accomplished without contaminating the wound area, without causing trauma to the wound, and without causing the patient to experience pain or discomfort.
- Patient's skin surrounding the wound is without signs of irritation, infection, and maceration; and the wound continues to show signs of healing progression.

IMPLEMENTATION

ACTION	RATIONALE
1. Review the medical orders for wound care or the nursing plan of care related to wound care.	Reviewing the order and plan of care validates the correct patient and correct procedure.
2. Gather the necessary supplies and bring to the bedside stand or overbed table.	Preparation promotes efficient time management and an organized approach to the task. Bringing everything to the bedside conserves time and energy. Arranging items nearby is convenient, saves time, and avoids unnecessary stretching and twisting of muscles on the part of the nurse.
3. Perform hand hygiene and put on PPE, if indicated. 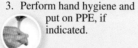	Hand hygiene and PPE prevent the spread of microorganisms. PPE is required based on transmission precautions.
4. Identify the patient.	Identifying the patient ensures the right patient receives the intervention and helps prevent errors.
5. Close curtains around bed and close the door to the room, if possible. Explain what you are going to do and why you are going to do it to the patient.	This ensures the patient's privacy. Explanation relieves anxiety and facilitates cooperation.
6. Assess the patient for possible need for nonpharmacologic pain-reducing interventions or analgesic medication before wound care dressing change. Administer appropriate prescribed analgesic. Allow sufficient time for the analgesic to achieve its effectiveness.	Pain is a subjective experience influenced by past experience. Wound care and dressing changes may cause pain for some patients.
7. Place a waste receptacle or bag at a convenient location for use during the procedure.	Having a waste container handy means the soiled dressing may be discarded easily, without the spread of microorganisms.

ACTION	RATIONALE
8. Adjust bed to comfortable working height, usually elbow height of the caregiver (VISN 8 Patient Safety Center, 2009).	Having the bed at the proper height prevents back and muscle strain.
9. Assist the patient to a comfortable position that provides easy access to the wound area. Position the patient so the wound cleanser or irrigation solution will flow from the clean end of the wound toward the dirtier end, if being used (See Skill 55 for wound cleansing and Skill 183 for irrigation techniques).Use the bath blanket to cover any exposed area other than the wound. Place a waterproof pad under the wound site.	Patient positioning and use of a bath blanket provide for comfort and warmth. Gravity directs the flow of liquid from the least contaminated to the most contaminated area. Waterproof pad protects underlying surfaces.
10. Put on clean gloves. Carefully and gently remove the soiled dressings. If there is resistance, use a silicone-based adhesive remover to help remove the tape. If any part of the dressing sticks to the underlying skin, use small amounts of sterile saline to help loosen and remove it.	Gloves protect the nurse from handling contaminated dressings. Cautious removal of the dressing is more comfortable for the patient and ensures that any drain present is not removed. A silicone-based adhesive remover allows for the easy, rapid, and painless removal without the associated problems of skin stripping (Rudoni, 2008; Stephen-Haynes, 2008). Sterile saline moistens the dressing for easier removal and minimizes damage and pain.
11. After removing the dressing, note the presence, amount, type, color, and odor of any drainage on the dressings. Place soiled dressings in the appropriate waste receptacle.	The presence of drainage should be documented. Discarding dressings appropriately prevents the spread of microorganisms.
12. Assess the wound for appearance, stage, the presence of	This information provides evidence about the wound healing

ACTION	RATIONALE
eschar, granulation tissue, epithelialization, undermining, tunneling, necrosis, sinus tract, and drainage. Assess the appearance of the surrounding tissue. Measure the wound.	process and/or the presence of infection.
13. Remove your gloves and put them in the receptacle.	Discarding gloves prevents the spread of microorganisms.
14. Using sterile technique, open the supplies and dressings. Place the fine-mesh gauze into the basin and pour the ordered solution over the mesh to saturate it.	Gauze touching the wound surface must be moistened to increase the absorptive ability and promote healing.
15. Put on the sterile gloves. Alternately, clean gloves (clean technique) may be used to clean a chronic wound.	Sterile gloves maintain surgical asepsis. Clean technique is appropriate when cleaning chronic wounds.
16. Clean the wound (See Skill 55). Alternately, irrigate the wound, as ordered or required (See Skill 183).	Cleaning the wound removes previous drainage and wound debris.
17. Dry the surrounding skin with sterile gauze dressings.	Moisture provides a medium for growth of microorganisms.
18. Apply a skin protectant to the surrounding skin, if needed.	A skin protectant prevents skin irritation and breakdown.
19. If not already on, put on sterile gloves. Squeeze excess fluid from the gauze dressing. Unfold and fluff the dressing.	Sterile gloves prevent contamination of the dressing material. The gauze provides a thin, moist layer to contact all the wound surfaces.
20. Gently press to loosely pack the moistened gauze into the wound. If necessary, use the forceps or cotton-tipped applicators to press the gauze into all wound surfaces.	The dressing provides a moist environment for all wound surfaces. Avoid overpacking the gauze; loosely pack to prevent too much pressure in the wound bed, which could impede wound healing.
21. Apply several dry, sterile gauze pads over the wet gauze.	Dry gauze absorbs excess moisture and drainage.

ACTION	RATIONALE
22. Place the ABD pad over the gauze.	The ABD pad prevents contamination.
23. Remove and discard gloves. Apply tape, Montgomery straps, or roller gauze to secure the dressings. Alternately, many commercial wound products are self-adhesive and do not require additional tape.	Proper disposal of gloves prevents the spread of microorganisms. Tape or other securing products are easier to apply after gloves have been removed.
24. After securing the dressing, label it with date and time. Remove all remaining equipment; place the patient in a comfortable position, with side rails up and bed in the lowest position.	Recording date and time provides communication and demonstrates adherence to plan of care. Proper patient and bed positioning promotes safety and comfort.
25. Remove PPE, if used. Perform hand hygiene.	Removing PPE properly reduces the risk for infection transmission and contamination of other items. Hand hygiene prevents the spread of microorganisms.
26. Check all wound dressings every shift. More frequent checks may be needed if the wound is more complex or dressings become saturated quickly.	Checking dressings ensures the assessment of changes in patient condition and timely intervention to prevent complications.

EVALUATION

• Procedure is accomplished without contaminating the wound area, without causing trauma to the wound, and without causing the patient to experience pain or discomfort.
• Sterile technique is maintained (if appropriate).
• Wound healing is promoted.
• Patient's skin surrounding the wound is without signs of irritation, infection, and maceration.
• Patient's wound continues to show signs of healing progression.

DOCUMENTATION

• Document the location of the wound and that the dressing was removed. Record assessment of the wound, including evidence of granulation tissue, presence of necrotic tissue, stage (if appropriate), and characteristics of drainage. Include the appearance of the surrounding skin. Document the cleansing or irrigation of the wound and solution used. Record the type of dressing that was reapplied. Note pertinent patient and family education and any patient reaction to this procedure, including patient's pain level and effectiveness of nonpharmacologic interventions or analgesia if administered.

GENERAL CONSIDERATIONS

- Make sure ancillary staff understand the importance of reporting excessive drainage from the dressing, and any soiled or loose dressings.
- Guidelines from the Wound, Ostomy, Continence Nurses Society (WOCN) and National Pressure Ulcer Advisory Panel (NPUAP) recommend that clean gloves may be used to treat chronic wounds and pressure ulcers as long as the infection-control procedures are followed. The *no-touch technique* may be used within these guidelines. Clean gloves are used to handle dressing material. Irrigants and dressings are sterile. The wound is re-dressed by picking up dressing materials by the corner and placing the untouched side over the wound (NPUAP, 2007b; Wooten & Hawkins, 2005).
- Many products are available to treat chronic wounds and pressure ulcers. Treatment varies based on facility policy, nursing protocol, clinical specialist referrals, primary care provider orders, and product in use.

Skill · 59   Instilling Ear Drops

Drugs are instilled into the auditory canal for their local effect. They are used to soften wax, relieve pain, apply local anesthesia, and treat infections.

The tympanic membrane separates the external ear from the middle ear. Normally, it is intact and closes the entrance to the middle ear completely. If it is ruptured or has been opened by surgical intervention, the middle ear and the inner ear have a direct passage to the external ear. When this occurs, perform instillations with the greatest of care to prevent forcing materials from the outer ear into the middle ear and the inner ear. Use sterile technique to prevent infection.

EQUIPMENT

- Medication (warmed to 37°C [98.6°F])
- Dropper
- Tissue
- Cotton ball (optional)
- Gloves
- Additional PPE, as indicated
- Washcloth (optional)

- Normal saline solution
- Computer-generated Medication Administration Record

(CMAR) or Medication Administration Record (MAR)

ASSESSMENT GUIDELINES

- Assess the affected ear for redness, erythema, edema, drainage, and
  tenderness.
- Assess the patient for allergies.
- Verify patient name, dose, route, and time of administration.
- Assess the patient's knowledge of medication and procedure. If the
  patient has a knowledge deficit about the medication, this may be an
  appropriate time to begin education about the medication.
- Assess the patient's ability to cooperate with the procedure.

NURSING DIAGNOSES

- Deficient Knowledge
- Acute Pain
- Anxiety
- Risk for Allergy Response
- Risk for Injury

OUTCOME IDENTIFICATION AND PLANNING

Expected outcomes may include:
- Drops are administered successfully into the ear.
- Patient understands the rationale for the eardrop instillation and has
  decreased anxiety.
- Patient remains free from pain.
- Patient experiences no allergic response or injury.

IMPLEMENTATION

ACTION

1. Gather equipment. Check
   medication order against the
   original order in the medical
   record, according to facility
   policy. Clarify any inconsistencies. Check the patient's
   chart for allergies.

2. Know the actions, special
   nursing considerations, safe
   dose ranges, purpose of
   administration, and adverse
   effects of the medication to
   be administered. Consider

RATIONALE

This comparison helps to identify errors that may have
occurred when orders were transcribed. The primary care provider's order is the legal record
of medication orders for each
facility.

This knowledge aids the nurse in
evaluating the therapeutic effect
of the medication in relation to
the patient's disorder and can
also be used to educate the
patient about the medication.

ACTION	RATIONALE
the appropriateness of the medication for this patient.	
3. Perform hand hygiene.	Hand hygiene prevents the spread of microorganisms.
4. Move the medication cart to the outside of the patient's room or prepare for administration in the medication area.	Organization facilitates error-free administration and saves time.
5. Unlock the medication cart or drawer. Enter pass code and scan employee identification, if required.	Locking of the cart or drawer safeguards each patient's medication supply. Hospital accrediting organizations require medication carts to be locked when not in use. Entering pass code and scanning ID allows only authorized users into the system and identifies user for documentation by the computer.
6. **Prepare medications for one patient at a time.**	This prevents errors in medication administration.
7. Read the CMAR/MAR and select the proper medication from the patient's medication drawer or unit stock.	This is the *first* check of the label.
8. Compare the label with the CMAR/MAR. Check expiration dates and perform calculations, if necessary. Scan the bar code on the package, if required.	This is the *second* check of the label. Verify calculations with another nurse to ensure safety, if necessary.
9. **When all medications for one patient have been prepared, recheck the label with the CMAR/MAR before taking them to the patient.**	This is a *third* check to ensure accuracy and to prevent errors. Some facilities require the third check to occur at the bedside, after identifying the patient and before administration.
10. Lock the medication cart before leaving it.	Locking the cart or drawer safeguards the patient's medication supply. Hospital accrediting

ACTION	RATIONALE
	organizations require medication carts to be locked when not in use.
11. Transport medications to the patient's bedside carefully, and keep the medications in sight at all times.	Careful handling and close observation prevent accidental or deliberate disarrangement of medications.
12. **Ensure that the patient receives the medications at the correct time.**	Check agency policy, which may allow for administration within a period of 30 minutes before or 30 minutes after the designated time.
13. Perform hand hygiene and put on PPE, if indicated.	Hand hygiene and PPE prevent the spread of microorganisms. PPE is required based on transmission precautions.
14. Identify the patient. Usually, the patient should be identified using two methods. Compare information with the CMAR/MAR.	Identifying the patient ensures the right patient receives the medications and helps prevent errors.
a. Check the name and identification number on the patient's identification band.	This is the most reliable method. Replace the identification band if it is missing or inaccurate in any way.
b. Ask the patient to state his or her name and birth date, based on facility policy.	This requires a response from the patient, but illness and strange surroundings often cause patients to be confused.
c. If the patient cannot identify himself or herself, verify the patient's identification with a staff member who knows the patient for the second source.	This is another way to double-check identity. Do not use the name on the door or over the bed, because these may be inaccurate.
15. Complete necessary assessments before administering medications. Check the patient's allergy bracelet or ask the patient about allergies. Explain the purpose and	Assessment is a prerequisite to administration of medications.

ACTION	RATIONALE

action of each medication to
the patient.

16. Scan the patient's bar code
on the identification band, if
required.

Provides an additional check to
ensure that the medication is
given to the right patient.

17. Put on gloves.

Gloves protect the nurse from
potential contact with contaminants and body fluids.

18. Cleanse external ear of any
drainage with cotton ball or
washcloth moistened with
normal saline.

Debris and drainage may prevent
some of the medication from
entering the ear canal.

19. Place patient on his or her
unaffected side in bed, or, if
ambulatory, have the patient
sit with the head well tilted to
the side so that the affected
ear is uppermost.

This positioning prevents the
drops from escaping from the
ear.

20. Draw up the amount of solution needed in the dropper.
Do not return excess medication to stock bottle. A prepackaged monodrip plastic
container may also be used.

Risk for contamination is
increased when medication is
returned to the stock bottle.

21. Straighten auditory canal by
pulling cartilaginous portion
of pinna up and back for an
adult.

Pulling on the pinna as described
helps to straighten the canal
properly for eardrop instillation.

22. Hold dropper in the ear with
its tip above the auditory
canal. Do not touch the dropper to the ear. For an infant
or an irrational or confused
patient, protect the dropper
with a piece of soft tubing to
help prevent injury to the ear.

By holding the dropper in the
ear, most of the medication will
enter the ear canal. Touching the
dropper to the ear contaminates
the dropper and medication. The
hard tip of the dropper can damage the tympanic membrane if it
is jabbed into the ear.

23. **Allow drops to fall on the
side of the canal.**

It is uncomfortable for the
patient if the drops fall directly
onto the tympanic membrane.

24. Release pinna after instilling
drops, and have patient maintain the position to prevent
escape of medication.

Medication should remain in ear
canal for at least 5 minutes.

ACTION	RATIONALE
25. Gently press on the tragus a few times.	Pressing on the tragus causes medication from the canal to move toward the tympanic membrane.
26. If ordered, loosely insert a cotton ball into the ear canal.	A cotton ball can help prevent medication from leaking out of the ear canal.
27. Remove gloves. Assist the patient to a comfortable position.	This ensures patient comfort.
28. Remove additional PPE, if used. Perform hand hygiene.	Removing PPE properly reduces the risk for infection transmission and contamination of other items. Hand hygiene prevents the spread of microorganisms.
29. Document the administration of the medication immediately after administration. See Documentation section below.	Timely documentation helps to ensure patient safety.
30. Evaluate the patient's response to medication within appropriate time frame.	The patient needs to be evaluated for therapeutic and adverse effects from the medication.

EVALUATION

• Patient receives the eardrops successfully.
• Patient understands the rationale for ear drop instillation and exhibits no or decreased anxiety.
• Patient experiences no or minimal pain.
• Patient experiences no allergic response or injury.

DOCUMENTATION

• Document the administration of the medication immediately after administration, including date, time, dose, route of administration, and site of administration, specifically right, left, or both ears, on the CMAR/MAR or record, using the required format. If using a bar-code system, medication administration is automatically recorded when the bar code is scanned. PRN medications require documentation of the reason for administration. Prompt recording avoids the possibility of accidentally repeating the administration of the drug. Document pre- and postadministration assessments, characteristics of any drainage, and the patient's response to the treatment, if appropriate. If the drug was refused or omitted, record this in the appropriate area on the medication record and notify the primary care provider. This verifies the reason the medication was omitted and ensures that the primary care provider is aware of the patient's condition.

GENERAL CONSIDERATIONS

- If both ears are to be treated, wait 5 minutes before instilling drops into the second ear.
- Ongoing assessment is an important part of nursing care to evaluate patient response to administered treatments and early detection of adverse effects. If an adverse effect is suspected, notify the patient's primary healthcare provider. Additional intervention is based on type of reaction and patient assessment.
- Pull pinna straight back for a child more than 3 years of age and down and back for an infant or a child younger than 3 years.

Skill · 60   Administering an Ear Irrigation

Irrigations of the external auditory canal are ordinarily performed for cleaning purposes or to apply heat to the area. Typically, normal saline solution is used, although an antiseptic solution may be indicated for local action. To prevent pain, the irrigation solution should be at least room temperature. Usually, an irrigation syringe is used; however, an irrigating container with tubing and an ear tip may also be used, especially if the purpose of the irrigation is to apply heat to the area.

EQUIPMENT

- Prescribed irrigating solution (warmed to 98.6°F)
- Irrigation set (container and irrigating or bulb syringe)
- Waterproof pad
- Emesis basin
- Cotton-tipped applicators
- Disposable gloves
- Additional PPE, as indicated
- Cotton balls
- Computer-generated Medication Administration Record (CMAR) or Medication Administration Record (MAR)

ASSESSMENT GUIDELINES

- Assess the affected ear for redness, erythema, edema, drainage, and tenderness.
- Assess the patient's ability to hear.
- Assess the patient for allergies.

- Verify patient name, dose, route, and time of administration.
- Assess the patient's knowledge of medication and procedure. If the patient has a knowledge deficit about the medication, this may be an appropriate time to begin education about the medication.
- Assess the patient's ability to cooperate with the procedure.

NURSING DIAGNOSES
- Acute Pain
- Impaired Skin Integrity
- Risk for Injury
- Deficient Knowledge

OUTCOME IDENTIFICATION AND PLANNING
Expected outcomes may include:
- Irrigation is administered successfully.
- Patient remains free from pain and injury.
- Patient will experience improved hearing.
- Patient understands the rationale for the procedure.

IMPLEMENTATION

ACTION	RATIONALE
1. Gather equipment. Check medication order against the original order in the medical record, according to facility policy. Clarify any inconsistencies. Check the patient's chart for allergies.	This comparison helps to identify errors that may have occurred when orders were transcribed. The primary care provider's order is the legal record of medication orders for each facility.
2. Know the actions, special nursing considerations, safe dose ranges, purpose of administration, and adverse effects of the medication to be administered. Consider the appropriateness of the medication for this patient.	This knowledge aids the nurse in evaluating the therapeutic effect of the medication in relation to the patient's disorder and can also be used to educate the patient about the medication.
3. Perform hand hygiene.	Hand hygiene prevents the spread of microorganisms.
4. Move the medication cart to the outside of the patient's	Organization facilitates error-free administration and saves time.

ACTION	RATIONALE

room or prepare for administration in the medication area.

5. Unlock the medication cart or drawer. Enter pass code and scan employee identification, if required.

Locking of the cart or drawer safeguards each patient's medication supply. Hospital accrediting organizations require medication carts to be locked when not in use. Entering pass code and scanning ID allows only authorized users into the system and identifies user for documentation by the computer.

6. **Prepare medications for one patient at a time.**

This prevents errors in medication administration.

7. Read the CMAR/MAR and select the proper medication from the patient's medication drawer or unit stock.

This is the *first* check of the label.

8. Compare the label with the CMAR/MAR. Check expiration dates and perform calculations, if necessary. Scan the bar code on the package, if required.

This is the *second* check of the label. Verify calculations with another nurse to ensure safety, if necessary.

9. **When all medications for one patient have been prepared, recheck the label with the CMAR/MAR before taking them to the patient.**

This is a *third* check to ensure accuracy and to prevent errors. Some facilities require the third check to occur at the bedside, after identifying the patient and before administration.

10. Lock the medication cart before leaving it.

Locking the cart or drawer safeguards the patient's medication supply. Hospital accrediting organizations require medication carts to be locked when not in use.

11. Transport medications to the patient's bedside carefully, and keep the medications in sight at all times.

Careful handling and close observation prevent accidental or deliberate disarrangement of medications.

12. **Ensure that the patient receives the medications at the correct time.**

Check agency policy, which may allow for administration within a period of 30 minutes before or 30 minutes after designated time.

ACTION	RATIONALE

13. Perform hand hygiene and put on PPE, if indicated.

Hand hygiene and PPE prevent the spread of microorganisms. PPE is required based on transmission precautions.

14. Identify the patient. Usually, the patient should be identified using two methods. Compare information with the CMAR or MAR.

Identifying the patient ensures the right patient receives the medications and helps prevent errors.

   a. Check the name and identification number on the patient's identification band.

This is the most reliable method. Replace the identification band if it is missing or inaccurate in any way.

   b. Ask the patient to state his or her name and birth date, based on facility policy.

This requires a response from the patient, but illness and strange surroundings often cause patients to be confused.

   c. If the patient cannot identify himself or herself, verify the patient's identification with a staff member who knows the patient for the second source.

This is another way to double-check identity. Do not use the name on the door or over the bed, because these may be inaccurate.

15. Explain the procedure to the patient.

Explanation facilitates cooperation and reassures the patient.

16. Assemble equipment at the patient's bedside.

This provides for an organized approach to the task.

17. Put on gloves.

Gloves protect the nurse from potential contact with contaminants and body fluids.

18. Have the patient sit up or lie with head tilted toward side of the affected ear. Protect the patient and bed with a waterproof pad. Have the patient support the basin under the ear to receive the irrigating solution.

Gravity causes the irrigating solution to flow from the ear to the basin.

19. Clean pinna and meatus of auditory canal, as necessary, with moistened cotton-tipped

Materials lodged on the pinna and at the meatus may be washed into the ear.

ACTION	RATIONALE
applicators dipped in warm tap water or the irrigating solution.	
20. Fill bulb syringe with warm solution. If an irrigating container is used, prime the tubing.	Priming the tubing allows air to escape from the tubing. Air forced into the ear canal is noisy and therefore unpleasant for the patient.
21. Straighten the auditory canal by pulling the cartilaginous portion of the pinna up and back for an adult.	Straightening the ear canal allows the solution to reach all areas of the canal easily.
22. **Direct a steady, slow stream of solution against the roof of the auditory canal, using only enough force to remove secretions. Do not occlude the auditory canal with the irrigating nozzle. Allow solution to flow out unimpeded.**	Directing the solution at the roof of the canal helps prevent injury to the tympanic membrane. Continuous in-and-out flow of the irrigating solution helps to prevent pressure in the canal.
23. When irrigation is complete, place cotton ball loosely in auditory meatus and have the patient lie on side of affected ear on a towel or absorbent pad.	The cotton ball absorbs excess fluid, and gravity allows the remaining solution in the canal to escape from the ear.
24. Remove gloves. Assist the patient to a comfortable position.	This ensures patient comfort.
25. Remove additional PPE, if used. Perform hand hygiene.	Removing PPE properly reduces the risk for infection transmission and contamination of other items. Hand hygiene prevents the spread of microorganisms.
26. Document the administration of the medication immediately after administration. See Documentation section below.	Timely documentation helps to ensure patient safety.
27. Evaluate patient's response to the procedure. Return in 10 to 15 minutes and remove cotton ball and assess drainage. Evaluate patient's response to medication within appropriate time frame.	The patient needs to be evaluated for any adverse effects from the procedure. Drainage or pain may indicate injury to the tympanic membrane. The patient needs to be evaluated for therapeutic and adverse effects from the medication.

EVALUATION
- Ear canal is irrigated successfully.
- Patient experiences no or minimal pain or discomfort.
- Patient's hearing is improved.
- Patient understands the rationale for the ear irrigation procedure.

DOCUMENTATION
- Document the administration of the medication immediately after administration, including date, time, dose, route of administration, and site of administration, specifically right, left, or both ears, on the CMAR/MAR or record using the required format. If using a bar-code system, medication administration is automatically recorded when it is scanned. PRN medications require documentation of the reason for administration. Prompt recording avoids the possibility of accidentally repeating the administration of the drug. Document the procedure, site, the type of solution and volume used, and length of time irrigation performed. Document pre- and postadministration assessments, characteristics of any drainage, and the patient's response to the treatment, if appropriate. If the drug was refused or omitted, record this in the appropriate area on the medication record and notify the primary care provider. This verifies the reason medication was omitted and ensures that the primary care provider is aware of the patient's condition.

GENERAL CONSIDERATIONS
- Ongoing assessment is an important part of nursing care to evaluate patient response to administered treatments and early detection of adverse effects. If an adverse effect is suspected, notify the patient's primary healthcare provider. Additional intervention is based on type of reaction and patient assessment.
- Pull pinna straight back for a child more than 3 years of age and down and back for an infant or a child younger than 3 years.

Skill · 61   Assisting a Patient with Eating

Depending on the patient's condition, the physician will order a diet for the patient. Many patients are independently able to meet their nutritional needs by feeding themselves. Other patients, especially the very young and some elderly patients, such as those individuals with arthritis of the hands, may have some difficulty opening juice containers, and so on. Patients with paralysis of the hands or advanced dementia may be unable to feed themselves. For these patients, it is necessary for the nurse to provide whatever assistance is needed. This skill is frequently delegated to nursing assistants. However, the nurse is responsible for the initial and ongoing assessment of the patient for potential complications related to feeding. Before this skill can be delegated, it is paramount for the nurse to make sure that the nursing assistant has been educated to observe for any swallowing difficulties and has knowledge of aspiration precautions.

EQUIPMENT

- Patient tray of food, based on prescribed diet
- Wet wipes for hand hygiene
- Mouth care materials
- Patient's dentures, eyeglasses, hearing aid, if needed
- Special adaptive utensils as needed
- Napkins, protective covering, or towel
- PPE, as indicated

ASSESSMENT GUIDELINES

- Validate the type of diet that has been ordered for the patient.
- Assess for any food allergies and religious or cultural preferences, as appropriate.
- Check to make sure the patient does not have any scheduled laboratory or diagnostic studies that may have an impact on whether he or she is able to eat a meal.
- Assess for any swallowing difficulties.

NURSING DIAGNOSES

- Deficient Knowledge
- Anxiety
- Risk for Aspiration
- Impaired Swallowing
- Feeding Self-Care Deficit

OUTCOME IDENTIFICATION AND PLANNING

Expected outcomes may include:
- Patient consumes 50% to 60% of the contents of the meal tray.
- Patient does not aspirate during or after the meal.
- Patient expresses contentment related to eating, as appropriate.

IMPLEMENTATION

ACTION	RATIONALE
1. Check the medical order for the type of diet prescribed for the patient.	Ensures the correct diet for the patient.

ACTION	RATIONALE
2. Perform hand hygiene and put on PPE, if indicated.	Hand hygiene and PPE prevent the spread of microorganisms. PPE is required based on transmission precautions.
3. Identify the patient.	Identifying the patient ensures the right patient receives the intervention and helps prevent errors.
4. Explain the procedure to the patient.	Explanations provide reassurance and facilitate cooperation of the patient.
5. **Assess level of consciousness, for any physical limitations, and decreased hearing or visual acuity. If the patient uses a hearing aid or wears glasses or dentures, provide as needed. Ask if the patient has any cultural or religious preferences and food likes and dislikes, if possible.**	Alertness is necessary for a patient to swallow and consume food. Using a hearing aid, glasses, and dentures for chewing facilitates the intake of food. Patient preferences should be considered in food selection as much as possible to increase the intake of food and maximize the benefit of the meal.
6. Pull the patient's bedside curtain. Assess the abdomen. Ask the patient if he or she has any nausea or has any difficulty swallowing. Assess the patient for nausea or pain and administer an antiemetic or analgesic, as needed.	Provide for privacy. A functioning GI tract is essential for digestion. The presence of pain or nausea will diminish appetite. If the patient is medicated, wait for the appropriate time for absorption of the medication before beginning the feeding.
7. Offer to assist the patient with any elimination needs.	Promotes comfort and may avoid interruptions for toileting during meals.
8. Provide hand hygiene and mouth care, as needed.	May improve appetite and promote comfort.
9. Remove any bedpans or undesirable equipment and odors from the vicinity where meal will be eaten, if possible.	Unpleasant odors and equipment may decrease the appetite of the patient.
10. Open the patient's bedside curtain. Assist to, or position	Proper positioning improves swallowing ability and reduces the risk of aspiration.

ACTION	RATIONALE
the patient in, a high Fowler's or sitting position in the bed or chair. Position the bed in the low position, if the patient remains in bed.	
11. Place protective covering or towel over the patient, if desired.	Prevents soiling of the patient's gown.
12. Check tray to make sure that it is the correct tray before serving. Place tray on the overbed table so patient can see food if able. Ensure that hot foods are hot and cold foods are cold. Use caution with hot beverages, allowing sufficient time for cooling if needed. Ask the patient for his or her preference related to what foods are desired first. Cut food into small pieces, as needed. Observe swallowing ability throughout the meal.	Ensures that the correct tray is given to the patient. Encouraging the patient's choice promotes patient dignity and respect. Close observation is necessary to assess for signs of aspiration or difficulty with the meal.
13. If possible, sit facing the patient while feeding is taking place. If patient is able, encourage him or her to hold finger foods and feed self as much as possible. Converse with patient during the meal, as appropriate. If, however, the patient has dysphagia, limit questioning or conversation that would require a response from the patient during eating. Play relaxation music if patient desires.	In general, optimal meal time involves social interaction and conversation. Talking during eating is contraindicated for patients with dysphagia, because of an increased risk for aspiration.
14. Allow enough time for the patient to chew and swallow the food adequately. The patient may need to rest for short periods during eating.	Eating requires energy and many medical conditions can weaken patients. Rest can restore energy for eating.

ACTION	RATIONALE
15. When the meal is completed or the patient is unable to eat any more, remove the tray from the room. **Note the amount and types of food consumed. Note the volume of liquid consumed.**	Nutrition plays an important role in healing and overall health. If the patient is not eating enough to meet nutritional requirements, alternative methods need to be considered.
16. Reposition the overbed table, remove the protective covering, offer hand hygiene, as needed, and offer the bedpan. Assist the patient to a position of comfort and relaxation.	Promotes the comfort of the patient, meets possible elimination needs, and facilitates digestion.
17. Remove PPE, if used. Perform hand hygiene.	Removing PPE properly reduces the risk for infection transmission and contamination of other items. Hand hygiene prevents the spread of microorganisms.

EVALUATION

- Patient consumes an adequate amount of nutrients.
- Patient expresses an appetite for the food, relating likes and dislikes.
- Patient experiences no nausea, vomiting, or aspiration episodes.

DOCUMENTATION

- Document the condition of the abdomen. Record that the head of the bed was elevated at least 30 to 45 degrees. Note any swallowing difficulties and the patient's response to the meal. Document the percentage of the intake from the meal. If the patient had a poor intake, document the need for further consultation with the physician and dietitian, as needed. Record any pertinent teaching that was conducted.

GENERAL CONSIDERATIONS

- For patients with arthritis of the hands, special utensils with modified handles that facilitate an easier grip are available. Contact an occupational therapist for guidance on adaptive equipment.
- A visually impaired patient may be guided to feed himself or herself through use of a 'clock' pattern. For example, the chicken is placed at 6 o'clock; the vegetables at 3 o'clock.
- For the patient with dysphagia, suggest small bites of food such as puddings, ground meat, or cooked vegetables. Advise the patient not to talk while swallowing and to swallow twice after each bite.

Skill · 62   Obtaining an Electrocardiogram (ECG)

Electrocardiography (ECG [also abbreviated as EKG in some references]) measures the heart's electrical activity. Impulses moving through the heart's conduction system create electric currents that can be monitored on the body's surface. Electrodes attached to the skin can detect these electric currents and transmit them to an instrument that produces a record (the electrocardiogram) of cardiac activity. The data are graphed as waveforms. ECG can be used to identify myocardial ischemia and infarction, rhythm and conduction disturbances, chamber enlargement, electrolyte imbalances, and drug toxicity.

The standard 12-lead ECG uses a series of electrodes placed on the extremities and the chest wall to assess the heart from 12 different views. The 12 leads consist of three standard bipolar limb leads (designated I, II, III), three unipolar augmented leads (aV_R, aV_L, aV_F), and six unipolar precordial leads (V_1 to V_6). The exact location on the extremities does not matter as long as skin contact is good and bone is avoided. The chest leads are placed in specific locations to ensure accurate recording. The limb leads and augmented leads show the heart from the frontal plane. The precordial leads show the heart from the horizontal plane.

Each lead overlies a specific area of the myocardium and provides an electrographic snapshot of electrochemical activity of the cell membrane. The ECG device measures and averages the differences between the electrical potential of the electrode sites for each lead and graphs them over time, creating the standard ECG complex, called PQRST.

Interpreting the ECG requires the following:

• Determine the rhythm.
• Determine the rate.
• Evaluate the P wave.
• Determine the duration of the PR interval.
• Determine the duration of the QRS complex.
• Evaluate the T waves.
• Determine the duration of the QT interval.
• Evaluate any other components.

An ECG is typically accomplished using a multichannel method. All electrodes are attached to the patient at once and the machine prints a simultaneous view of all leads. It is important to reassure the patient that the leads just sense and record and do not transmit any electricity. The patient must be able to lie still and refrain from speaking to prevent body movement from creating artifact in the ECG. Variations of standard ECGs include exercise ECG (stress ECG) and ambulatory ECG (Holter monitoring).

EQUIPMENT
• ECG machine
• Recording paper
• Disposable pregelled electrodes
• Adhesive remover swabs

- 4 × 4 gauze pads
- Soap and water, if necessary
- PPE, as indicated
- Bath blanket

ASSESSMENT GUIDELINES

- Review the patient's medical record and plan of care for information about the patient's need for an ECG.
- Assess the patient's cardiac status, including heart rate, blood pressure, and auscultation of heart sounds.
- If the patient is already connected to a cardiac monitor, remove the electrodes to accommodate the precordial leads and minimize electrical interference on the ECG tracing.
- Keep the patient away from objects that might cause electrical interference, such as equipment, fixtures, and power cords.
- Inspect the patient's chest for areas of irritation, breakdown, or excessive hair that might interfere with electrode placement.

NURSING DIAGNOSES

- Decreased Cardiac Output
- Acute Pain
- Excess Fluid Volume
- Deficient Knowledge
- Ineffective Health Maintenance
- Activity Intolerance
- Anxiety

OUTCOME IDENTIFICATION AND PLANNING

Expected outcomes may include:
- Cardiac electrical tracing is obtained without any complications.
- Patient displays an increased understanding about the ECG.

IMPLEMENTATION

ACTION	RATIONALE
1. Verify the order for an ECG on the patient's medical record.	This ensures that the correct intervention is performed on the correct patient.
2. Gather all equipment and bring to bedside.	Having equipment available saves time and facilitates accomplishment of the procedure.
3. Perform hand hygiene and put on PPE, if indicated.	Hand hygiene and PPE prevent the spread of microorganisms. PPE is required based on transmission precautions.

ACTION	RATIONALE
4. Identify the patient. 	Identifying the patient ensures the right patient receives the intervention and helps prevent errors.
5. Close curtains around bed and close the door to the room, if possible. As you set up the machine to record a 12-lead ECG, explain the procedure to the patient. Tell the patient that the test records the heart's electrical activity, and it may be repeated at certain intervals. Emphasize that no electrical current will enter his or her body. Tell the patient the test typically takes about 5 minutes. Ask the patient about allergies to adhesive, as appropriate.	This ensures the patient's privacy. Explanation relieves anxiety and facilitates cooperation. Possible allergies may exist related to adhesive on ECG leads.
6. Place the ECG machine close to the patient's bed, and plug the power cord into the wall outlet.	Having equipment available saves time and facilitates accomplishment of the task.
7. If bed is adjustable, raise bed to comfortable working height, usually elbow height of the caregiver (VISN 8 Patient Safety Center, 2009).	Having the bed at the proper height prevents back and muscle strain.
8. Have the patient lie supine in the center of the bed with the arms at the sides. Raise the head of the bed, if necessary, to promote comfort. Expose the patient's arms and legs, and drape appropriately. Encourage the patient to relax the arms and legs. If the bed is too narrow, place the patient's hands under the buttocks to prevent muscle tension. Also use this technique	This helps increase patient comfort and will produce a better tracing. Having the arms and legs relaxed minimizes muscle trembling, which can cause electrical interference.

ACTION	RATIONALE
if the patient is shivering or trembling. Make sure the feet do not touch the bed's footboard.	
9. Select flat, fleshy areas on which to place the electrodes. Avoid muscular and bony areas. If the patient has an amputated limb, choose a site on the stump.	Tissue conducts the current more effectively than bone, producing a better tracing.
10. If an area is excessively hairy, clip the hair. **Do not shave hair.** Clean excess oil or other substances from the skin with soap and water and dry it completely.	Shaving causes microabrasions on the chest skin. Oils and excess hair interfere with electrode contact and function. Alcohol, benzoin, and antiperspirant are not recommended to prepare the skin.
11. Refer to FIGURE 1 for lead placement (FIGURE 1). Apply the limb lead electrodes. The tip of each lead wire is lettered and color-coded for easy identification. The white (or RA) lead goes to the right arm; the green (or RL) lead to the right leg; the red (or LL) lead to the left leg; the black (or LA) lead to the left arm. Peel the contact paper off the self-sticking disposable electrode and apply directly to the prepared site, as recommended by the manufacturer. Position disposable electrodes on the legs with the lead connection pointing superiorly.	Having the lead connection pointing superiorly guarantees the best connection to the lead wire.
12. Connect the limb lead wires to the electrodes. Make sure the metal parts of the electrodes are clean and bright.	Dirty or corroded electrodes prevent a good electrical connection.
13. Expose the patient's chest. Apply the precordial lead electrodes. The tip of each lead wire is lettered and	Proper lead placement is necessary for accurate test results.

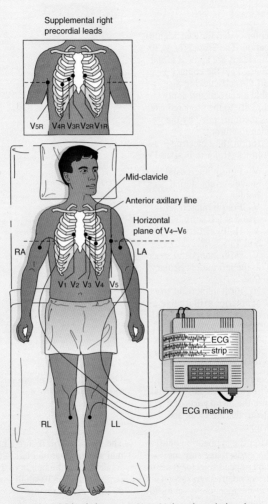

FIGURE 1 ECG lead placement. *Note*: V₆ (not shown) placed at midaxillary line, level with V₄. (From Smeltzer, S. C., Bare, B. G., et al. (2010). *Brunner and Suddarth's textbook of medical-surgical nursing*. 12th ed. Philadelphia, PA: Lippincott Williams & Wilkins, with permission).

color-coded for easy identification. The brown (or V_1 to
V_6) leads are applied to the
chest. Peel the contact paper
off the self-sticking disposable electrode and apply
directly to the prepared site,
as recommended by the
manufacturer.

Position chest electrodes as
follows (Refer to FIGURE 1):

- V_1: Fourth intercostal
  space at right sternal
  border
- V_2: Fourth intercostal
  space at left sternal border
- V_3: Halfway between V_2
  and V_4
- V_4: Fifth intercostal space
  at the left midclavicular
  line
- V_5: Fifth intercostal space
  at anterior axillary line
  (halfway between V_4 and
  V_6)
- V_6: Fifth intercostal space
  at midaxillary line, level
  with V_4

14. Connect the precordial lead
    wires to the electrodes. Make
    sure the metal parts of the
    electrodes are clean and
    bright.

    Dirty or corroded electrodes pre-
    vent a good electrical
    connection.

15. After the application of all
    the leads, make sure the
    paper-speed selector is set to
    the standard 25 m/second and
    that the machine is set to full
    voltage.

    The machine will record a nor-
    mal standardization mark—a
    square that is the height of 2
    large squares or 10 small squares
    on the recording paper.

16. If necessary, enter the appro-
    priate patient identification
    data into the machine.

    This allows for proper identifica-
    tion of the ECG strip.

17. Ask the patient to relax
    and breathe normally.

    Lying still and not talking pro-
    duces a better tracing.

ACTION	RATIONALE
Instruct the patient to lie still and not to talk while you record the ECG.	
18. Press the AUTO button. Observe the tracing quality. The machine will record all 12 leads automatically, recording three consecutive leads simultaneously. Some machines have a display screen so you can preview waveforms before the machine records them on paper. Adjust waveform, if necessary. If any part of the waveform extends beyond the paper when you record the ECG, adjust the normal standardization to half-standardization and repeat. Note this adjustment on the ECG strip, because this will need to be considered in interpreting the results.	Observation of tracing quality allows for adjustments to be made, if necessary. Notation of adjustments ensures accurate interpretation of results.
19. When the machine finishes recording the 12-lead ECG, remove the electrodes and clean the patient's skin, if necessary, with adhesive remover for sticky residue.	Removal and cleaning promote patient comfort.
20. After disconnecting the lead wires from the electrodes, dispose of the electrodes. Return the patient to a comfortable position. Lower bed height and adjust head of bed to a comfortable position.	Proper disposal deters the spread of microorganisms. Promotes patient comfort. Promotes patient safety.
21. Clean ECG machine, per facility policy. If not done electronically from data entered into machine, label the ECG with the patient's name, date of birth, location, date and time of recording,	Cleaning equipment between patient uses decreases the risk for transmission of microorganisms. Accurate labeling ensures the ECG is recorded for the correct patient.

ACTION	RATIONALE
and other relevant information, such as symptoms that occurred during the recording (Jevon, 2007b).	
22. Remove additional PPE, if used. Perform hand hygiene.	Removing PPE properly reduces the risk for infection transmission and contamination of other items. Hand hygiene prevents transmission of microorganisms.

EVALUATION

• A quality ECG reading is obtained without any undue patient anxiety, complications, or injury.
• Patient verbalizes an understanding of the reason for the ECG.

DOCUMENTATION

• Document significant assessment findings, the date and time that the ECG was obtained, and the patient's response to the procedure. Label the ECG recording with the patient's name, room number, and facility identification number, if this was not done by the machine. Record the date and time, as well as any appropriate clinical information on the ECG, such as blood pressure measurement, if the patient was experiencing chest pain.

GENERAL CONSIDERATIONS

• If self-sticking disposable electrodes are not used, apply electrode paste or gel to the patient's skin at the appropriate sites. Rub the gel or paste into the skin. The paste or gel facilitates electrode contact and enhances tracing. Secure electrodes promptly after applying the paste or gel. This prevents drying of the medium, which could impair ECG quality. Never use alcohol or acetone pads in place of the electrode paste or gel. Acetone and alcohol impair electrode contact with the skin and diminish the transmission of electrical impulses. The use of alcohol as a conducting material can result in burns. After disconnecting the lead wires from the electrodes, dispose of, or clean, the electrodes, as indicated. Proper cleaning after use ensures that the machine will be ready for next use.
• For female patients, place the electrodes below the breast tissue. In a large-breasted woman, you may need to displace the breast tissue laterally and/or superiorly.
• If necessary, trim small areas of hair on the patient's chest or extremities, but this usually is not necessary.

- If the patient's skin is exceptionally oily, scaly, or diaphoretic, rub the electrode site with a dry 4 × 4 gauze or soap and water before applying the electrode to help reduce interference in the tracing. Alcohol, benzoin, and antiperspirant are not recommended to prepare skin.
- If the patient has a pacemaker, perform an ECG with or without a magnet, according to the primary care provider's orders. Note the presence of a pacemaker and the use of the magnet on the strip.
- Be aware that a new 80-lead ECG system (body surface mapping) is available, which looks at a patient's heart from 80 views. It can detect up to 15% more patients with myocardial infarction than a standard 12-lead ECG. Additional education regarding use of this technology is required. ECGs obtained with body surface mapping can be interpreted in about 5 minutes, using the same skills as the standard 12-lead ECG (Self et al., 2006).

Skill · 63   Securing an Endotracheal Tube

Endotracheal tubes provide an airway for patients who cannot maintain a sufficient airway on their own. A tube is passed through the mouth or nose into the trachea. Patients who have an endotracheal tube have a high risk for skin breakdown related to securing the endotracheal tube, compounded by the risk of increased secretions. The endotracheal tube should be retaped every 24 hours to prevent skin breakdown and to ensure that the tube is secured properly. Retaping an endotracheal tube requires two people. There are other ways of securing an endotracheal tube besides tape. Endotracheal tube holders are commercially available. To secure with one of these devices, follow the manufacturer's recommendations. However, the literature suggests using tape to secure an endotracheal tube may be the best method (Carlson et al., 2007). One example of taping an endotracheal tube is provided below, but this skill might be performed differently in your institution. Always refer to specific agency policy.

EQUIPMENT

- Assistant (nurse or respiratory therapist)
- Portable or wall suction unit with tubing
- Sterile suction catheter with Y-port
- 1-inch tape (adhesive or waterproof tape)
- Disposable gloves
- Mask and goggles or face shield
- Additional PPE, as indicated
- Sterile suctioning kit
- Oral suction catheter
- Two 3-mL syringes or tongue blade
- Scissors
- Washcloth and cleaning agent

- Skin barrier (e.g., 3M or Skin Prep)
- Adhesive remover swab
- Towel
- Razor (optional)
- Shaving cream (optional)
- Sterile saline or water
- Handheld pressure gauge

ASSESSMENT GUIDELINES

- Assess the need for retaping, which may include loose or soiled tape, pressure on mucous membranes, or repositioning of tube.
- Assess endotracheal tube length. The tube has markings on the side to ensure it is not moved during the retaping.
- Assess lung sounds to obtain a baseline. Ensure that the lung sounds are still heard throughout the lobes.
- Assess oxygen saturation level. If the tube is dislodged, the oxygen saturation level may change.
- Assess the chest for symmetric rise and fall during respiration. If the tube is dislodged, the rise and fall of the chest will change.
- Assess the patient's need for pain medication or sedation. The patient should be calm, free of pain, and relaxed during the retaping so that he or she does not move and cause an accidental extubation.

NURSING DIAGNOSES

- Risk for Impaired Skin Integrity
- Impaired Oral Mucous Membrane
- Risk for Injury
- Risk for Infection

OUTCOME IDENTIFICATION AND PLANNING

Expected outcomes may include:
- Patient's endotracheal tube remains in place.
- Patient maintains bilaterally equal and clear lung sounds.
- Patient demonstrates understanding about the reason for the endotracheal tube.
- Patient's skin remains intact.
- Patient's oxygen saturation remains greater than 95%, chest rises symmetrically, and airway remains clear.

IMPLEMENTATION

ACTION

RATIONALE

1. Bring necessary equipment to the bedside stand or over-bed table.

Bringing everything to the bedside conserves time and energy. Arranging items nearby is convenient, saves time, and avoids unnecessary stretching and

ACTION	RATIONALE

<table>
<tr><td></td><td>twisting of muscles on the part of the nurse.</td></tr>
<tr><td>2. Perform hand hygiene and put on PPE, if indicated. </td><td>Hand hygiene and PPE prevent the spread of microorganisms. PPE is required based on transmission precautions.</td></tr>
<tr><td>3. Identify the patient.</td><td>Identifying the patient ensures the right patient receives the intervention and helps prevent errors.</td></tr>
<tr><td>4. Close curtains around bed and close the door to the room, if possible.</td><td>This ensures the patient's privacy.</td></tr>
<tr><td>5. Assess the need for endotracheal tube retaping. **Administer pain medication or sedation, as prescribed, before attempting to retape the endotracheal tube.** Explain the procedure to the patient.</td><td>Retaping the endotracheal tube can stimulate coughing, which may be painful for patients, particularly those with surgical incisions. Explanation facilitates cooperation and provides reassurance for the patient. Any procedure that compromises respiration is frightening for the patient.</td></tr>
<tr><td>6. Obtain the assistance of a second individual to hold the endotracheal tube in place while the old tape is removed and the new tape is placed.</td><td>This prevents accidental extubation.</td></tr>
<tr><td>7. Adjust the bed to a comfortable working position, usually elbow height of the caregiver (VISN 8, Patient Safety Center, 2009). Lower side rail closest to you. **If patient is conscious, place him or her in a semi-Fowler's position. If patient is unconscious, place him or her in the lateral position, facing you. Move the overbed table close to your**</td><td>Having the bed at the proper height prevents back and muscle strain. A sitting position helps the patient to cough and makes breathing easier. Gravity also facilitates catheter insertion. The lateral position prevents the airway from becoming obstructed and promotes drainage of secretions. The overbed table provides work surface and maintains sterility of objects on the work surface. Placing the trash receptacle</td></tr>
</table>

ACTION	RATIONALE
work area and raise it to waist height. Place a trash receptacle within easy reach of work area.	within reach allows for an organized approach to care.
8. Put on face shield or goggles and mask. Suction patient as described in Skills 64 and 65.	Personal protective equipment prevents exposure to contaminants. Suctioning decreases the likelihood of patient coughing during the retaping of the endotracheal tube. If the patient coughs, the tube may become dislodged.
9. Measure a piece of tape for the length needed to reach around the patient's neck to the mouth plus 8 inches. Cut tape. Lay it adhesive-side up on the table.	Extra length is needed so that tape can be wrapped around the endotracheal tube.
10. Cut another piece of tape long enough to reach from one jaw around the back of the neck to the other jaw. Lay this piece on the center of the longer piece on the table, matching the tapes' adhesive sides together.	This prevents the tape from sticking to the patient's hair and the back of the neck.
11. Take one 3-mL syringe or tongue blade and wrap the sticky tape around the syringe until the nonsticky area is reached. Do this for the other side as well.	This helps the nurse or respiratory therapist to manage the tape without it sticking to the sheets or the patient's hair.
12. Take one of the 3-mL syringes or tongue blades and pass it under the patient's neck so that there is a 3-mL syringe on either side of the patient's head.	This makes the tape easy to access when retaping the tube.
13. Put on disposable gloves. Have the assistant put on gloves as well.	Gloves protect the hands from exposure to contaminants.
14. **Provide oral care, including suctioning the oral cavity.**	This helps to decrease secretions in the oral cavity and pharynx region.

ACTION	RATIONALE
15. Take note of the 'cm' position markings on the tube. Begin to unwrap old tape from around the endotracheal tube. After one side is unwrapped, have an assistant hold the endotracheal tube as close to the lips or nares as possible to offer stabilization.	Assistant should hold the tube to prevent accidental extubation. Holding the tube as close to lips or nares as possible prevents accidental dislodgement of tube.
16. Carefully remove the remaining tape from the endotracheal tube. **After the tape is removed, have the assistant gently and slowly move the endotracheal tube (if orally intubated) to the other side of the mouth. Assess mouth for any skin breakdown. Before applying new tape, make sure that markings on the endotracheal tube are at the same spot as when retaping began.**	The endotracheal tube may cause pressure ulcers if left in the same place over time. By moving the tube, the risk for pressure ulcers is reduced.
17. Remove old tape from cheeks and side of face. Use adhesive remover to remove excess adhesive from tape. Clean the face and neck with washcloth and cleanser. If patient has facial hair, consider shaving cheeks. Pat cheeks dry with the towel.	To prevent skin breakdown, remove old adhesive. Shaving helps to decrease pain when tape is removed. Cheeks must be dry before new tape is applied to ensure that it sticks.
18. Apply the skin barrier to the patient's face (under the nose, cheeks, and lower lip) where the tape will sit. Unroll one side of the tape. Ensure that the nonstick part of the tape remains behind the patient's neck while pulling firmly on the tape. **Place the adhesive portion of the tape snugly against the patient's cheek. Split the**	Skin barrier protects the skin from injury with subsequent tape removal and helps the tape adhere better to the skin. The tape should be snug to the side of the patient's face to prevent accidental extubation.

ACTION	RATIONALE

tape in half from the end to the corner of the mouth.

By placing one piece of tape on the lip and the other piece of tape on the tube, the tube remains secure. Tab makes tape removal easier.

19. Place the top half piece of tape under the patient's nose (FIGURE 1). Wrap the lower half around the tube in one direction, such as over and around the tube. Fold over tab on end of tape.

By placing one piece of tape on the lip and the other piece of tape on the tube, the tube remains secure. Tab makes tape removal easier.

20. Unwrap second side of tape. Split to corner of the mouth. Place the bottom half piece of tape along the patient's lower lip. Wrap the top half around the tube in the opposite direction, such as below and around the tube. Fold over tab on end of tape. Ensure tape is secure (FIGURE 2).

Alternating the placement of the top and bottom pieces of tape provides more anchorage for the tube. Wrapping the tape in an alternating manner ensures that the tape will not accidentally be unwound.

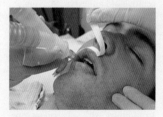

FIGURE 1 Putting new tape in place.

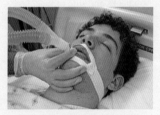

FIGURE 2 Ensuring tape is securely stabilizing the tube.

21. **Auscultate lung sounds. Assess for cyanosis, oxygen saturation, chest symmetry, and stability of the endotracheal tube. Again check to ensure that the tube is at the correct depth.**

If the tube has been moved from its original place, the lung sounds may change, as well as oxygen saturation and chest symmetry. The tube should be stable and should not move with each respiration cycle.

ACTION	RATIONALE
22. **If the endotracheal tube is cuffed, check pressure of the balloon pressure by attaching a handheld pressure gauge to the pilot balloon of the endotracheal tube.**	Maximal cuff pressures should not exceed 24 to 30 cm H_2O to prevent tracheal ischemia and necrosis.
23. Assist patient to a comfortable position. Raise the bed rail and place the bed in the lowest position.	Ensures patient comfort. Proper positioning with raised side rails and proper bed height provide for patient comfort and safety.
24. Remove face shield or goggles and mask. Remove additional PPE, if used. Perform hand hygiene.	Removing PPE properly reduces the risk for infection transmission and contamination of other items. Hand hygiene prevents the spread of microorganisms.

EVALUATION

- Patient's endotracheal tube tape is changed without dislodgement or a change in tube depth.
- Patient's lung sounds remain equal.
- No pressure ulcers are noted.
- Patient's airway remains clear.
- Patient's oxygen saturation remains greater than 95%, chest rises symmetrically, and skin remains acyanotic.
- Endotracheal tube cuff pressure is maintained at 20 to 25 cm H_2O.

DOCUMENTATION

- Document the procedure, including the depth of the endotracheal tube from teeth or lips; the amount, consistency, and color of secretions suctioned; presence of any skin or mucous membrane changes or pressure ulcers; and pre- and postassessment, including lung sounds, oxygen saturation, skin color, cuff pressure, and chest symmetry.

GENERAL CONSIDERATIONS

- Emergency equipment should be easily accessible at the bedside. Keep bag-valve mask, oxygen, and suction equipment at the bedside of a patient with an endotracheal tube at all times.

Skill · 64 Suctioning an Endotracheal Tube: Closed System

The purpose of suctioning is to maintain a patent airway and remove pulmonary secretions, blood, vomitus, or foreign material from the airway. When suctioning via an endotracheal tube, the goal is to remove secretions that are not accessible to cilia bypassed by the tube itself. Tracheal suctioning can lead to hypoxemia, cardiac dysrhythmias, trauma, atelectasis, infection, bleeding, and pain. It is imperative to be diligent in maintaining aseptic technique and following facility guidelines and procedures to prevent potential hazards. Suctioning frequency is based on clinical assessment to determine the need for suctioning.

Suctioning removes secretions not accessible to bypassed cilia, so the catheter should be inserted only as far as the end of the endotracheal tube. Catheter contact and suction cause tracheal mucosal damage, loss of cilia, edema, and fibrosis, as well as increased risk of infection and bleeding for the patient. Insertion of the suction catheter to a predetermined distance, no more than 1 cm past the length of the endotracheal tube, avoids contact with the trachea and carina, reducing the effects of tracheal mucosal damage (Ireton, 2007; Pate, 2004; Pate & Zapata, 2002).

Closed system suction (FIGURE 1) may be used routinely or when a patient must be frequently and quickly suctioned due to an excess of secretions, depending on the policies of the institution. One drawback of closed suctioning is thought to be the hindrance of the sheath when rotating the suction catheter upon removal.

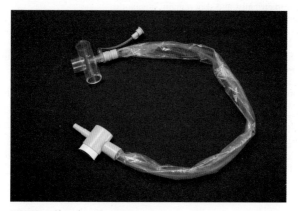

FIGURE 1 Closed suction system.

EQUIPMENT

- Portable or wall suction unit with tubing
- Closed suction device of appropriate size for patient
- 3-mL or 5-mL normal saline solution in dosette or syringe
- Sterile gloves
- Additional PPE, as indicated

ASSESSMENT GUIDELINES

- Assess lung sounds. Patients who need to be suctioned may have wheezes, crackles, or gurgling.
- Assess oxygenation saturation level. Oxygen saturation usually decreases when a patient needs to be suctioned.
- Assess respiratory status, including respiratory rate and depth. Patients may become tachypneic when they need to be suctioned. Assess patient for signs of respiratory distress, such as nasal flaring, retractions, or grunting.
- Additional indications for suctioning via an endotracheal tube include secretions in the tube, acute respiratory distress, and frequent or sustained coughing.
- Also assess for pain and the potential to cause pain during the intervention. Perform individualized pain management in response to the patient's needs (Arroyo-Novoa et al., 2007). If the patient has had abdominal surgery or other procedures, administer pain medication before suctioning.
- Assess appropriate suction catheter depth.

NURSING DIAGNOSES

- Ineffective Airway Clearance
- Risk for Aspiration
- Impaired Gas Exchange
- Risk for Infection

OUTCOME IDENTIFICATION AND PLANNING

Expected outcomes may include:
- Patient will exhibit improved breath sounds and a clear, patent airway.
- Patient will exhibit an oxygen saturation level within acceptable parameters.
- Patient will demonstrate a respiratory rate and depth within age-acceptable range.
- Patient will remain free of any signs of respiratory distress.

IMPLEMENTATION

ACTION	RATIONALE
1. Bring necessary equipment to the bedside stand or over-bed table.	Bringing everything to the bedside conserves time and energy. Arranging items nearby is convenient, saves time, and avoids unnecessary stretching and twisting of muscles on the part of the nurse.
2. Perform hand hygiene and put on PPE, if indicated.	Hand hygiene and PPE prevent the spread of microorganisms. PPE is required based on transmission precautions.
3. Identify the patient.	Identifying the patient ensures the right patient receives the intervention and helps prevent errors.
4. Close curtains around bed and close the door to the room, if possible.	This ensures the patient's privacy.
5. Determine the need for suctioning. Verify the suction order in the patient's chart. **Assess for pain or the potential to cause pain. Administer pain medication, as prescribed, before suctioning.**	To minimize trauma to airway mucosa, suctioning should be done only when secretions have accumulated or adventitious breath sounds are audible. Suctioning can cause moderate to severe pain for patients. Individualized pain management is imperative (Arroyo-Novoa et al., 2007). Suctioning stimulates coughing, which is painful for patients with surgical incisions.
6. Explain what you are going to do and the reason for doing it to the patient, even if the patient does not appear to be alert. Reassure the patient you will interrupt the procedure if he or she indicates respiratory difficulty.	Explanation alleviates fears. Even if the patient appears unconscious, the nurse should explain what is happening. Any procedure that compromises respiration is frightening for the patient.
7. Adjust bed to comfortable working position, usually	Having the bed at the proper height prevents back and muscle

ACTION	RATIONALE

elbow height of the caregiver (VISN 8 Patient Safety Center, 2009). Lower side rail closest to you. **If patient is conscious, place him or her in a semi-Fowler's position. If patient is unconscious, place him or her in the lateral position, facing you. Move the overbed table close to your work area and raise to waist height.**

strain. A sitting position helps the patient to cough and makes breathing easier. Gravity also facilitates catheter insertion. The lateral position prevents the airway from becoming obstructed and promotes drainage of secretions. The overbed table provides work surface and maintains sterility of objects on it.

8. **Turn suction to appropriate pressure.**

Higher pressures can cause excessive trauma, hypoxemia, and atelectasis.

For a wall unit for an adult: 100–120 mm Hg (Roman, 2005); neonates: 60–80 mm Hg; infants: 80–100 mm Hg; children: 80–100 mm Hg; adolescents: 80–120 mm Hg (Ireton, 2007).

For a portable unit for an adult: 10–15 cm Hg; neonates: 6–8 cm Hg; infants: 8–10 cm Hg; children: 8–10 cm Hg; adolescents: 8–10 cm Hg.

9. **Open the package of the closed suction device using aseptic technique. Make sure that the device remains sterile.**

The device must remain sterile to prevent a nosocomial infection.

10. Put on sterile gloves.

Gloves deter the spread of microorganisms.

11. Using nondominant hand, disconnect the ventilator from the endotracheal tube. **Place ventilator tubing in a convenient location so that the inside of the tubing remains sterile or continue to hold the tubing in your nondominant hand.**

This provides access to the endotracheal tube while keeping one hand sterile. The inside of the ventilator tubing should remain sterile to prevent a nosocomial infection.

ACTION	RATIONALE
12. **Using dominant hand and keeping device sterile, connect the closed suctioning device so that the suctioning catheter is in line with the endotracheal tube.**	Keeping the device sterile decreases the risk for a nosocomial infection.
13. **Keeping the inside of the ventilator tubing sterile, attach ventilator tubing to the port perpendicular to the endotracheal tube.** Attach suction tubing to the suction catheter.	The inside of the ventilator tubing must remain sterile to prevent a nosocomial infection. By connecting the ventilator tubing to the port, the patient does not need to be disconnected from the ventilator to be suctioned.
14. Pop top off sterile normal saline dosette. Open plug to port by suction catheter and insert saline dosette or syringe.	The saline will help to clean the catheter between suctioning.
15. **Hyperventilate the patient by using the 'sigh' button on the ventilator before suctioning.** Turn on the safety cap suction button of catheter so that button is depressed easily.	Hyperoxygenating and hyperventilating before suctioning helps to decrease the effects of oxygen removal during suctioning. The safety button keeps the patient from accidentally depressing the button and decreasing the oxygen saturation.
16. Grasp the suction catheter through protective sheath, about 6 inches (15 cm) from the endotracheal tube. Gently insert the catheter into the endotracheal tube (FIGURE 2). Release the catheter while holding on to the protective	The sheath keeps the suction catheter sterile. Catheter contact and suction cause tracheal mucosal damage, loss of cilia, edema, and fibrosis, as well as increasing the risk of infection and bleeding for the patient. Insertion of the suction catheter

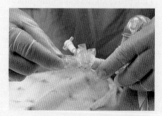

FIGURE 2 Inserting catheter through sheath and into the endotracheal tube.

ACTION	RATIONALE
sheath. Move the hand farther back on the catheter. **Grasp catheter through sheath and repeat movement, advancing the catheter to the predetermined length. Do not occlude the Y-port when inserting the catheter.**	to a predetermined distance, no more than 1 cm past the length of the endotracheal tube, avoids contact with the trachea and carina, reducing the effects of tracheal mucosal damage (Ireton, 2007; Pate, 2004; Pate & Zapata, 2002). If resistance is met, the carina or tracheal mucosa has been hit. Withdraw the catheter at least ½ inch before applying suction. Suctioning when inserting the catheter increases the risk for trauma to airway mucosa and increases risk of hypoxemia.
17. Apply intermittent suction by depressing the suction button with the thumb of the nondominant hand. Gently rotate the catheter with the thumb and index finger of the dominant hand as catheter is being withdrawn. **Do not suction for more than 10 to 15 seconds at a time.** Hyperoxygenate or hyperventilate with the 'sigh' button on the ventilator, as ordered.	Turning the catheter while withdrawing it helps clean surfaces of respiratory tract and prevents injury to tracheal mucosa. Suctioning for longer than 10 to 15 seconds robs the respiratory tract of oxygen, which may result in hypoxemia. Suctioning too quickly may be ineffective at clearing all secretions. Hyperoxygenation and hyperventilation reoxygenate the lungs.
18. Once the catheter is withdrawn back into the sheath (FIGURE 3), depress the suction button while gently squeezing the normal saline dosette until the catheter is clean. **Allow at least**	Flushing cleans and clears catheter and lubricates it for next insertion. Allowing time interval and replacing oxygen delivery setup help compensate for hypoxia induced by the suctioning.

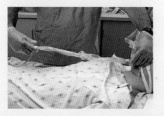

FIGURE 3 Removing suction catheter by pulling back into sheath.

ACTION	RATIONALE
a 30-second to 1-minute interval if additional suctioning is needed. No more than three suction passes should be made per suctioning episode.	Excessive suction passes contribute to complications.
19. When the procedure is completed, ensure that catheter is withdrawn into sheath, and turn safety button. Remove normal saline dosette and apply cap to port.	By turning the safety button, the suction is blocked at the catheter so the suction cannot remove oxygen from the endotracheal tube.
20. Suction the oral cavity with a separate single-use, disposable catheter and perform oral hygiene. Remove gloves. Turn off suction.	Suctioning of the oral cavity removes secretions that may be stagnant in the mouth and pharynx, reducing the risk for infection. Oral hygiene offers comfort to the patient. Removing PPE properly reduces the risk for infection transmission and contamination of other items.
21. Assist the patient to a comfortable position. Raise the bed rail and place the bed in the lowest position.	Ensures patient comfort. Proper positioning with raised side rails and proper bed height provide for patient comfort and safety.
22. Reassess patient's respiratory status, including respiratory rate, effort, oxygen saturation, and lung sounds.	Assesses effectiveness of suctioning and the presence of complications.
23. Remove additional PPE, if used. Perform hand hygiene.	Removing PPE properly reduces the risk for infection transmission and contamination of other items. Hand hygiene prevents the spread of microorganisms.

EVALUATION

• Patient exhibits improved breath sounds and a clear and patent airway.
• Patient's oxygen saturation level is within acceptable parameters.
• Patient does not exhibit signs or symptoms of respiratory distress or complications.

DOCUMENTATION

- Document the time of suctioning, pre- and postintervention assessment, reason for suctioning, oxygen saturation levels, and the characteristics and amount of secretions.

GENERAL CONSIDERATIONS

- Determine the catheter size to be used by the size of the endotracheal tube. The external diameter of the suction catheter should not exceed half of the internal diameter of the endotracheal tube. Larger catheters can contribute to trauma and hypoxemia.
- Make sure emergency equipment is easily accessible at the bedside. Keep a bag-valve mask, oxygen, and suction equipment at the bedside of a patient with an endotracheal tube at all times.

Skill · 65 **Suctioning an Endotracheal Tube: Open System**

The purpose of suctioning is to maintain a patent airway and remove pulmonary secretions, blood, vomitus, or foreign material from the airway. When suctioning via an endotracheal tube, the goal is to remove secretions that are not accessible to cilia bypassed by the tube itself. Remember, tracheal suctioning can lead to hypoxemia, cardiac dysrhythmias, trauma, atelectasis, infection, bleeding, and pain, so it is imperative to be diligent in maintaining aseptic technique and following facility guidelines and procedures to prevent potential hazards. Frequency of suctioning is based on clinical assessment.

Because suctioning removes secretions not accessible to bypassed cilia, the catheter should be inserted only as far as the end of the endotracheal tube. Catheter contact and suction cause tracheal mucosal damage, loss of cilia, edema, and fibrosis, as well as increasing the risk of infection and bleeding for the patient. Insertion of the suction catheter to a predetermined distance, no more than 1 cm past the length of the endotracheal tube, avoids contact with the trachea and carina, reducing the effects of tracheal mucosal damage (Ireton, 2007; Pate, 2004; Pate & Zapata, 2002).

Some consider open system suctioning to be the most efficient way to suction the endotracheal tube, arguing that there are no limitations to the movement of the suction catheter while suctioning. However, the nurse may unknowingly contaminate an open system during the procedure. In addition, with the open system, the patient must be removed from the ventilator during suctioning.

EQUIPMENT

- Portable or wall suction unit with tubing
- A commercially prepared suction kit with an appropriate size catheter (see General Considerations) or
  - Sterile suction catheter with Y-port in the appropriate size
  - Sterile disposable container
- Sterile gloves
- Towel or waterproof pad
- Goggles and mask or face shield
- Additional PPE, as indicated
- Disposable, clean glove
- Resuscitation bag connected to 100% oxygen
- Assistant (optional)

ASSESSMENT GUIDELINES

- Assess lung sounds. Patients who need to be suctioned may have wheezes, crackles, or gurgling present.
- Assess oxygenation saturation level. Oxygen saturation usually decreases when a patient needs to be suctioned.
- Assess respiratory status, including respiratory rate and depth. Patients may become tachypneic when they need to be suctioned. Assess patient for signs of respiratory distress, such as nasal flaring, retractions, or grunting.
- Additional indications for suctioning via an endotracheal tube include secretions in the tube, acute respiratory distress, and frequent or sustained coughing.
- Also assess for pain and the potential to cause pain during the intervention. Perform individualized pain management in response to the patient's needs (Arroyo-Novoa et al., 2007). If patient has had abdominal surgery or other procedures, administer pain medication before suctioning.
- Assess appropriate suction catheter depth.

NURSING DIAGNOSES

- Ineffective Airway Clearance
- Risk for Aspiration
- Impaired Gas Exchange
- Risk for Infection

OUTCOME IDENTIFICATION AND PLANNING

Expected outcomes may include:
- Patient will exhibit improved breath sounds and a clear, patent airway.
- Patient will exhibit an oxygen saturation level within acceptable parameters.
- Patient will demonstrate a respiratory rate and depth within age-acceptable range.
- Patient will remain free of any signs of respiratory distress.

IMPLEMENTATION

ACTION | RATIONALE

1. Bring necessary equipment to the bedside stand or over-bed table.

Bringing everything to the bed-side conserves time and energy. Arranging items nearby is convenient, saves time, and avoids unnecessary stretching and twisting of muscles on the part of the nurse.

2. Perform hand hygiene and put on PPE, if indicated.

Hand hygiene and PPE prevent the spread of microorganisms. PPE is required based on transmission precautions.

3. Identify the patient.

Identifying the patient ensures the right patient receives the intervention and helps prevent errors.

4. Close curtains around bed and close the door to the room, if possible.

This ensures the patient's privacy.

5. Determine the need for suctioning. Verify the suction order in the patient's chart. Assess for pain or the potential to cause pain. Administer pain medication, as prescribed, before suctioning.

To minimize trauma to airway mucosa, suctioning should be done only when secretions have accumulated or adventitious breath sounds are audible. Suctioning can cause moderate to severe pain for patients. Individualized pain management is imperative (Arroyo-Novoa et al., 2007). Suctioning stimulates coughing, which is painful for patients with surgical incisions.

6. Explain what you are going to do and the reason for doing it to the patient, even if the patient does not appear to be alert. Reassure the patient you will interrupt the procedure if he or she indicates respiratory difficulty.

Explanation alleviates fears. Even if the patient appears unconscious, the nurse should explain what is happening. Any procedure that compromises respiration is frightening for the patient.

7. Adjust bed to comfortable working position, usually

Having the bed at the proper height prevents back and muscle

ACTION	RATIONALE
elbow height of the caregiver (VISN 8, Patient Safety Center, 2009). Lower side rail closest to you. If the patient is conscious, place him or her in a semi-Fowler's position. **If patient is unconscious, place him or her in the lateral position, facing you. Move the overbed table close to your work area and raise it to waist height.**	strain. A sitting position helps the patient to cough and makes breathing easier. Gravity also facilitates catheter insertion. The lateral position prevents the airway from becoming obstructed and promotes drainage of secretions. The overbed table provides work surface and maintains sterility of objects on it.
8. Place towel or waterproof pad across patient's chest.	This protects bed linens and the patient.
9. **Turn suction to appropriate pressure.**	Higher pressures can cause excessive trauma, hypoxemia, and atelectasis.
For a wall unit for an adult: 100–120 mm Hg (Roman, 2005); neonates: 60–80 mm Hg; infants: 80–100 mm Hg; children: 80–100 mm Hg; adolescents: 80–120 mm Hg (Ireton, 2007).	
For a portable unit for an adult: 10–15 cm Hg; neonates: 6–8 cm Hg; infants: 8–10 cm Hg; children: 8–10 cm Hg; adolescents: 8–10 cm Hg.	
10. Put on a disposable, clean glove and occlude the end of the connecting tubing to check suction pressure. Place the connecting tubing in a convenient location. Place the resuscitation bag connected to oxygen within convenient reach, if using.	Glove prevents contact with blood and body fluids. Checking pressure ensures equipment is working properly. Allows for an organized approach to procedure.
11. Open sterile suction package using aseptic technique. The open wrapper becomes a sterile field to hold other	Sterile normal saline or water is used to lubricate the outside of the catheter, minimizing irritation of mucosa during

ACTION	RATIONALE
supplies. Carefully remove the sterile container, touching only the outside surface. Set it up on the work surface and pour sterile saline into it.	introduction. It is also used to clear the catheter between suction attempts.
12. Put on face shield or goggles and mask. Put on sterile gloves. **The dominant hand will manipulate the catheter and must remain sterile. The nondominant hand is considered clean rather than sterile and will control the suction valve (Y-port) on the catheter.**	Handling the sterile catheter using a sterile glove helps prevent introducing organisms into the respiratory tract; the clean glove protects the nurse from microorganisms.
13. With dominant gloved hand, pick up sterile catheter. Pick up the connecting tubing with the nondominant hand and connect the tubing and suction catheter.	Sterility of the suction catheter is maintained.
14. Moisten the catheter by dipping it into the container of sterile saline, unless it is a silicone catheter. Occlude Y-tube to check suction.	Lubricating the inside of the catheter with saline helps move secretions in the catheter. Silicone catheters do not require lubrication. Checking suction ensures equipment is working properly.
15. Hyperventilate the patient using your nondominant hand and a manual resuscitation bag and delivering three to six breaths or use the 'sigh' mechanism on a mechanical ventilator.	Hyperventilation and hyperoxygenation aid in preventing hypoxemia during suctioning.
16. Open the adapter on the mechanical ventilator tubing or remove the manual resuscitation bag with your nondominant hand.	This exposes the tracheostomy tube without contaminating sterile gloved hand.

ACTION	RATIONALE

17. Using your dominant hand, gently and quickly insert catheter into trachea (FIGURE 1). **Advance the catheter to the predetermined length. Do not occlude the Y-port when inserting the catheter.**

Catheter contact and suction cause tracheal mucosal damage, loss of cilia, edema, and fibrosis, as well as increasing the risk of infection and bleeding for the patient. Insertion of the suction catheter to a predetermined distance, no more than 1 cm past the length of the endotracheal tube, avoids contact with the trachea and carina, reducing the effects of tracheal mucosal damage (Ireton, 2007; Pate, 2004; Pate & Zapata, 2002). If resistance is met, the carina or tracheal mucosa has been hit. Withdraw the catheter at least ½ inch before applying suction. Occluding the Y-port (i.e., suctioning) when inserting catheter increases the risk for trauma to airway mucosa and increases risk of hypoxemia.

18. Apply suction by intermittently occluding the Y-port on the catheter with the thumb of your nondominant hand, and gently rotate the catheter as it is being withdrawn (FIGURE 2).

Turning the catheter as it is withdrawn minimizes trauma to the mucosa. Suctioning for longer than 10 to 15 seconds robs the respiratory tract of oxygen, which may result in hypoxemia. Suctioning too quickly may be

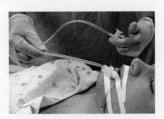

FIGURE 1 Inserting suction catheter into endotracheal tube.

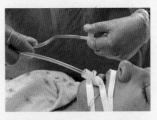

FIGURE 2 Withdrawing suction catheter and intermittently occluding Y-port with thumb to apply suction.

ACTION	RATIONALE
Do not suction for more than 10 to 15 seconds at a time.	ineffective at clearing all secretions.
19. Hyperventilate the patient using your nondominant hand and a manual resuscitation bag and delivering 3 to 6 breaths. Replace the oxygen delivery device, if applicable, using your nondominant hand and have the patient take several deep breaths. If the patient is mechanically ventilated, close the adapter on the mechanical ventilator tubing or replace ventilator tubing and use the 'sigh' mechanism on a mechanical ventilator.	Suctioning removes air from the patient's airway and can cause hypoxemia. Hyperventilation and hyperoxygenation can help prevent suction-induced hypoxemia.
20. Flush catheter with saline. Assess effectiveness of suctioning and repeat, as needed, and according to patient's tolerance.	Flushing clears catheter and lubricates it for next insertion. Reassessment determines need for additional suctioning.
Wrap the suction catheter around your dominant hand between attempts.	Wrapping the catheter prevents inadvertent contamination of catheter.
21. Allow at least a 30-second to 1-minute interval if additional suctioning is needed. No more than three suction passes should be made per suctioning episode. Suction the oropharynx after suctioning the trachea. Do not reinsert in the endotracheal tube after suctioning the mouth.	The interval allows for reventilation and reoxygenation of airways. Excessive suction passes contribute to complications. Suctioning the oropharynx clears the mouth of secretions. More microorganisms are usually present in the mouth, so it is suctioned last to prevent transmission of contaminants.
22. When suctioning is completed, remove gloves from dominant hand over the coiled catheter, pulling it off inside-out. Remove glove from nondominant hand and dispose of gloves, catheter, and container with solution in the appropriate receptacle. Assist patient	This technique of glove removal and disposal of equipment reduces transmission of microorganisms. Proper positioning with raised side rails and proper bed height provide for patient comfort and safety.

ACTION	RATIONALE

to a comfortable position.
Raise bed rail and place bed
in the lowest position.

23. Turn off suction. Remove
    face shield or goggles
    and mask. Perform
    hand hygiene.

Removing face shield or goggles
and mask properly reduces the
risk for infection transmission
and contamination of other
items. Hand hygiene prevents
transmission of microorganisms.

24. Offer oral hygiene after
    suctioning.

Respiratory secretions that are
allowed to accumulate in the
mouth are irritating to mucous
membranes and unpleasant for
the patient.

25. Reassess the patient's respi-
    ratory status, including respi-
    ratory rate, effort, oxygen
    saturation, and lung sounds.

Assesses the effectiveness of
suctioning and the presence of
complications.

26. Remove additional PPE, if
    used. Perform hand
    hygiene.

Removing PPE properly reduces
the risk for infection transmission and contamination of other
items. Hand hygiene prevents the
spread of microorganisms.

EVALUATION

- Patient exhibits improved breath sounds and a clear and patent airway.
- Patient's oxygen saturation level is within acceptable parameters.
- Patient does not exhibit signs or symptoms of respiratory distress or
  complications.

DOCUMENTATION

- Document the time of suctioning, pre- and postintervention assessment, reason for suctioning, oxygen saturation levels, and the characteristics and amount of secretions.

GENERAL CONSIDERATIONS

- Determine the size of catheter to use by the size of the endotracheal
  tube. The external diameter of the suction catheter should not exceed
  half of the internal diameter of the endotracheal tube. Larger catheters
  can contribute to trauma and hypoxemia.
- Make sure emergency equipment is easily accessible at the bedside.
  Keep a bag-valve mask, oxygen, and suction equipment at the bedside of a patient with an endotracheal tube at all times.

Skill · 66   **Administering a Large-Volume Cleansing Enema**

Cleansing enemas are given to remove feces from the colon. Some of the reasons for administering a cleansing enema include relieving constipation or fecal impaction, preventing involuntary escape of fecal material during surgical procedures, promoting visualization of the intestinal tract by radiographic or instrument examination, and helping to establish regular bowel function during a bowel training program. Cleansing enemas are classified as either large-volume or small-volume. This Skill addresses administering a large-volume enema. Large-volume enemas are known as hypotonic or isotonic, depending on the solution used. Hypotonic (tap water) and isotonic (normal saline solution) enemas are large-volume enemas that result in rapid colonic emptying. However, using such large volumes of solution (adults: 500 to 1,000 mL; infants: 150 to 250 mL) may be dangerous for patients with weakened intestinal walls, such as those with bowel inflammation or bowel infection. These solutions often require special preparation and equipment. Small-volume enemas are addressed in Skill 69.

EQUIPMENT

- Solution as ordered by the physician at a temperature of 105°F to 110°F (40°C to 43°C) for adults in the prescribed amount. (Amount will vary depending on type of solution, patient's age, and patient's ability to retain the solution. Average cleansing enema for an adult may range from 750 to 1,000 mL.)
- Disposable enema set, which includes a solution container and tubing
- Water-soluble lubricant
- IV pole
- Necessary additives, as ordered
- Waterproof pad
- Bath thermometer (if available)
- Bath blanket
- Bedpan and toilet tissue
- Disposable gloves
- Additional PPE, as indicated
- Paper towel
- Washcloth, soap, and towel

ASSESSMENT GUIDELINES

- Ask the patient when he or she had the last bowel movement.
- Assess the patient's abdomen, including auscultating for bowel sounds, percussing, and palpating. Because the goal of a cleansing enema is to increase peristalsis, which should increase bowel sounds, assess the abdomen before and after the enema.
- Assess the rectal area for any fissures, hemorrhoids, sores, or rectal tears. If present, added care should be taken while inserting the tube.
- Assess the results of the patient's laboratory work, specifically the platelet count and white blood cell (WBC) count. An enema is contraindicated for patients with a low platelet count or low WBC count.

An enema may irritate or traumatize the gastrointestinal mucosa, causing bleeding, bowel perforation, or infection. Any unnecessary procedures that would place the patient at risk for bleeding or infection should not be performed.
• Assess for dizziness, light-headedness, diaphoresis, and clammy skin. The enema may stimulate a vagal response, which increases parasympathetic stimulation, causing a decrease in heart rate.
• Do not administer enemas to patients who have severe abdominal pain, bowel obstruction, bowel inflammation or bowel infection, or after rectal, prostate, or colon surgery.

NURSING DIAGNOSES
• Acute Pain
• Constipation
• Risk for Injury
• Risk for Constipation

OUTCOME IDENTIFICATION AND PLANNING
Expected outcomes may include:
• Patient expels feces.
• Patient verbalizes decreased discomfort.
• Abdominal distention is absent.
• Patient remains free of any evidence of trauma to the rectal mucosa or other adverse effects.

IMPLEMENTATION

ACTION	RATIONALE
1. Verify the order for the enema. Bring necessary equipment to the bedside stand or overbed table.	Verifying the physician's order is crucial to ensuring that the proper enema is administered to the right patient. Bringing everything to the bedside conserves time and energy. Arranging items nearby is convenient, saves time, and avoids unnecessary stretching and twisting of muscles on the part of the nurse.
2. Perform hand hygiene and put on PPE, if indicated.	Hand hygiene and PPE prevent the spread of microorganisms. PPE is required based on transmission precautions.

ACTION	RATIONALE
3. Identify the patient.	Identifying the patient ensures the right patient receives the intervention and helps prevent errors.
4. Close curtains around the bed and close the door to the room, if possible. Explain what you are going to do and why you are going to do it to the patient. Discuss where the patient will defecate. Have a bedpan, commode, or nearby bathroom ready for use.	This ensures the patient's privacy. Explanation relieves anxiety and facilitates cooperation. The patient is better able to relax and cooperate if he or she is familiar with the procedure and knows everything is in readiness when the urge to defecate is felt. Defecation usually occurs within 5 to 15 minutes.
5. Warm solution in amount ordered, and check temperature with a bath thermometer, if available. If bath thermometer is not available, warm to room temperature or slightly higher, and test on inner wrist. If tap water is used, adjust temperature as it flows from faucet.	Warming the solution prevents chilling the patient, which would add to the discomfort of the procedure. Cold solution could cause cramping; too warm solution could cause trauma to intestinal mucosa.
6. Add enema solution to container. Release clamp and allow fluid to progress through tube before reclamping.	This causes any air to be expelled from the tubing. Although allowing air to enter the intestine is not harmful, it may further distend the intestine.
7. Adjust bed to comfortable working height, usually elbow height of the caregiver (VISN 8 Patient Safety Center, 2009). Position the patient on the left side (Sims' position), as dictated by patient comfort and condition. Fold top linen back just enough to allow access to the patient's rectal area. Place a waterproof pad under the patient's hip.	Having the bed at the proper height prevents back and muscle strain. Sims' position facilitates flow of solution via gravity into the rectum and colon, optimizing retention of solution. Folding back the linen in this manner minimizes unnecessary exposure and promotes the patient's comfort and warmth. The waterproof pad will protect the bed.
8. Put on nonsterile gloves.	Gloves prevent contact with contaminants and body fluids.

ACTION	RATIONALE
9. Elevate solution so that it is no higher than 18 inches (45 cm) above level of anus. Plan to give the solution slowly over a period of 5 to 10 minutes. Hang the container on an IV pole or hold it at the proper height.	Gravity forces the solution to enter the intestine. The amount of pressure determines the rate of flow and pressure exerted on the intestinal wall. Giving the solution too quickly causes rapid distention and pressure, poor defecation, or damage to the mucous membrane.
10. Generously lubricate end of rectal tube 2 to 3 inches (5 to 7 cm). A disposable enema set may have a prelubricated rectal tube.	Lubrication facilitates passage of the rectal tube through the anal sphincter and prevents injury to the mucosa.
11. Lift buttock to expose anus. Slowly and gently insert the enema tube 3 to 4 to inches (7 to 10 cm) for an adult. Direct it at an angle pointing toward the umbilicus, not bladder. Ask the patient to take several deep breaths.	Good visualization of the anus helps prevent injury to tissues. The anal canal is about 1 to 2 inches (2½ to 5 cm) long. The tube should be inserted past the external and internal sphincters, but further insertion may damage intestinal mucous membrane. The suggested angle follows the normal intestinal contour and thus will help to prevent perforation of the bowel. Slow insertion of the tube minimizes spasms of the intestinal wall and sphincters. Deep breathing helps relax the anal sphincters.
12. If resistance is met while inserting tube, permit a small amount of solution to enter, withdraw tube slightly, and then continue to insert it. **Do not force entry of the tube.** Ask the patient to take several deep breaths.	Resistance may be due to spasms of the intestine or failure of the internal sphincter to open. The solution may help to reduce spasms and relax the sphincter, thus making continued insertion of the tube safe. Forcing a tube may injure the intestinal mucosa wall. Taking deep breaths helps relax the anal sphincter.
13. Introduce solution slowly over a period of 5 to 10 minutes. Hold tubing all the time that solution is being instilled.	Introducing the solution slowly helps prevent rapid distention of the intestine and a desire to defecate.

ACTION	RATIONALE
14. Clamp tubing or lower container if patient has desire to defecate or cramping occurs. Instruct the patient to take small, fast breaths or to pant.	These techniques help relax muscles and prevent premature expulsion of the solution.
15. After the solution has been given, clamp tubing and remove tube. Have paper towel ready to receive tube as it is withdrawn.	Wrapping tube in paper towel prevents dripping of solution.
16. Return the patient to a comfortable position. Encourage the patient to hold the solution until the urge to defecate is strong, usually in about 5 to 15 minutes. Make sure the linens under the patient are dry. Remove your gloves and ensure that the patient is covered.	This amount of time usually allows muscle contractions to become sufficient to produce good results. Promotes patient comfort. Removing contaminated gloves prevents spread of microorganisms.
17. Raise side rail. Lower bed height and adjust head of bed to a comfortable position.	Promotes patient safety.
18. Remove additional PPE, if used. Perform hand hygiene.	Removing PPE properly reduces the risk for infection transmission and contamination of other items. Hand hygiene prevents the spread of microorganisms.
19. When patient has a strong urge to defecate, place him or her in a sitting position on a bedpan or assist to commode or bathroom. Offer toilet tissue, if not in patient's reach. Stay with patient or have call bell readily accessible.	The sitting position is most natural and facilitates defecation. Fall prevention is a high priority due to the urgency of reaching the commode.
20. Remind patient not to flush commode before nurse inspects results of enema.	The nurse needs to observe and record the results. Additional enemas may be necessary if the physician has ordered enemas "until clear."
21. Put on gloves and assist patient, if necessary, with cleaning of anal area. Offer	Gloves prevent contact with contaminants and body fluids. Cleaning the anal area and

ACTION	RATIONALE
washcloths, soap, and water for handwashing. Remove gloves.	proper hygiene deter the spread of microorganisms.
22. Leave the patient clean and comfortable. Care for equipment properly.	Bacteria that grow in the intestine can be spread to others if equipment is not properly cleaned.
23. Perform hand hygiene.	Hand hygiene deters the spread of microorganisms.

EVALUATION

- Patient expels feces.
- Patient verbalizes decreased discomfort.
- Abdominal distention is absent.
- Patient remains free of any evidence of trauma to the rectal mucosa or other adverse effect.

DOCUMENTATION

- Document the amount and type of enema solution used; amount, consistency, and color of stool. Record abdominal assessment, pain assessment, and assessment of perineal area. Document patient's reaction to the procedure.

GENERAL CONSIDERATIONS

- Rectal agents and rectal manipulation, including enemas, should not be used with myelosuppressed patients and/or patients at risk for myelosuppression and mucositis. These interventions can lead to development of bleeding, anal fissures, or abscesses, which are portals for infection.
- If the patient experiences fullness or pain or if fluid escapes around the tube, stop administration. Wait 30 seconds to a minute and then restart the flow at a slower rate. If symptoms persist, stop administration and contact the patient's physician.
- If the enema has been ordered to be given "until clear," check with the physician before administering more than three enemas. Severe fluid and electrolyte imbalances may occur if the patient receives more than three cleansing enemas. Results are considered clear

whenever there are no more pieces of stool in enema return. The solution may be colored but still considered a clear return.
• Older adult patients who cannot retain the enema solution should receive the enema while on the bedpan in the supine position. For comfort, the head of the bed can be elevated 30 degrees, if necessary, and pillows used appropriately.

Skill · 67   Administering a Retention Enema

Retention enemas are ordered for various reasons. *Oil-retention* enemas help to lubricate the stool and intestinal mucosa, making defecation easier. *Carminative* enemas help to expel flatus from the rectum and relieve distention secondary to flatus. *Medicated* enemas are used to administer a medication rectally. *Anthelmintic* enemas are administered to destroy intestinal parasites. *Nutritive* enemas are administered to replenish fluids and nutrition rectally.

EQUIPMENT

• Enema solution (varies, depending on reason for enema), often prepackaged, commercially prepared solutions
• Nonsterile gloves
• Additional PPE, as indicated
• Waterproof pad
• Bath blanket
• Washcloth, soap, and towel
• Bedpan or commode
• Toilet tissue
• Water-soluble lubricant

ASSESSMENT GUIDELINES

• Ask the patient when he or she had the last bowel movement.
• Assess the patient's abdomen, including auscultating for bowel sounds, percussing, and palpating. Because the goal of a cleansing enema is to increase peristalsis, which should increase bowel sounds, assess the abdomen before and after the enema.
• Assess the rectal area for any fissures, hemorrhoids, sores, or rectal tears. If present, added care should be taken while inserting the tube.
• Assess the results of the patient's laboratory work, specifically the platelet count and white blood cell (WBC) count. An enema is contraindicated for patients with a low platelet count or low WBC count. An enema may irritate or traumatize the gastrointestinal mucosa, causing bleeding, bowel perforation, or infection. Any unnecessary procedures that would place the patient at risk for bleeding or infection should not be performed.
• Assess for dizziness, light-headedness, diaphoresis, and clammy skin. The enema may stimulate a vagal response, which increases parasympathetic stimulation, causing a decrease in heart rate.

• Enemas should not be administered to patients who have severe abdominal pain, bowel obstruction, bowel inflammation or bowel infection, or after rectal, prostate, and colon surgery.

NURSING DIAGNOSES
• Constipation
• Risk for Injury
• Risk for Infection
• Acute Pain
• Imbalanced Nutrition, Less than Body Requirements

OUTCOME IDENTIFICATION AND PLANNING
Expected outcomes may include:
• Patient retains the solution for the prescribed, appropriate length of time and experiences the expected therapeutic effect of the solution.
• Patient verbalizes decreased discomfort.
• Abdominal distention is absent.
• Patient demonstrates signs and symptoms indicative of a resolving infection.
• Patient exhibits signs and symptoms of adequate nutrition.
• Patient remains free of any evidence of trauma to the rectal mucosa or other adverse effect.

IMPLEMENTATION

ACTION	RATIONALE
1. Verify the order for the enema. Bring necessary equipment to the bedside stand or overbed table. Warm the solution to body temperature in a bowl of warm water.	Verifying the physician's order is crucial to ensuring that the proper enema is administered to the right patient. Bringing everything to the bedside conserves time and energy. Arranging items nearby is convenient, saves time, and avoids unnecessary stretching and twisting of muscles on the part of the nurse. A cold solution can cause intestinal cramping.
2. Perform hand hygiene and put on PPE, if indicated.	Hand hygiene and PPE prevent the spread of microorganisms. PPE is required based on transmission precautions.

ACTION	RATIONALE

3. Identify the patient.

Identifying the patient ensures the right patient receives the intervention and helps prevent errors.

4. Close curtains around bed and close the door to the room, if possible. Explain what you are going to do and why you are going to do it to the patient. Have a bedpan, commode, or nearby bathroom ready for use.

This ensures the patient's privacy. Explanation relieves anxiety and facilitates cooperation. The patient is better able to relax and cooperate if he or she is familiar with the procedure and knows everything is in readiness if the urge to dispel the enema is felt.

5. Adjust bed to comfortable working height, usually elbow height of the caregiver (VISN 8 Patient Safety Center, 2009). Position the patient on the left side (Sims' position), as dictated by patient comfort and condition. Fold top linen back just enough to allow access to the patient's rectal area. Place a waterproof pad under the patient's hip.

Having the bed at the proper height prevents back and muscle strain. Sims' position facilitates flow of solution via gravity into the rectum and colon, optimizing solution retention. Folding back the linen in this manner minimizes unnecessary exposure and promotes the patient's comfort and warmth. The waterproof pad will protect the bed.

6. Put on nonsterile gloves.

Gloves prevent contact with blood and body fluids.

7. Remove cap of prepackaged enema solution. Apply a generous amount of lubricant to the tube.

Lubrication is necessary to minimize trauma on insertion.

8. Lift buttock to expose anus. Slowly and gently insert rectal tube 3 to 4 inches (7 to 10 cm) for an adult. Direct it at an angle pointing toward the umbilicus. Ask the patient to take several deep breaths.

Good visualization of the anus helps prevent injury to tissues. The anal canal is about 1 to 2 inches (2.5 to 5 cm) long. The tube should be inserted past the external and internal sphincters, but further insertion may damage the intestinal mucous membrane. The suggested angle follows the normal intestinal contour and thus helps to prevent perforation

ACTION	RATIONALE

of the bowel. Slow insertion of the tube minimizes spasms of the intestinal wall and sphincters. Deep breathing helps relax the anal sphincters.

9. If resistance is met while inserting the tube, permit a small amount of solution to enter, withdraw tube slightly, and then continue to insert it. **Do not force entry of tube.**

Resistance may be due to spasms of the intestine or failure of the internal sphincter to open. The solution may help to reduce spasms and relax the sphincter, thus making continued insertion of the tube safe. Forcing a tube may injure the intestinal mucosa wall.

10. Slowly squeeze enema container, emptying entire contents.

Compressing the container slowly allows the solution to enter the rectum and prevents rapid distention of the intestine and a desire to defecate.

11. **Remove container while keeping it compressed.** Have paper towel ready to receive tube as it is withdrawn.

If container is released, a vacuum will form, allowing some of the enema solution to re-enter the container.

12. **Instruct the patient to retain the enema solution for at least 30 minutes or as indicated, per manufacturer's direction.**

Solution needs to dwell for at least 30 minutes, or per manufacturer's direction, to allow for optimal action of the solution.

13. Remove your gloves. Return the patient to a comfortable position. Make sure the linens under the patient are dry and ensure that the patient is covered.

Removing contaminated gloves prevents spread of microorganisms and promotes patient comfort. Removing contaminated gloves prevents spread of microorganisms.

14. Raise side rail. Lower bed height and adjust head of bed to a comfortable position.

Promotes patient safety.

15. Remove additional PPE, if used. Perform hand hygiene.

Removing PPE properly reduces the risk for infection transmission and contamination of other items. Hand hygiene prevents the spread of microorganisms.

ACTION	RATIONALE
16. If the patient has a strong urge to dispel the solution, place him or her in a sitting position on bedpan or assist to commode or bathroom. Stay with patient or have call bell readily accessible.	The sitting position is most natural and facilitates defecation. Fall prevention is a high priority due to the urgency of reaching the commode.
17. Remind patient not to flush the commode before nurse inspects results of enema, if used for bowel evacuation. Record character of stool, as appropriate, and patient's reaction to enema.	The nurse needs to observe and record the results.
18. Put on gloves and assist patient, if necessary, with cleaning of anal area. Offer washcloths, soap, and water for handwashing. Remove gloves.	Cleaning the anal area and proper hygiene deter the spread of microorganisms. Removing PPE properly reduces the risk for infection transmission and contamination of other items.
19. Leave patient clean and comfortable. Care for equipment properly.	Bacteria that grow in the intestine can be spread to others if equipment is not properly cleaned.
20. Perform hand hygiene.	Hand hygiene deters the spread of microorganisms.

EVALUATION
- Patient expels feces without evidence of trauma to the rectal mucosa.
- Patient verbalizes a decrease in pain.
- Patient demonstrates signs and symptoms indicative of a resolving infection.
- Patient exhibits signs and symptoms of adequate nutrition.

DOCUMENTATION
- Document the amount and type of enema solution used and length of time retained by the patient. Record the amount, consistency, and color of stool, as appropriate. Record pain assessment and assessment of perianal area. Document patient's reaction to procedure.

GENERAL CONSIDERATIONS

- In myelosuppressed patients and/or patients at risk for myelosuppression and mucositis, rectal agents and manipulation, including enemas, are discouraged because they can lead to development of bleeding, anal fissures, or abscesses, which are portals for infection (NCI, 2006).

| Skill · 68 | **Administering a Small-Volume Cleansing Enema** |

Cleansing enemas are given to remove feces from the colon. Some of the reasons for administering a cleansing enema include relieving constipation or fecal impaction, preventing involuntary escape of fecal material during surgical procedures, promoting visualization of the intestinal tract by radiographic or instrument examination, and helping to establish regular bowel function during a bowel training program. Small-volume enemas are also known as hypertonic enemas. Hypertonic solution preparations are available commercially and are administered in smaller volumes (adult, 70 to 130 mL). These solutions draw water into the colon, which stimulates the defecation reflex. They may be contraindicated in patients for whom sodium retention is a problem. They are also contraindicated for patients with renal impairment or reduced renal clearance, because these patients have compromised ability to excrete phosphate adequately, with resulting hyperphosphatemia (Bowers, 2006). Large-volume enemas are addressed in Skill 68.

EQUIPMENT

- Commercially prepared enema with rectal tip
- Water-soluble lubricant
- Waterproof pad
- Bath blanket
- Bedpan and toilet tissue
- Disposable gloves
- Additional PPE, as indicated
- Paper towel
- Washcloth, soap, and towel

ASSESSMENT GUIDELINES

- Assess the patient's abdomen, including auscultating for bowel sounds, percussing, and palpating. Because the goal of a cleansing enema is to increase peristalsis, which should increase bowel sounds, assess the abdomen before and after the enema.
- Inspect the rectal area for any fissures, hemorrhoids, sores, or rectal tears. If any of these are noted, added care should be taken while administering the enema.
- Check the results of the patient's laboratory work, specifically the platelet count and white blood cell (WBC) count. A normal platelet count ranges from 150,000 to 400,000/mm^3. A platelet count of less

than 20,000 may seriously compromise the patient's ability to clot blood. Therefore, any unnecessary procedures that would place the patient at risk for bleeding or infection should not be performed. A low WBC count places the patient at risk for infection.
- Do not administer enemas to patients who have severe abdominal pain, bowel obstruction, bowel inflammation or bowel infection, or after rectal, prostate, and colon surgery.

NURSING DIAGNOSES
- Acute Pain
- Constipation
- Risk for Injury
- Risk for Constipation

OUTCOME IDENTIFICATION AND PLANNING
Expected outcomes may include:
- Patient expels feces and reports a decrease in pain and discomfort.
- Patient remains free of any evidence of trauma to the rectal mucosa.

IMPLEMENTATION

ACTION	RATIONALE
1. Verify the order for the enema. Bring necessary equipment to the bedside stand or over-bed table. Warm the solution to body temperature in a bowl of warm water.	Verifying the physician's order is crucial to ensuring that the proper enema is administered to the right patient. Bringing everything to the bedside conserves time and energy. Arranging items nearby is convenient, saves time, and avoids unnecessary stretching and twisting of muscles on the part of the nurse. A cold solution can cause intestinal cramping.
2. Perform hand hygiene and 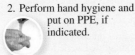 put on PPE, if indicated.	Hand hygiene and PPE prevent the spread of microorganisms. PPE is required based on transmission precautions.
3. Identify the patient.	Identifying the patient ensures the right patient receives the intervention and helps prevent errors.

ACTION	RATIONALE
4. Close curtains around bed and close the door to the room, if possible. Explain what you are going to do and why you are going to do it to the patient. Discuss where the patient will defecate. Have a bedpan, commode, or nearby bathroom ready for use.	This ensures the patient's privacy. Explanation relieves anxiety and facilitates cooperation. The patient is better able to relax and cooperate if he or she is familiar with the procedure and knows everything is in readiness when the urge to defecate is felt. Defecation usually occurs within 5 to 15 minutes.
5. Adjust bed to comfortable working height, usually elbow height of the caregiver (VISN 8 Patient Safety Center, 2009). Position the patient on the left side (Sims' position), as dictated by patient comfort and condition. Fold top linen back just enough to allow access to the patient's rectal area. Place a waterproof pad under the patient's hip.	Having the bed at the proper height prevents back and muscle strain. Sims' position facilitates flow of solution via gravity into the rectum and colon, optimizing retention of the solution. Folding back the linen in this manner minimizes unnecessary exposure and promotes the patient's comfort and warmth. The waterproof pad will protect the bed.
6. Put on nonsterile gloves.	Gloves prevent contact with contaminants and body fluids.
7. Remove the cap and generously lubricate end of rectal tube 2 to 3 inches (5 to 7 cm).	Lubrication facilitates passage of the rectal tube through the anal sphincter and prevents injury to the mucosa.
8. Lift buttock to expose anus. Slowly and gently insert the rectal tube 3 to 4 inches (7 to 10 cm) for an adult. Direct it at an angle pointing toward the umbilicus, not bladder. **Do not force entry of the tube.** Ask the patient to take several deep breaths.	Good visualization helps prevent injury to tissues. The anal canal is about 1 to 2 inches (2.5 to 5 cm) long. Insert the tube past the external and internal sphincters; further insertion may damage the intestinal mucous membrane. The suggested angle follows the normal intestinal contour, helping prevent bowel perforation. Forcing a tube may injure the intestinal mucosa wall. Taking deep breaths helps relax the anal sphincter.

ACTION	RATIONALE
9. Compress the container with your hands. Roll the end up on itself, toward the rectal tip. Administer all the solution in the container.	Rolling the container aids administration of all of the contents of the container.
10. After the solution has been given, remove the tube, keeping the container compressed. Have paper towel ready to receive tube as it is withdrawn. Encourage the patient to hold the solution until the urge to defecate is strong, usually in about 5 to 15 minutes.	This amount of time usually allows muscle contractions to become sufficient to produce good results.
11. Remove gloves. Return the patient to a comfortable position. Make sure the linens under the patient are dry. Ensure that the patient is covered.	Promotes patient comfort. Removing contaminated gloves prevents spread of microorganisms.
12. Raise side rail. Lower bed height and adjust head of bed to a comfortable position.	Promotes patient safety.
13. Remove additional PPE, if used. Perform hand hygiene.	Removing PPE properly reduces the risk for infection transmission and contamination of other items. Hand hygiene prevents the spread of microorganisms.
14. When patient has a strong urge to defecate, place him or her in a sitting position on a bedpan or assist to commode or bathroom. Stay with the patient or have call bell readily accessible.	The sitting position is most natural and facilitates defecation. Fall prevention is a high priority due to the urgency of reaching the commode.
15. Remind the patient not to flush commode before nurse inspects results of enema.	The nurse needs to observe and record the results. Additional enemas may be necessary if physician has ordered enemas "until clear."

ACTION	RATIONALE
16. Put on gloves and assist patient, if necessary, with cleaning of anal area. Offer washcloths, soap, and water for handwashing. Remove gloves.	Cleaning the anal area and proper hygiene deter the spread of microorganisms.
17. Leave the patient clean and comfortable. Care for equipment properly.	Bacteria that grow in the intestine can be spread to others if equipment is not properly cleaned.
18. Perform hand hygiene.	Hand hygiene deters the spread of microorganisms.

EVALUATION

• Patient expels feces and verbalizes decreased discomfort.
• Abdominal distention is absent.
• Patient remains free of any evidence of trauma to the rectal mucosa or other adverse effect.

DOCUMENTATION

• Document the amount and type of enema solution used; amount, consistency, and color of stool. Record abdominal assessment, pain assessment, and assessment of the perineal area. Document the patient's reaction to procedure.

GENERAL CONSIDERATIONS

• In myelosuppressed patients and/or patients at risk for myelosuppression and mucositis, rectal agents and manipulation, including enemas, are discouraged because they can lead to development of bleeding, anal fissures, or abscesses, which are portals for infection (NCI, 2006).
• Enemas containing phosphates should be used with caution in frail older patients due to the potential for dehydration, electrolyte imbalances, and sodium phosphate toxicity (Bowers, 2006).

Skill · 69   Caring for a Patient Receiving Epidural Analgesia

Epidural analgesia is being used more commonly to provide pain relief during the immediate postoperative phase (particularly after thoracic, abdominal, orthopedic, and vascular surgery) and for chronic pain situations. Epidural pain management is also being used with infants and children (Ellis et al., 2007). The anesthesiologist or radiologist usually inserts the catheter in the mid-lumbar region into the epidural space that exists between the walls of the vertebral canal and the dura mater or outermost connective tissue membrane surrounding the spinal cord. For temporary therapy, the catheter exits directly over the spine, and the tubing is positioned over the patient's shoulder with the end of the catheter taped to the chest. For long-term therapy, the catheter is usually tunneled subcutaneously and exits on the side of the body or on the abdomen.

The epidural analgesia can be administered as a bolus dose (either one time or intermittent), via a continuous infusion pump, or by a patient-controlled epidural analgesia (PCEA) pump (D'Arcy, 2005a; Ellis et al., 2007; Pasero, 2003b; Roman & Cabaj, 2005). Additional information specific to PCA administration is discussed in Skill 130. Epidural catheters used for the management of acute pain are typically removed 36 to 72 hours after surgery, when oral medication can be substituted for pain relief.

EQUIPMENT

- Volume infusion device
- Epidural infusion tubing
- Prescribed epidural analgesic solutions
- Computerized medication administration record (CMAR) or medication administration record (MAR)
- Pain assessment tool and/or scale
- Transparent dressing or gauze pads
- Labels for epidural infusion line
- Tape
- Emergency drugs and equipment, such as naloxone, oxygen, endotracheal intubation set, handheld resuscitation bag, per facility policy
- Nonsterile gloves
- Additional PPE, as indicated

ASSESSMENT GUIDELINES

- Review the patient's medical record and plan of care for specific instructions related to epidural analgesia therapy, including the medical order for the drug and conditions indicating the need for therapy.
- Review the patient's history for conditions that might contraindicate therapy, such as local or systemic infections, neurologic disease, coagulopathy or use of anticoagulant therapy, spinal arthritis or spinal deformity, hypotension, marked hypertension, allergy to the prescribed medication, or psychiatric disorder.
- Check to ensure proper functioning of the unit.

- Assess the patient's level of consciousness and understanding of epi-dural analgesia therapy and the rationale for its use.
- Assess the patient's level of discomfort and pain using an appropriate assessment tool. Assess the characteristics of any pain. Assess for other symptoms that often occur with the pain, such as headache or restlessness. Ask the patient what interventions have and have not been successful in the past to promote comfort and relieve pain.
- Assess the patient's vital signs and respiratory status, including rate, depth, and rhythm, and oxygen saturation level using pulse oximetry.
- Assess the patient's sedation score.
- Assess the patient's response to the intervention to evaluate effective-ness and for the presence of adverse effects.

NURSING DIAGNOSES

- Acute Pain
- Ineffective Coping
- Chronic Pain
- Anxiety
- Fear
- Deficient Knowledge
- Risk for Infection
- Risk for Injury

OUTCOME IDENTIFICATION AND PLANNING

Expected outcomes may include:
- Patient reports increased comfort and/or decreased pain, without adverse effects, oversedation, and respiratory depression.
- Patient displays decreased anxiety.
- Patient displays improved coping skills.
- Patient remains free from infection.
- Patient verbalizes an understanding of the therapy and the reason for its use.

IMPLEMENTATION

ACTION	RATIONALE
1. Check the medication order against the original medical order according to agency policy. Clarify any inconsis-tencies. Check the patient's chart for allergies.	This comparison helps to identify errors that may have occurred when orders were transcribed. The medical order is the legal record of medication orders for each agency.
2. Know the actions, special nursing considerations, safe	This knowledge aids the nurse in evaluating the therapeutic effect

ACTION	RATIONALE
dose ranges, purpose of administration, and adverse effects of the medications to be administered. Consider the appropriateness of the medication for this patient.	of the medication in relation to the patient's disorder and can also be used to educate the patient about the medication.
3. Prepare the medication syringe or other container, based on facility policy, for administration.	Proper preparation and administration procedure prevents errors.
4. Perform hand hygiene and put on PPE, if indicated.	Hand hygiene and PPE prevent the spread of microorganisms. PPE is required based on transmission precautions.
5. Identify the patient.	Identifying the patient ensures the right patient receives the intervention and helps prevent errors.
6. Show the patient the device, and explain the function of the device and reason for use. Explain the purpose and action of the medication to the patient.	Explanation encourages patient understanding and cooperation and reduces apprehension.
7. Close curtains around the bed and close the door to the room, if possible.	Closing the door or curtain provides patient privacy.
8. Complete necessary assessments before administering medication. Check allergy bracelet or ask patient about allergies. Assess the patient's pain, using an appropriate assessment tool and measurement scale. Put on gloves.	Assessment is a prerequisite to administration of medications. Accurate assessment is necessary to guide treatment/relief interventions and to evaluate the effectiveness of pain control measures. Gloves are indicated for potential contact with blood or body fluids.
9. **Have an ampule of 0.4 mg naloxone (Narcan) and a syringe at the bedside.**	Naloxone reverses the respiratory depressant effect of opioids.

ACTION	RATIONALE
10. After the catheter has been inserted and the infusion initiated by the anesthesiologist or radiologist, **check the label on the medication container and the rate of infusion with the medication record and patient identification.** Obtain verification of information from a second nurse, according to facility policy. If using a barcode administration system, scan the barcode on the medication label, if required.	This action verifies that the correct drug and dosage will be administered to the correct patient. Confirmation of information by a second nurse helps prevent errors. Scanning the barcode provides an additional check to ensure that the medication is given to the right patient.
11. Tape all connection sites. Label the bag, tubing, and pump apparatus "For Epidural Infusion Only." **Do not administer any other narcotics or adjuvant drugs without the approval of the clinician responsible for the epidural injection.**	Taping prevents accidental dislodgement. Labeling prevents inadvertent administration of other intravenous medications through this setup. Additional medication may potentiate the action of the opioid, increasing the risk for respiratory depression.
12. Assess the catheter exit site and apply a transparent dressing over the catheter insertion site, if not already in place (FIGURE 1). Remove gloves and additional PPE, if used. Perform hand hygiene.	The transparent dressing protects the site while still allowing assessment. Removing PPE properly reduces the risk for infection transmission and contamination of other items. Hand hygiene reduces transmission of microorganisms.

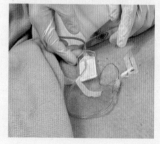

FIGURE 1 Assessing the catheter exit site.

ACTION	RATIONALE
13. Monitor the infusion rate according to facility policy. Assess and record sedation level and respiratory status every hour for the first 24 hours, then at 4-hour intervals (or according to agency policy). **Notify the primary care provider if the sedation rating is 3 or 4, the respiratory depth decreases, or the respiratory rate falls below 8 breaths per minute.**	Monitoring the infusion rate prevents incorrect administration of the medication. Opioids can depress the respiratory center in the medulla. A change in the level of consciousness is usually the first sign of altered respiratory function.
14. Keep the head of bed elevated 30 degrees unless contraindicated.	Elevation of the patient's head minimizes upward migration of the opioid in the spinal cord, thus decreasing the risk for respiratory depression.
15. Assess the patient's level of pain and the effectiveness of pain relief.	This information helps in determining the need for subsequent "breakthrough" pain medication.
16. Monitor urinary output and assess for bladder distention.	Opioids can cause urinary retention.
17. Assess motor strength and sensation every 4 hours.	The catheter may migrate into the intrathecal space and allow opioids to block the transmission of nerve impulses completely through the spinal cord to the brain.
18. Monitor for adverse effects (pruritus, nausea, and vomiting).	Opioids may spread into the trigeminal nerve, causing itching, or resulting in nausea and vomiting due to slowed gastrointestinal function or stimulation of a chemoreceptor trigger zone in the brain. Medications are available to treat these adverse effects.
19. Assess for signs of infection at the insertion site.	Inflammation or local infection may develop at the catheter insertion site.

ACTION	RATIONALE
20. Change the dressing over the catheter exit site every 24 to 48 hours or as needed per agency policy using aseptic technique. Change the infusion tubing every 48 hours or as specified by agency policy.	Dressing and tubing changes using aseptic technique reduce the risk for infection.

EVALUATION

- Patient verbalizes pain relief.
- Patient exhibits a dry, intact dressing, and the catheter exit site is free of signs and symptoms of complications, injury, or infection.
- Patient reports a decrease in anxiety and increased ability to cope with pain.
- Patient verbalizes information related to the functioning of the epidural catheter and the reasons for its use.

DOCUMENTATION

- Document catheter patency, the condition of the insertion site and dressing, vital signs and assessment information, any change in infusion rate, solution or tubing, analgesics administered, and the patient's response.

GENERAL CONSIDERATIONS

- Notify the anesthesiologist/pain management team immediately if the patient exhibits any of the following: respiratory rate below 10 breaths per minute, continued complaints of unmanaged pain, leakage at the insertion site, fever, inability to void, paresthesia, itching, or headache (Roman & Cabaj, 2005).
- Do not administer other sedatives or analgesics unless ordered by the anesthesiologist/pain management team to avoid oversedation (Roman & Cabaj, 2005).
- Always ensure that the patient receiving epidural analgesia has a peripheral IV line in place, either as a continuous IV infusion or as an intermittent infusion device, to allow immediate administration of emergency drugs if warranted.
- Keep in mind that drugs given via the epidural route diffuse slowly and may cause adverse reactions, including excessive sedation, for up to 12 hours after the infusion has been discontinued.
- Typically, an anesthesiologist orders analgesics and removes the catheter. However, facility policy may allow a specially trained nurse to remove the catheter.
- Be aware that no resistance should be felt during the removal of an epidural catheter.

Skill · 70   Caring for a Patient with an External Fixation Device

External fixation devices are used to manage open fractures with soft-tissue damage. They consist of one of a variety of frames to hold pins that are drilled into or through bones. External fixators provide stable support for severe crushed or splintered fractures and access to and treatment for soft-tissue injuries. The use of these devices allows treatment of the fracture and damaged soft tissues while promoting patient comfort, early mobility, and active exercise of adjacent uninvolved joints. Complications related to disuse and immobility are minimized. Nursing responsibilities include reassuring the patient, maintaining the device, monitoring neurovascular status, promoting exercise, preventing complications from the therapy, preventing infection by providing pin site care, and providing teaching to ensure compliance and self-care. Pin site care is performed frequently in the first 48 to 72 hours after application, when drainage may be heavy. Thereafter, pin site care may be done daily or weekly. Dressings are often applied for the first 48 to 72 hours, and then sites may be left open to air. There is little research evidence on which to base the management of pin sites (Baird Holmes & Brown, 2005). Pin site care varies based on primary care provider and facility policy. Refer to specific patient medical orders and facility guidelines. Nurses play a major role in preparing the patient psychologically for the application of an external fixator. The devices appear clumsy and large. In addition, the nurse needs to clarify misconceptions regarding pain and discomfort associated with the device.

EQUIPMENT

- Sterile applicators
- Cleansing solution, usually sterile normal saline or chlorhexidine, per primary care provider or facility policy
- Ice bag
- Sterile gauze
- Foam, nonstick, or gauze dressing, per medical order or facility policy
- Analgesic, per physician order
- Antimicrobial ointment, per primary care provider order or facility policy

ASSESSMENT GUIDELINES

- Review the patient's medical record and the nursing plan of care to determine the type of device being used and prescribed care.
- Assess the external fixator to ensure proper function and position.
- Perform a skin assessment and neurovascular assessment. Inspect the pin insertion sites for signs of inflammation and infection, including swelling, cloudy or offensive drainage, pain, or redness.
- Assess the patient's knowledge regarding the device and self-care activities and responsibilities.

NURSING DIAGNOSES
- Risk for Infection
- Impaired Physical Mobility
- Impaired Skin Integrity
- Risk for Injury
- Anxiety
- Deficient Knowledge
- Acute Pain
- Self-Care Deficit (toileting, bathing, or dressing)

OUTCOME IDENTIFICATION AND PLANNING
Expected outcomes may include:
- Patient shows no evidence of complication, such as infection, contractures, venous stasis, thrombus formation, or skin breakdown.
- Patient maintains proper body alignment.
- Patient reports an increased level of comfort.
- Patient is free from injury.

IMPLEMENTATION

ACTION	RATIONALE
1. Review the medical record and the nursing plan of care to determine the type of device being used and prescribed care.	Reviewing the medical record and plan of care validates the correct patient and correct procedure.
2. Perform hand hygiene. Put on PPE, as indicated.	Hand hygiene and PPE prevent the spread of microorganisms. PPE is required based on transmission precautions.
3. Identify the patient. Explain the procedure to the patient. Assure the patient that there will be little pain after the fixation device is in place. Reinforce that the patient will be able to adjust to the device and to move about with the device, allowing him or her to resume normal activities more quickly.	Patient identification validates the correct patient and correct procedure. Discussion and explanation allay anxiety and prepare the patient psychologically for the application of the device.

ACTION	RATIONALE
4. **After the fixation device is in place, apply ice to the surgical site as ordered or per facility policy. Elevate the affected body part if appropriate.**	Ice and elevation help reduce swelling, relieve pain, and reduce bleeding.
5. Perform a pain assessment and assess for muscle spasm. Administer prescribed medications in sufficient time to allow for the full effect of the analgesic and/or muscle relaxant.	Pain assessment and analgesic administration help promote patient comfort.
6. Administer analgesics as ordered before exercising or mobilizing the affected body part.	Administration of analgesics promotes patient comfort and facilitates movement.
7. Perform neurovascular assessments per facility policy or physician's order, usually every 2 to 4 hours for 24 hours, then every 4 to 8 hours. Assess the affected body part for color, motion, sensation, edema, capillary refill, and pulses. If appropriate, compare with the unaffected side. Assess for pain not relieved by analgesics, burning, tingling, and numbness.	Assessment promotes early detection and prompt intervention of abnormal neurovascular function, nerve damage, or circulatory impairment. Assessment of neurovascular status determines the circulation and oxygenation of tissues.
8. Close curtains around the bed and close the door to the room, if possible. Place the bed at an appropriate and comfortable working height, usually elbow height of the caregiver (VISN 8 Patient Safety Center, 2009).	Closing the door or curtains provides for privacy. Proper bed height prevents back and muscle strain.
9. Assess the pin site for redness, tenting of the skin, prolonged or purulent drainage, swelling, and bowing, bending, or loosening of the pins. Monitor body temperature.	Assessing pin sites aids in early detection of infection and stress on the skin and allows for appropriate intervention.

ACTION	RATIONALE
10. Perform pin site care.	Performing pin site care prevents crusting at the site that could lead to fluid buildup, infection, and osteomyelitis.
a. Using sterile technique, open the applicator package and pour the cleansing agent into the sterile container.	Using sterile technique reduces the risk for transmission of microorganisms.
b. Put on the sterile gloves.	Gloves prevent contact with blood and/or body fluids.
c. Place the applicators into the solution.	
d. Clean the pin site starting at the insertion area and working outward, away from the pin site (FIGURE 1).	Cleaning from the center outward promotes movement from the least to most contaminated area.
e. Use each applicator once. Use a new applicator for each pin site.	Using each applicator only once prevents transfer of microorganisms.

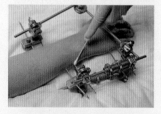

FIGURE 1 Cleaning around pin sites with normal saline on an applicator.

ACTION	RATIONALE
11. Depending on primary care provider order and facility policy, apply the antimicrobial ointment to the pin sites and apply a dressing.	Antimicrobial ointment prevents infection; applying a dressing helps contain drainage.
12. Place the bed in the lowest position, with the side rails up. Make sure the call bell and other necessary items are within easy reach.	Having the bed at proper height and leaving the call bell and other items within reach ensure patient safety.
13. Remove gloves and any other PPE, if used. Perform hand hygiene.	Removing PPE properly decreases the risk for infection transmission and contamination of other items. Hand hygiene deters the spread of microorganisms.

EVALUATION

- Patient exhibits an external fixation device in place with pin sites that are clean, dry, and intact, without evidence of infection.
- Patient remains free of complications, such as contractures, venous stasis, thrombus formation, or skin breakdown.
- Patient verbalizes pain relief.
- Patient demonstrates knowledge of pin site care.

DOCUMENTATION

- Document the time, date, and type of device in place. Include the skin assessment, pin site assessment, and pin site care. Document the patient's response to the device and the neurovascular status of the affected area.

GENERAL CONSIDERATIONS

- Teach the patient and significant others how to provide pin site care and how to recognize the signs of pin site infection. External fixator devices are in place for prolonged periods of time. Clean technique can be used at home instead of sterile technique.
- Teach the patient and significant others to identify early signs of infection, signs of a loose pin, and how to contact the orthopedic team, if necessary.
- Encourage the patient to refrain from smoking, if appropriate, to avoid delayed bone healing (Baird Holmes & Brown, 2005).
- Reinforce the importance of keeping the affected body part elevated when sitting or lying down to prevent edema.
- Do not adjust the clamps on the external fixator frame. It is the physician's or advanced practice professional's responsibility to adjust the clamps.
- Fractures often require additional treatment and stabilization with a cast or molded splint after the fixator device is removed.

Skill · 71   Instilling Eye Drops

Eye drops are instilled for their local effects, such as for pupil dilation or constriction when examining the eye, for infection treatment, or for controlling intraocular pressure (for patients with glaucoma). The type and amount of solution depend on the purpose of the instillation.

The eye is a delicate organ, highly susceptible to infection and injury. Although the eye is never free of microorganisms, the secretions of the conjunctiva protect against many pathogens. For maximal safety for the patient, the equipment, solutions, and ointments introduced into the conjunctival sac should be sterile. If this is not possible, follow careful guidelines for medical asepsis.

EQUIPMENT

- Gloves
- Additional PPE, as indicated
- Medication
- Tissues
- Normal saline solution
- Washcloth, cotton balls, or gauze squares
- Computer-generated Medication Administration Record (CMAR) or Medication Administration Record (MAR)

ASSESSMENT GUIDELINES

- Assess the patient for any allergies.
- Check the expiration date before administering the medication.
- Assess the appropriateness of the drug for the patient. Review assessment and laboratory data that may influence drug administration.
- Verify patient name, dose, route, and time of administration.
- Assess the affected eye for any drainage, erythema, or swelling.
- Assess the patient's knowledge of the medication. If the patient has a knowledge deficit about the medication, this may be the appropriate time to begin education about the medication.

NURSING DIAGNOSES

- Risk for Allergy Response
- Risk for Injury
- Deficient Knowledge

OUTCOME IDENTIFICATION AND PLANNING

Expected outcomes may include:
- Medication is delivered successfully into the eye.
- Patient experiences no allergy response.
- Patient does not exhibit systemic effects of the medication.
- Patient's eye remains free from injury.
- Patient understands the rationale for medication administration.

IMPLEMENTATION

ACTION	RATIONALE
1. Gather equipment. Check medication order against the original order in the medical record, according to facility policy. Clarify any inconsistencies. Check the patient's chart for allergies.	This comparison helps to identify errors that may have occurred when orders were transcribed. The primary care provider's order is the legal record of medication orders for each facility.
2. Know the actions, special nursing considerations, safe	This knowledge aids the nurse in evaluating the therapeutic effect

ACTION	**RATIONALE**
dose ranges, purpose of administration, and adverse effects of the medication to be administered. Consider the appropriateness of the medication for this patient.	of the medication in relation to the patient's disorder and can also be used to educate the patient about the medication.
3. Perform hand hygiene.	Hand hygiene prevents the spread of microorganisms.
4. Move the medication cart to the outside of the patient's room or prepare for administration in the medication area.	Organization facilitates error-free administration and saves time.
5. Unlock the medication cart or drawer. Enter pass code and scan employee identification, if required.	Locking of the cart or drawer safeguards each patient's medication supply. Hospital accrediting organizations require medication carts to be locked when not in use. Entering pass code and scanning ID allows only authorized users into the system and identifies the user for documentation by the computer.
6. **Prepare medications for one patient at a time.**	This prevents errors in medication administration.
7. Read the CMAR/MAR and select the proper medication from the patient's medication drawer or unit stock.	This is the *first* check of the label.
8. Compare the label with the CMAR/MAR. Check expiration dates and perform calculations, if necessary. Scan the barcode on the package, if required.	This is the *second* check of the label. Verify calculations with another nurse to ensure safety, if necessary.
9. **When all medications for one patient have been prepared, recheck the label with the CMAR/MAR before taking them to the patient.**	This is a *third* check to ensure accuracy and to prevent errors. Some facilities require the third check to occur at the bedside, after identifying the patient and before administration.

ACTION	RATIONALE
10. Lock the medication cart before leaving it.	Locking the cart or drawer safeguards the patient's medication supply. Hospital accrediting organizations require medication carts to be locked when not in use.
11. Transport medications to the patient's bedside carefully, and keep the medications in sight at all times.	Careful handling and close observation prevent accidental or deliberate disarrangement of medications.
12. **Ensure that the patient receives the medications at the correct time.**	Check agency policy, which may allow for administration within a period of 30 minutes before or 30 minutes after designated time.
13. Perform hand hygiene and put on PPE, if indicated.	Hand hygiene and PPE prevent the spread of microorganisms. PPE is required based on transmission precautions.
14. Identify the patient. Usually, 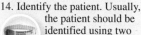 the patient should be identified using two methods. Compare information with the CMAR/MAR.	Identifying the patient ensures the right patient receives the medications and helps prevent errors.
a. Check the name and identification number on the patient's identification band.	This is the most reliable method. Replace the identification band if it is missing or inaccurate in any way.
b. Ask the patient to state his or her name and birth date, based on facility policy.	This requires a response from the patient, but illness and strange surroundings often cause patients to be confused.
c. If the patient cannot identify himself or herself, verify the patient's identification with a staff member who knows the patient for the second source.	This is another way to double-check identity. Do not use the name on the door or over the bed, because these may be inaccurate.
15. Complete necessary assessments before administering medications. Check the patient's allergy bracelet or ask the patient about	Assessment is a prerequisite to administration of medications.

ACTION	RATIONALE
allergies. Explain the purpose and action of each medication to the patient.	
16. Scan the patient's bar code on the identification band, if required.	Provides additional check to ensure that the medication is given to the right patient.
17. Put on gloves.	Gloves protect the nurse from potential contact with mucous membranes and body fluids.
18. Offer tissue to patient.	Solution and tears may spill from the eye during the procedure.
19. Cleanse the eyelids and eyelashes of any drainage with a washcloth, cotton balls, or gauze squares moistened with normal saline solution. Use each area of the cleaning surface once, moving from the inner toward the outer canthus.	Debris can be carried into the eye when the conjunctival sac is exposed. Using each area of the gauze once and moving from the inner canthus to the outer canthus prevent carrying debris to the lacrimal ducts.
20. Tilt the patient's head back slightly if sitting, or place the patient's head over a pillow if lying down. The head may be turned slightly to the affected side to prevent solution or tears from flowing toward the opposite eye.	Tilting patient's head back slightly makes it easier to reach the conjunctival sac. This should be avoided if the patient has a cervical spine injury. Turning the head to the affected side helps to prevent solution or tears from flowing toward the opposite eye.
21. Remove the cap from the medication bottle, being careful not to touch the inner side of the cap.	Touching the inner side of the cap may contaminate the bottle of medication.
22. Invert the monodrip plastic container that is commonly used to instill eye drops. Have the patient look up and focus on something on the ceiling.	By having the patient look up and focus on something else, the procedure is less traumatic and keeps the eye still.
23. Place thumb or two fingers near the margin of the lower eyelid immediately below the eyelashes, and exert pressure downward over the bony	The eye drop should be placed in the conjunctival sac, not directly on the eyeball.

ACTION	RATIONALE

prominence of cheek. Lower conjunctival sac is exposed as lower lid is pulled down (FIGURE 1).

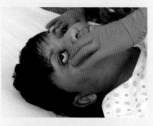

FIGURE 1 Exerting pressure downward to expose lower conjunctival sac.

ACTION	RATIONALE
24. **Hold dropper close to eye, but avoid touching eyelids or lashes.** Squeeze container and allow prescribed number of drops to fall in lower conjunctival sac.	Touching the eye, eyelids, or lashes can contaminate the medication in the bottle; startle the patient, causing blinking; or injure the eye. Do not allow medication to fall onto the cornea. This may injure the cornea or cause the patient to have an unpleasant sensation.
25. Release lower lid after eye drops are instilled. Ask the patient to close eyes gently.	This allows the medication to be distributed over the entire eye.
26. Apply gentle pressure over inner canthus to prevent eye drops from flowing into tear duct.	This minimizes the risk of systemic effects from the medication.
27. Instruct patient not to rub affected eye.	This prevents injury and irritation to eye.
28. Remove gloves. Assist the patient to a comfortable position.	This ensures patient comfort.
29. Remove additional PPE, if used. Perform hand hygiene.	Removing PPE properly reduces the risk for infection transmission and contamination of other items. Hand hygiene prevents the spread of microorganisms.

ACTION	RATIONALE
30. Document the administration of the medication immediately after administration. See Documentation section below.	Timely documentation helps to ensure patient safety.
31. Evaluate the patient's response to medication within appropriate time frame.	The patient needs to be evaluated for therapeutic and adverse effects from the medication.

EVALUATION

- Patient receives the eye drops.
- Patient experienced no adverse effects, including allergy response, systemic effect, or injury.
- Patient verbalizes an understanding of the rationale for the medication administration.

DOCUMENTATION

- Document the administration of the medication immediately after administration, including date, time, dose, route of administration, and site of administration, specifically right, left, or both eyes, on the CMAR/MAR or record using the required format. If using a bar-code system, medication administration is automatically recorded when scanned. PRN medications require documentation of the reason for administration. Prompt recording avoids the possibility of accidentally repeating the administration of the drug. If the drug was refused or omitted, record this in the appropriate area on the medication record and notify the primary care provider. This verifies the reason medication was omitted and ensures that the primary care provider is aware of the patient's condition.

GENERAL CONSIDERATIONS

- Ongoing assessment is an important part of nursing care to evaluate patient response to administered medications and early detection of adverse effects. If an adverse effect is suspected, withhold further medication doses and notify the patient's primary healthcare provider. Additional intervention is based on type of reaction and patient assessment.

Skill · 72 Administering an Eye Irrigation

Eye irrigation is performed to remove secretions or foreign bodies or to cleanse and soothe the eye. When irrigating one eye, take care that the overflowing irrigation fluid does not contaminate the other eye.

EQUIPMENT
- Sterile irrigation solution (warmed to 37°C [98.6°F])
- Sterile irrigation set (sterile container and irrigating or bulb syringe)
- Emesis basin or irrigation basin
- Washcloth
- Waterproof pad
- Towel
- Disposable gloves
- Additional PPE, as indicated
- Computer-generated Medication Administration Record (CMAR) or Medication Administration Record (MAR)

ASSESSMENT GUIDELINES
- Assess the patient's eyes for redness, erythema, edema, drainage, or tenderness.
- Assess the patient for allergies.
- Verify patient name, dose, route, and time of administration.
- Assess the patient's knowledge of the procedure. If patient has a knowledge deficit about the procedure, this may be an appropriate time to begin patient education.
- Assess the patient's ability to cooperate with the procedure.

NURSING DIAGNOSES
- Deficient Knowledge
- Risk for Injury
- Acute Pain

OUTCOME IDENTIFICATION AND PLANNING
Expected outcomes may include:
- Eye is cleansed successfully.
- Patient understands the rationale for the procedure and is able to participate.
- Patient's eye remains free from injury.
- Patient remains free from pain.

IMPLEMENTATION

ACTION	RATIONALE
1. Gather equipment. Check the original order in the medical record for the irrigation, according to facility policy. Clarify any inconsistencies. Check the patient's chart for allergies.	This comparison helps to identify errors that may have occurred when orders were transcribed. The primary care provider's order is the legal record of medication orders for each facility.
2. Perform hand hygiene and put on PPE, if indicated.	Hand hygiene and PPE prevent the spread of microorganisms. PPE is required based on transmission precautions.
3. Identify the patient. Usually, the patient should be identified using two methods. Compare information with the CMAR or MAR.	Identifying the patient ensures the right patient receives the medications and helps prevent errors.
a. Check the name and identification number on the patient's identification band.	This is the most reliable method. Replace the identification band if it is missing or inaccurate in any way.
b. Ask the patient to state his or her name and birth date, based on facility policy.	This requires a response from the patient, but illness and strange surroundings often cause patients to be confused.
c. If the patient cannot identify himself or herself, verify the patient's identification with a staff member who knows the patient for the second source.	This is another way to double-check identity. Do not use the name on the door or over the bed, because these may be inaccurate.
4. Explain procedure to patient.	Explanation facilitates cooperation and reassures the patient.
5. Assemble equipment at the patient's bedside.	This provides for an organized approach to the task.
6. Have patient sit or lie with head tilted toward side of affected eye. Protect the patient and bed with a waterproof pad.	Gravity aids flow of solution away from the unaffected eye and from the inner canthus of the affected eye toward the outer canthus.

ACTION	RATIONALE
7. Put on gloves. Clean lids and lashes with washcloth moistened with normal saline or the solution ordered for the irrigation. Wipe from inner canthus to outer canthus. Use a different corner of washcloth with each wipe.	Gloves protect the nurse from contact with mucous membranes, body fluids, and contaminants. Materials lodged on lids or in lashes may be washed into the eye. This cleaning motion protects the nasolacrimal duct and other eye.
8. Place curved basin at cheek on the side of the affected eye to receive irrigating solution. If patient is able, ask him or her to support the basin.	Gravity aids flow of solution.
9. Expose lower conjunctival sac and hold upper lid open with your nondominant hand.	Solution is directed into lower conjunctival sac because the cornea is sensitive and easily injured. This also prevents reflex blinking.
10. Fill the irrigation syringe with the prescribed fluid. **Hold irrigation syringe about 2.5 cm (1 inch) from the eye. Direct flow of solution from inner to outer canthus along conjunctival sac.**	This minimizes the risk for injury to the cornea. Directing the solution toward the outer canthus helps to prevent the spread of contamination from the eye to the lacrimal sac, the lacrimal duct, and the nose.
11. Irrigate until the solution is clear or all the solution has been used. **Use only enough force to remove secretions gently from the conjunctiva. Avoid touching any part of the eye with the irrigating tip.**	Directing solutions with force may cause injury to the tissues of the eye as well as to the conjunctiva. Touching the eye is uncomfortable for the patient and may cause damage to the cornea.
12. Pause irrigation and have patient close the eye periodically during procedure.	Movement of the eye when the lids are closed helps to move secretions from the upper to the lower conjunctival sac.
13. Dry the periorbital area with gauze sponge after irrigation. Offer a towel to the patient if face and neck are wet.	Leaving the skin moist after irrigation is uncomfortable for the patient.

ACTION	RATIONALE
14. Remove gloves. Assist the patient to a comfortable position.	This ensures patient comfort.
15. Remove additional PPE, if used. Perform hand hygiene.	Removing PPE properly reduces the risk for infection transmission and contamination of other items. Hand hygiene prevents the spread of microorganisms.
16. Evaluate the patient's response to the procedure within appropriate time frame.	The patient needs to be evaluated for therapeutic and adverse affects from the procedure.

EVALUATION
- Eye has been irrigated successfully.
- Patient understands the rationale for the procedure and is able to comply with the procedure.
- Eye is not injured.
- Patient experiences minimal discomfort.

DOCUMENTATION
- Document the procedure, site, the type of solution and volume used, length of time irrigation performed, pre- and postprocedure assessments, characteristics of any drainage, and the patient's response to the treatment.

GENERAL CONSIDERATIONS
- Ongoing assessment is an important part of nursing care to evaluate patient response to administered treatments and early detection of adverse effects. If an adverse effect is suspected, notify the patient's primary healthcare provider. Provide additional intervention based on type of reaction and patient assessment.

Skill · 73   Fall Prevention

Falls are associated with physical and psychological trauma, especially in older people. Fall-related injuries are often serious and can be fatal. Falls are caused by, and associated with, multiple factors. Primary causes of falls include a change in balance or gait disturbance, muscle weakness, dizziness, syncope, vertigo, cardiovascular changes (e.g., postural hypotension), change in vision or vision impairment, physical environment/environmental hazards, acute illness, neurologic disease (e.g., dementia or depression), language disorders that impair communication, and polypharmacy. (American Geriatrics Society, British Geriatrics Society, and American Academy of Orthopaedic Surgeons Panel on Falls Prevention [AGS, BGS, AAOS]. [2001; updated 2008]; MacCulloch, P., Gardner, T., & Bonner, A. [2007]; Rao, S. [2005]).

Many of these causes are within the realm of nursing responsibility. Identifying at-risk patients is crucial to planning appropriate interventions to prevent a fall. The combination of an assessment tool with a care/intervention plan sets the stage for best practice (AGS, BGS, AAOS, 2008; Ferris, 2008; Gray-Micelli, 2008; Hendrich, 2007; MacCulloch, et al., 2007; and Nadzam, 2008). Accurate assessment and use of appropriate fall interventions leads to maximal prevention. Fall risk assessment is discussed in the following Assessment section. Providing patient education and a safer patient environment can reduce the incidence and severity of falls. The ultimate goal is to reduce the physical and psychological trauma experienced by patients and their significant others.

EQUIPMENT

- Fall-risk assessment tool, if available
- PPE, as indicated
- Additional intervention tools, as appropriate (refer to sample intervention equipment following in this skill)

ASSESSMENT GUIDELINES

- At a minimum, fall-risk assessment needs to occur on admission to a facility, following a change in the patient's condition, after a fall, and when the patient is transferred. If it is determined that the patient is at risk for falling, regular assessment must continue (Nadzam, 2008).
- Assess the patient and the medical record for factors that increase the patient's risk for falling. The use of an objective, systematic fall assessment is made easier by the use of a fall assessment tool.
- Assess for a history of falls. If the patient has experienced a previous fall, assess the circumstances surrounding the fall and any associated symptoms.
- Review the patient's medication history and medication record for medications that may increase the risk for falls.
- Assess for the following additional risk factors for falls (Ferris, 2008; Gray-Micelli, 2008; Hendrich, 2007; Kratz, 2008; MacCulloch, et al., 2007; Rao, 2005; Swann, 2008):
- Lower extremity muscle weakness
- Use of four or more medications
- Gait or balance deficit
- Depression
- Restraint use
- Visual deficit

- Use of an assistive device
- Arthritis
- Presence of Intravenous Therapy
- History of Cerebrovascular Accident
- Impaired Activities of Daily Living
- Cognitive Impairment
- Age 75 Years or Older
- Secondary Diagnosis/Chronic Disease
- Altered Elimination
- History of Falls
- Administration of high risk drugs, such as narcotic analgesics, anti-epileptics, benzodiazepines, and drugs with anticholinergic effects (Hendrich, 2007; Kratz, 2008)

NURSING DIAGNOSES

- Risk for Falls
- Activity Intolerance
- Risk for Injury
- Impaired Home Maintenance
- Impaired Urinary Elimination
- Impaired Physical Mobility
- Deficient Knowledge Related to Safety Precautions

OUTCOME IDENTIFICATION AND PLANNING

Expected outcomes may include:
- Patient does not experience a fall and remains free of injury.
- Patient's environment is free from hazards.
- Patient and/or caregiver demonstrates an understanding of appropriate interventions to prevent falls.
- Patient uses assistive devices correctly.
- Patient uses safe transfer procedures.
- Appropriate precautions are implemented related to the use of medications that increase the risk for falls.

IMPLEMENTATION

 ACTION

 RATIONALE

ACTION	RATIONALE
1. Perform hand hygiene and put on PPE, if indicated.	Hand hygiene and PPE prevent the spread of microorganisms. PPE is required based on transmission precautions.
2. Identify the patient.	Identifying the patient ensures the right patient receives the intervention and helps prevent errors.

ACTION	RATIONALE
3. Explain the rationale for fall prevention interventions to the patient and family/significant others.	Explanation helps reduce anxiety and promotes compliance and understanding.
4. Include the patient's family and/or significant others in the plan of care.	This promotes continuity of care and cooperation.
5. Provide adequate lighting. Use a night light during sleeping hours.	Good lighting reduces accidental tripping over and bumping into objects that may not be seen. Night light provides illumination in an unfamiliar environment.
6. Remove excess equipment, supplies, furniture, and other objects from rooms and walkways. Pay particular attention to high traffic areas and the route to the bathroom.	All are possible hazards.
7. Orient patient and significant others to new surroundings, including use of the telephone, call bell, patient bed, and room illumination. Indicate the location of the patient bathroom.	Knowledge of surroundings and proper use of equipment relieve anxiety and promote compliance.
8. Provide a 'low bed' to replace regular hospital bed.	Low beds are 14 inches from floor, reducing the risk of injury related to falling out of the bed.
9. Use floor mats if patient is at risk for serious injury.	Floor mats cushion fall and may prevent serious injury to patients at risk, such as those with osteoporosis (Gray-Micelli, 2008).
10. Provide nonskid footwear and/or walking shoes.	Nonskid footwear prevents slipping and walking shoes improve balance when ambulating or transferring.
11. Institute a toileting regimen and/or continence program, if appropriate.	Toileting on a regular basis decreases risk for falls.
12. Provide a bedside commode and/ or urinal/bedpan, if	This prevents falls related to incontinence or trying to get to the bathroom.

ACTION	RATIONALE
appropriate. Ensure that it is near the bed at all times.	
13. Ensure that the call bell, bedside table, telephone, and other personal items are within the patient's reach at all times.	This prevents the patient from having to overreach for device or items, and/or possibly attempt ambulation or transfer unassisted.
14. Confer with primary care provider regarding appropriate exercise and physical therapy.	Exercise programs, such as muscle strengthening, balance training, and walking plans, decrease falls and fall-related injuries.
15. Confer with primary care provider regarding appropriate mobility aids, such as a cane or walker.	Mobility aids can help improve balance and steady the patient's gait.
16. Confer with primary care provider regarding the use of bone-strengthening medications, such as calcium, vitamin D, and drugs to prevent/treat osteoporosis.	Bone strengthening has been suggested to reduce fracture rates with falls (AGS, BGS, AAOS, 2008; Nadzam, 2008).
17. Encourage the patient to rise or change position slowly and sit for several minutes before standing.	Gradual position changes reduce the risk of falls related to orthostatic hypotension.
18. Evaluate the appropriateness of elastic stockings for lower extremities.	Elastic stockings minimize venous pooling and promote venous return.
19. Review medications for potential hazards.	Certain medications and combinations of medications have been associated with increased risk for falls.
20. Keep the bed in the lowest position during use. If elevated to provide care (to reduce caregiver strain), ensure that it is lowered when care is completed.	Keeping bed in lowest position reduces risk of fall-related injury.
21. Make sure locks on the bed or wheelchair are secured at all times.	Locking prevents the bed or wheelchair from moving out from under the patient.

ACTION	RATIONALE
22. Use bed rails according to facility policy, when appropriate.	Inappropriate bed-rail use has been associated with patient injury and increased fall risk. Side rails may be considered a restraint when used to prevent an ambulatory patient from getting out of bed.
23. Anticipate patient needs and provide assistance with activities instead of waiting for the patient to ask.	Patients whose needs are met sustain fewer falls.
24. Consider the use of an electronic personal alarm or pressure sensor alarm for the bed or chair.	The alarm helps alert staff to unassisted changes in position by the patient.
25. Discuss the possibility of appropriate family member(s) staying with patient.	The presence of a family member provides familiarity and companionship.
26. Consider the use of patient attendant or sitter.	Attendant or sitter can provide companionship and supervision.
27. Increase the frequency of patient observation and surveillance; 1-hour or 2-hour nursing rounds, including pain assessment, toileting assistance, patient comfort, personal items in reach, and patient needs.	Patient care rounds/nursing rounds can reduce patient falls (Meade, et al., 2006; Weisgram & Raymond, 2008).
28. Remove PPE, if used. Perform hand hygiene.	Removing PPE properly reduces the risk for infection transmission and contamination of other items. Hand hygiene prevents transmission of microorganisms.

EVALUATION

• Patient remains free of falls.
• Interventions are implemented to minimize risk factors that might precipitate a fall.
• Patient's environment is free from hazards.
• Patient and/or caregiver demonstrates an understanding of appropriate interventions to prevent falls.

- Patient uses assistive devices correctly.
- Patient uses safe transfer procedures.
- Appropriate precautions are implemented related to use of medications that increase the risk for falls.

DOCUMENTATION

- Document patient fall-risk assessment. Include appropriate interventions to reduce fall risk in nursing care plan. Document patient and family teaching relative to fall-risk reduction. Document interventions included in care.

GENERAL CONSIDERATIONS

- Patients are at risk for falls in their home settings. Assess for risk factors and home environment. Include patient teaching regarding falls as part of nursing plan of care.

Skill · 74   Applying a Fecal Incontinence Pouch

A fecal incontinence pouch is used to protect the perianal skin from excoriation due to repeated exposure to liquid stool. A skin barrier is applied before the pouch to protect the patient's skin and improve adhesion. If excoriation is already present, the skin barrier should be applied before applying a pouch.

EQUIPMENT

- Fecal incontinence pouch
- Disposable gloves
- Additional PPE, as indicated
- Washcloth and towel
- Urinary drainage (Foley) bag
- Scissors (optional)
- Skin protectant or barrier
- Bath blanket

ASSESSMENT GUIDELINES

- Assess the amount and consistency of stool being passed. Also assess the frequency. Inspect the perianal area for any excoriation, wounds, or hemorrhoids.

NURSING DIAGNOSES

- Bowel Incontinence
- Risk for Impaired Skin Integrity
- Risk for Infection
- Impaired Skin Integrity

OUTCOME IDENTIFICATION AND PLANNING

Expected outcomes may include:

- Patient expels feces into the pouch and maintains intact perianal skin.
- Patient demonstrates a decrease in the amount and severity of excoriation.
- Patient verbalizes decreased discomfort.
- Patient remains free of any signs and symptoms of infection.

IMPLEMENTATION

ACTION	RATIONALE
1. Bring necessary equipment to the bedside stand or over-bed table.	Bringing everything to the bedside conserves time and energy. Arranging items nearby is convenient, saves time, and avoids unnecessary stretching and twisting of muscles on the part of the nurse.
2. Perform hand hygiene and put on PPE, if indicated.	Hand hygiene and PPE prevent the spread of microorganisms. PPE is required based on transmission precautions.
3. Identify the patient.	Identifying the patient ensures the right patient receives the intervention and helps prevent errors.
4. Close curtains around bed and close the door to the room, if possible. Explain what you are going to do and why you are going to do it to the patient.	This ensures the patient's privacy. Explanation relieves anxiety and facilitates cooperation. Discussion promotes cooperation and helps to minimize anxiety.
5. Adjust bed to comfortable working height, usually elbow height of the caregiver (VISN 8 Patient Safety Center, 2009). Position the patient on the left side (Sims' position), as dictated by patient comfort and condition. Fold top linen back just enough to allow access to the patient's rectal area. Place a waterproof pad under the patient's hip.	Having the bed at the proper height prevents back and muscle strain. Sims' position facilitates access into the rectum and colon, optimizing retention of solution. Folding back the linen in this manner minimizes unnecessary exposure and promotes the patient's comfort and warmth. The waterproof pad will protect the bed.

ACTION	RATIONALE
6. Put on nonsterile gloves. Cleanse perianal area. Pat dry thoroughly.	Gloves protect the nurse from microorganisms in feces. The GI tract is not a sterile environment. Skin must be dry for the pouch to adhere securely.
7. Trim perianal hair with scissors, if needed.	It may be uncomfortable if the perianal hair is pulled by adhesive from the fecal pouch. Trimming with scissors minimizes the risk for infection compared with shaving.
8. Apply a skin protectant or barrier and allow to dry.	Skin protectant aids in adhesion of pouch and protects the skin from irritation and injury from the adhesive. Skin must be dry for the pouch to adhere securely.
9. Remove paper backing from adhesive of pouch.	Removing the paper backing is necessary so that the pouch can adhere to the skin.
10. With nondominant hand, separate buttocks. Apply fecal pouch to anal area with dominant hand, ensuring that the bag opening is over the anus (FIGURE 1).	Opening should be over the anus so that stool empties into the bag and does not stay on the patient's skin, which could lead to skin breakdown.

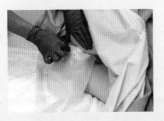

FIGURE 1 Applying pouch over anal opening.

11. Release buttocks. Attach connector of fecal incontinence pouch to urinary drainage bag. Hang drainage bag below patient.	Bag must be dependent for stool to drain into bag.
12. Remove gloves. Return the patient to a comfortable position. Make sure the linens	Promotes patient comfort. Removing contaminated gloves prevents spread of microorganisms.

ACTION	RATIONALE
under the patient are dry. Ensure that the patient is covered.	
13. Raise side rail. Lower bed height and adjust head of bed to a comfortable position.	Promotes patient safety.
14. Remove additional PPE, if used. Perform hand hygiene.	Removing PPE properly reduces the risk for infection transmission and contamination of other items. Hand hygiene prevents the spread of microorganisms.

EVALUATION
• Patient expels feces into the pouch and maintains intact perianal skin.
• Patient demonstrates a decrease in the amount and severity of excoriation.
• Patient verbalizes decreased discomfort.
• Patient remains free of any signs and symptoms of infection.

DOCUMENTATION
• Document the date and time the fecal pouch was applied. Document assessment of the perianal area. Record the color of stool, intake, and output (amount of stool out), and patient's reaction to the procedure.

GENERAL CONSIDERATIONS
• Remove fecal pouch at least every 72 hours to check for signs of skin breakdown.

Skill · 75   **Caring for a Patient with a Fiber Optic Intracranial Catheter**

Fiber optic catheters are another method used to monitor intracranial pressure (ICP). Fiber optic catheters directly monitor ICP using an intracranial transducer located in the tip of the catheter. A miniature transducer in the catheter tip is coupled by a long, continuous wire or fiber optic cable to an external electronic module. This device can be inserted into the lateral ventricle, subarachnoid space, subdural space, or brain parenchyma, or under a bone flap. The dura is perforated, and the transducer probe is threaded through the cerebral tissue to the desired depth and fixed in position (Hickey, 2009). Fiber optic catheters can be used to monitor the ICP and cerebral perfusion pressure (CPP). Some versions of catheters can also be used to drain cerebral spinal fluid (CSF). These devices are calibrated by the manufacturer and zero-balanced only once at the time of insertion.

An ICP measurement is used to calculate CPP, an estimate of the adequacy of cerebral blood supply. CPP is the pressure difference across the brain. It is the difference between the incoming systemic mean arterial pressure (MAP) and the ICP. It is calculated by finding the difference between the MAP and the ICP (Blissitt, 2006).

EQUIPMENT
- PPE, as indicated

ASSESSMENT GUIDELINES
- Perform a neurologic assessment. Assess the patient's level of consciousness. If the patient is awake, assess the patient's orientation to person, place, and time. If the patient's level of consciousness is decreased, note the patient's ability to respond and be aroused. Inspect pupil size and response to light. Pupils should be equal and round and should react to light bilaterally. Any changes in level of consciousness or pupillary response may suggest a neurologic problem. If the patient can move the extremities, assess strength of hands and feet. A change in strength or a difference in strength on one side compared with the other may indicate a neurologic problem.
- Assess vital signs, because changes in vital signs can reflect a neurologic problem.
- Assess the patient's pain level. The patient may be experiencing pain at the fiber optic catheter insertion site.

NURSING DIAGNOSES
- Risk for Infection
- Risk for Injury
- Ineffective Tissue Perfusion: Cerebral
- Pain

OUTCOME IDENTIFICATION AND PLANNING
Expected outcomes may include:
- Patient maintains ICP less than 10 to 15 mm Hg (Arbour, 2004) and CPP 60 to 90 mm Hg (Hickey, 2009).
- Patient is free from infection and injury.
- Patient is free from pain.
- Patient/significant others understand the need for the catheter and monitoring.

IMPLEMENTATION

ACTION	RATIONALE
1. Review the medical orders for specific information about monitoring parameters.	The nurse needs to know the most recent order for acceptable ICP and CPP values.
2. Gather the necessary supplies and bring to the bedside stand or overbed table.	Preparation promotes efficient time management and an organized approach to the task. Bringing everything to the bedside conserves time and energy. Arranging items nearby is convenient, saves time, and avoids unnecessary stretching and twisting of muscles on the part of the nurse.
3. Perform hand hygiene and put on PPE, if indicated.	Hand hygiene and PPE prevent the spread of microorganisms. PPE is required based on transmission precautions.
4. Identify the patient.	Identifying the patient ensures the right patient receives the intervention and helps prevent errors.
5. Close curtains around bed and close the door to the room, if possible. Explain what you are going to do and why you are going to do it to the patient.	This ensures the patient's privacy. Explanation relieves anxiety and facilitates cooperation.
6. Assess the patient for any changes in neurologic status.	Patients with ventriculostomies are at risk for problems with the neurologic system.
7. Assess ICP, MAP, and CPP at least hourly. Note ICP waveforms as shown on the monitor. **Notify the primary care provider if A- or B-waves are present.**	Frequent assessment provides valuable indicators for identifying subtle trends that may suggest developing problems. A- and B-waves are indicators of clinically significant problems.
8. Care for the insertion site according to the institution's policy. Assess the site for any	Site care varies, possibly ranging from leaving the site open to air to applying antibiotic ointment

ACTION	RATIONALE
signs of infection, such as drainage, redness, or warmth. Ensure the catheter is secured at the site per facility policy.	and gauze. Site care aids in reducing the risk for infection. Securing the catheters after insertion prevents dislodgement and breakage of the device.
9. Calculate the CPP, if necessary. Calculate the difference between the systemic MAP and the ICP.	CPP is an estimate of the adequacy of the blood supply to the brain.
10. Remove PPE, if used. Perform hand hygiene.	Removing PPE properly reduces the risk for infection transmission and contamination of other items. Hand hygiene prevents the spread of microorganisms.

EVALUATION

- Patient demonstrates a CPP and an ICP within identified parameters.
- Patient remains free from infection.
- Patient/significant other verbalizes an understanding of the need for the catheter and monitoring.
- Patient reports no pain.

DOCUMENTATION

- Document the neurologic assessment; ICP and CPP measurement readings; vital signs; pain; and the appearance of the insertion site.

GENERAL CONSIDERATIONS

- Secure the catheters according to facility policy after insertion and use care when moving patients to prevent dislodgement and breakage of these devices (March, 2005).
- Keep in mind that several independent nursing activities, such as turning and positioning, have been shown to increase ICP. Take precautions when caring for patients with ICP monitoring to manage factors known to increase ICP. Turn and position the patient in proper body alignment, avoiding angulation of body parts. Extreme hip flexion or flexion of upper legs can increase intra-abdominal pressure, leading to increased ICP. Use logrolling. Maintain the neck in a neutral position at all times to avoid neck vein compression, which can interfere with venous return. Maintain the head of the bed in the flat position or elevated to 30 degrees, depending on medical orders and facility procedure. Avoid noxious stimuli, using soft voices or music and a gentle touch. Plan care to avoid grouping activities and procedures

known to increase ICP. Bathing, turning, and other routine care often have a cumulative effect to increase ICP when performed in succession. Allow rest periods between procedures and carefully assess the patient's response to interventions (Hickey, 2009; Hockenberry, 2009).

Skill · 76   Applying a Figure-Eight Bandage

Bandages are used to apply pressure over an area, immobilize a body part, prevent or reduce edema, and secure splints and dressings. Bandages can be elasticized or made of gauze, flannel, or muslin. In general, narrow bandages are used to wrap feet, the lower legs, hands, and arms, and wider bandages are used for the thighs and trunk. A roller bandage is a continuous strip of material wound on itself to form a roll. The free end is anchored and the roll is passed or rolled around the body part, maintaining equal tension with all turns. The bandage is unwound gradually and only as needed. The bandage should overlap itself evenly and by one-half to two-thirds the width the bandage. The figure-eight turn consists of oblique overlapping turns that ascend and descend alternately. It is used around the knee, elbow, ankle, and wrist.

EQUIPMENT
- Elastic or other bandage of the appropriate width
- Tape, pins, or self-closures
- Gauze pads
- Nonsterile gloves and/or other PPE, as indicated

ASSESSMENT GUIDELINES
- Review the medical record, physician's orders, and nursing plan of care and assess the situation to determine the need for a bandage.
- Assess the affected limb for pain and edema. Perform a neurovascular assessment of the affected extremity. Assess body parts distal to the site for evidence of cyanosis, pallor, coolness, numbness, tingling, and swelling and absent or diminished pulses. Assess the distal circulation of the extremity after the bandage is in place and reassess at least every 4 hours.

NURSING DIAGNOSES
- Impaired Physical Mobility
- Acute Pain
- Risk for Impaired Skin Integrity
- Risk for Injury
- Dressing Self-Care Deficit
- Risk for Peripheral Neurovascular Dysfunction

OUTCOME IDENTIFICATION AND PLANNING

Expected outcomes may include:
- The bandage is applied correctly without injury or complications.
- The patient maintains circulation to the affected part and remains free of neurovascular complications.

IMPLEMENTATION

ACTION	RATIONALE
1. Review the medical record and nursing plan of care to determine the need for a figure-eight bandage.	Reviewing the medical record and plan of care validates the correct patient and correct procedure and reduces risk for injury.
2. Perform hand hygiene. Put on PPE, as indicated.	Hand hygiene and PPE prevent the spread of microorganisms. PPE is required based on transmission precautions.
3. Identify the patient. Explain the procedure to the patient.	Patient identification validates the correct patient and correct procedure. Discussion and explanation help allay anxiety and prepare the patient for what to expect.
4. Close curtain around the bed and close the door to the room, if possible. Place the bed at an appropriate and comfortable working height, usually elbow height of the caregiver (VISN8 Patient Safety Center, 2009).	Closing the door or curtains provides privacy. Proper bed height helps reduce back strain.
5. Assist the patient to a comfortable position, with the affected body part in a normal functioning position.	Keeping the body part in a normal functioning position promotes circulation and prevents deformity and discomfort.
6. Hold the bandage roll with the roll facing upward in one hand while holding the free end of the roll in the other hand. Make sure to hold the bandage roll so it is close to the affected body part.	Proper handling of the bandage allows application of even tension and pressure.

ACTION

RATIONALE

7. Wrap the bandage around the limb twice, below the joint, to anchor it (FIGURE 1).

Anchoring the bandage ensures that it will stay in place.

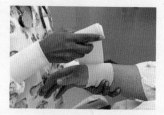

FIGURE 1 Wrapping the bandage around the patient's limb twice, below the joint, to anchor it.

8. Use alternating ascending and descending turns to form a figure eight (FIGURE 2). Overlap each turn of the bandage by one-half to two-thirds the width of the strip (FIGURE 3).

Making alternating ascending and descending turns helps to ensure the bandage will stay in place on a moving body part.

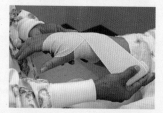

FIGURE 2 Using alternating ascending and descending turns to form a figure eight.

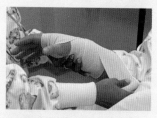

FIGURE 3 Overlapping each turn of the bandage by one-half to two-thirds the width of the strip.

9. Unroll the bandage as you wrap, not before wrapping.

Unrolling the bandage with wrapping prevents uneven pressure, which could interfere with blood circulation.

10. Wrap firmly, but not tightly. Assess the patient's comfort as you wrap. If the patient reports tingling, itching, numbness, or pain, loosen the bandage.

Firm wrapping is necessary to provide support and prevent injury, but wrapping too tightly interferes with circulation. Patient complaints are helpful indicators of possible circulatory compromise.

ACTION	RATIONALE
11. After the area is covered, wrap the bandage around the limb twice, above the joint, to anchor it. Secure the end of the bandage with tape, pins, or self-closures. Avoid metal clips.	Anchoring at the end ensures the bandage will stay in place. Metal clips can cause injury.
12. Place the bed in the lowest position, with the side rails up. Make sure the call bell and other necessary items are within easy reach.	Repositioning the bed and having items nearby ensure patient safety.
13. Remove PPE, if used. Perform hand hygiene.	Removing PPE properly reduces the risk for infection transmission and contamination of other items. Hand hygiene prevents the spread of microorganisms.
14. Elevate the wrapped extremity for 15 to 30 minutes after application of the bandage.	Elevation promotes venous return and reduces edema.
15. Assess the distal circulation after the bandage is in place.	Elastic may tighten as it is wrapped. Frequent assessment of distal circulation ensures patient safety and prevents injury.
16. Lift the distal end of the bandage and assess the skin for color, temperature, and integrity. Assess for pain and perform a neurovascular assessment of the affected extremity after applying the bandage and reassess at least every 4 hours, or per facility policy.	Assessment aids in prompt detection of compromised circulation and allows for early intervention for skin irritation and other complications.
17. Perform hand hygiene.	Hand hygiene prevents the spread of microorganisms.

EVALUATION

- Patient exhibits a bandage that is applied correctly, without causing injury or neurovascular compromise.
- Patient demonstrates proper alignment of the bandaged body part.

- Patient remains free of evidence of complications.
- Patient demonstrates understanding of signs and symptoms to report immediately.

DOCUMENTATION

- Document the time, date, and site that the bandage was applied and the size of the bandage used. Include the skin assessment and care provided before application. Document the patient's response to the bandage and the neurovascular status of the extremity.

GENERAL CONSIDERATIONS

- Keep in mind that a figure-eight bandage may be contraindicated if skin breakdown or lesions are present on the area to be wrapped.
- When wrapping an extremity, elevate it for 15 to 30 minutes before applying the bandage, if possible. This promotes venous return and prevents edema. Avoid applying the bandage to a dependent extremity.
- Place gauze pads or cotton between skin surfaces, such as toes and fingers, to prevent skin irritation. Skin surfaces should not touch after the bandage is applied.
- Include the heel when wrapping the foot, but do not wrap the toes or fingers unless necessary. Assess distal body parts to detect impaired circulation.
- Avoid leaving gaps in bandage layers or leaving skin exposed, which may result in uneven pressure on the body part.
- Remove and change the bandage at least once a day, or per physician order or facility policy. Cleanse the skin and dry thoroughly before applying a new bandage. Assess the skin for irritation and breakdown.

Skill · 77 Applying a Forced-Air Warming Device

Patients returning from surgery are often hypothermic. The application of a forced-air warming device is a more effective way of warming the patient than using warm blankets. This device circulates warm air around the patient.

EQUIPMENT

- Forced-air warming device unit
- Forced-air blanket
- Electronic thermometer
- PPE, as indicated

ASSESSMENT GUIDELINES

- Assess patient's temperature and skin color and perfusion. Patients who are hypothermic are generally pale to dusky and cool to the touch and have decreased peripheral perfusion.

• Inspect nail beds and mucous membranes of patients with darker skin tones for signs of decreased perfusion.

NURSING DIAGNOSES
• Risk for Imbalanced Body Temperature
• Hypothermia

OUTCOME IDENTIFICATION AND PLANNING
Expected outcomes may include:
• Patient will return to and maintain a temperature of 97.7°F to 99.5°F (36.5°C to 37.5°C).
• Patient's skin will become warm, capillary refill will be less than 2 to 3 seconds, and patient will not experience shivering.

IMPLEMENTATION

ACTION	RATIONALE
1. Check patient's chart for the medical order for the use of a forced-air warming device.	Reviewing the order validates the correct patient and correct procedure. Organization facilitates performance of task.
2. Gather the necessary supplies and bring to the bedside stand or overbed table.	Preparation promotes efficient time management and an organized approach to the task. Bringing everything to the bedside conserves time and energy. Arranging items nearby is convenient, saves time, and avoids unnecessary stretching and twisting of muscles on the part of the nurse.
3. Perform hand hygiene and put on PPE, if indicated.	Hand hygiene and PPE prevent the spread of microorganisms. PPE is required based on transmission precautions.
4. Identify the patient.	Identifying the patient ensures the right patient receives the intervention and helps prevent errors.
5. Close curtains around bed and close the door to the room, if possible. Explain	This ensures the patient's privacy. Explanation relieves anxiety and facilitates cooperation.

ACTION	RATIONALE

what you are going to do and why you are going to do it to the patient.

6. **Assess patient's temperature.**

Baseline temperature validates the need for use of the device and provides baseline information for future comparison.

7. Plug forced-air warming device into an electrical outlet. Place blanket over patient, with plastic side up. Keep air-hose inlet at foot of bed (FIGURE 1).

Blanket should always be used with device. Do not place air hose under cotton blankets with airflow blanket to avoid causing burns.

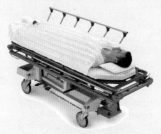

FIGURE 1 Forced-air blanket on patient, plastic side up, with air hose inlet at foot of bed. *Photo is used with permission. © 2009 Arizant Healthcare Inc. All rights reserved.*

8. Securely insert air hose into inlet. Place a lightweight fabric blanket over forced-air blanket, according to manufacturer's instructions. Turn on machine and adjust temperature of air to desired effect.

Air hose must be properly inserted to ensure that it will not fall out. Blanket will help keep warmed air near patient. Adjust air temperature, depending on desired patient temperature. If blanket is being used to maintain an already stable temperature, it may be turned down lower than if needed to raise the patient's temperature.

9. Remove PPE, if used. Perform hand hygiene.

Removing PPE properly reduces the risk for infection transmission and contamination of other items. Hand hygiene prevents transmission of microorganisms.

10. **Monitor patient's temperature at least every 30 minutes while using the forced-air**

Monitoring the patient's temperature ensures that the patient

ACTION	RATIONALE
device. If rewarming a patient with hypothermia, do not raise temperature more than 1°C per hour to prevent a rapid vasodilation effect.	does not experience too rapid a rise in body temperature, resulting in vasodilation.
11. Discontinue use of forced-air device once patient's temperature is adequate and patient can maintain the temperature without assistance.	Forced-air device is not needed once the patient is warm and sufficiently stable to maintain temperature.
12. Remove device and clean according to agency policy and manufacturer's instructions.	Proper care of equipment helps to maintain function of the device.

EVALUATION

- Patient's temperature returns to the normal range of 97.7°F to 99.5°F (36.5°C to 37.5°C) and the patient is able to maintain this temperature.
- Patient's skin is warm.
- Patient is free from shivering.

DOCUMENTATION

- Document the patient's temperature and the route used for measurement. Record that the forced-air warming device was applied to the patient. Document appearance of the skin and that the patient did not experience any adverse effects from the warming device. Record that the patient's temperature was monitored every 30 minutes, as well as the actual temperature after 30 minutes.

Skill · 78   Administering a Tube Feeding

Depending on the patient's physical and psychosocial condition and nutritional requirements, a feeding through the NG tube or other GI tube might be ordered. The steps for administering feedings are similar regardless of the tube used. Feeding can be provided on an intermittent or continuous basis. Intermittent feedings are delivered at regular intervals, using gravity for instillation or a feeding pump to administer the formula over a set period of time. Intermittent feedings might also be given as a bolus, using a syringe to instill the formula quickly in one large amount. An intermittent feeding is the preferred method of introducing the formula over a set period of time via gravity or pump. If the order calls for continuous feeding, an external feeding pump is needed to regulate the flow of formula. Continuous feedings permit gradual introduction of the formula into the GI tract, promoting maximal absorption. However, there is a risk of both reflux and aspiration with this method. Feeding intolerance is less likely to occur with smaller volumes. Hanging smaller amounts of feeding also reduces the risk for bacteria growth and contamination of feeding at room temperature (when using open systems).

The procedure below describes using open systems and a feeding pump; the skill variation at the end of the skill describes using a closed system.

EQUIPMENT
- Prescribed tube feeding formula at room temperature
- Feeding bag or prefilled tube feeding set
- Stethoscope
- Nonsterile gloves
- Additional PPE, as indicated
- Alcohol preps
- Disposable pad or towel
- Asepto or Toomey syringe
- Enteral feeding pump (if ordered)
- Rubber band
- Clamp (Hoffman or butterfly)
- IV pole
- Water for irrigation and hydration, as needed
- pH paper
- Tape measure, or other measuring device

ASSESSMENT GUIDELINES
- Assess the patient's abdomen by inspecting for presence of distention, auscultating for bowel sounds, and palpating the abdomen for firmness or tenderness. If the abdomen is distended, consider measuring the abdominal girth at the umbilicus.
- If the patient reports any tenderness or nausea, exhibits any rigidity or firmness of the abdomen, and if there is an absence of bowel sounds, confer with primary care provider before administering the tube feeding.
- Assess for patient and/or family understanding, if appropriate, for the rationale for the tube feeding and address any questions or concerns expressed by the patient and family members. Consult primary care provider if needed for further explanation.

NURSING DIAGNOSES

- Risk for Aspiration
- Deficient Knowledge
- Risk for Impaired Social Interaction
- Risk for Alteration in Nutrition
- Risk for Body Image Disturbance

OUTCOME IDENTIFICATION AND PLANNING

Expected outcomes may include:
- Patient will receive the tube feeding without complaints of nausea or episodes of vomiting.
- Patient demonstrates an increase in weight.
- Patient exhibits no signs and symptoms of aspiration.
- Patient verbalizes knowledge related to tube feeding.

IMPLEMENTATION

ACTION	RATIONALE
1. Assemble equipment. Check amount, concentration, type, and frequency of tube feeding on patient's chart. Check expiration date of formula.	This provides an organized approach to the task. Checking ensures that correct feeding will be administered. Outdated formula may be contaminated.
2. Perform hand hygiene and put on PPE, if indicated.	Hand hygiene and PPE prevent the spread of microorganisms. PPE is required based on transmission precautions.
3. Identify the patient.	Identifying the patient ensures the right patient receives the intervention and helps prevent errors.
4. Explain the procedure to the patient and why this intervention is needed. Answer any questions as needed.	Explanation facilitates patient cooperation.
5. Assemble equipment on overbed table within reach.	Organization facilitates performance of task.
6. Close curtains around bed and close the door to the room, if possible. Raise bed to a comfortable working	Closing curtains or door provides for patient privacy. Having the bed at the proper height prevents back and muscle strain. Due to

ACTION	RATIONALE
position, usually elbow height of the caregiver (VISN 8 Patient Safety Center, 2009). Perform key abdominal assessments as described above.	changes in patient's condition, assessment is vital before initiating the intervention.
7. **Position patient with head of bed elevated at least 30 to 45 degrees or as near normal position for eating as possible.**	This position minimizes the possibility of aspiration into trachea. Patients who are considered at high risk for aspiration should be assisted to at least a 45-degree position.
8. Put on gloves. Unpin tube from patient's gown. Verify the position of the marking on the tube at the nostril. Measure length of exposed tube and compare with the documented length.	Gloves prevent contact with blood and body fluids. The tube should be marked with an indelible marker at the nostril. This marking should be assessed each time the tube is used to ensure the tube has not become displaced. Tube length should be checked and compared with this initial measurement, in conjunction with pH measurement and visual assessment of aspirate. An increase in the length of the exposed tube may indicate dislodgement (Bourgault, et al., 2007; Smeltzer et al., 2010).
9. Attach syringe to end of tube and aspirate a small amount of stomach contents, as described in Skill 113.	The tube is in the stomach if its contents can be aspirated: pH of aspirate can then be tested to determine gastric placement. If unable to obtain a specimen, reposition the patient and flush the tube with 30 mL of air. This action may be necessary several times. Current literature recommends that the nurse ensures proper placement of the NG tube by relying on multiple methods and not on one method alone.

ACTION	RATIONALE
10. Check the pH as described in Skill 113.	Current research demonstrates that the use of pH is predictive of correct placement. The pH of gastric contents is acidic (less than 5.5). If the patient is taking an acid-inhibiting agent, the range may be 4.0 to 6.0. The pH of intestinal fluid is 7.0 or higher. The pH of respiratory fluid is 6.0 or higher. This method will not effectively differentiate between intestinal fluid and pleural fluid. The testing for pH before the next feeding in intermittent feedings is conducted since the stomach has been emtied of the feeding formula. However, if the patient is receiving continuous feedings, the pH measurement is not as useful, because the formula raises the pH.
11. Visualize aspirated contents, checking for color and consistency.	Gastric fluid can be green with particles, off-white, or brown if old blood is present. Intestinal aspirate tends to look clear or straw-colored to a deep golden-yellow color. Also, intestinal aspirate may be greenish-brown if stained with bile. Respiratory or tracheobronchial fluid is usually off-white to tan and may be tinged with mucus. A small amount of blood-tinged fluid may be seen immediately after NG insertion.
12. If it is not possible to aspirate contents; assessments to check placement are inconclusive; the exposed tube length has changed; or there are any other indications that the tube is not in place, check placement by x-ray.	The x-ray is considered the most reliable method for identifying the position of the NG tube.

ACTION	RATIONALE

13. After multiple steps have been taken to ensure that the feeding tube is located in the stomach or small intestine, **aspirate all gastric contents with the syringe and measure to check for the residual amount of feeding in the stomach.** Return the residual based on facility policy. Proceed with feeding if amount of residual does not exceed agency policy or the limit indicated in the medical record.

Checking for residual before each feeding or every 4 to 6 hours during a continuous feeding according to institutional policy is done to identify delayed gastric emptying. Research suggests continuing the feedings with residuals up to 400 mL. If greater than 400 mL, confer with physician or hold feedings according to agency policy. For patients who are experiencing gastric dysfunction or decreased level of consciousness, feedings may be held for smaller residual amounts (<400 mL) (Bourgault et al., 2007; Keithley & Swanson, 2004; Metheny, 2008). Research findings are inconclusive on the benefit of returning gastric volumes to the stomach or intestine to avoid fluid or electrolyte imbalance, which has been accepted practice. Consult agency policy concerning this practice.

14. Flush tube with 30 mL of water for irrigation. Disconnect syringe from tubing and cap end of tubing while preparing the formula feeding equipment. Remove gloves.

Flushing tube prevents occlusion. Capping the tube deters the entry of microorganisms and prevents leakage onto the bed linens.

15. Put on gloves before preparing, assembling and handling any part of the feeding system.

Gloves prevent contact with blood and body fluids and deter transmission of contaminants to feeding equipment and/or formula.

16. Administer feeding.

When Using a Feeding Bag (Open System)

   a. Label bag and/or tubing with date and time. Hang bag on IV pole and adjust to about 12 inches above

Labeling date and time of first use allows for disposal within 24 hours, to deter growth of microorganisms. Proper feeding

ACTION	RATIONALE

the stomach. Clamp tubing.

bag height reduces risk of formula being introduced too quickly.

b. Check the expiration date of the formula. Cleanse top of feeding container with a disinfectant before opening it. Pour formula into feeding bag and allow solution to run through the tubing. Close clamp.

Cleansing container top with alcohol minimizes risk for contaminants entering feeding bag (Padula, et al., 2004). Formula displaces air in tubing.

c. Attach feeding setup to feeding tube, open clamp, and regulate drip according to the medical order, or allow feeding to run in over 30 minutes.

Introducing formula at a slow, regular rate allows the stomach to accommodate to the feeding and decreases GI distress.

d. **Add 30 to 60 mL (1 to 2 oz) of water for irrigation to the feeding bag when feeding is almost completed and allow it to run through the tube.**

Water rinses the feeding from the tube and helps to keep it patent.

e. Clamp tubing immediately after water has been instilled. Disconnect **feeding setup** from feeding tube. Clamp tube and cover end with cap.

Clamping the tube prevents air from entering the stomach. Capping the tube deters entry of microorganisms and covering the end of the tube protects patient and linens from fluid leakage from tube.

When Using a Large Syringe (Open System)

a. Remove plunger from 30- or 60-mL syringe.

b. Attach syringe to feeding tube, pour premeasured amount of tube feeding formula into syringe, open clamp, and allow food to enter tube. **Regulate rate, fast or slow, by height of the syringe. Do not push formula with syringe plunger.**

Introducing the formula at a slow, regular rate allows the stomach to accommodate to the feeding and decreases GI distress. The higher the syringe is held, the faster the formula flows.

ACTION	RATIONALE

c. Add 30 to 60 mL (1 to 2 oz) of water for irrigation to the syringe when feeding is almost completed, and allow it to run through the tube.

Water rinses the feeding from the tube and helps to keep it patent.

d. When the syringe has emptied, hold it high and disconnect it from the tube. Clamp the tube and cover end with cap.

By holding the syringe high, the formula will not backflow out of tube and onto the patient. Clamping the tube prevents air from entering the stomach. Capping the tube end deters entry of microorganisms. Covering the end protects patient and linens from fluid leakage from tube.

When Using an Enteral Feeding Pump

a. Close flow-regulator clamp on tubing and fill feeding bag with prescribed formula. Amount used depends on agency policy. Place label on container with patient's name, date, and time the feeding was hung.

Closing the clamp prevents formula from moving through tubing until nurse is ready. Labeling date and time of first use allows for disposal within 24 hours, to deter growth of microorganisms.

b. Hang feeding container on IV pole. **Allow solution to flow through tubing.**

This prevents air from being forced into the stomach or intestines.

c. Connect to feeding pump following manufacturer's directions. Set rate. Maintain the patient in the upright position throughout the feeding. If the patient temporarily needs to lie flat, the feeding should be paused. The feeding may be resumed after the patient's position has been changed back to at least 30 to 45 degrees.

Feeding pumps vary. Some of the newer pumps have built-in safeguards that protect the patient from complications. Safety features include cassettes that prevent free flow of formula, automatic tube flush, safety tips that prevent accidental attachment to an IV setup, and various audible and visible alarms. Feedings are started at full strength rather than diluting the feeding, which was recommended previously. A smaller volume, 10 to 40 mL, of feeding infused per

ACTION	RATIONALE
	hour and gradually increased has been shown to be more easily tolerated by patients.
d. **Check placement of tube and gastric residual every 4 to 6 hours.**	Checking placement verifies the tube has not moved out of the stomach. Checking gastric residual monitors absorption of the feeding and prevents distention, which could lead to aspiration. However, presence of large amounts of residual, such as more than 250 to 400 mL, should not be the sole criterion for stopping the enteral feeding (Bourgault, et al., 2007; Metheny, 2008).
17. Observe the patient's response during and after tube feeding and assess the abdomen at least once a shift.	Pain or nausea may indicate stomach distention, which may lead to vomiting. Physical signs, such as abdominal distention and firmness, or regurgitation of tube feeding may indicate intolerance.
18. **Have patient remain upright for at least 1 hour after feeding.**	This position minimizes the risk for backflow and discourages aspiration, if any reflux or vomiting should occur.
19. Remove equipment and return the patient to a position of comfort. Remove gloves. Raise side rail and lower bed.	Promotes patient comfort and safety. Removing gloves properly reduces the risk for infection transmission and contamination of other items.
20. Put on gloves. Wash and clean equipment or replace according to agency policy. Remove gloves.	This prevents contamination and deters spread of microorganisms. Reusable systems are cleansed with soap and water with each use and replaced every 24 hours. Refer to agency's policy and manufacturer's guidelines for specifics on equipment care.
21. Remove additional PPE, if used. Perform hand hygiene.	Removing PPE properly reduces the risk for infection transmission and contamination of other items. Hand hygiene prevents transmission of microorganisms.

EVALUATION

• Patient receives the ordered tube feeding without complaints of nausea or episodes of vomiting.
• Patient demonstrates an increase in weight.
• Patient remains free of any signs and symptoms of aspiration.
• Patient voices knowledge related to tube feeding.

DOCUMENTATION

• Document the type of nasogastric tube or gastrostomy/jejunostomy tube that is present. Record the criteria that were used to confirm proper placement before feeding was initiated, such as the tube length in inches or centimeters compared with the length on initial insertion. Document the aspiration of gastric contents and pH of the gastric contents when intermittent feeding is used. Note the components of the abdominal assessment, such as observation of the abdomen, presence of distention or firmness, and presence of bowel sounds. Include subjective data, such as any reports from the patient (e.g., abdominal pain or nausea) or any other patient response. Record the amount of residual volume that was obtained. Document the position of the patient, the type of feeding, and the method and the amount of feeding. Include any relevant patient teaching.

GENERAL CONSIDERATIONS

• Research suggests continuing the feedings with residuals up to 400 mL. If greater than 400 mL, confer with the physician or hold feedings according to agency policy. For patients who are experiencing gastric dysfunction or decreased level of consciousness, feedings may be held for smaller residual amounts (<400 mL) (Borugault, et al., 2007; Keithley & Swanson, 2004; Metheny, 2008). Also, research findings are inconclusive on the benefit of returning gastric volumes to the stomach or intestine to avoid fluid or electrolyte imbalance, which has been accepted practice. Consult agency policy concerning this practice. Some researchers point out that high residual volumes are not indicative of intolerance to the tube feeding. In contrast, low residual volumes do not guarantee that patients are tolerating enteral tube feedings and are not at risk for aspiration (McClave et al., 2005). Monitoring for trends in gradually increasing amounts of residual volumes and assessing for other signs of intolerance, such as gastric pain or distention, should be implemented (Metheny, 2008).
• When a patient with dementia and/or family is deciding on whether to agree to tube feeding nutrition, inform them that research is recommending that tube feedings not be used for this population of patients because they do not increase survival or prevent malnutrition or aspiration. It is suggested to use such methods as increasing feeding assistance and changing food consistency, as well as respecting patient preferences, as needed (American Dietetic Association [ADA], 2008).

| **Skill Variation** | **Using a Prefilled Tube-Feeding Set (Closed System)** |

Prefilled tube feeding solutions, which are considered closed systems, are frequently used to provide patient nourishment. Closed systems contain sterile feeding solutions in ready-to-hang containers. This method reduces the opportunity for bacterial contamination of the feeding formula. In general, these prefilled feedings are administered via an enteral pump.

1. Verify the medical order.
2. Gather all equipment, checking the feeding solution and container for correct solution and expiration date. Label with patient's name, type of solution, and prescribed rate.
3. Perform hand hygiene.

4. Identify the patient and explain the procedure.

5. Put on gloves and additional PPE, as indicated.
6. Ensure the correct placement of the feeding tube by checking marking on tube at nose (if NG tube), checking length of exposed tube, aspiration of stomach contents, and checking for gastric or intestinal pH.
7. Check for residual amount of feeding in the stomach and return residual, as ordered.

8. Flush tube with 30 mL of water.
9. Remove screw on cap, and attach administration setup with drip chamber and tubing.
10. Hang feeding container on IV pole and connect to feeding pump, allowing solution to flow through tubing, following manufacturer's directions.
11. Attach the feeding setup to the patient's feeding tube.
12. Open the clamp of the patient's feeding tube.
13. Turn on the pump.
14. Set the pump at the prescribed rate of flow and remove the nonsterile gloves.
15. Observe the patient's response during the tube feeding.
16. Continue to assess the patient for signs and symptoms of gastrointestinal distress, such as nausea, abdominal distention, or absence of bowel sounds.
17. Have patient remain in the upright position throughout the feeding and for at least 1 hour after feeding. If the patient's position needs to be changed to a supine position or the patient needs to be turned in bed, pause the feeding pump during this time.
18. After the prescribed amount of feeding has been administrated or according

(continued on page 428)

**Using a Prefilled Tube Feeding Set
(Closed System)** *continued*

to agency policy, turn off the pump, put on nonsterile gloves, clamp the feeding tube, and disconnect the feeding tube from the feeding set tube, capping the end of the feeding set.

19. Draw up 30 to 60 mL of water using a syringe.

20. Attach the syringe to the feeding tube, unclamp the feeding tube, and instill the 30 to 60 mL of water into the feeding tube.

21. Clamp the feeding tube.

22. Remove equipment according to agency policy.

23. Provide for any patient needs.

24. Remove gloves and additional PPE, if used. Perform hand hygiene.

Skill · 79   **Caring for a Gastrostomy Tube**

When enteral feeding is required for a long-term period, an enterostomal tube may be placed through an opening created into the stomach (gastrostomy) or into the jejunum (jejunostomy) (Smeltzer, et al., 2010). Placement of a tube into the stomach can be accomplished by a surgeon or gastroenterologist via a percutaneous endoscopic gastrostomy (PEG) or a surgically (open or laparoscopically) placed gastrostomy tube. PEG tube insertion is often used because, unlike a traditional, surgically placed gastrostomy tube, it usually does not require general anesthesia. Use of a PEG tube or other type of gastrostomy tube requires an intact, functional GI tract. Providing care at the insertion site is a nursing responsibility.

EQUIPMENT
- Nonsterile gloves
- Additional PPE, as indicated
- Washcloth, towel, and soap
- Cotton-tipped applicators
- Sterile saline solution
- Gauze (if needed)

ASSESSMENT GUIDELINES
- Assess gastrostomy or jejunostomy tube site, noting any drainage, skin breakdown, or erythema.
- Measure the length of exposed tube, comparing with the initial measurement after insertion. Alternately, the tube may be marked at the skin with an indelible marker; mark should be at skin level at the insertion site.

- Check to ensure that the tube is securely stabilized and has not become dislodged.
- Assess the tension of the tube. If there is not sufficient tension, the tube may leak gastric or intestinal drainage around exit site. If the tension is too great, the internal anchoring device may erode through the skin.

NURSING DIAGNOSES

- Imbalanced Nutrition, Less than Body Requirements
- Nausea
- Risk for Infection
- Impaired Skin Integrity
- Deficient Knowledge
- Alteration in Comfort

OUTCOME IDENTIFICATION AND PLANNING

Expected outcomes may include:
- Patient ingests an adequate diet and exhibits no signs and symptoms of irritation, excoriation, or infection at the tube insertion site.
- Patient verbalizes little discomfort related to tube placement.
- Patient will be able to verbalize the care needed for the gastrostomy tube.

IMPLEMENTATION

ACTION	RATIONALE
1. Assemble equipment. Verify the medical order or facility policy and procedure regarding site care.	Assembling equipment provides for an organized approach to the task. Verification ensures the patient receives correct intervention.
2. Perform hand hygiene and put on PPE, if indicated.	Hand hygiene and PPE prevent the spread of microorganisms. PPE is required based on transmission precautions.
3. Identify the patient.	Identifying the patient ensures the right patient receives the intervention and helps prevent errors.
4. Explain the procedure to the patient and why this intervention is needed. Answer any questions, as needed.	Explanation facilitates patient cooperation.

ACTION	RATIONALE
5. Assess the patient for presence of pain at the tube insertion site. If pain is present, offer patient analgesic medication, per physician's order, and wait for medication absorption before beginning insertion site care.	Feeding tubes can be uncomfortable, especially the first few days after insertion. Analgesic medication may permit the patient to tolerate the insertion site care more easily. After the first few days, it has been reported that the need for pain medication decreases.
6. Pull the patient's bedside curtain. Raise bed to a comfortable working position, usually elbow height of the caregiver (VISN 8 Patient Safety Center, 2009).	Provide for privacy. Appropriate working height facilitates comfort and proper body mechanics for the nurse.
7. Put on gloves. If gastrostomy tube is new and still has sutures holding it in place, dip cotton-tipped applicator into sterile saline solution and gently clean around the insertion site, removing any crust or drainage. Avoid adjusting or lifting the external disk for the first few days after placement except to clean the area. If the gastric tube insertion site has healed and the sutures are removed, wet a washcloth and apply a small amount of soap onto washcloth. Gently cleanse around the insertion, removing any crust or drainage. **Rinse site, removing all soap.**	Cleaning a new site with sterile saline solution prevents the introduction of microorganisms into the wound. Crust and drainage can harbor bacteria and lead to skin breakdown. Removing soap helps to prevent skin irritation. If able, the patient may shower and cleanse the site with soap and water.
8. Pat skin around insertion site dry.	Drying the skin thoroughly prevents skin breakdown.
9. If the sutures have been removed, **gently rotate the guard or external bumper 90 degrees at least once a day.** Assess that the guard or external bumper is not	Rotation of the guard or external bumper prevents skin breakdown and pressure ulcers. The risk of dislodgement is decreased when the tube has an

ACTION	RATIONALE
digging into the surrounding skin. Avoid placing any tension on the feeding tube.	external anchoring or bumper device.
10. Leave the site open to air unless there is drainage. If drainage is present, place one thickness of precut gauze pad or drain sponge under the external bumper and change, as needed, to keep the area dry. Use a skin protectant or substance, such as zinc oxide, to prevent skin breakdown.	The digestive enzymes from the gastric secretions may cause skin breakdown. Under normal conditions, expect only a minimal amount of drainage on a feeding tube dressing. Increased amounts of drainage should be explored for a cause, such as a possible gastric fluid leak.
11. Remove gloves. Lower the bed and assist the patient to a position of comfort, as needed.	Removing gloves reduces the risk for infection transmission and contamination of other items. Lowering the bed and assisting the patient ensure patient safety and comfort.
12. Remove additional PPE, if used. Perform hand hygiene.	Removing PPE properly reduces the risk for infection transmission and contamination of other items. Hand hygiene prevents transmission of microorganisms.

EVALUATION

- Patient exhibits a clean, dry, intact gastrostomy tube site without evidence of irritation, excoriation, or infection.
- Patient verbalizes no pain when the guard is rotated.
- Patient's skin is without any sign of skin breakdown.
- Patient verbalizes an understanding of gastrostomy tube care.
- Patient participates in care measures.

DOCUMENTATION

- Document the care that was given, including the substance used to cleanse the tube site. Record the condition of the site, including the surrounding skin. Note if any drainage was present, recording the amount and color. Note the rotation of the guard. Comment on the patient's response to the care, if the patient experienced any pain, and if an analgesic was given. Record any patient instruction that was given.

GENERAL CONSIDERATIONS

- Do not place a dressing between the skin and external fixation device unless drainage is present. Change the dressing immediately when soiled, to prevent skin complications.
- If the exposed tube length has changed or marking on tube is not visible, do not use the tube. Notify the patient's primary care provider of the finding.
- Instruct patient on appropriate actions if tube comes out. In the event the gastrostomy tube is pulled out, teach the patient to clean the area with water, cover the opening with a clean dressing, tape in place, and call the primary care provider immediately (Tracey & Patterson, 2006).

Skill · 80 **Putting on Sterile Gloves and Removing Soiled Gloves**

When applying and wearing sterile gloves, keep hands above waist level and away from nonsterile surfaces. Replace gloves if they develop an opening or tear, the integrity of the material becomes compromised, or the gloves come in contact with any unsterile surface or unsterile item. It is a good idea to bring an extra pair of gloves with you when gathering supplies, according to facility policy. That way, if the first pair is contaminated in some way and needs to be replaced, you will not have to leave the procedure to get a new pair.

EQUIPMENT

- Sterile gloves of the appropriate size
- PPE, as indicated

ASSESSMENT GUIDELINES

- Assess the situation to determine the necessity for sterile gloves.
- Check the patient's chart for information about a possible latex allergy. Question the patient about any history of allergy, including latex allergy or sensitivity and signs and symptoms that have occurred. If the patient has a latex allergy, anticipate the need for latex-free gloves.

NURSING DIAGNOSES

- Ineffective Protection
- Risk for Latex Allergy Response

OUTCOME IDENTIFICATION AND PLANNING

Expected outcomes may include:
- Gloves are applied and removed without contamination.

- Patient remains free of exposure to infectious microorganisms.
- Patient does not exhibit signs and symptoms of a latex allergy response.

IMPLEMENTATION

ACTION	RATIONALE

1. Perform hand hygiene and put on PPE, if indicated.

Hand hygiene and PPE prevent the spread of microorganisms. PPE is required based on transmission precautions.

2. Identify the patient. Explain the procedure to the patient.

Patient identification validates the correct patient and correct procedure. Discussion and explanation help allay anxiety and prepare the patient for what to expect.

3. Check that the sterile glove package is dry and unopened. Also note expiration date, making sure that the date is still valid.

Moisture contaminates a sterile package. Expiration date indicates period that package remains sterile.

4. Place sterile glove package on clean, dry surface at, or above, your waist.

Moisture could contaminate the sterile gloves. Any sterile object held below the waist is considered contaminated.

5. Open the outside wrapper by carefully peeling the top layer back. Remove inner package, handling only the outside of it.

This maintains sterility of gloves in the inner packet.

6. Place the inner package on the work surface with the side labeled "cuff end" closest to the body.

Allows for ease of glove application.

7. Carefully open the inner package. Fold open the top flap, then the bottom and sides. Take care not to touch the inner surface of the package or the gloves.

The inner surface of the package is considered sterile. The outer 1 inch border of the inner package is considered contaminated. The sterile gloves are exposed with the cuff end closest to you.

8. With the thumb and forefinger of the nondominant hand, grasp the folded cuff of the

Unsterile hand touches only inside of glove. Outside remains sterile.

| ACTION | RATIONALE |

glove for your dominant hand, touching only the exposed inside of the glove (FIGURE 1).

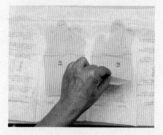

FIGURE 1 Grasping cuff of glove for dominant hand.

9. Keeping the hands above the waistline, lift and hold the glove up and off the inner package with fingers down. **Be careful it does not touch any unsterile object.**

Glove is contaminated if it touches any unsterile objects.

10. Carefully insert your dominant hand palm up into the glove and pull it on. Leave the cuff folded until the opposite hand is gloved.

Attempting to turn upward with unsterile hand may result in contamination of the sterile glove.

11. Hold the thumb of the gloved hand outward. Place the fingers of the gloved hand inside the cuff of the remaining glove (FIGURE 2). Lift it from the wrapper, taking care not to touch anything with the gloves or hands.

Thumb is less likely to become contaminated if held outward. Sterile surface touching sterile surface prevents contamination.

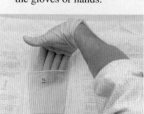

FIGURE 2 Sliding fingers under cuff of glove for nondominant hand.

ACTION	RATIONALE
12. Carefully insert your non-dominant hand into glove. Pull the glove on, taking care that the skin does not touch any of the outer surfaces of the gloves.	Sterile surface touching sterile surface prevents contamination.
13. **Slide the fingers of one hand under the cuff of the other and fully extend the cuff down the arm, touching only the sterile outside of the glove (FIGURE 3). Repeat for the remaining hand.**	Sterile surface touching sterile surface prevents contamination.

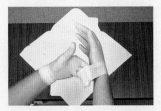

FIGURE 3 Sliding fingers of one hand under cuff of other hand and extending cuff down the arm.

14. **Adjust gloves on both hands if necessary, touching only sterile areas with other sterile areas.**	Sterile surface touching sterile surface prevents contamination.
15. Continue with procedure as indicated.	

Removing Soiled Gloves

16. Use your dominant hand to grasp the opposite glove near cuff end on the outside exposed area. Remove it by pulling it off, inverting it as it is pulled, keeping the contaminated area on the inside. Hold the removed glove in the remaining gloved hand.	Contaminated area does not come in contact with hands or wrists.
17. Slide fingers of ungloved hand between the remaining glove and the wrist. **Take care to avoid touching the outside surface of the glove.**	Contaminated area does not come in contact with hands or wrists.

ACTION	RATIONALE
Remove it by pulling it off, inverting it as it is pulled, keeping the contaminated area on the inside, and securing the first glove inside the second.	
18. Discard gloves in appropriate container. Remove additional PPE, if used. Perform hand hygiene.	Proper disposal and removal of PPE reduces the risk for infection transmission and contamination of other items. Hand hygiene prevents the spread of microorganisms.

EVALUATION

• Gloves are applied and removed without contamination.
• Patient remains free of exposure to potential infection-causing microorganisms.
• Patient does not exhibit signs and symptoms of a latex-allergy response.

DOCUMENTATION

• It is not usually necessary to document the application of sterile gloves. However, documentation should be recorded regarding the use of sterile technique for any procedure performed using sterile technique.

Skill · 81   Performing Hand Hygiene Using an Alcohol-Based Hand Rub

Alcohol-based hand rubs can be used in the healthcare setting and they take less time to use than traditional handwashing. When using these products, check the product labeling for correct amount of product needed. Alcohol-based hand rubs (CDC, 2002a; 2002b):

• May be used if hands are not visibly soiled, or have not come in contact with blood or body fluids
• Should be used before and after each patient contact, or contact with surfaces in the patient's environment
• Significantly reduce the number of microorganisms on skin, are fast acting, and cause less skin irritation.

EQUIPMENT
* Alcohol-based hand rub
* Oil-free lotion (optional)

ASSESSMENT GUIDELINES
* Assess hands for any visible soiling or contact with blood or body fluids. Alcohol-based hand rubs may be used if hands are not visibly soiled, or have not come in contact with blood or body fluids. If food is to be eaten, or the nurse has used the restroom, hands must be washed with soap and water. If hands are visibly soiled, proceed with washing the hands with soap and water. If hands have been in contact with blood or body fluids, even if there is no visible soiling, proceed with washing the hands with soap and water.

NURSING DIAGNOSES
* Risk for Infection

OUTCOME IDENTIFICATION AND PLANNING
Expected outcomes may include:
* Hands will be free of visible soiling and transient microorganisms will be eliminated.

IMPLEMENTATION

ACTION	RATIONALE
1. Remove jewelry, if possible, and secure in a safe place. A plain wedding band may remain in place.	Removal of jewelry facilitates proper cleansing. Microorganisms may accumulate in settings of jewelry. If jewelry was worn during care, it should be left on during handwashing.
2. Check the product labeling for correct amount of product needed.	Amount of product required to be effective varies from manufacturer to manufacturer, but is usually 1 to 3 mL.
3. Apply the correct amount of product to the palm of one hand. Rub hands together, covering all surfaces of hands and fingers, and between fingers. Also clean the fingertips and the area beneath the fingernails.	Adequate amount of product is required to cover hand surfaces thoroughly. All surfaces must be treated to prevent disease transmission.

ACTION	RATIONALE
4. Rub hands together until they are dry (at least 15 seconds).	Drying ensures antiseptic effect.
5. Use oil-free lotion on hands if desired.	Oil-free lotion helps to keep the skin soft and prevents chapping. It is best applied after patient care is complete and from small, personal containers. Oil-based lotions should be avoided because they can cause deterioration of gloves.

EVALUATION

• Hands are free of visible soiling and transient microorganisms are eliminated.

DOCUMENTATION

• The performance of hand hygiene using an alcohol-based hand rub is not generally documented.

Skill · 82   **Performing Hand Hygiene Using Soap and Water (Handwashing)**

Handwashing remains the best method to decontaminate hands. Handwashing, as opposed to hand hygiene with an alcohol-based rub, is required (CDC, 2002a):

• When hands are visibly dirty
• When hands are visibly soiled with or in contact with blood or other body fluids
• Before eating and after using the restroom
• If exposure to certain organisms, such as those causing anthrax or *Clostridium difficile,* is known or suspected. (Other agents have poor activity against these organisms.)

EQUIPMENT

• Antimicrobial or non-antimicrobial soap (if in bar form, soap must be placed on a soap rack)
• Paper towels
• Oil-free lotion (optional)

ASSESSMENT GUIDELINES

• Assess for any of the above requirements for handwashing. If no requirements are fulfilled, the caregiver has the option of decontaminating hands with soap and water or using an alcohol-based hand rub.

NURSING DIAGNOSES

• Risk for Infection

OUTCOME IDENTIFICATION AND PLANNING

Expected outcomes may include:
• Hands will be free of visible soiling and transient microorganisms will be eliminated.

IMPLEMENTATION

ACTION	RATIONALE
1. Gather the necessary supplies. Stand in front of the sink. Do not allow your clothing to touch the sink during the washing procedure.	The sink is considered contaminated. Clothing may carry organisms from place to place.
2. Remove jewelry, if possible, and secure in a safe place. A plain wedding band may remain in place.	Removal of jewelry facilitates proper cleansing. Microorganisms may accumulate in settings of jewelry. If jewelry was worn during care, it should be left on during handwashing.
3. Turn on water and adjust force. Regulate the temperature until the water is warm.	Water splashed from the contaminated sink will contaminate clothing. Warm water is more comfortable and is less likely to open pores and remove oils from the skin. Organisms can lodge in roughened and broken areas of chapped skin.
4. Wet the hands and wrist area. Keep hands lower than elbows to allow water to flow toward fingertips.	Water should flow from the cleaner area toward the more contaminated area. Hands are more contaminated than forearms.

ACTION	RATIONALE
5. Use about 1 teaspoon liquid soap from dispenser or rinse bar of soap and lather thoroughly. Cover all areas of the hands with the soap product. Rinse soap bar again and return to soap rack.	Rinsing the soap before and after use removes the lather, which may contain microorganisms.
6. With firm rubbing and circular motions, wash the palms and backs of the hands, each finger, the areas between the fingers, and the knuckles, wrists, and forearms. **Wash at least 1 inch above the area of contamination.** If hands are not visibly soiled, wash to 1 inch above the wrists.	Friction caused by firm rubbing and circular motions helps to loosen dirt and organisms that can lodge between the fingers, in skin crevices of knuckles, on the palms and backs of the hands, and on the wrists and forearms. Cleaning less contaminated areas (forearms and wrists) after hands are clean prevents spreading microorganisms from the hands to the forearms and wrists.
7. Continue this friction motion for at least 15 seconds.	Length of handwashing is determined by degree of contamination.
8. Use fingernails of the opposite hand or a clean orangewood stick to clean under fingernails.	Area under nails has a high microorganism count, and organisms may remain under the nails, where the organisms can grow and be spread to other persons.
9. Rinse thoroughly with water flowing toward the fingertips.	Running water rinses microorganisms and dirt into the sink.
10. Pat hands dry with a paper towel, beginning with the fingers and moving upward toward forearms, and discard it immediately. Use another clean towel to turn off the faucet. Discard towel immediately without touching other clean hand.	Patting the skin dry prevents chapping. Dry hands first because they are considered the cleanest and least contaminated area. Turning off the faucet with a clean paper towel protects the clean hands from contact with a soiled surface.
11. Use oil-free lotion on hands if desired.	Oil-free lotion helps to keep the skin soft and prevents chapping. It is best applied after patient care is complete and from small, personal containers. Oil-based lotions should be avoided because they can cause deterioration of gloves.

EVALUATION

- Hands are free of visible soiling and transient microorganisms are eliminated.

DOCUMENTATION

- The performance of handwashing is not generally documented.

GENERAL CONSIDERATIONS

- An antimicrobial soap product is recommended for use with handwashing before participating in an invasive procedure and after exposure to blood or body fluids. The length of the scrub will vary based on need. Liquid or bar soap, granules, or leaflets are all acceptable forms of non-antimicrobial soap.

Skill · 83   Applying an External Heating Pad

Heat applications accelerate the inflammatory response, promoting healing. Heat is also used to reduce muscle tension, and to relieve muscle spasm and joint stiffness. Heat also helps relieve pain. It is used to treat infections, surgical wounds, inflammation, arthritis, joint pain, muscle pain, and chronic pain.

Heat is applied by moist and dry methods. The medical order should include the type of application, the body area to be treated, the frequency of application, and the length of time for the applications. Water used for heat applications needs to be at the appropriate temperature to avoid skin damage: 115°F to 125°F for older children and adults and 105°F to 110°F for infants, young children, older adults, and patients with diabetes or those who are unconscious.

Common types of external heating devices include Aquathermia pads (one brand) and crushable, microwaveable hot packs. Aquathermia pads are used in healthcare agencies and are safer to use than heating pads. The temperature setting for an Aquathermia pad should not exceed 105°F to 109.4°F, depending on facility policy. Microwaveable packs are easy and inexpensive to use but have several disadvantages. They may leak and pose a danger from burns related to improper use. They are used most often in the home setting.

EQUIPMENT

- Aquathermia heating pad (or other brand) with electronic unit
- Distilled water
- Cover for the pad, if not part of pad
- Gauze bandage or tape to secure the pad
- Bath blanket
- PPE, as indicated

ASSESSMENT GUIDELINES

- Assess the situation to determine the appropriateness for the application of heat.
- Assess the patient's physical and mental status and the condition of the body area to be treated with heat.
- Confirm the medical order for heat therapy, including frequency, type of therapy, body area to be treated, and length of time for the application.
- Check the equipment to be used, including the condition of cords, plugs, and heating elements. Look for fluid leaks. Once the equipment is turned on, make sure there is a consistent distribution of heat and the temperature is within safe limits.

NURSING DIAGNOSES

- Chronic Pain
- Acute Pain
- Impaired Skin Integrity
- Risk for Impaired Skin Integrity
- Delayed Surgical Recovery
- Impaired Tissue Integrity
- Risk for Injury

OUTCOME IDENTIFICATION AND PLANNING

Expected outcomes may include:
- Patient experiences increased comfort.
- Patient experiences decreased muscle spasms.
- Patient exhibits improved wound healing.
- Patient demonstrates a reduction in inflammation.
- Patient remains free from injury.

IMPLEMENTATION

ACTION	RATIONALE
1. Review the medical order for the application of heat therapy, including frequency, type of therapy, body area to be treated, and length of time for the application.	Reviewing the order and plan of care validates the correct patient and correct procedure.
2. Gather the necessary supplies and bring to the bedside stand or overbed table.	Preparation promotes efficient time management and an organized approach to the task. Bringing everything to the bedside conserves time and energy. Arranging items nearby is

ACTION	RATIONALE
	convenient, saves time, and avoids unnecessary stretching and twisting of muscles on the part of the nurse.
3. Perform hand hygiene and put on PPE, if indicated.	Hand hygiene and PPE prevent the spread of microorganisms. PPE is required based on transmission precautions.
4. Identify the patient.	Identifying the patient ensures the right patient receives the intervention and helps prevent errors.
5. Close curtains around bed and close the door to the room, if possible. Explain what you are going to do and why you are going to do it to the patient.	This ensures the patient's privacy. Explanation relieves anxiety and facilitates cooperation.
6. Adjust bed to comfortable working height, usually elbow height of the caregiver (VISN 8 Patient Safety Center, 2009).	Having the bed at the proper height prevents back and muscle strain.
7. Assist the patient to a comfortable position that provides easy access to the area where the heat will be applied; use a bath blanket to cover any other exposed area.	Patient positioning and use of a bath blanket provide for comfort and warmth.
8. Assess the condition of the skin where the heat is to be applied.	Assessment supplies baseline data for post-treatment comparison and identifies conditions that may contraindicate the application.
9. Check that the water in the electronic unit is at the appropriate level. Fill the unit two-thirds full or to the fill mark, with distilled water, if necessary. Check the temperature setting on the unit to ensure it is within the safe range.	Sufficient water in the unit is necessary to ensure proper function of the unit. Tap water leaves mineral deposits in the unit. Checking the temperature setting helps to prevent skin or tissue damage.

ACTION	RATIONALE
10. Attach pad tubing to the electronic unit tubing.	Allows flow of warmed water through heating pad.
11. Plug in the unit and warm the pad before use. Apply the heating pad to the prescribed area. Secure with gauze bandage or tape.	Plugging in the pad readies it for use. Heat travels by conduction from one object to another. Gauze bandage or tape holds the pad in position; **do not use pins, because they may puncture and damage the pad.**
12. **Assess the condition of the skin and the patient's response to the heat at frequent intervals, according to facility policy. Do not exceed the prescribed length of time for the application of heat.**	Maximal vasodilation and therapeutic effects from the application of heat occur within 20 to 30 minutes. Using heat for more than 45 minutes results in tissue congestion and vasoconstriction, known as the rebound phenomenon. Also, prolonged heat application may result in an increased risk of burns.
13. Remove gloves and discard. Remove all remaining equipment; place the patient in a comfortable position, with side rails up and bed in the lowest position.	Proper removal of gloves prevents spread of microorganisms. Proper patient and bed positioning promotes safety and comfort.
14. Remove additional PPE, if used. Perform hand hygiene.	Removing PPE properly reduces the risk for infection transmission and contamination of other items. Hand hygiene prevents the spread of microorganisms.
15. Remove pad after the prescribed amount of time. Reassess the patient and area of application, noting the effect and presence of adverse effects.	Removal reduces the risk of injury due to prolonged heat application. Heat applications are used to promote healing; reduce muscle tension; relieve muscle spasm, joint stiffness, and pain; and to treat infections, surgical wounds, inflammation, arthritis, joint pain, muscle pain, and chronic pain. Assessment provides input to the effectiveness of the treatment.

EVALUATION

- Patient exhibits increased comfort, decreased muscle spasm, decreased pain, improved wound healing, and/or decreased inflammation.
- Patient remains free of injury.

DOCUMENTATION

- Document the rationale for application of heat therapy. If the patient is receiving heat therapy for pain, document the assessment of pain pre- and postintervention. Specify the type of heat therapy and location where it is applied, as well as length of time applied. Record the condition of the skin, noting any redness or irritation before and after the heat application. Document the patient's reaction to the heat therapy. Record any appropriate patient or family education.

GENERAL CONSIDERATIONS

- Direct heat treatment is contraindicated for patients at risk for bleeding, patients with a sprained limb in the acute stage, or patients with a condition associated with acute inflammation. Use cautiously with children and older adults. Patients with diabetes, stroke, spinal cord injury, and peripheral neuropathy are at risk for thermal injury, as are patients with very thin or damaged skin. Be extremely careful when applying to heat-sensitive areas, such as scar tissue and stomas.
- Instruct the patient not to lean or lie directly on the heating device, because this reduces air space and increases the risk of burns.
- Check the water level in the Aquathermia unit periodically. Evaporation may occur. If the unit runs dry, it could become damaged. Refill with distilled water periodically.

Skill · 84 Caring for a Hemodialysis Access (Arteriovenous Fistula or Graft)

Hemodialysis, a method of removing fluid and wastes from the body, requires access to the patient's vascular system. This is done via the insertion of a catheter into a vein or the creation of a fistula or graft. If a catheter is used, it is cared for in the same manner as a central venous access device (See Skill 29). An arteriovenous fistula is a surgically created passage that connects an artery and vein. An arteriovenous graft is a surgically created connection between an artery and vein using a synthetic material. Accessing a hemodialysis arteriovenous graft or fistula should be done only by specially trained healthcare team members.

EQUIPMENT

- Stethoscope
- PPE, as indicated

ASSESSMENT GUIDELINES

- Ask the patient how much he or she knows about caring for the site. Ask the patient to describe important observations to be made.
- Note the location of the access site.
- Assess the site for signs of infection, including inflammation, edema, and drainage, and healing of the incision.
- Assess for patency by assessing for presence of bruit and thrill (refer to rationale in Step 4).

NURSING DIAGNOSES

- Deficient Knowledge
- Risk for Injury

OUTCOME IDENTIFICATION AND PLANNING

Expected outcomes may include:

- Patient verbalizes appropriate care measures and observations to be made.
- Patient demonstrates care measures.
- Graft or fistula remains patent.

IMPLEMENTATION

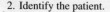 **ACTION**

ACTION	RATIONALE
1. Perform hand hygiene and put on PPE, if indicated.	Hand hygiene and PPE prevent the spread of microorganisms. PPE is required based on transmission precautions.
2. Identify the patient.	Identifying the patient ensures the right patient receives the intervention and helps prevent errors.
3. Close curtains around bed and close the door to the room, if possible. Explain what you are going to do, and why you are going to do it, to the patient.	This ensures the patient's privacy. Explanation relieves anxiety and facilitates cooperation. Discussion promotes cooperation and helps to minimize anxiety.
4. Inspect the area over the access site for any redness,	Inspection, palpation, and auscultation aid in determining the

ACTION	RATIONALE
warmth, tenderness, or blemishes. **Palpate over the access site, feeling for a thrill or vibration. Palpate pulses distal to the site. Auscultate over the access site with bell of stethoscope, listening for a bruit or vibration.**	patency of the hemodialysis access. Assessment of distal pulse aids in determining the adequacy of circulation.
5. Ensure that a sign is placed over the head of the bed informing the healthcare team which arm is affected. **Do not measure blood pressure, perform a venipuncture, or start an IV on the access arm.**	The affected arm should not be used for any other procedures such as obtaining blood pressure, which could lead to clotting of the graft or fistula. Venipuncture or IV access could lead to an infection of the affected arm and could cause the loss of the graft or fistula.
6. Instruct the patient not to sleep with the arm with the access site under head or body.	This could lead to clotting of the fistula or graft.
7. Instruct the patient not to lift heavy objects with, or put pressure on, the arm with the access site. Advise the patient not to carry heavy bags (including purses) on the shoulder of that arm.	This could lead to clotting of the fistula or graft.
8. Remove PPE, if used. Perform hand hygiene.	Removing PPE properly reduces the risk for infection transmission and contamination of other items. Hand hygiene prevents the spread of microorganisms.

EVALUATION

- Access site has an audible bruit and a palpable thrill.
- Access site is without erythema, warmth, skin blemishes, or pain.
- Patient verbalizes appropriate information about caring for the access site and observations to report.

DOCUMENTATION

- Document assessment findings, including the presence or absence of a bruit and thrill. Document any patient education and patient response.

Teaching Patient to Use an Incentive Spirometer

Incentive spirometry provides visual reinforcement for deep breathing by the patient. It assists the patient to breathe slowly and deeply, and to sustain maximal inspiration, while providing immediate positive reinforcement. Incentive spirometry encourages the patient to maximize lung inflation and prevent or reduce atelectasis. Optimal gas exchange is supported and secretions can be cleared and expectorated.

EQUIPMENT

- Incentive spirometer
- Stethoscope
- Folded blanket or pillow for splinting of chest or
- abdominal incision, if appropriate
- PPE, as indicated

ASSESSMENT GUIDELINES

- Assess the patient for pain and administer pain medication as prescribed if deep breathing may cause pain. Presence of pain may interfere with learning and performing required activities.
- Assess lung sounds before and after use to establish a baseline and to determine the effectiveness of incentive spirometry. Incentive spirometry encourages patients to take deep breaths, and lung sounds may be diminished before using the incentive spirometer.
- Assess vital signs and oxygen saturation to provide baseline data to evaluate patient response. Oxygen saturation may increase due to reinflation of alveoli.

NURSING DIAGNOSES

- Ineffective Breathing Pattern
- Risk for Injury
- Risk for Infection
- Deficient Knowledge
- Impaired Gas Exchange
- Activity Intolerance
- Acute Pain

OUTCOME IDENTIFICATION AND PLANNING

Expected outcomes may include:
- Patient accurately demonstrates the procedure for using the spirometer.
- Patient demonstrates increased oxygen saturation level.
- Patient reports adequate control of pain during use of incentive spirometer.
- Patient demonstrates increased lung expansion with clear breath sounds.

IMPLEMENTATION

ACTION

RATIONALE

1. Review chart for any health problems that would affect the patient's oxygenation status.

Identifying influencing factors aids in interpretation of results.

2. Bring necessary equipment to the bedside stand or over-bed table.

Bringing everything to the bedside conserves time and energy. Arranging items nearby is convenient, saves time, and avoids unnecessary stretching and twisting of muscles on the part of the nurse.

3. Perform hand hygiene and put on PPE, if indicated.

Hand hygiene and PPE prevent the spread of microorganisms. PPE is required based on transmission precautions.

4. Identify the patient.

Identifying the patient ensures the right patient receives the intervention and helps prevent errors.

5. Close curtains around bed and close the door to the room, if possible. Explain what you are going to do and why you are going to do it to the patient.

This ensures the patient's privacy. Explanation relieves anxiety and facilitates cooperation.

6. Assist patient to an upright or semi-Fowler's position if possible. Remove dentures if they fit poorly. Assess the patient's level of pain. Administer pain medication as prescribed, if needed. Wait the appropriate amount of time for the medication to take effect. **If the patient has recently undergone abdominal or chest surgery, place a pillow or folded blanket over a chest or abdominal incision for splinting.**

Upright position facilitates lung expansion. Dentures may inhibit the patient from taking deep breaths if he or she is concerned that dentures may fall out. Pain may decrease the patient's ability to take deep breaths. Deep breaths may cause the patient to cough. Splinting the incision supports the area and helps reduce pain from the incision.

ACTION	RATIONALE
7. Demonstrate how to steady the device with one hand and hold the mouthpiece with the other hand (FIGURE 1). If the patient cannot use hands, assist the patient with the incentive spirometer.	This allows the patient to remain upright, visualize the volume of each breath, and stabilize the device.

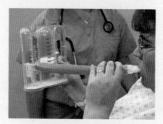

FIGURE 1 Patient using incentive spirometer.

ACTION	RATIONALE
8. Instruct the patient to exhale normally and then place lips securely around the mouthpiece.	Patient should fully empty lungs so that maximal volume may be inhaled. A tight seal allows for maximal use of the device.
9. Instruct the patient to inhale slowly and as deeply as possible through the mouthpiece without using nose (if desired, a nose clip may be used).	Inhaling through the nose would provide an inaccurate measurement of inhalation volume.
10. When the patient cannot inhale anymore, the patient should hold his or her breath and count to three. Check position of gauge to determine progress and level attained. If patient begins to cough, splint an abdominal or chest incision.	Holding breath for 3 seconds helps the alveoli to re-expand. Volume on incentive spirometry should increase with practice.
11. Instruct the patient to remove lips from mouthpiece and exhale normally. If the patient becomes lightheaded during the process, tell him or her to stop and take a few	Deep breaths may change the CO_2 level, leading to light-headedness.

ACTION	RATIONALE

normal breaths before
resuming incentive
spirometry.

12. Encourage the patient to perform incentive spirometry 5 to 10 times every 1 to 2 hours, if possible.

This helps to reinflate the alveoli and prevent atelectasis due to hypoventilation.

13. Clean the mouthpiece with water and shake to dry. Remove PPE, if used. Perform hand hygiene.

Cleaning equipment deters the spread of microorganisms and contaminants. Removing PPE properly reduces the risk for infection transmission and contamination of other items. Hand hygiene prevents the spread of microorganisms.

EVALUATION

- Patient demonstrates the steps for use of the incentive spirometer correctly and exhibits lung sounds that are clear and equal in all lobes.
- Patient demonstrates an increase in oxygen saturation levels.
- Patient verbalizes adequate pain control.
- Patient verbalizes an understanding of the importance of, and need for, incentive spirometry.

DOCUMENTATION

- Document that the incentive spirometer was used by the patient, the number of repetitions, and the average volume reached. Document patient teaching and patient response, if appropriate. If the patient coughs, document whether the cough is productive or nonproductive. If productive cough is present, include the characteristics of the sputum, including consistency, amount, and color.

GENERAL CONSIDERATIONS

- Reinforce importance of continued use by postoperative patients upon discharge.
- Older adults have decreased muscle function and fatigue more easily. Encourage rest periods between repetitions.

Skill · 86 Administering Medication via a Dry Powder Inhaler

Dry powder inhalers (DPI) are another type of delivery method for inhaled medications. The medication is supplied in a powder form, either in a small capsule or disk inserted into the DPI, or in a compartment inside the DPI. DPIs are breath activated. A quick breath by the patient activates the flow of medication, eliminating the need to coordinate activating the inhaler (spraying the medicine) while inhaling the medicine However, the drug output and size distribution of the aerosol from a DPI is more or less dependent on the flow rate through the device, so the patient must be able to take a powerful, deep inspiration (Lannefors, 2006). Many types of DPIs are available, with distinctive operating instructions. Some have to be loaded with a dose of medication each time they are used and some hold a preloaded number of doses. It is important to understand the particular instructions for the medication and particular delivery device being used.

EQUIPMENT
- Stethoscope
- DPI and appropriate medication
- Computer-generated Medication Administration Record
- (CMAR) or Medication Administration Record (MAR)
- PPE, as indicated

ASSESSMENT GUIDELINES
- Assess lung sounds before and after use to establish a baseline and determine the effectiveness of the medication.
- If appropriate, assess oxygen saturation level before medication administration.
- Assess patient's ability to manage the DPI.
- Verify patient name, dose, route, and time of administration.
- Assess the patient's knowledge and understanding of the medication's purpose and action.

NURSING DIAGNOSES
- Ineffective Airway Clearance
- Ineffective Breathing Pattern
- Impaired Gas Exchange
- Deficient Knowledge
- Risk for Activity Intolerance

OUTCOME IDENTIFICATION AND PLANNING
Expected outcomes may include:
- Patient receives the medication via inhalation.
- Patient demonstrates improved lung expansion and breath sounds.
- Patient's respiratory status is within acceptable parameters.

• Patient verbalizes an understanding of medication purpose and action.
• Patient demonstrates correct use of DPI.

IMPLEMENTATION

ACTION	RATIONALE
1. Gather equipment. Check each medication order against the original order in the medical record, according to facility policy. Clarify any inconsistencies. Check the patient's chart for allergies.	This comparison helps to identify errors that may have occurred when orders were transcribed. The primary care provider's order is the legal record of medication orders for each facility.
2. Know the actions, special nursing considerations, safe dose ranges, purpose of administration, and adverse effects of the medications to be administered. Consider the appropriateness of the medication for this patient.	This knowledge aids the nurse in evaluating the therapeutic effect of the medication in relation to the patient's disorder and can also be used to educate the patient about the medication.
3. Perform hand hygiene.	Hand hygiene prevents the spread of microorganisms.
4. Move the medication cart to the outside of the patient's room or prepare for administration in the medication area.	Organization facilitates error-free administration and saves time.
5. Unlock the medication cart or drawer. Enter pass code and scan employee identification, if required.	Locking the cart or drawer safeguards each patient's medication supply. Hospital accrediting organizations require medication carts to be locked when not in use. Entering pass code and scanning ID allows only authorized users into the system and identifies user for documentation by the computer.
6. **Prepare medications for one patient at a time.**	This prevents errors in medication administration.

ACTION	RATIONALE
7. Read the CMAR/MAR and select the proper medication from the patient's medication drawer or unit stock.	This is the *first* check of the label.
8. Compare the label with the CMAR/MAR. Check expiration dates and perform calculations, if necessary. Scan the bar code on the package, if required.	This is the *second* check of the label. Verify calculations with another nurse to ensure safety, if necessary.
9. **When all medications for one patient have been prepared, recheck the label with the CMAR/MAR before taking them to the patient.**	This is a *third* check to ensure accuracy and to prevent errors. Some facilities require the third check to occur at the bedside, after identifying the patient and before administration.
10. Lock the medication cart before leaving it.	Locking the cart or drawer safeguards the patient's medication supply. Hospital accrediting organizations require medication carts to be locked when not in use.
11. Transport medications to the patient's bedside carefully, and keep the medications in sight at all times.	Careful handling and close observation prevent accidental or deliberate disarrangement of medications.
12. **Ensure that the patient receives the medications at the correct time.**	Check agency policy, which may allow for administration within a period of 30 minutes before or 30 minutes after designated time.
13. Perform hand hygiene and 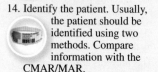 put on PPE, if indicated.	Hand hygiene and PPE prevent the spread of microorganisms. PPE is required based on transmission precautions.
14. Identify the patient. Usually, the patient should be identified using two methods. Compare information with the CMAR/MAR.	Identifying the patient ensures the right patient receives the medications and helps prevent errors.

ACTION	RATIONALE
a. Check the name and identification number on the patient's identification band.	This is the most reliable method. Replace the identification band if it is missing or inaccurate in any way.
b. Ask the patient to state his or her name and birth date, based on facility policy.	This requires a response from the patient, but illness and strange surroundings often cause patients to be confused.
c. If the patient cannot identify himself or herself, verify the patient's identification with a staff member who knows the patient for the second source.	This is another way to double-check identity. Do not use the name on the door or over the bed, because these may be inaccurate.
15. Complete necessary assessments before administering medications. Check the patient's allergy bracelet or ask the patient about allergies. Explain what you are going to do, and the reason for doing it, to the patient.	Assessment is a prerequisite to administration of medications. Explanation relieves anxiety and facilitates cooperation.
16. Scan the patient's bar code on the identification band, if required.	Provides additional check to ensure that the medication is given to the right patient.
17. Remove the mouthpiece cover or remove from storage container. Load a dose into the device as directed by the manufacturer, if necessary. Alternately, activate the inhaler, if necessary, according to manufacturer's directions.	This is necessary to deliver the medication.
18. Have the patient breathe out slowly and completely, without breathing into the DPI.	This allows for deeper inhalation with the medication dose. Moisture from the patient's breath can clog the inhaler.
19. Patient should place teeth over, and seal lips around, the mouthpiece. Do not block the opening with the tongue or teeth.	Prevents medication from escaping and allows for a tight seal, ensuring maximal dosing of medication. Blocking of opening interferes with medication delivery.

ACTION	RATIONALE
20. **Patient should breathe in quickly and deeply through the mouth, for longer than 2 to 3 seconds.**	Activates the flow of medication. Deep inhalation allows for maximal distribution of medication to lung tissue.
21. Remove inhaler from mouth. **Instruct patient to hold the breath for 5 to 10 seconds, or as long as possible, and then to exhale slowly through pursed lips.**	This allows better distribution and longer absorption time for the medication.
22. **Wait 1 to 5 minutes, as prescribed, before administering the next puff.**	This ensures that both puffs are absorbed as much as possible. Bronchodilation after the first puff allows for deeper penetration by subsequent puffs.
23. After the prescribed amount of puffs has been administered, have patient replace the cap or storage container.	By replacing the cap, the patient is preventing any dust or dirt from entering and being propelled into the bronchioles with later doses or clogging the inhaler.
24. Have the patient gargle and rinse with tap water after using DPI, as necessary. Clean the DPI according to the manufacturer's directions.	Rinsing is necessary when using inhaled steroids, because oral fungal infections can occur. Rinsing removes medication residue from the mouth. The buildup of medication in the device can affect how the medication is delivered, as well as attract bacteria.
25. Remove gloves and additional PPE, if used. Perform hand hygiene.	Removing PPE properly reduces the risk for infection transmission and contamination of other items. Hand hygiene prevents the spread of microorganisms.
26. Document the administration of the medication immediately after administration. See Documentation section below.	Timely documentation helps to ensure patient safety.
27. Evaluate patient's response to medication within appropriate time frame. **Reassess lung sounds, oxygenation saturation, if ordered, and respirations.**	The patient needs to be evaluated for therapeutic and adverse effects from the medication. Lung sounds and oxygenation saturation may improve after DPI use. Respirations may decrease after DPI use.

EVALUATION

• Patient receives the medication via inhalation.
• Patient demonstrates improved lung sounds and ease of breathing.
• Patient demonstrates correct use of DPI and verbalizes correct information about medication therapy associated with DPI use.

DOCUMENTATION

• Document the administration of the medication immediately after administration, including date, time, dose, and route of administration on the CMAR/MAR or record using the required format. If using a bar-code system, medication administration is automatically recorded when it is scanned. PRN medications require documentation of the reason for administration. Prompt recording avoids the possibility of accidentally repeating the administration of the drug. Document respiratory rate, oxygen saturation, if applicable, lung assessment, and the patient's response to the treatment, if appropriate. If the drug was refused or omitted, record this in the appropriate area on the medication record and notify the primary care provider. This verifies the reason medication was omitted and ensures that the primary care provider is aware of the patient's condition.

GENERAL CONSIDERATIONS

• Instruct the patient never to exhale into the mouthpiece.
• If mist can be seen from the mouth or nose, the DPI is being used incorrectly.
• Follow the manufacturer's directions to clean the DPI.
• Store inhaler, capsules, and discs away from moisture.
• Ongoing assessment is an important part of nursing care to evaluate patient response to administered medications and early detection of adverse effects. If an adverse effect is suspected, withhold further medication doses and notify the patient's primary healthcare provider. Additional intervention is based on type of reaction and patient assessment.
• Teach the patient how to tell when medication levels are getting low. The most reliable method is to look on the package and see how many doses the DPI contains. Divide this number by the number of doses used daily to ascertain how many days the DPI will last. Keep a diary or record of DPI use and discard the DPI on reaching the labeled number of doses.
• Many DPIs have dosage counters to keep track of remaining doses.

Skill · 87   Administering Medication via a Metered-Dose Inhaler (MDI)

Many medications for respiratory problems are delivered via the respiratory system. A metered-dose inhaler (MDI) is a handheld inhaler that uses an aerosol spray or mist to deliver a controlled dose of medication with each compression of the canister. The medication is then absorbed rapidly through the lung tissue, resulting in local and systemic effects.

EQUIPMENT

- Stethoscope
- Medication in an MDI
- Spacer or holding chamber (optional but recommended for many medications)
- Computerized-generated Medication Administration Record (CMAR) or Medication Administration Record (MAR)
- PPE, as indicated

ASSESSMENT GUIDELINES

- Assess lung sounds before and after use to establish a baseline and determine the effectiveness of the medication. Frequently, patients will have wheezes or coarse lung sounds before medication administration.
- If ordered, assess oxygen saturation level before medication administration. The oxygenation level usually increases after the medication is administered.
- Verify patient name, dose, route, and time of administration.
- Assess patient's ability to manage an MDI; young and older patients may have dexterity problems.
- Assess the patient's knowledge and understanding of the medication's purpose and action.

NURSING DIAGNOSES

- Ineffective Airway Clearance
- Ineffective Breathing Pattern
- Impaired Gas Exchange
- Deficient Knowledge
- Risk for Activity Intolerance

OUTCOME IDENTIFICATION AND PLANNING

Expected outcomes may include:
- Patient receives the medication via inhalation.
- Patient demonstrates improved lung expansion and breath sounds.
- Patient's respiratory status is within acceptable parameters.
- Patient verbalizes an understanding of medication purpose and action.
- Patient demonstrates correct use of MDI.

IMPLEMENTATION

ACTION	RATIONALE
1. Gather equipment. Check each medication order against the original order in the medical record, according to facility policy. Clarify any inconsistencies. Check the patient's chart for allergies.	This comparison helps to identify errors that may have occurred when orders were transcribed. The primary care provider's order is the legal record of medication orders for each facility.
2. Know the actions, special nursing considerations, safe dose ranges, purpose of administration, and adverse effects of the medications to be administered. Consider the appropriateness of the medication for this patient.	This knowledge aids the nurse in evaluating the therapeutic effect of the medication in relation to the patient's disorder and can also be used to educate the patient about the medication.
3. Perform hand hygiene.	Hand hygiene prevents the spread of microorganisms.
4. Move the medication cart to the outside of the patient's room or prepare for administration in the medication area.	Organization facilitates error-free administration and saves time.
5. Unlock the medication cart or drawer. Enter pass code and scan employee identification, if required.	Locking the cart or drawer safeguards each patient's medication supply. Hospital accrediting organizations require medication carts to be locked when not in use. Entering pass code and scanning ID allows only authorized users into the system and identifies user for documentation by the computer.
6. **Prepare medications for one patient at a time.**	This prevents errors in medication administration.
7. Read the CMAR/MAR and select the proper medication from the patient's medication drawer or unit stock.	This is the *first* check of the label.

ACTION	RATIONALE
8. Compare the label with the CMAR/MAR. Check expiration dates and perform calculations, if necessary. Scan the bar code on the package, if required.	This is the *second* check of the label. Verify calculations with another nurse to ensure safety, if necessary.
9. **When all medications for one patient have been prepared, recheck the label with the MAR before taking them to the patient.**	This is a *third* check to ensure accuracy and to prevent errors. Some facilities require the third check to occur at the bedside, after identifying the patient and before administration.
10. Lock the medication cart before leaving it.	Locking the cart or drawer safeguards the patient's medication supply. Hospital accrediting organizations require medication carts to be locked when not in use.
11. Transport medications to the patient's bedside carefully, and keep the medications in sight at all times.	Careful handling and close observation prevent accidental or deliberate disarrangement of medications.
12. **Ensure that the patient receives the medications at the correct time.**	Check agency policy, which may allow for administration within a period of 30 minutes before or 30 minutes after designated time.
13. Perform hand hygiene and 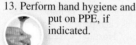 put on PPE, if indicated.	Hand hygiene and PPE prevent the spread of microorganisms. PPE is required based on transmission precautions.
14. Identify the patient. Usually, 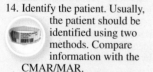 the patient should be identified using two methods. Compare information with the CMAR/MAR.	Identifying the patient ensures the right patient receives the medications and helps prevent errors.
a. Check the name and identification number on the patient's identification band.	This is the most reliable method. Replace the identification band if it is missing or inaccurate in any way.

ACTION	RATIONALE

b. Ask the patient to state his or her name and birth date, based on facility policy.

This requires a response from the patient, but illness and strange surroundings often cause patients to be confused.

c. If the patient cannot identify himself or herself, verify the patient's identification with a staff member who knows the patient for the second source.

This is another way to double-check identity. Do not use the name on the door or over the bed, because these may be inaccurate.

15. Complete necessary assessments before administering medications. Check the patient's allergy bracelet or ask the patient about allergies. Explain what you are going to do and the reason for doing it to the patient.

Assessment is a prerequisite to administration of medications. Explanation relieves anxiety and facilitates cooperation.

16. Scan the patient's bar code on the identification band, if required.

Provides additional check to ensure that the medication is given to the right patient.

17. Perform hand hygiene.

Hand hygiene deters the spread of microorganisms.

18. Remove the mouthpiece cover from the MDI and the spacer. Attach the MDI to the spacer.

The use of a spacer is preferred because it traps the medication and aids in delivery of the correct dose.

19. Shake the inhaler and spacer well.

The medication and propellant may separate when the canister is not in use. Shaking well ensures that the patient is receiving the correct dosage of medication.

20. Have patient place the spacer's mouthpiece into the mouth, grasping securely with teeth and lips. Have patient breathe normally through the spacer.

Medication should not leak out around the mouthpiece.

ACTION	RATIONALE
21. Patient should depress the canister, releasing one puff into the spacer, then inhale slowly and deeply through the mouth.	The spacer will hold the medication in suspension for a short period so that the patient can receive more of the prescribed medication than if it had been projected into the air. Breathing slowly and deeply distributes the medication deep into the airways.
22. **Instruct patient to hold his or her breath for 5 to 10 seconds, or as long as possible, and then to exhale slowly through pursed lips.**	This allows better distribution and longer absorption time for the medication.
23. **Wait 1 to 5 minutes, as prescribed, before administering the next puff.**	This ensures that both puffs are absorbed as much as possible. Bronchodilation after the first puff allows for deeper penetration by subsequent puffs.
24. After the prescribed amount of puffs has been administered, have patient remove the MDI from the spacer and replace the caps on both.	By replacing the caps, the patient is preventing any dust or dirt from entering and being propelled into the bronchioles with later doses.
25. Have the patient gargle and rinse with tap water after using MDI, as necessary. Clean the MDI according to the manufacturer's directions.	Rinsing removes medication residue from the mouth. Rinsing is necessary when using inhaled steroids because oral fungal infections can occur. The buildup of medication in the device can attract bacteria and affect how the medication is delivered.
26. Remove gloves and additional PPE, if used. Perform hand hygiene.	Removing PPE properly reduces the risk for infection transmission and contamination of other items. Hand hygiene prevents the spread of microorganisms.
27. Document the administration of the medication immediately after administration. See Documentation section below.	Timely documentation helps to ensure patient safety.

ACTION	RATIONALE
28. Evaluate the patient's response to the medication within an appropriate time frame. **Reassess lung sounds, oxygenation saturation, if ordered, and respirations.**	The patient needs to be evaluated for therapeutic and adverse effects from the medication. Lung sounds and oxygenation saturation may improve after MDI use. Respirations may decrease after MDI use.

EVALUATION

• Patient receives the medication via inhalation.
• Patient demonstrates improved lung sounds and ease of breathing.
• Patient demonstrates correct use of MDI and verbalizes correct information about medication therapy associated with MDI use.

DOCUMENTATION

• Document the administration of the medication immediately after administration, including date, time, dose, and route of administration on the CMAR/MAR or record using the required format. If using a bar-code system, medication administration is recorded automatically when it is scanned. PRN medications require documentation of the reason for administration. Prompt recording avoids the possibility of accidentally repeating the administration of the drug. Document respiratory rate, oxygen saturation, if applicable, lung assessment, and the patient's response to the treatment, if appropriate. If the drug was refused or omitted, record this in the appropriate area on the medication record and notify the primary care provider. This verifies the reason medication was omitted and ensures that the primary care provider is aware of the patient's condition.

GENERAL CONSIDERATIONS

• Spacers and inhalers should be cleaned at least weekly with warm water or soaked in a vinegar solution (1 pint of water to 2 oz white vinegar) for 20 minutes. Rinse with clean water and allow to air-dry.
• If the medication being administered is a steroid, the patient should rinse the mouth with water after administration to prevent a thrush infection.
• Ongoing assessment is an important part of nursing care to evaluate patient response to administered medications and early detection of adverse effects. If an adverse effect is suspected, withhold further medication doses and notify the patient's primary healthcare provider. Additional intervention is based on type of reaction and patient assessment.

Intradermal injections are administered into the dermis, just below the epidermis. The intradermal route has the longest absorption time of all parenteral routes. For this reason, intradermal injections are used for sensitivity tests, such as tuberculin and allergy tests, and local anesthesia. The advantage of the intradermal route for these tests is that the body's reaction to substances is easily visible, and the degrees of reaction are discernible by comparative study.

Sites commonly used are the inner surface of the forearm and the upper back, under the scapula. Equipment used for an intradermal injection includes a tuberculin syringe calibrated in tenths and hundredths of a milliliter and a ¼ to ½ inch, 26- or 27-gauge needle. The dosage given intradermally is small, usually less than 0.5 mL. The angle of administration for an intradermal injection is 5 to 15 degrees.

EQUIPMENT

- Prescribed medication
- Sterile syringe, usually a tuberculin syringe calibrated in tenths and hundredths, and needle, ¼ to ½ inch, 26- or 27-gauge
- Antimicrobial swab
- Disposable gloves
- Small gauze square
- Computer-generated Medication Administration Record (CMAR) or Medication Administration Record (MAR)
- PPE, as indicated

ASSESSMENT GUIDELINES

- Assess the patient for any allergies.
- Check expiration date before administering medication.
- Assess the appropriateness of the drug for the patient.
- Review assessment and laboratory data that may influence drug administration.
- Assess the site on the patient where the injection is to be given. Avoid areas of broken or open skin. Avoid areas that are highly pigmented; have lesions, bruises, or scars; and are hairy.
- Assess the patient's knowledge of the medication. This may provide an opportune time for patient education.
- Verify the patient's name, dose, route, and time of administration.

NURSING DIAGNOSES

- Deficient Knowledge
- Risk for Allergy Response
- Risk for Infection
- Risk for Injury
- Anxiety

OUTCOME IDENTIFICATION AND PLANNING

Expected outcomes may include:
- Medication will be administered with the appearance of a wheal at the site of injection.
- Patient refrains from rubbing the site.
- Patient's anxiety is decreased.
- Patient does not experience adverse effects.
- Patient understands and complies with the medication regimen.

IMPLEMENTATION

ACTION	RATIONALE
1. Gather equipment. Check each medication order against the original order in the medical record, according to facility policy. Clarify any inconsistencies. Check the patient's chart for allergies.	This comparison helps to identify errors that may have occurred when orders were transcribed. The primary care provider's order is the legal record of medication orders for each facility.
2. Know the actions, special nursing considerations, safe dose ranges, purpose of administration, and adverse effects of the medication to be administered. Consider the appropriateness of the medication for this patient.	This knowledge aids the nurse in evaluating the therapeutic effect of the medication in relation to the patient's disorder and can also be used to educate the patient about the medication.
3. Perform hand hygiene.	Hand hygiene prevents the spread of microorganisms.
4. Move the medication cart to the outside of the patient's room or prepare for administration in the medication area.	Organization facilitates error-free administration and saves time.
5. Unlock the medication cart or drawer. Enter pass code and scan employee identification, if required.	Locking the cart or drawer safeguards each patient's medication supply. Hospital accrediting organizations require medication carts to be locked when not in use. Entering pass code and scanning ID allows only authorized users into the system and identifies user for documentation by the computer.

ACTION	RATIONALE
6. **Prepare medications for one patient at a time.**	This prevents errors in medication administration.
7. Read the CMAR/MAR and select the proper medication from the patient's medication drawer or unit stock.	This is the *first* check of the label.
8. Compare the label with the CMAR/MAR. Check expiration dates and perform calculations, if necessary. Scan the bar code on the package, if required.	This is the *second* check of the label. Verify calculations with another nurse to ensure safety.
9. If necessary, withdraw medication from an ampule or vial as described in Skill 105 and Skill 106.	
10. **When all medications for one patient have been prepared, recheck the label with the CMAR/MAR before taking them to the patient.**	This is a *third* check to ensure accuracy and to prevent errors. Some facilities require the third check to occur at the bedside, after identifying the patient and before administration.
11. Lock the medication cart before leaving it.	Locking the cart or drawer safeguards the patient's medication supply. Hospital accrediting organizations require medication carts to be locked when not in use.
12. Transport medications to the patient's bedside carefully, and keep the medications in sight at all times.	Careful handling and close observation prevent accidental or deliberate disarrangement of medications.
13. **Ensure that the patient receives the medications at the correct time.**	Check agency policy, which may allow for administration within a period of 30 minutes before or 30 minutes after the designated time.
14. Perform hand hygiene and put on PPE, if indicated.	Hand hygiene and PPE prevent the spread of microorganisms. PPE is required based on transmission precautions.

ACTION	RATIONALE

15. Identify the patient. Usually, the patient should be identified using two methods. Compare information with the CMAR/MAR.

Identifying the patient ensures the right patient receives the medications and helps prevent errors.

   a. Check the name and identification number on the patient's identification band.

This is the most reliable method. Replace the identification band if it is missing or inaccurate in any way.

   b. Ask the patient to state his or her name and birth date, based on facility policy.

This requires a response from the patient, but illness and strange surroundings often cause patients to be confused.

   c. If the patient cannot identify himself or herself, verify the patient's identification with a staff member who knows the patient for the second source.

This is another way to double-check identity. Do not use the name on the door or over the bed, because these may be inaccurate.

16. Close curtains around bed and close the door to the room, if possible.

This provides patient privacy.

17. Complete necessary assessments before administering medications. Check allergy bracelet or ask the patient about allergies. Explain the purpose and action of the medication to the patient.

Assessment is a prerequisite to administration of medications. Explanation provides rationale, increases knowledge, and reduces anxiety.

18. Scan the patient's bar code on the identification band, if required.

Provides additional check to ensure that the medication is given to the right patient.

19. Put on clean gloves.

Gloves help prevent exposure to contaminants.

20. Select an appropriate administration site. Assist the patient to the appropriate position for the site chosen. Drape, as needed, to expose only area of site to be used.

Appropriate site prevents injury and allows for accurate reading of the test site at the appropriate time. Draping provides privacy and warmth.

21. Cleanse the site with an antimicrobial swab while wiping

Pathogens on the skin can be forced into the tissues by the

ACTION	RATIONALE
with a firm, circular motion and moving outward from the injection site. Allow the skin to dry.	needle. Moving from the center outward prevents contamination of the site. Allowing skin to dry prevents introducing alcohol into the tissue, which can be irritating and uncomfortable.
22. Remove the needle cap with the nondominant hand by pulling it straight off.	This technique lessens the risk of an accidental needlestick.
23. Use the nondominant hand to spread the skin taut over the injection site.	Taut skin provides an easy entrance into intradermal tissue.
24. Hold the syringe in the dominant hand, between the thumb and forefinger with the bevel of the needle up.	Using the dominant hand allows for easy, appropriate handling of syringe. Having the bevel up allows for smooth piercing of the skin and introduction of medication into the dermis.
25. Hold the syringe at a 5- to 15-degree angle from the site. **Place the needle almost flat against the patient's skin (FIGURE 1), bevel side up, and insert the needle into the skin. Insert the needle only about ¹⁄₈ inch with entire bevel under the skin.**	The dermis is entered when the needle is held as nearly parallel to the skin as possible and is inserted about ⅛ inch.

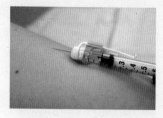

FIGURE 1 Inserting the needle almost level with the skin.

ACTION	RATIONALE
26. Once the needle is in place, steady the lower end of the syringe. Slide your dominant hand to the end of the plunger.	Prevents injury and inadvertent advancement or withdrawal of needle.

ACTION	RATIONALE
27. Slowly inject the agent while watching for a small wheal or blister to appear (FIGURE 2).	The appearance of a wheal indicates the medication is in the dermis.

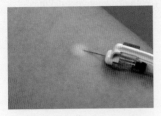

FIGURE 2 Observing for wheal while injecting medication.

ACTION	RATIONALE
28. Withdraw the needle quickly at the same angle that it was inserted. Do not recap the used needle. Engage the safety shield or needle guard.	Withdrawing the needle quickly and at the angle at which it entered the skin minimizes tissue damage and discomfort for the patient. Safety shield or needle guard prevents accidental needle stick injury.
29. **Do not massage the area after removing the needle. Tell the patient not to rub or scratch the site. If necessary, gently blot the site with a dry gauze square. Do not apply pressure or rub the site.**	Massaging the area where an intradermal injection is given may spread the medication to underlying subcutaneous tissue.
30. Assist the patient to a position of comfort.	This provides for the well-being of the patient.
31. Discard the needle and syringe in the appropriate receptacle.	Proper disposal of the needle prevents injury.
32. Remove gloves and additional PPE, if used. Perform hand hygiene.	Removing PPE properly reduces the risk for infection transmission and contamination of other items. Hand hygiene prevents the spread of microorganisms.
33. Document the administration of the medication immediately after administration. See Documentation section below.	Timely documentation helps to ensure patient safety.

ACTION	RATIONALE
34. Evaluate patient's response to medication within appropriate time frame.	The patient needs to be evaluated for therapeutic and adverse effects from the medication.
35. Observe the area for signs of a reaction at determined intervals after administration. Inform the patient of the need for inspection.	With many intradermal injections, the nurse needs to look for a localized reaction in the injection area at the appropriate interval(s) determined by the type of medication and purpose. Explaining this to the patient increases compliance.

EVALUATION

• Outcome is met when nurse notes a wheal at site of injection.
• Patients refrains from rubbing the site.
• Patient's anxiety is decreased.
• Patient did not experience adverse effects.
• Patient verbalizes an understanding of, and complies with, the medication regime.

DOCUMENTATION

• Record each medication administered on the CMAR/MAR or record using the required format, including date, time, and the site of administration, immediately after administration. Some facilities recommend circling the injection site with ink. Circling the injection site easily identifies the site of the intradermal injection and allows for future careful observation of the exact area. If using a bar-code system, medication administration is automatically recorded when it is scanned. PRN medications require documentation of the reason for administration. Prompt recording avoids the possibility of accidentally repeating the administration of the drug. If the drug was refused or omitted, record this in the appropriate area on the medication record and notify the primary care provider. This verifies the reason medication was omitted and ensures that the primary care provider is aware of the patient's condition.

GENERAL CONSIDERATIONS

• Ongoing assessment is an important part of nursing care to evaluate patient response to administered medications and early detection of adverse effects. If an adverse effect is suspected, withhold further medication doses and notify the patient's primary healthcare provider. Additional intervention is based on type of reaction and patient assessment.

- Aspiration, pulling back on the plunger after insertion and before administration, is not recommended for an intradermal injection. The dermis does not contain large blood vessels.
- Some agencies recommend administering intradermal injections with the bevel down instead of the bevel up. Check facility policy.

Skill · 89   Administering an Intramuscular Injection

Intramuscular injections deliver medication through the skin and subcutaneous tissues into certain muscles. Muscles have larger and a greater number of blood vessels than subcutaneous tissue, allowing faster onset of action than with subcutaneous injections.

It is important to choose the right needle length for a particular intramuscular injection. Needle length should be based on the site for injection and the patient's age. Patients who are obese may require a longer needle, and emaciated patients may require a shorter needle. Appropriate gauge is determined by the medication being administered.

Site/Age	Needle Length
Vastus lateralis	$5/8''$ to $1''$
Deltoid (children)	$5/8''$ to $1\frac{1}{4}''$
Deltoid (adults)	$1''$ to $1\frac{1}{2}''$
Ventrogluteal (adults)	$1\frac{1}{2}''$

To avoid complications, be able to identify anatomic landmarks and site boundaries. Consider the age of the patient, medication type, and medication volume when selecting a site for intramuscular injection. Rotate the sites used to administer intramuscular medications when therapy requires repeated injections. Administer the intramuscular injection so that the needle is perpendicular to the patient's body. This ensures it is given using an angle of injection between 72 and 90 degrees (Nicoll & Hesby, 2002).

The volume of medication that can be administered intramuscularly varies based on the intended site. Generally, 1 to 4 mL is the accepted volume range, with no more than 1 to 2 mL given at the deltoid site. The less-developed muscles of children and elderly people limit the intramuscular injection to 1 to 2 mL.

A previously included practice associated with intramuscular injections is the inclusion of aspiration; the process of pulling back on the plunger of the syringe before injection to ensure the medication is not injected into a blood vessel. According to the CDC (2009), aspiration is not required.

EQUIPMENT

- Disposable gloves
- Medication
- Sterile syringe and needle of appropriate size and gauge
- Antimicrobial swab

- Small gauze square
- Computer-generated Medication Administration Record (CMAR) or Medication Administration Record (MAR)
- Additional PPE, as indicated

ASSESSMENT GUIDELINES

- Assess the patient for any allergies.
- Check the expiration date before administering medication.
- Assess the appropriateness of the drug for the patient. Verify patient name, dose, route, and time of administration.
- Review assessment and laboratory data that may influence drug administration.
- Assess the site on the patient where the injection is to be given. Avoid any site that is bruised, tender, hard, swollen, inflamed, or scarred.
- Assess the patient's knowledge of the medication. If the patient has deficient knowledge about the medication, this may be the appropriate time to begin education about the medication.
- If the medication may affect the patient's vital signs, assess them before administration.

NURSING DIAGNOSES

- Deficient Knowledge
- Risk for Allergy Response
- Acute Pain
- Risk for Injury
- Anxiety

OUTCOME IDENTIFICATION AND PLANNING

Expected outcomes may include:
- Patient receives the medication via the intramuscular route.
- Patient's anxiety is decreased.
- Patient does not experience adverse effects.
- Patient understands and complies with the medication regimen.

IMPLEMENTATION

ACTION	RATIONALE
1. Gather equipment. Check each medication order against the original order in the medical record according to facility policy. Clarify any	This comparison helps to identify errors that may have occurred when orders were transcribed. The primary care provider's order is the legal record

ACTION	RATIONALE

inconsistencies. Check the patient's chart for allergies.

of medication orders for each facility.

2. Know the actions, special nursing considerations, safe dose ranges, purpose of administration, and adverse effects of the medications to be administered. Consider the appropriateness of the medication for this patient.

This knowledge aids the nurse in evaluating the therapeutic effect of the medication in relation to the patient's disorder and can also be used to educate the patient about the medication.

3. Perform hand hygiene.

Hand hygiene prevents the spread of microorganisms.

4. Move the medication cart to the outside of the patient's room or prepare for administration in the medication area.

Organization facilitates error-free administration and saves time.

5. Unlock the medication cart or drawer. Enter pass code and scan employee identification, if required.

Locking the cart or drawer safeguards each patient's medication supply. Hospital accrediting organizations require medication carts to be locked when not in use. Entering pass code and scanning ID allows only authorized users into the system and identifies user for documentation by the computer.

6. **Prepare medications for one patient at a time.**

This prevents errors in medication administration.

7. Read the CMAR/MAR and select the proper medication from the patient's medication drawer or unit stock.

This is the *first* check of the label.

8. Compare the label with the CMAR/MAR. Check expiration dates and perform calculations, if necessary. Scan the bar code on the package, if required.

This is the *second* check of the label. Verify calculations with another nurse to ensure safety, if necessary.

9. If necessary, withdraw medication from an ampule or vial

ACTION	RATIONALE
as described in Skills 105 and 106.	
10. **When all medications for one patient have been prepared, recheck the label with the MAR before taking them to the patient.**	This is a *third* check to ensure accuracy and to prevent errors. Some facilities require the third check to occur at the bedside, after identifying the patient and before administration.
11. Lock the medication cart before leaving it.	Locking the cart or drawer safeguards the patient's medication supply. Hospital accrediting organizations require medication carts to be locked when not in use.
12. Transport medications to the patient's bedside carefully, and keep the medications in sight at all times.	Careful handling and close observation prevent accidental or deliberate disarrangement of medications.
13. **Ensure that the patient receives the medications at the correct time.**	Check agency policy, which may allow for administration within a period of 30 minutes before or 30 minutes after designated time.
14. Perform hand hygiene and put on PPE, if indicated.	Hand hygiene and PPE prevent the spread of microorganisms. PPE is required based on transmission precautions.
15. Identify the patient. Usually, 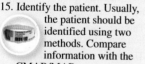 the patient should be identified using two methods. Compare information with the CMAR/MAR.	Identifying the patient ensures the right patient receives the medications and helps prevent errors.
a. Check the name and identification number on the patient's identification band.	This is the most reliable method. Replace the identification band if it is missing or inaccurate in any way.
b. Ask the patient to state his or her name and birth date, based on facility policy.	This requires a response from the patient, but illness and strange surroundings often cause patients to be confused.

ACTION	RATIONALE
c. If the patient cannot identify himself or herself, verify the patient's identification with a staff member who knows the patient for the second source.	This is another way to double-check identity. Do not use the name on the door or over the bed, because these may be inaccurate.
16. Close the curtain around the bed and close the door to the room, if possible.	This provides patient privacy.
17. Complete necessary assessments before administering medications. Check the patient's allergy bracelet or ask the patient about allergies. Explain the purpose and action of the medication to the patient.	Assessment is a prerequisite to administration of medications. Explanation provides rationale, increases knowledge, and reduces anxiety.
18. Scan the patient's bar code on the identification band, if required.	Provides additional check to ensure that the medication is given to the right patient.
19. Put on clean gloves.	Gloves help prevent exposure to contaminants.
20. Select an appropriate administration site.	Selecting the appropriate site prevents injury.
21. Assist the patient to the appropriate position for the site chosen. Drape, as needed, to expose only the site area being used.	Appropriate positioning for the site chosen prevents injury. Draping helps maintain the patient's privacy.
22. **Identify the appropriate landmarks for the site chosen.**	Good visualization is necessary to establish the correct location of the site and to avoid damage to tissues.
23. Cleanse the area around the injection site with an antimicrobial swab. Use a firm, circular motion while moving outward from the injection site. Allow area to dry.	Pathogens on the skin can be forced into the tissues by the needle. Moving from the center outward prevents contamination of the site. Allowing skin to dry prevents introducing alcohol into the tissue, which can be irritating and uncomfortable.

ACTION	RATIONALE
24. Remove the needle cap by pulling it straight off. Hold the syringe in your dominant hand between the thumb and forefinger.	This technique lessens the risk of an accidental needlestick and also prevents inadvertently unscrewing the needle from the barrel of the syringe.
25. Displace the skin in a Z-track manner by pulling the skin down or to one side about 1 inch (2.5 cm) with your non-dominant hand and hold the skin and tissue in this position.	This ensures medication does not leak back along the needle track and into the subcutaneous tissue.
26. Quickly dart the needle into the tissue so that the needle is perpendicular to the patient's body. This should ensure that it is given using an angle of injection between 72 and 90 degrees.	A quick injection is less painful. Inserting the needle at a 72- to 90-degree angle facilitates entry into muscle tissue (Nicoll & Hesby, 2002).
27. As soon as the needle is in place, use the thumb and forefinger of your nondominant hand to hold the lower end of the syringe. Slide your dominant hand to the end of the plunger. Inject the solution slowly (10 seconds per milliliter of medication).	Moving the syringe could cause damage to the tissues and inadvertent administration into an incorrect area. Rapid injection of the solution creates pressure in the tissues, resulting in discomfort. An outdated practice is the inclusion of aspiration (process of pulling back on the plunger of the syringe before injection to ensure the medication is not injected into a blood vessel) has been part of this procedure in the past. According to the CDC (2009), this procedure is not required.
28. Once the medication has been instilled, wait 10 seconds before withdrawing the needle.	Allows medication to begin to diffuse into the surrounding muscle tissue (Nicoll & Hesby, 2002).
29. Withdraw the needle smoothly and steadily at the same angle at which it was inserted, supporting tissue around the injection site with your nondominant hand.	Slow withdrawal of the needle pulls the tissues and causes discomfort. Applying counter traction around the injection site helps to prevent pulling on the tissue as the needle is withdrawn. Removing the needle at the same

ACTION	RATIONALE
	angle at which it was inserted minimizes tissue damage and discomfort for the patient.
30. **Apply gentle pressure at the site with a dry gauze.** Do not massage the site.	Light pressure causes less trauma and irritation to the tissues. Massaging can force medication into subcutaneous tissues.
31. Do not recap the used needle. Engage the safety shield or needle guard, if present. Discard the needle and syringe in the appropriate receptacle.	Proper disposal of the needle prevents injury.
32. Assist the patient to a position of comfort.	This provides for the well-being of the patient.
33. Remove gloves and additional PPE, if used. Perform hand hygiene.	Removing PPE properly reduces the risk for infection transmission and contamination of other items. Hand hygiene prevents the spread of microorganisms.
34. Document the administration of the medication immediately after administration (see Documentation section below).	Timely documentation helps to ensure patient safety.
35. Evaluate the patient's response to medication within an appropriate time frame. Assess site, if possible, within 2 to 4 hours after administration.	The patient needs to be evaluated for therapeutic and adverse effects from the medication. Visualization of the site allows for assessment of any untoward effects.

EVALUATION

- Patient receives the medication via the intramuscular route.
- Patient's anxiety is decreased.
- Patient does not experience adverse effects or injury.
- Patient understands and complies with the medication regimen.

DOCUMENTATION

- Record each medication given on the CMAR/MAR or record using the required format, including date, time, and the site of administration, immediately after administration. If using a bar-code system, medication administration is automatically recorded when scanned. PRN medications require documentation of the reason for administration.

Prompt recording avoids the possibility of accidentally repeating the administration of the drug. If the drug was refused or omitted, record this in the appropriate area on the medication record and notify the primary care provider. This verifies the reason medication was omitted and ensures that the primary care provider is aware of the patient's condition.

GENERAL CONSIDERATIONS

- Ongoing assessment is an important part of nursing care to evaluate patient response to administered medications and early detection of adverse effects. If an adverse effect is suspected, withhold further medication doses and notify the patient's primary healthcare provider. Additional intervention is based on the type of reaction and patient assessment.
- The vastus lateralis is the preferred site for infants.
- Muscle mass atrophies as a person ages. Take care to evaluate the patient's muscle mass and body composition. Use appropriate needle length and gauge for patient's body composition. Choose appropriate site based on the patient's body composition.

Skill · 90   **Administering a Subcutaneous Injection**

Subcutaneous injections are administered into the adipose tissue layer just below the epidermis and dermis. This tissue has few blood vessels, so drugs administered here have a slow, sustained rate of absorption into the capillaries.

It is important to choose the right equipment to ensure depositing the medication into the intended tissue layer and not the underlying muscle. Equipment used for a subcutaneous injection includes a syringe of appropriate volume for the amount of drug being administered. An insulin pen may be used for subcutaneous injection of insulin. A 25- to 30-gauge, ³⁄₈- to 1-inch needle can be used; ³⁄₈- and ⁵⁄₈-inch sized needles are most commonly used. Some medications are packaged in prefilled cartridges with a needle attached. Confirm that the provided needle is appropriate for the patient before use. If not, the medication will have to be transferred to another syringe and the appropriate needle attached.

Review the specifics of the particular medication before administrating it to the patient. Various sites may be used for subcutaneous injections, including the outer aspect of the upper arm, the abdomen (from below the costal margin to the iliac crests), the anterior aspects of the thigh, the upper back, and the upper ventral gluteal area. Absorption rates are different from the different sites. Injections in the abdomen are absorbed most rapidly, absorbed somewhat slower from the arms, even slower from the thighs, and slowest from the upper ventral gluteal areas (ADA, 2004; Caffrey, 2003).

Subcutaneous injections are administered at a 45- to 90-degree angle. Choose the angle of needle insertion based on the amount of subcutaneous tissue present and the length of the needle. Choose the needle length based on the amount of subcutaneous tissue present, based on the patient's body weight and build (Annersten & Willman, 2005). Generally, insert the shorter, ³/₈-inch needle at a 90-degree angle and the longer, ⁵/₈-inch needle at a 45-degree angle.

Recommendations differ regarding pinching or bunching of a skin fold for administration. Pinching is advised for thinner patients and when a longer needle is used, to lift the adipose tissue away from underlying muscle and tissue. If pinching is used, once the needle is inserted, release the skin to avoid injecting into compressed tissue (Rushing, 2004).

Aspiration, or pulling back on the plunger to check that a blood vessel has been entered, is not necessary and has not proved to be a reliable indicator of needle placement. The likelihood of injecting into a blood vessel is small (Rushing, 2004). The American Diabetes Association (2004) has stated that routine aspiration is not necessary when injecting insulin. Aspiration is definitely contraindicated with administration of heparin because this action can result in hematoma formation.

Usually, no more than 1 mL of solution is given subcutaneously. Giving larger amounts adds to the patient's discomfort and may predispose to poor absorption.

EQUIPMENT

- Prescribed medication
- Sterile syringe and needle. Needle size depends on the medication administered and patient body type (see previous discussion).
- Antimicrobial swab
- Disposable gloves
- Small gauze square
- Computer-generated Medication Administration Record (CMAR) or Medication Administration Record (MAR)
- PPE, as indicated

ASSESSMENT GUIDELINES

- Assess the patient for any allergies.
- Check expiration date before administering medication.
- Assess the appropriateness of the drug for the patient.
- Verify patient name, dose, route, and time of administration.
- Review assessment and laboratory data that may influence drug administration.
- Assess the site on the patient where the injection is to be given. Avoid sites that are bruised, tender, hard, swollen, inflamed, or scarred. These conditions could affect absorption or cause discomfort and injury (Hunter, 2008).
- Assess the patient's knowledge of the medication. If the patient has deficient knowledge about the medication, this may be the appropriate time to begin education about the medication.

- If the medication may affect the patient's vital signs, assess them before administration.
- If the medication is for pain relief, assess the patient's pain before and after administration.

NURSING DIAGNOSES
- Deficient Knowledge
- Risk for Allergy Response
- Risk for Infection
- Risk for Injury
- Anxiety

OUTCOME IDENTIFICATION AND PLANNING
Expected outcomes may include:
- Patient receives medication via the subcutaneous route.
- Patient's anxiety is decreased.
- Patient does not experience adverse effects.
- Patient understands and complies with the medication regimen.

IMPLEMENTATION

ACTION	RATIONALE
1. Gather equipment. Check each medication order against the original order in the medical record, according to facility policy. Clarify any inconsistencies. Check the patient's chart for allergies.	This comparison helps to identify errors that may have occurred when orders were transcribed. The primary care provider's order is the legal record of medication orders for each facility.
2. Know the actions, special nursing considerations, safe dose ranges, purpose of administration, and adverse effects of the medication to be administered. Consider the appropriateness of the medication for this patient.	This knowledge aids the nurse in evaluating the therapeutic effect of the medication in relation to the patient's disorder and can also be used to educate the patient about the medication.
3. Perform hand hygiene.	Hand hygiene prevents the spread of microorganisms.
4. Move the medication cart to the outside of the patient's	Organization facilitates error-free administration and saves time.

ACTION	RATIONALE
room or prepare for administration in the medication area.	
5. Unlock the medication cart or drawer. Enter pass code and scan employee identification, if required.	Locking the cart or drawer safeguards each patient's medication supply. Hospital accrediting organizations require medication carts to be locked when not in use. Entering pass code and scanning ID allows only authorized users into the system and identifies user for documentation by the computer.
6. **Prepare medications for one patient at a time.**	This prevents errors in medication administration.
7. Read the CMAR/MAR and select the proper medication from the patient's medication drawer or unit stock.	This is the *first* check of the label.
8. Compare the label with the CMAR/MAR. Check expiration dates and perform calculations, if necessary. Scan the bar code on the package, if required.	This is the *second* check of the label. Verify calculations with another nurse to ensure safety, if necessary.
9. If necessary, withdraw medication from an ampule or vial as described in Skill 105 and Skill 106.	
10. **When all medications for one patient have been prepared, recheck the label with the MAR before taking them to the patient.**	This is a *third* check to ensure accuracy and to prevent errors. Some facilities require the third check to occur at the bedside, after identifying the patient and before administration.
11. Lock the medication cart before leaving it.	Locking the cart or drawer safeguards the patient's medication supply. Hospital accrediting organizations require medication carts to be locked when not in use.
12. Transport medications to the patient's bedside carefully,	Careful handling and close observation prevent accidental or

ACTION	RATIONALE
and keep the medications in sight at all times.	deliberate disarrangement of medications.
13. **Ensure that the patient receives the medications at the correct time.**	Check agency policy, which may allow for administration within a period of 30 minutes before or 30 minutes after the designated time.
14. Perform hand hygiene and put on PPE, if indicated.	Hand hygiene and PPE prevent the spread of microorganisms. PPE is required based on transmission precautions.
15. Identify the patient. Usually, 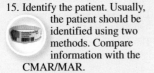 the patient should be identified using two methods. Compare information with the CMAR/MAR.	Identifying the patient ensures the right patient receives the medication and helps prevent errors.
a. Check the name and identification number on the patient's identification band.	This is the most reliable method. Replace the identification band if it is missing or inaccurate in any way.
b. Ask the patient to state his or her name and birth date, based on facility policy.	This requires a response from the patient, but illness and strange surroundings often cause patients to be confused.
c. If the patient cannot identify himself or herself, verify the patient's identification with a staff member who knows the patient for the second source.	This is another way to double-check identity. Do not use the name on the door or over the bed, because these may be inaccurate.
16. Close curtains around bed and close the door to the room, if possible.	This provides patient privacy.
17. Complete necessary assessments before administering medication. Check the patient's allergy bracelet or ask the patient about allergies. Explain the purpose and action of the medication to the patient.	Assessment is a prerequisite to administration of medications. Explanation provides rationale, increases knowledge, and reduces anxiety.

ACTION	RATIONALE
18. Scan the patient's bar code on the identification band, if required.	Scanning provides additional check to ensure that the medication is given to the right patient.
19. Put on clean gloves.	Gloves help prevent exposure to contaminants.
20. Select an appropriate administration site.	Appropriate site prevents injury and allows for accurate reading of the test site at the appropriate time.
21. Assist the patient to the appropriate position for the site chosen. Drape, as needed, to expose only area of site to be used.	Appropriate site prevents injury. Draping helps maintain the patient's privacy.
22. Identify the appropriate landmarks for the site chosen.	Good visualization is necessary to establish the correct site location and to avoid damage to tissues.
23. Cleanse the area around the injection site with an antimicrobial swab. Use a firm, circular motion while moving outward from the injection site. Allow area to dry.	Pathogens on the skin can be forced into the tissues by the needle. Moving from the center outward prevents contamination of the site. Allowing skin to dry prevents introducing alcohol into the tissue, which can be irritating and uncomfortable.
24. Remove the needle cap with the nondominant hand, pulling it straight off.	The cap protects the needle from contact with microorganisms. This technique lessens the risk of an accidental needlestick.
25. Grasp and bunch the area surrounding the injection site or spread the skin taut at the site.	Decision to create a skin fold is based on the nurse's assessment of the patient and needle length used. Pinching is advised for thinner patients and when a longer needle is used, to lift the adipose tissue away from underlying muscle and tissue. If pinching is used, once the needle is inserted, release the skin to avoid injecting into compressed tissue. If skin is pulled taut, it provides easy, less-painful entry into the subcutaneous tissue.

ACTION	RATIONALE
26. **Hold the syringe in the dominant hand between the thumb and forefinger. Inject the needle quickly at a 45- to 90-degree angle.**	Inserting the needle quickly causes less pain to the patient. Subcutaneous tissue is abundant in well-nourished, well-hydrated people and spare in emaciated, dehydrated, or very thin persons. For a person with little subcutaneous tissue, it is best to insert the needle at a 45-degree angle.
27. After the needle is in place, release the tissue. If you have a large skin fold pinched up, ensure that the needle stays in place as the skin is released. Immediately move your nondominant hand to steady the lower end of the syringe. Slide your dominant hand to the end of the plunger. Avoid moving the syringe.	Injecting the solution into compressed tissues results in pressure against nerve fibers and creates discomfort. If there is a large skin fold, the skin may retract away from the needle. The nondominant hand secures the syringe. Moving the syringe could cause damage to the tissues and inadvertent administration into an incorrect area.
28. Inject the medication slowly (at a rate of 10 sec/mL).	Rapid injection of the solution creates pressure in the tissues, resulting in discomfort.
29. Withdraw the needle quickly at the same angle at which it was inserted, while supporting the surrounding tissue with your nondominant hand.	Slow withdrawal of the needle pulls the tissues and causes discomfort. Applying counter traction around the injection site helps to prevent pulling on the tissue as the needle is withdrawn. Removing the needle at the same angle at which it was inserted minimizes tissue damage and discomfort for the patient.
30. Using a gauze square, apply gentle pressure to the site after the needle is withdrawn. Do not massage the site.	Massaging the site is not necessary and can damage underlying tissue and increase the absorption of the medication. Massaging after heparin administration can contribute to hematoma formation. Massaging after an insulin injection may contribute to unpredictable absorption of the medication.

ACTION	RATIONALE
31. Do not recap the used needle. Engage the safety shield or needle guard. Discard the needle and syringe in the appropriate receptacle.	Safety shield or needle guard prevents accidental needlestick. Proper disposal of the needle prevents injury.
32. Assist the patient to a position of comfort.	This provides for the well-being of the patient.
33. Remove gloves and additional PPE, if used. Perform hand hygiene.	Removing PPE properly reduces the risk for infection transmission and contamination of other items. Hand hygiene prevents the spread of microorganisms.
34. Document the administration of the medication immediately after administration. See Documentation section below.	Timely documentation helps to ensure patient safety.
35. Evaluate the response of the patient to the medication within an appropriate time frame for the particular medication.	The patient needs to be evaluated for therapeutic and adverse effects from the medication.

EVALUATION

- Patient receives the medication via the subcutaneous route.
- Patient's anxiety is decreased.
- Patient does not experience adverse effects.
- Patient understands and complies with the medication regimen.

DOCUMENTATION

- Record each medication given on the CMAR/MAR or record using the required format, including date, dose, time, and the site of administration, immediately after administration. If using a bar-code system, medication administration is automatically recorded when it is scanned. PRN medications require documentation of the reason for administration. Prompt recording avoids the possibility of accidentally repeating the administration of the drug. If the drug was refused or omitted, record this in the appropriate area on the medication record and notify the primary care provider. This verifies the reason medication was omitted and ensures that the primary care provider is aware of the patient's condition.

GENERAL CONSIDERATIONS

- Ongoing assessment is an important part of nursing care to evaluate patient response to administered medications and early detection of adverse effects. If an adverse effect is suspected, withhold further medication doses and notify the patient's primary healthcare provider. Additional intervention is based on type of reaction and patient assessment.
- Heparin is also administered subcutaneously. The abdomen is the most commonly used site. Avoid the area 2 inches around the umbilicus and the belt line. The manufacturer's (Sanofi Aventis, 2007) directions for subcutaneous administration of low–molecular-weight heparin preparations, such as enoxaparin (Lovenox), include specific instructions regarding administration site and technique. Administer enoxaparin in an area on the abdomen between the left or right anterolateral and left or right posterolateral abdominal wall. To administer the medication, pinch the tissue gently and insert the needle at a 90-degree angle. In addition, enoxaparin is packaged in a prefilled syringe with an air bubble. Do not expel the air bubble before administration.
- Many elderly patients have less adipose tissue. Adjust the angle of the needle and angle of insertion accordingly to avoid inadvertently intramuscular administration.

Skill · 91	**Administering Continuous Subcutaneous Infusion: Applying an Insulin Pump**

Some medications, such as insulin and morphine, may be administered continuously via the subcutaneous route. Continuous subcutaneous insulin infusion (CSII or insulin pump) allows for multiple preset rates of insulin delivery. This system uses a small computerized reservoir that delivers insulin via tubing through a needle inserted into the subcutaneous tissue. The pump is programmed to deliver multiple preset rates of insulin delivery. The settings can be adjusted for exercise and illness, and bolus dose delivery can be timed in relation to meals. Change sites every 2 to 3 days to prevent tissue damage or absorption problems (Olohan & Zappitelli, 2003). Advantages of continuous subcutaneous medication infusion include the longer rate of absorption via the subcutaneous route and convenience for the patient.

EQUIPMENT

- Insulin pump
- Pump syringe and vial of insulin or prefilled cartridge, as ordered
- Sterile infusion set
- Insertion (triggering) device
- Needle (24- or 22-gauge, or blunt-ended needle)

* Antimicrobial swabs
* Sterile nonocclusive dressing
* Computer-generated Medication Administration Record

(CMAR) or Medication Administration Record (MAR)
* Clean gloves
* Additional PPE, as indicated

ASSESSMENT GUIDELINES

* Assess the patient for any allergies. Check the expiration date before administering medication.
* Assess the appropriateness of the drug for the patient.
* Review assessment and laboratory data that may influence drug administration.
* Verify patient name, dose, route, and time of administration.
* Assess the infusion site. Typical infusion sites include those areas used for subcutaneous insulin injection.
* Assess the area where the pump is to be applied. Do not place the pump on skin that is irritated or broken down.
* Assess the patient's knowledge of the medication. If the patient has a knowledge deficit about the medication, this may be the appropriate time to begin education about it.
* Assess the patient's blood glucose level, as appropriate, or as ordered.

NURSING DIAGNOSES

* Deficient Knowledge
* Risk for Allergy Response
* Risk for Impaired Skin Integrity
* Acute Pain
* Risk for Infection

OUTCOME IDENTIFICATION AND PLANNING

Expected outcomes may include:
* Device is applied successfully and medication is administered.
* Patient understands the rationale for the pump use and mechanism of action.
* Patient experiences no allergy response.
* Patient's skin remains intact.
* Pump is applied using aseptic technique.
* Patient does not experience adverse effect.

IMPLEMENTATION

ACTION	RATIONALE
1. Gather equipment. Check each medication order against the original order in the medical record, according	This comparison helps to identify errors that may have occurred when orders were transcribed. The primary care

ACTION	RATIONALE
to facility policy. Clarify any inconsistencies. Check the patient's chart for allergies.	provider's order is the legal record of medication orders for each facility.
2. Know the actions, special nursing considerations, safe dose ranges, purpose of administration, and adverse effects of the medications to be administered. Consider the appropriateness of the medication for this patient.	This knowledge aids the nurse in evaluating the therapeutic effect of the medication in relation to the patient's disorder and can also be used to educate the patient about the medication.
3. Perform hand hygiene.	Hand hygiene prevents the spread of microorganisms.
4. Move the medication cart to the outside of the patient's room or prepare for administration in the medication area.	Organization facilitates error-free administration and saves time.
5. Unlock the medication cart or drawer. Enter pass code and scan employee identification, if required.	Locking the cart or drawer safeguards each patient's medication supply. Hospital accrediting organizations require medication carts to be locked when not in use. Entering pass code and scanning ID allows only authorized users into the system and identifies user for documentation by the computer.
6. **Prepare medications for one patient at a time.**	This prevents errors in medication administration.
7. Read the CMAR/MAR and select the proper medication from the patient's medication drawer or unit stock.	This is the *first* check of the label.
8. Compare the label with the CMAR/MAR. Check expiration dates and perform calculations, if necessary. Scan the bar code on the package, if required.	This is the *second* check of the label. Verify calculations with another nurse to ensure safety, if necessary.

ACTION	RATIONALE
9. Attach a blunt-ended needle or a small-gauge needle to a syringe. Follow Skill 106 to remove insulin from the vial. Remove enough insulin to last patient 2 to 3 days, plus 30 units for priming tubing. If using insulin cartridge, remove from packaging.	Patient will wear pump for up to 3 days without changing syringe or tubing.
10. **When all medications for one patient have been prepared, recheck the label with the MAR before taking them to the patient.**	This is a *third* check to ensure accuracy and to prevent errors. Some facilities require the third check to occur at the bedside, after identifying the patient and before administration.
11. Lock the medication cart before leaving it.	Locking the cart or drawer safeguards the patient's medication supply. Hospital accrediting organizations require medication carts to be locked when not in use.
12. Transport medications to the patient's bedside carefully, and keep the medications in sight at all times.	Careful handling and close observation prevent accidental or deliberate disarrangement of medications.
13. **Ensure that the patient receives the medications at the correct time.**	Check agency policy, which may allow for administration within a period of 30 minutes before or 30 minutes after designated time.
14. Perform hand hygiene and put on PPE, if indicated.	Hand hygiene and PPE prevent the spread of microorganisms. PPE is required based on transmission precautions.
15. Identify the patient. Usually, the patient should be identified using two methods. Compare information with the CMAR/MAR.	Identifying the patient ensures the right patient receives the medication and helps prevent errors.
a. Check the name and identification number on the patient's identification band.	This is the most reliable method. Replace the identification band if it is missing or inaccurate in any way.

ACTION	RATIONALE
b. Ask the patient to state his or her name and birth date, based on facility policy.	This requires a response from the patient, but illness and strange surroundings often cause patients to be confused.
c. If the patient cannot identify himself or herself, verify the patient's identification with a staff member who knows the patient.	This is another way to double-check identity. Do not use the name on the door or over the bed, because these may be inaccurate.
16. Close curtains around bed and close the door to the room, if possible.	This provides patient privacy.
17. Complete necessary assessments before administering medications. Check the patient's allergy bracelet or ask the patient about allergies. Explain the purpose and action of the medication to the patient.	Assessment is a prerequisite to administration of medications. Explanation provides rationale, increases knowledge, and reduces anxiety.
18. Scan the patient's bar code on the identification band, if required.	Provides an additional check to ensure that the medication is given to the right patient.
19. Perform hand hygiene. Put on clean gloves.	Hand hygiene prevents the spread of microorganisms.
20. Remove the cap from the syringe of insulin cartridge. Attach sterile tubing to syringe or insulin cartridge. Open the pump and place the syringe or cartridge in compartment according to manufacturer's directions. Close the pump.	
21. Initiate priming of tubing, according to manufacturer's directions. Program the pump according to manufacturer's recommendations following primary care provider's	Syringe must be placed in pump correctly for delivery of insulin.

ACTION	RATIONALE
orders. **Check for any bubbles in the tubing.**	
22. Activate the delivery device. Place the needle between prongs of the insertion device with the sharp edge facing out. Push insertion set down until a click is heard.	To ensure correct placement of the insulin pump needle, an insertion device must be used.
23. Select an appropriate administration site.	Appropriate site prevents injury.
24. Assist the patient to the appropriate position for the site chosen. Drape, as needed, to expose only area of site to be used.	Appropriate site prevents injury. Draping maintains privacy and warmth.
25. Identify the appropriate landmarks for the site chosen.	Good visualization is necessary to establish the correct location of the site and avoid damage to tissues.
26. Cleanse area around the injection site with an antimicrobial swab. Use a firm, circular motion while moving outward from the insertion site. Allow antiseptic to dry.	Pathogens on the skin can be forced into the tissues by the needle. Moving from the center outward prevents contamination of the site. Allowing skin to dry prevents introducing alcohol into the tissue, which can be irritating and uncomfortable.
27. Remove paper from adhesive backing. Remove the needle guard. Pinch skin at insertion site, press insertion device on site, and press release button to insert needle. Remove triggering device.	To ensure delivery of insulin into subcutaneous tissue, a skin fold is made with a pinch *before* insertion of the medication.
28. Apply sterile occlusive dressing over the insertion site, if not part of the insertion device. Attach the pump to the patient's clothing, as desired.	Dressing prevents contamination of site. Pump can be dislodged easily if not attached securely to patient.
29. Assist the patient to a position of comfort.	This provides for the well-being of the patient.

ACTION	RATIONALE
30. Discard the needle and syringe in the appropriate receptacle.	Proper disposal of the needle prevents injury.
31. Remove gloves and additional PPE, if used. Perform hand hygiene.	Removing PPE properly reduces the risk for infection transmission and contamination of other items. Hand hygiene prevents the spread of microorganisms.
32. Document the administration of the medication immediately after administration. See Documentation section below.	Timely documentation helps to ensure patient safety.
33. Evaluate patient's response to medication within appropriate time frame. Monitor the patient's blood glucose levels, as appropriate, or as ordered.	Patient needs to be evaluated to ensure that the pump is delivering the drug appropriately. The patient needs to be evaluated for therapeutic and adverse effects from the medication.

EVALUATION

- Patient receives insulin from the attached pump successfully without hypo- or hyperglycemic effects noted.
- Patient understands the rationale for the pump.
- Patient experiences no allergy response.
- Patient's skin remained intact.
- Patient remains infection free.
- Patient experiences no or minimal pain.

DOCUMENTATION

- Document the application of the pump, the type of insulin used, pump settings, insertion site, and any teaching done with the patient on the CMAR/MAR or record using the required format, including date, time, and the site of administration, immediately after administration. If using a bar-code system, medication administration is automatically recorded when it is scanned. Prompt recording avoids the possibility of accidentally repeating the administration of the drug. If the drug was refused or omitted, record this in the appropriate area on the medication record and notify the primary care provider. This verifies the reason medication was omitted and ensures that the primary care provider is aware of the patient's condition.

GENERAL CONSIDERATIONS

- Assess infusion site areas routinely for inflammation, allergic reactions, infection, and lipodystrophy.
- Good hygiene and frequent catheter site changes reduce risk of site complications. Change catheter site every 2 to 3 days.
- Contact dermatitis is sometimes a problem at the catheter site area. The primary care provider may order topical antibiotics, aloe, vitamin E, or corticosteroids to treat a contact dermatitis.
- Insulin self-administered by the patient through the insulin pump should be communicated to the nurse at the time of administration. This allows for accurate documentation of insulin requirements.
- Ongoing assessment is an important part of nursing care to evaluate patient response to administered medications and early detection of adverse effects. If an adverse effect is suspected, withhold further medication doses and notify the patient's primary healthcare provider. Additional intervention is based on type of reaction and patient assessment.

Skill · 92 | **Initiating a Peripheral Venous Access IV Infusion**

Administering and monitoring IV fluids is an essential part of routine patient care. The primary care provider often orders IV therapy to prevent or correct problems in fluid and electrolyte balance. For IV therapy to be administered, an IV must be inserted. The nurse must also verify the amount and type of solution to be administered, as well as the prescribed infusion rate. Follow the facility's policies and guidelines to determine if the infusion should be administered by electronic pump or by gravity.

EQUIPMENT

- IV solution, as prescribed
- Medication administration record (MAR) or computer-generated MAR (CMAR)
- Towel or disposable pad
- Nonallergenic tape
- IV administration set
- Label for infusion set (for next change date)
- Transparent site dressing
- Electronic infusion device (if appropriate)
- Tourniquet
- Time tape and/or label (for IV container)

- Cleansing swabs (chlorhexidine preferred)
- IV securement/stabilization device, as appropriate
- Clean gloves
- Additional PPE, as indicated
- IV pole
- Local anesthetic (if ordered)
- IV catheter (over the needle, Angiocath) or butterfly needle
- Short extension tubing
- End cap for extension tubing
- Alcohol wipes
- Skin protectant wipe (e.g., SkinPrep)
- Prefilled 2-mL syringe with sterile normal saline for injection

ASSESSMENT GUIDELINES

- Review the patient's record for baseline data, such as vital signs, intake and output balance, and pertinent laboratory values, such as serum electrolytes.
- Assess the appropriateness of the solution for the patient. Review assessment and laboratory data that may influence solution administration.
- Assess arms and hands for potential sites for initiating the IV.
- Determine the most desirable accessible vein. The cephalic vein, accessory cephalic vein, metacarpal, and basilic vein are appropriate sites for infusion (INS, 2006). The superficial veins on the dorsal aspect of the hand can also be used successfully for some people, but can be more painful (I.V. Rounds, 2008). Initiate venipuncture at least 2 inches (5 cm) above the crease of the wrist in an adult patient (Masoorli, 2007). Initiate venous access in the distal areas of the upper extremities, because this allows for future sites proximal to the previous insertion site (INS, 2006). Either arm may be used for IV therapy. If the patient is right-handed and both arms appear equally usable, select the left arm to free the right arm for the patient's use.
- Determine accessibility based on the patient's condition. For example, a person with severe burns on both forearms does not have vessels available in these areas, or a patient with a history of axillary node dissection should not have venipuncture in the affected arm.
- Do not use the antecubital veins if another vein is available. They are not a good choice for infusion because flexion of the patient's arm can displace the IV catheter over time. By avoiding the antecubital veins for peripheral venous catheters, a PICC line may be inserted at a later time, if needed.
- Do not use veins in the leg, unless other sites are inaccessible, because of the danger of stagnation of peripheral circulation and possible serious complications. The cannulation of the lower extremities is associated with risk of embolism and thrombophlebitis (INS, 2006). Some institutions require a physician's order to insert an IV catheter in an adult patient's lower extremity.

• Do not use veins in surgical areas. For example, infusions in the arm should not be given on the same side as recent extensive breast surgery, because of vascular disturbances in the area, or in an arm that has a device inserted for dialysis (e.g., fistula or shunt).

NURSING DIAGNOSES
• Deficient Fluid Volume
• Impaired Skin Integrity
• Risk for Injury
• Risk for Deficient Fluid Volume
• Risk for Infection

OUTCOME IDENTIFICATION AND PLANNING
Expected outcomes may include:
• Access device is inserted using sterile technique on the first attempt.
• Patient experiences minimal trauma and the IV solution infuses without difficulty.

IMPLEMENTATION

ACTION	RATIONALE
1. Verify the IV solution order on the MAR/CMAR with the medical order. Clarify any inconsistencies. Check the patient's chart for allergies. Check for color, leaking, and expiration date. Know techniques for IV insertion, precautions, purpose of the IV administration, and medications if ordered.	This ensures that the correct IV solution and rate of infusion, and/or medication will be administered. This knowledge and skill is essential for safe and accurate IV and medication administration.
2. Gather all equipment and bring to the bedside.	Having equipment available saves time and facilitates accomplishment of procedure.
3. Perform hand hygiene and put on PPE, if indicated.	Hand hygiene and PPE prevent the spread of microorganisms. PPE is required based on transmission precautions.

ACTION	RATIONALE
4. Identify the patient.	Identifying the patient ensures the right patient receives the intervention and helps prevent errors.
5. Close curtains around bed and close the door to the room, if possible. Explain what you are going to do and why you are going to do it to the patient. Ask the patient about allergies to medications, tape, or skin antiseptics, as appropriate. If considering using a local anesthetic, inquire about allergies for these substances as well.	This ensures the patient's privacy. Explanation relieves anxiety and facilitates cooperation. Possible allergies may exist related to medications, tape, or local anesthetic. Injectable anesthetic can result in allergic reactions and tissue damage.
6. If using a local anesthetic, explain the rationale and procedure to the patient. Apply the anesthetic to a few potential insertion sites. Allow sufficient time for the anesthetic to take effect.	Explanations provide reassurance and facilitate cooperation of the patient. Local anesthetic decreases the amount of pain felt at the insertion site. Some of the anesthetics take up to an hour to become effective.

Prepare the IV Solution and Administration Set

7. Compare the IV container label with the MAR/CMAR. Remove the outer wrapper from the IV bag, if indicated. Check expiration dates. Scan bar code on the container, if necessary. Compare on patient identification band with the MAR/CMAR. Alternately, label the solution container with the patient's name, solution type, additives, date, and time. Complete a time strip for the infusion and apply to the IV container.	Checking label with MAR/CMAR ensures correct IV solution will be administered. Identifying the patient ensures the right patient receives the medications and helps prevent errors. Time strip allows for quick visual reference by the nurse to monitor infusion accuracy.

ACTION	RATIONALE
8. Maintain aseptic technique when opening sterile packages and IV solution. Remove administration set from package. Apply label to tubing reflecting the day/date for next set change, per facility guidelines.	Asepsis is essential for preventing the spread of microorganisms. Labeling tubing ensures adherence to facility policy regarding administration set changes and reduces the risk of spread of microorganisms. In general, IV tubing is changed every 72 to 96 hours.
9. Close the roller clamp or slide clamp on the IV administration set. Invert the IV solution container and remove the cap on the entry site, taking care not to touch the exposed entry site. Remove the cap from the spike on the administration set. Using a twisting and pushing motion, insert the administration set spike into the entry site of the IV container. Alternately, follow the manufacturer's directions for insertion.	Clamping the IV tubing prevents air and fluid from entering the IV tubing at this time. Inverting the container allows easy access to the entry site. Touching the opened entry site on the IV container and/or the spike on the administration set results in contamination and the container/administration set would have to be discarded. Inserting the spike punctures the seal in the IV container and allows access to contents.
10. Hang the IV container on the IV pole. Squeeze the drip chamber and fill it at least halfway.	Suction causes fluid to move into the drip chamber. Fluid prevents air from moving down the tubing.
11. Open the IV tubing clamp, and allow fluid to move through tubing. Follow additional manufacturer's instructions for specific electronic infusion pump, as indicated. **Allow fluid to flow until all air bubbles have disappeared and the entire length of the tubing is primed (filled) with IV solution.** Close clamp. Alternately, some brands of tubing may require cap removal at the end of the IV tubing to	This technique prepares for IV fluid administration and removes air from the tubing. In large amounts, if air is not removed from the tubing, it can act as an embolus. Touching the open end of the tubing results in contamination and the administration set would have to be discarded.

ACTION	RATIONALE
allow fluid to flow. Maintain its sterility. After fluid has filled the tubing, recap end of tubing.	
12. If an electronic device is to be used, follow manufacturer's instructions for inserting tubing into the device.	This ensures proper use of equipment.

Initiate Peripheral Venous Access

ACTION	RATIONALE
13. Place patient in low Fowler's position in bed. Place protective towel or pad under the patient's arm.	The supine position permits either arm to be used and allows for good body alignment. Towel protects underlying surface from blood contamination.
14. Provide emotional support as needed.	Patient may experience anxiety because he or she may fear needlestick or IV infusion in general.
15. Open the short extension tubing package. Attach end cap, if not in place. Clean end cap with alcohol wipe. Insert syringe with normal saline into extension tubing. Fill extension tubing with normal saline and apply slide clamp. Remove the syringe and place extension tubing and syringe back on package, within easy reach.	Priming extension tubing removes air from tubing and prevents administration of air when connected to venous access. Having tubing within easy reach facilitates accomplishment of procedure.
16. Select and palpate for an appropriate vein. Refer to guidelines in previous Assessment section.	The use of an appropriate vein decreases discomfort for the patient and reduces the risk for damage to body tissues.
17. If the site is hairy and agency policy permits, clip a 2-inch area around the intended site of entry.	Hair can harbor microorganisms and inhibit adhesion of site dressing.
18. Put on gloves.	Gloves prevent contact with blood and body fluids.

ACTION	RATIONALE
19. Apply a tourniquet 3 to 4 inches above the venipuncture site to obstruct venous blood flow and distend the vein. Direct the ends of the tourniquet away from the site of entry. Make sure the radial pulse is still present.	Interrupting the blood flow to the heart causes the vein to distend. Distended veins are easy to see, palpate, and enter. The end of the tourniquet could contaminate the area of injection if directed toward the site of entry.
	Tourniquet may be applied too tightly so assessment for radial pulse is important.
	Checking radial pulse ensures arterial supply is not compromised.
20. Instruct the patient to hold the arm lower than the heart.	Lowering the arm below the heart level helps distend the veins by filling them.
21. Ask the patient to open and close the fist. Observe and palpate for a suitable vein. Try the following techniques if a vein cannot be felt:	Contracting the muscles of the forearm forces blood into the veins, thereby distending them further.
a. Massage the patient's arm from proximal to distal end and gently tap over intended vein.	Massaging and tapping the vein help distend veins by filling them with blood.
b. Remove tourniquet and place warm, moist compresses over intended vein for 10 to 15 minutes.	Warm, moist compresses help dilate veins.
22. **Cleanse site with an antiseptic solution such as chlorhexidine or according to facility policy. Press applicator against the skin and apply chlorhexidine using a back and forth friction scrub for at least 30 seconds. Do not wipe or blot. Allow to dry completely.**	Scrubbing motion and length of time (minimum 30 seconds) is necessary for chlorhexidine to be effective (ICT, 2005). Organisms on the skin can be introduced into the tissues or the bloodstream with the needle. Chlorhexidine is the preferred antiseptic solution, but iodine, povidone-iodine, and 70% alcohol are considered acceptable alternatives (INS, 2006).
23. Use the nondominant hand, placed about 1 or 2 inches below the entry site, to hold	Pressure on the vein and surrounding tissues helps prevent movement of the vein as the

ACTION	RATIONALE

the skin taut against the vein. **Avoid touching the prepared site.** Ask the patient to remain still while performing the venipuncture.

needle or catheter is being inserted. The needle entry site must remain untouched to prevent contamination from unsterile hands. Patient movement may prevent proper technique for IV insertion.

24. Enter the skin gently, holding the catheter by the hub in your dominant hand, bevel side up, at a 10- to 15-degree angle (FIGURE 1). Insert the catheter from directly over the vein or from the side of the vein. While following the course of the vein, advance the needle or catheter into the vein. A sensation of "give" can be felt when the needle enters the vein.

This allows needle or catheter to enter the vein with minimal trauma and deters passage of the needle through the vein.

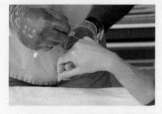

FIGURE 1 Stretching skin taut and inserting needle.

25. When blood returns through the lumen of the needle or the flashback chamber of the catheter, advance either device into the vein until the hub is at the venipuncture site. The exact technique depends on the type of device used.

The tourniquet causes increased venous pressure, resulting in automatic backflow. Placing the access device well into the vein helps to prevent dislodgement.

26. Release the tourniquet. Quickly remove the protective cap from the extension tubing and attach it to the

Bleeding is minimized and the patency of the vein is maintained if the connection is made smoothly between the catheter and tubing.

ACTION	RATIONALE
catheter or needle. Stabilize the catheter or needle with your nondominant hand.	
27. Continue to stabilize the catheter or needle and flush gently with the saline, observing the site for infiltration and leaking.	Infiltration and/or leaking and patient reports of pain and/or discomfort indicate that the insertion into the vein is not successful and should be discontinued.
28. Open the skin protectant wipe. Apply the skin protectant to the site, making sure to cover—at minimum—the area to be covered with the dressing. Place sterile transparent dressing or catheter securing/stabilization device over venipuncture site. Loop the tubing near the entry site, and anchor it with tape (nonallergenic) close to the site.	Skin protectant aids in adhesion of the dressing and decreases the risk for skin trauma when the dressing is removed. Transparent dressing allows easy visualization and protects the site. Stabilization/securing devices preserve the integrity of the access device and prevent catheter migration and loss of access (INS, 2006, p. S44). Some stabilization devices act as a site dressing also. The weight of the tubing is sufficient to pull it out of the vein if it is not well anchored. Nonallergenic tape is less likely to tear fragile skin.
29. Label the IV dressing with the date, time, site, and type and size of catheter or needle used for the infusion.	Other personnel working with the infusion will know what type of device is being used, the site, and when it was inserted. IV insertion sites are changed every 48 to 72 hours or according to agency policy (Lavery, 2005).
30. Using an antimicrobial swab, cleanse the access cap on the extension tubing. Remove the end cap from the administration set. Insert the end of the administration set into the end cap. Loop the administration set tubing near the entry site, and anchor it with tape (nonallergenic) close to the site. Remove gloves.	Inserting the administration set allows initiation of the fluid infusion. The weight of the tubing is sufficient to pull it out of the vein if it is not well anchored. Nonallergenic tape is less likely to tear fragile skin. Removing gloves properly reduces the risk for infection transmission and contamination of other items.

ACTION	RATIONALE
31. Open the clamp on the administration set. Set the flow rate and begin the fluid infusion. Alternately, start the flow of solution by releasing the clamp on the tubing and counting the drops. Adjust until the correct drop rate is achieved. Assess the flow of the solution and function of the infusion device. Inspect the insertion site for signs of infiltration.	Verifying the rate and device settings ensures the patient receives the correct volume of solution. If the catheter or needle slips out of the vein, the solution will accumulate (infiltrate) into the surrounding tissue.
32. Apply an IV securement/ stabilization device if not already in place as part of dressing, as indicated, based on facility policy. Explain to the patient the purpose of the device and the importance of safeguarding the site when using the extremity.	These systems are recommended for use on all venous access sites, and particularly central venous access sites, to preserve the integrity of the access device and to prevent catheter migration and loss of access (INS, 2006, p. S44). Some devices act as a site dressing also and may already have been applied.
33. Remove equipment and return the patient to a position of comfort. Lower the bed, if not in lowest position.	Promotes patient comfort and safety.
34. Remove additional PPE, if used. Perform hand hygiene.	Removing PPE properly reduces the risk for infection transmission and contamination of other items. Hand hygiene prevents transmission of microorganisms.
35. Return to check flow rate and observe IV site for infiltration 30 minutes after starting the infusion, and at least hourly thereafter. Ask the patient if he or she is experiencing any pain or discomfort related to the IV infusion.	Continued monitoring is important to maintain correct flow rate. Early detection of problems ensures prompt intervention.

EVALUATION

- IV access is initiated on the first attempt.
- Fluid flows easily into the vein without any sign of infiltration.
- Patient verbalizes minimal discomfort related to insertion and demonstrates understanding of the reasons for the IV.

DOCUMENTATION

- Document the location where the IV access was placed, as well as the size of the IV catheter or needle, the type of IV solution, and the rate of the IV infusion, as well as the use of a securing or stabilization device. Document the condition of the site, such as presence of redness, swelling, or drainage. Record the patient's reaction to the procedure and pertinent patient teaching, such as alerting the nurse if the patient experiences any pain from the IV or notices any swelling at the site. If necessary, document the IV fluid solution on the intake and output record.

GENERAL CONSIDERATIONS

- Make only two venipuncture attempts when initiating venous access for a patient. If unsuccessful after two attempts, a colleague with advanced skills, such as a member of the nurse IV team, should attempt to initiate the venous access (Arbique & Arbique, 2007).
- Avoid using vigorous friction and too much alcohol at the insertion site. Both can traumatize fragile skin and veins in the elderly.
- Catheter stabilization/securing devices should be used routinely with older adults to preserve the integrity of the access device and to prevent catheter migration and loss of access (INS, 2006; Smith & Hannum, 2008).

Skill · 93   **Capping for Intermittent Use and Flushing a Peripheral Venous Access Device**

When the continuous infusion of IV solution is no longer necessary, it is often converted to an access point for intermittent or emergency use. A capped line consists of the IV catheter connected to a short length of extension tubing sealed with a cap. There are different ways to accomplish this. Refer to facility policy for the procedure to convert to an access for intermittent use. Intermittent peripheral venous access devices are flushed at periodic intervals with normal saline to keep the IV catheter patent and to prevent clots from forming in the catheter. Flushing with normal saline solution is generally done at least every 12 hours and before and after administering an IV medication. Refer to facility policy for specific guidelines.

The following skill describes converting a primary line when extension tubing is present; the accompanying skill variation describes converting a primary line when the administration set is connected directly to the hub of the IV catheter, without extension tubing.

EQUIPMENT
- End cap device
- Clean gloves
- Additional PPE, as indicated
- 4 × 4 gauze pad

- Normal saline flush prepared in a syringe (1–3 mL), according to facility policy
- Antimicrobial wipe
- Tape

ASSESSMENT GUIDELINES
- Assess insertion site for signs of any IV complications.
- Verify the medical order for discontinuation of IV fluid infusion.

NURSING DIAGNOSES
- Risk for Infection
- Risk for Injury

OUTCOME IDENTIFICATION AND PLANNING
Expected outcomes may include:
- Patient will remain free of injury and any signs and symptoms of IV complications.
- Capped venous access device will remain patent.

IMPLEMENTATION

ACTION	RATIONALE
1. Determine the need for conversion to an intermittent access. Verify medical order. Check facility policy. Gather all equipment and bring to bedside.	Ensures correct intervention for correct patient. Having equipment available saves time and facilitates accomplishment of procedure.
2. Perform hand hygiene and put on PPE, if indicated.	Hand hygiene and PPE prevent the spread of microorganisms. PPE is required based on transmission precautions.
3. Identify the patient.	Identifying the patient ensures the right patient receives the intervention and helps prevent errors.

ACTION	RATIONALE
4. Close curtains around bed and close the door to the room, if possible. Explain what you are going to do and why you are going to do it to the patient. Ask the patient about allergies to tape and skin antiseptics.	This ensures the patient's privacy. Explanation relieves anxiety and facilitates cooperation. Possible allergies may exist related to tape or antiseptics.
5. Assess the IV site. Refer to Skill 95.	Complications, such as infiltration, phlebitis, or infection, necessitate discontinuation of the IV infusion at that site.
6. If using an electronic infusion device, stop the device. Close the roller clamp on the administration set. If using gravity infusion, close the roller clamp on the administration set.	The action of the infusion device needs to be stopped and clamps closed to prevent fluid leaking when the tubing is disconnected.
7. Put on gloves. Close the clamp on the short extension tubing connected to the IV catheter in the patient's arm.	Clamping the tubing on the extension set prevents introduction of air into the extension tubing.
8. Remove the administration set tubing from the extension set. Cleanse the end cap with an antimicrobial swab.	Removing the infusion tubing discontinues the infusion. Cleaning the cap reduces the risk for contamination.
9. Insert the saline flush syringe into the cap on the extension tubing. Pull back on the syringe to aspirate the catheter for positive blood return. If positive, instill the solution over 1 minute or flush the line according to facility policy. Remove the syringe and reclamp the extension tubing.	Positive blood return confirms patency before administration of medications and solutions (INS, 2006). Flushing maintains patency of the IV line. Action of positive pressure end cap is maintained with removal of the syringe before the clamp is engaged. Clamping prevents air from entering the extension set.
10. If necessary, loop the extension tubing near the entry site, and anchor it with tape (nonallergenic) close to site.	The weight of the tubing is sufficient to pull it out of the vein if it is not well anchored. Nonallergenic tape is less likely to tear fragile skin.

ACTION	RATIONALE
11. Remove equipment. Ensure patient's comfort. Remove gloves. Lower bed, if not in lowest position.	Promotes patient comfort and safety. Removing gloves properly reduces the risk for infection transmission and contamination of other items.
12. Remove additional PPE, if used. Perform hand hygiene.	Removing PPE properly reduces the risk for infection transmission and contamination of other items. Hand hygiene prevents transmission of microorganisms.

EVALUATION

• Peripheral venous access device flushes without resistance.
• Patient exhibits an access site that is intact, and free of the signs and symptoms of infection, phlebitis, or infiltration.
• Site dressing is clean, dry, and intact.

DOCUMENTATION

• Document discontinuation of IV fluid infusion. Record the condition of the venous access site. Document the flushing of the venous access device. This is often done in the MAR. Record the patient's reaction to the procedure and any patient teaching that occurred.

GENERAL CONSIDERATIONS

• Some facilities may use end caps for venous access device that are not positive pressure devices. In this case, flush with the recommended volume of saline, ending with 0.5 mL of solution remaining in the syringe. While maintaining pressure on the syringe, clamp the extension tubing. This provides positive pressure, preventing backflow of blood into the catheter, decreasing risk for occlusion.

Skill Variation **Capping a Primary Line When No Extension Tube is in Place**

It is good practice to add a short extension tubing to decrease the risk of contact with blood, and for infection-control purposes if one was not placed during initiation of the peripheral venous access. After checking the medical order to convert the peripheral venous access, bring the end cap and the extension tubing to the

(continued on page 507)

**Capping a Primary Line When No
Extension Tube is in Place** *continued*

bedside, as well as other
required equipment.

1. Gather equipment and verify medical order.

2. Perform hand hygiene.

3. Put on PPE, as indicated.

4. Identify the patient.

5. Explain the procedure to the patient.

6. Fill the cap and extension tubing with normal saline.

7. Assess the IV site.

8. Put on gloves.

9. Place gauze 4 × 4 sponge underneath the IV connection hub, between the IV catheter and the tubing.

10. **Stabilize the hub of the IV catheter with nondominant**

hand. Use dominant hand to twist and disconnect IV tubing quickly from the catheter. Discard it. Attach the extension tubing to the IV catheter hub using aseptic technique.

11. Cleanse the cap with an antimicrobial solution.

12. Insert the syringe into the cap and gently flush with saline per facility policy. Remove the syringe. Engage the slide clamp on extension tubing.

13. Remove gloves.

14. Loop the extension tubing near the entry site, and anchor it with tape (nonallergenic) close to the site.

15. Ensure that the patient is comfortable. Perform hand hygiene.

16. Chart on IV administration record or MAR/CMAR, per institutional policy.

Skill · 94 | **Changing an IV Solution Container and Administration Set**

Intravenous fluid administration frequently involves multiple bags or bottles of fluid infusion. Verify the amount and type of solution to be administered, as well as the prescribed infusion rate. Follow the facility's policies and guidelines to determine if the infusion should be administered by electronic pump or by gravity. Focus on the following points:

• If more than one IV solution or medication is ordered, check facility policy and appropriate literature to make sure that the additional IV solution can be attached to the existing tubing.

- As one bag is infusing, prepare the next bag so it is ready for a change when less than 50 mL of fluid remains in the original container.
- Ongoing assessments related to the desired outcomes of the IV therapy, as well as assessing for both local and systemic IV infusion complications, are required.
- Before switching the IV solution containers, check the date and time of the infusion administration set to ensure it does not also need to be replaced. Check facility policy for guidelines for changing IV administration sets. For simple IV solutions, every 72 to 96 hours is recommended.

EQUIPMENT

For solution container change:
- IV solution, as prescribed
- Medication administration record (MAR) or computer-generated MAR (CMAR)
- Time tape and/or label (for IV container)
- PPE, as indicated

For tubing change:
- Administration set
- Label for administration set (for next change date)
- Sterile gauze
- Nonallergenic tape
- IV securement/stabilization device, as appropriate
- Clean gloves
- Additional PPE, as indicated
- Alcohol wipes

ASSESSMENT GUIDELINES

- Review the patient's record for baseline data, such as vital signs, intake and output balance, and pertinent laboratory values, such as serum electrolytes.
- Assess the appropriateness of the solution for the patient.
- Review assessment and laboratory data that may influence solution administration.
- Inspect the IV site. The dressing should be intact, adhering to the skin on all edges. Check to see if there are any leaks or fluid under or around the dressing.
- Inspect the tissue around the IV entry site for swelling, coolness, or pallor. These are signs of fluid infiltration into the tissue around the IV catheter. Also inspect the site for redness, swelling, and warmth. These signs might indicate the development of phlebitis or an inflammation of the blood vessel at the site.
- Ask the patient if he or she is experiencing any pain or discomfort related to the IV line. Pain or discomfort is sometimes associated with both infiltration and phlebitis.

NURSING DIAGNOSES

- Deficient Fluid Volume
- Impaired Skin Integrity
- Risk for Infection
- Risk for Deficient Fluid Volume

OUTCOME IDENTIFICATION AND PLANNING

Expected outcomes may include:
- Prescribed IV infusion continues without interruption and no infusion complications are identified.

IMPLEMENTATION

ACTION	RATIONALE
1. Verify IV solution order on MAR/CMAR with the medical order. Clarify any inconsistencies. Check the patient's chart for allergies. Check for color, leaking, and expiration date. Know the purpose of the IV administration and medications if ordered.	This ensures that the correct IV solution and rate of infusion, and/or medication will be administered. This knowledge and skill is essential for safe and accurate IV and medication administration.
2. Gather all equipment and bring to bedside.	Having equipment available saves time and facilitates accomplishment of procedure.
3. Perform hand hygiene and put on PPE, if indicated.	Hand hygiene and PPE prevent the spread of microorganisms. PPE is required based on transmission precautions.
4. Identify the patient.	Identifying the patient ensures the right patient receives the intervention and helps prevent errors.
5. Close curtains around bed and close the door to the room, if possible. Explain what you are going to do and why you are going to do it to the patient. Ask the patient about allergies to medications or tape, as appropriate.	This ensures the patient's privacy. Explanation relieves anxiety and facilitates cooperation. Possible allergies may exist related to IV solution additive or tape.
6. Compare IV container label with the MAR/CMAR. Remove IV bag from outer wrapper, if indicated. Check expiration dates. Scan bar	Checking the label with the MAR/CMAR ensures the correct IV solution will be administered. Identifying the patient ensures the right patient receives the

ACTION	RATIONALE
code on container, if necessary. Compare patient identification band with the MAR/CMAR. Alternately, label solution container with the patient's name, solution type, additives, date, and time. Complete a time strip for the infusion and apply it to the IV container.	medications and helps prevent errors. Time strip allows for quick visual reference by the nurse to monitor infusion accuracy.
7. Maintain aseptic technique when opening sterile packages and IV solution. Remove administration set from package. Apply label to tubing reflecting the day/date for next set change, per facility guidelines.	Asepsis is essential for preventing the spread of microorganisms. Labeling tubing ensures adherence to facility policy regarding administration set changes and reduces the risk of spread of microorganisms. In general, IV tubing is changed every 72 to 96 hours.

To Change IV Solution Container

ACTION	RATIONALE
8. If using an electronic infusion device, pause the device or put on "hold." Close the slide clamp on the administration set closest to the drip chamber. If using gravity infusion, close the roller clamp on the administration set.	The action of the infusion device needs to be paused while the solution container is changed. Closing the clamps prevents the fluid in the drip chamber from emptying and air from entering the tubing during the procedure.
9. Carefully remove the cap on the entry site of the new IV solution container and expose entry site, taking care not to touch the exposed entry site.	Touching the opened entry site on the IV container results in contamination and the container would have to be discarded.
10. Lift the empty container off the IV pole and invert it. Quickly remove the spike from the old IV container, being careful not to contaminate it. Discard the old IV container.	Touching the spike on the administration set results in contamination and the tubing would have to be discarded.

ACTION	RATIONALE
11. Using a twisting and pushing motion, insert the administration set spike into the entry site of the IV container. Alternately, follow the manufacturer's directions for insertion. Hang the container on the IV pole.	Inserting the spike punctures the seal in the IV container and allows access to the contents.
12. Alternately, hang the new IV fluid container on an open hook on the IV pole. Carefully remove the cap on the entry site of the new IV solution container and expose the entry site, taking care not to touch the exposed entry site. Lift the empty container off the IV pole and invert it. Quickly remove the spike from the old IV container, being careful not to contaminate it. Discard the old IV container. Using a twisting and pushing motion, insert the administration set spike into the entry port of the new IV container as it hangs on the IV pole.	Touching the opened entry site on the IV container or the administration set spike results in contamination and both would have to be discarded. Inserting the spike punctures the seal in the IV container and allows access to the contents.
13. If using an electronic infusion device, open the slide clamp, check the drip chamber of the administration set, verify the flow rate programmed in the infusion device, and turn the device to "run" or "infuse."	Verifying the rate and device settings ensures the patient receives the correct volume of solution.
14. If using gravity infusion, slowly open the roller clamp on the administration set and count the drops. Adjust until the correct drop rate is achieved.	Opening the clamp regulates the flow rate into the drip chamber. Verifying the rate ensures the patient receives the correct volume of solution.

ACTION	RATIONALE

To Change IV Solution Container and Administration Set

15. Prepare the IV solution and administration set. Refer to Skill 92, Steps 7–11.

16. Hang the IV container on an open hook on the IV pole. Close the clamp on the existing IV administration set. Also, close the clamp on the short extension tubing connected to the IV catheter in the patient's arm.

Clamping the existing IV tubing prevents leakage of fluid from the administration set after it is disconnected. Clamping the tubing on the extension set prevents introduction of air into the extension tubing.

17. If using an electronic infusion device, remove the current administration set from the device. Following manufacturer's directions, insert new administration set into the infusion device.

Administration set has to be removed in order to insert new tubing into device.

18. Put on gloves. Remove the current infusion tubing from the access cap on the short extension IV tubing. Using an antimicrobial swab, cleanse access cap on the extension tubing. Remove the end cap from the new administration set. Insert the end of the administration set into the access cap. Loop the administration set tubing near the entry site, and anchor it with tape (nonallergenic) close to the site.

Cleansing the cap or port reduces the risk of contamination. Inserting the administration set allows initiation of the fluid infusion. The weight of the tubing is sufficient to pull it out of the vein if it is not well anchored. Nonallergenic tape is less likely to tear fragile skin.

19. Open the clamp on the extension tubing. Open the clamp on the administration set.

Opening clamps allows the solution to flow to the patient.

20. If using an electronic infusion device, open the slide clamp, check the drip chamber of the administration set,

Verifying the rate and device settings ensures the patient receives the correct volume of solution.

ACTION	RATIONALE

verify the flow rate pro-
grammed in the infusion
device, and turn the device to
"run" or "infuse."

21. If using gravity infusion,
slowly open the roller clamp
on the administration set and
count the drops. Adjust until
the correct drop rate is
achieved.

Opening the clamp regulates the
flow rate into the drip chamber.
Verifying the rate and ensures the
patient receives the correct volume of solution.

22. Remove equipment. Ensure
patient's comfort. Remove
gloves. Lower bed, if not in
lowest position.

Promotes patient comfort and
safety. Removing gloves properly reduces the risk for infection
transmission and contamination
of other items.

23. Remove additional PPE, if
used. Perform hand
hygiene.

Removing PPE properly reduces
the risk for infection transmission and contamination of other
items. Hand hygiene prevents
transmission of microorganisms.

24. Return to check flow rate and
observe IV site for infiltration 30 minutes after starting
infusion, and at least hourly
thereafter. Ask the patient if
he or she is experiencing any
pain or discomfort related to
the IV infusion.

Continued monitoring is important to maintain correct flow rate.
Early detection of problems
ensures prompt intervention.

EVALUATION
• IV infusion continues without interruption.
• No infusion complications are identified.

DOCUMENTATION
• Document the type of IV solution and the rate of infusion; such as
presence of redness, swelling, or drainage. Record the patient's reaction to the procedure and pertinent patient teaching, such as alerting
the nurse if the patient experiences any pain from the IV or notices
any swelling at the site. If necessary, document the IV fluid solution
on the intake and output record.

Skill • 95 **Monitoring an IV Site and Infusion**

The nurse is responsible for monitoring the infusion rate and the IV site. This is routinely done as part of the initial patient assessment and at the beginning of a work shift. In addition, IV sites are checked at specific intervals and each time an IV medication is given, as dictated by the institution's policies. It is common to check IV sites every hour, but it is important to be familiar with the requirements of your institution. Monitoring the infusion rate is a very important part of the patient's overall management. If the patient does not receive the prescribed rate, he or she may experience a fluid volume deficit. In contrast, if the patient is administered too much fluid over a period of time, he or she may exhibit signs of fluid volume overload. Other responsibilities involve checking the IV site for possible complications and assessing for both the desired effects of an IV infusion as well as potential adverse reactions to IV therapy.

EQUIPMENT
• PPE, as indicated

ASSESSMENT GUIDELINES
• Inspect the IV infusion solution for any particulates and the IV label. Confirm it is the solution ordered.
• Assess the current flow rate by timing the drops if it is a gravity infusion or verifying the settings on the electronic infusion device.
• Check the tubing for kinks or anything that might clamp or interfere with the flow of solution.
• Inspect the IV site. The dressing should be intact, adhering to the skin on all edges.
• Assess fluid intake and output.
• Assess for complications associated with IV infusions.
• Assess the patient's knowledge of IV therapy.

NURSING DIAGNOSES
• Excess Fluid Volume
• Risk for Infection
• Deficient Fluid Volume
• Risk for Deficient Fluid Volume
• Risk for Injury

OUTCOME IDENTIFICATION AND PLANNING
Expected outcomes may include:
• Patient remains free from complications and demonstrates signs and symptoms of fluid balance.

IMPLEMENTATION

ACTION	RATIONALE
1. Verify IV solution order on MAR/CMAR with the medical order. Clarify any inconsistencies. Check the patient's chart for allergies. Check for color, leaking, and expiration date. Know the purpose of the IV administration and medications if ordered.	This ensures that the correct IV solution and rate of infusion, and/or medication will be administered. This knowledge and skill is essential for safe and accurate IV and medication administration.
2. **Monitor IV infusion every hour or per agency policy. More frequent checks may be necessary if medication is being infused.**	Promotes safe administration of IV fluids and medication.
3. Perform hand hygiene and put on PPE, if indicated.	Hand hygiene and PPE prevent the spread of microorganisms. PPE is required based on transmission precautions.
4. Identify the patient.	Identifying the patient ensures the right patient receives the intervention and helps prevent errors.
5. Close curtains around bed and close the door to the room, if possible. Explain what you are going to do to the patient.	This ensures the patient's privacy. Explanation relieves anxiety and facilitates cooperation.
6. If an electronic infusion device is being used, check settings, alarm, and indicator lights. Check set infusion rate. Note position of fluid in IV container in relation to time tape. Teach the patient about the alarm features on the electronic infusion device.	Observation ensures that the infusion control device is functioning and that the alarm is functioning. Lack of knowledge about "alarms" may create anxiety for the patient.
7. If IV is infusing via gravity, check the drip chamber and time the drops.	This ensures that the flow rate is correct.

ACTION	RATIONALE
	Use a watch with a second hand for counting the drops in regulating a gravity drip IV infusion.
8. Check tubing for anything that might interfere with the flow. Be sure clamps are in the open position.	Any kink or pressure on the tubing may interfere with flow.
9. Observe dressing for leakage of IV solution.	Leakage may occur at the connection of the tubing with the hub of the needle or catheter and allow for loss of IV solution.
10. Inspect the site for swelling, leakage at the site, coolness, or pallor, which may indicate infiltration. Ask patient if he or she is experiencing any pain or discomfort. If any of these symptoms are present, the IV will need to be removed and restarted at another site. Check facility policy for treating infiltration.	Catheter may become dislodged from the vein, and IV solution may flow into subcutaneous tissue.
11. Inspect the site for redness, swelling, and heat. Palpate for induration. Ask patient if he or she is experiencing pain. These findings may indicate phlebitis. Notify primary care provider if phlebitis is suspected. IV will need to be discontinued and restarted at another site. Check facility policy for treatment of phlebitis.	Chemical irritation or mechanical trauma causes injury to the vein and can lead to phlebitis. Phlebitis is the most common complication related to IV therapy (Lavery & Ingram, 2005).
12. Check for local manifestations (redness, pus, warmth, induration, and pain) that may indicate an infection is present at the site, or systemic manifestations (chills, fever, tachycardia, hypotension) that may accompany local	Poor aseptic technique may allow bacteria to enter the needle or catheter insertion site or tubing connection and may occur with manipulation of equipment.

ACTION	RATIONALE
infection at the site. If signs of infection are present, discontinue the IV and notify the primary care provider. Be careful not to disconnect IV tubing when putting on patient's hospital gown or assisting the patient with movement.	
13. Be alert for additional complications of IV therapy.	Infusing too much IV solution results in an increased volume of circulating fluid volume.
a. **Fluid overload can result in signs of cardiac and/or respiratory failure. Monitor intake and output and vital signs. Assess for edema and auscultate lung sounds. Ask patient if he or she is experiencing any shortness of breath.**	Elderly patients are most at risk for this complication due to possible decrease in cardiac and/or renal functions.
b. Check for bleeding at the site.	Bleeding may be caused by anticoagulant medication. Bleeding at the site is most likely to occur when the IV is discontinued.
14. If possible, instruct the patient to call for assistance if any discomfort is noted at site, solution container is nearly empty, flow has changed in any way, or if the electronic pump alarm sounds.	This facilitates cooperation of patient and safe administration of IV solution.
15. Ensure patient's comfort. Remove gloves. Lower bed, if not in lowest position.	Promotes patient comfort and safety. Removing gloves properly reduces the risk for infection transmission and contamination of other items.
16. Remove PPE, if used. Perform hand hygiene.	Removing PPE properly reduces the risk for infection transmission and contamination of other items. Hand hygiene prevents transmission of microorganisms.

EVALUATION
- Patient remains free of injury (specifically, complications related to IV therapy).
- Patient exhibits patent IV site.
- IV solution infuses at the prescribed flow rate.

DOCUMENTATION
- Document the type of IV solution as well as the infusion rate. Note the insertion site location and site assessment. Document the patient's reaction to the IV therapy as well as absence of subjective reports that he or she is not experiencing any pain or other discomfort, such as coolness or heat associated with the infusion. Record that the patient is not demonstrating any other IV complications, such as signs or symptoms of fluid overload. Record on the intake and output documents, as needed.

Skill · 96   Leg Exercises

During surgery, venous blood return from the legs slows; in addition some surgical positions decrease venous return. Thrombophlebitis and resultant emboli are potential complications from this circulatory stasis in the legs. Leg exercises increase venous return through flexion and contraction of the quadriceps and gastrocnemius muscles. Leg exercises must be individualized to patient needs, physical condition, primary care provider preference, and facility protocol.

EQUIPMENT
- PPE, as indicated

ASSESSMENT GUIDELINES
- Identify patients who are considered at greater risk, such as the patients with chronic disease; patients who are obese or have underlying cardiovascular disease; patients who have decreased mobility; and patients who are at risk for decreased compliance with postoperative activities, such as those with alterations in cognitive function. Depending on the particular at-risk patient, specific assessments and interventions may be warranted.
- Assess the patient's current level of knowledge regarding leg exercises.

IMPLEMENTATION

ACTION	RATIONALE
1. Check the patient's chart for the type of surgery and review the medical orders.	This check ensures that the care will be provided for the right patient and any specific teaching based on the type of surgery will be addressed.
2. Gather the necessary supplies and bring to the bedside stand or overbed table.	Preparation promotes efficient time management and organized approach to the task. Bringing everything to the bedside conserves time and energy. Arranging items nearby is convenient, saves time, and avoids unnecessary stretching and twisting of muscles on the part of the nurse.
3. Perform hand hygiene and put on PPE, if indicated.	Hand hygiene and PPE prevent the spread of microorganisms. PPE is required based on transmission precautions.
4. Identify the patient.	Identifying the patient ensures the right patient receives the intervention and helps prevent errors.
5. Close curtains around bed and close door to room, if possible. Explain what you are going to do and why you are going to do it to the patient.	This ensures the patient's privacy. Explanation relieves anxiety and facilitates cooperation.
6. Identify the patient's learning needs. Identify the patient's level of knowledge regarding leg exercises. If the patient has had surgery before, ask about this experience.	Identification of baseline knowledge contributes to individualized teaching. Previous surgical experience may impact preoperative/postoperative care positively or negatively, depending on this past experience.
7. Explain the rationale for performing leg exercises.	Explanation facilitates patient cooperation. An understanding of rationale may contribute to increased compliance.

ACTION	RATIONALE
8. Provide teaching regarding leg exercises.	Leg exercises assist in preventing muscle weakness, promote venous return, and decrease complications related to venous stasis.
a. Assist or ask the patient to sit up (semi-Fowler's position), and explain to the patient that you will first demonstrate, and then coach him/her to exercise one leg at a time.	
b. Straighten the patient's knee, raise the foot, extend the lower leg, and hold this position for a few seconds. Lower the entire leg. Practice this exercise with the other leg.	
c. Assist or ask the patient to point the toes of both legs toward the foot of the bed, then relax them. Next, flex or pull the toes toward the chin.	
d. Assist or ask the patient to keep legs extended and to make circles with both ankles, first circling to the left and then to the right. Instruct the patient to repeat these exercises three times.	
9. Validate the patient's understanding of information. Ask the patient to give a return demonstration. Ask the patient if he or she has any questions. Encourage the patient to practice the activities and ask questions, if necessary.	Validation facilitates the patient's understanding of information and performance of activities.
10. Remove PPE, if used. Perform hand hygiene.	Removing PPE properly reduces the risk for infection transmission and contamination of other items. Hand hygiene prevents the spread of microorganisms.

EVALUATION

• Patient and/or significant other verbalizes an understanding of the instructions related to leg exercises and is able to demonstrate the activities.

DOCUMENTATION

• Document the components of teaching related to leg exercises that were reviewed with the patient and family, if present. Record the patient's ability to demonstrate the leg exercises, coughing, and splinting and response to the teaching, and note if any follow-up instruction needs to be performed.

GENERAL CONSIDERATIONS

• Cardiovascular disorders, such as thrombocytopenia, hemophilia, myocardial infarction or cardiac surgery, and dysrhythmias increase the risk for venous stasis and thrombophlebitis
• Certain types of surgeries are associated with higher risk of deep vein thrombosis and pulmonary embolism, including major orthopedic surgery, major cardiothoracic, vascular, and neurosurgery (Joanna Briggs, 2008a).

Skill · 97   Logrolling a Patient

The "logrolling" technique is a maneuver that involves moving the patient's body as one unit so that the spine is kept in alignment, without twisting or bending. This technique is commonly used to reposition patients who have had spinal or back surgery or who have suffered back or neck injuries. If the patient is being logrolled due to a neck injury, do not use a fluffy pillow under the patient's head. However, the patient may need a cervical collar in place for the move; a bath blanket or small pillow under the head may be used to keep the spinal column straight. The patient's neck should remain straight during the procedure and after positioning. The use of logrolling when repositioning the patient helps to maintain the alignment of the neck and spine. Three caregivers, or more as appropriate, are needed to accomplish this safely. Do not try to logroll the patient without sufficient help. Do not twist the patient's head, spine, shoulders, knees, or hips while logrolling.

EQUIPMENT

• At least two additional persons to help
• Friction-reducing sheet to facilitate smooth movement, if not already in place; a drawsheet may be substituted if not available
• Small pillow for placement between the legs

• Wedge pillow or two pillows
  for behind the patient's back

• PPE, as indicated

ASSESSMENT GUIDELINES

• Assess for conditions that would contraindicate logrolling, such as
  unstable neurologic status, severe pain, or the presence of drains.
• Assess the patient's baseline neurologic status.
• Assess for paresthesia and pain.
• Assess for the need to use a cervical collar.
• If the patient is complaining of pain, consider medicating the patient
  before repositioning.

NURSING DIAGNOSES

• Risk for Injury
• Acute Pain
• Impaired Physical Mobility
• Impaired Tissue Integrity
• Risk for Impaired Skin Integrity
• Impaired Skin Integrity

OUTCOME IDENTIFICATION AND PLANNING

Expected outcomes may include:
• Patient's spine remains in proper alignment, thereby reducing the risk
  for injury.
• Patient verbalizes relief of pain.
• Patient maintains joint mobility.
• Patient remains free of alterations in skin and tissue integrity.

IMPLEMENTATION

ACTION	RATIONALE
1. Review the medical record and nursing plan of care for activity orders and conditions that may influence the patient's ability to move or to be positioned. Assess for tubes, IV lines, incisions, or equipment that may alter the positioning procedure. Identify any movement limitations.	Reviewing the medical record and care plan validates the correct patient and correct procedure. Checking for equipment and limitations reduces the risk for injury during the transfer.
2. Perform hand hygiene and put on PPE, if indicated.	Hand hygiene and PPE prevent the spread of microorganisms. PPE is required based on transmission precautions.

ACTION	RATIONALE
3. Identify the patient.	Identifying the patient ensures the right patient receives the intervention and helps prevent errors.
4. Close curtains around bed and close the door to the room, if possible. Explain the purpose of the logrolling technique and what you are going to do, even if the patient is not conscious. Answer any questions.	This ensures the patient's privacy. Explanation relieves anxiety and facilitates cooperation.
5. Place the bed at an appropriate and comfortable working height, usually elbow height of the caregiver (VISN 8 Patient Safety Center, 2009).	Having the bed at the proper height prevents back and muscle strain.
6. Position at least one caregiver on one side of the bed and the two other caregivers on the opposite side of the bed. If a cervical collar is not in place, position one caregiver at the top of the bed, at the patient's head. Place the bed in flat position. Lower the side rails. Place a small pillow between the patient's knees.	Using four or more people to turn the patient helps ensure that the spinal column will remain in straight alignment. A pillow placed between the knees helps keep the spinal column aligned.
7. If a friction-reducing sheet is not in place under the patient, take the time to place one at this time, to facilitate future movement of the patient.	Use of a friction-reducing sheet facilitates smooth movement in unison and minimizes pulling on the patient's body. A drawsheet may be used if friction-reducing sheets are not available.
8. If the patient can move the arms, ask the patient to cross the arms on the chest. Roll or fanfold the friction-reducing sheet close to the patient's sides and grasp it. In unison, gently slide the patient to the side of the bed opposite that	Crossing arms across the chest keeps the arms out of the way while rolling the patient. This also encourages the patient not to help by pulling on the side rails. Moving the patient to the side opposite that to which the patient will be turned prevents the

ACTION	RATIONALE
to which the patient will be turned.	patient from being uncomfortably close to the side rail. If the patient is large, more assistants may be needed to prevent injury to the patient.
9. Make sure the friction-reducing sheet under the patient is straight and wrinkle free.	Drawsheet should be wrinkle free to prevent skin breakdown. Rolling the drawsheet strengthens the sheet and helps the nurse hold on to the sheet.
10. If necessary, reposition personnel to ensure two nurses stand on the side of the bed to which the patient is turning. The third helper stands on the other side. **Grasp the friction-reducing sheet at hip and shoulder level.**	Proper positioning of personnel provides even division of support and pulling forces on the patient to maintain alignment.
11. Have all caregivers face the patient. On a predetermined signal, turn the patient by holding the friction-reducing sheet taut to support the body. The caregiver at the patient's head should firmly hold the patient's head on either side, directly above the ears. Turn the patient as a unit in one smooth motion toward the side of the bed with the two nurses. The patient's head, shoulders, spine, hips, and knees should turn simultaneously.	Holding the patient's head stabilizes the cervical spine. The patient's spine should not twist during the turn. The spine should move as one unit.
12. **Once the patient has been turned, use pillows to support the patient's neck, back, buttocks, and legs in straight alignment in a side-lying position.** Raise the side rails as appropriate.	The pillows or wedge provide support and ensure continued spinal alignment after turning.
13. **Stand at the foot of the bed and assess the spinal column. It should be straight,**	Inspection of the spinal column ensures that the patient's back is not twisted or bent. Lowering the bed ensures patient safety.

ACTION	RATIONALE
without any twisting or bending. Place the bed in the lowest position. Ensure that the call bell and telephone are within reach. Replace covers. Lower bed height.	
14. Reassess the patient's neurologic status and comfort level.	Reassessment helps to evaluate the effects of movement on the patient.
15. Remove PPE, if used. Perform hand hygiene.	Removing PPE properly reduces the risk for infection transmission and contamination of other items. Hand hygiene prevents transmission of microorganisms.

EVALUATION

- Patient remains free of injury during and after turning and exhibits proper spinal alignment in the side-lying position.
- Patient states that pain was minimal on turning.
- Patient demonstrates adequate joint mobility.
- Patient exhibits no signs or symptoms of skin breakdown.

DOCUMENTATION

- Document the time of the patient's change of position, use of supports, and any pertinent observations, including neurologic and skin assessments. Document the patient's tolerance of the position change. Many facilities provide areas on bedside flow sheets to document repositioning.

Skill · 98   Administering Medications via a Gastric Tube

Patients with a gastrointestinal tube (nasogastric, nasointestinal, percutaneous endoscopic gastrostomy [PEG], or jejunostomy [J] tube) often receive medication through the tube. Use liquid medications when possible, because they are readily absorbed and less likely to cause tube occlusions. Certain solid dosage medications can be crushed and combined with liquid. Medications should be crushed to a fine powder and mixed with 15 to 30 mL of water before delivery through the tube. Certain capsules may be opened, emptied into liquid, and administered through the tube (Toedter Williams, 2008). Check manufacturer recommendations and/or with a pharmacist to verify.

EQUIPMENT
- Irrigation set (60-mL syringe and irrigation container)
- Medications
- Water (gastrostomy tubes) or sterile water (nasogastric
- tubes), according to facility policy
- Gloves
- Additional PPE, as indicated

ASSESSMENT GUIDELINES
- Research each medication to be given, especially for mode of action, side effects, nursing implications, ability to be crushed, and whether medication should be given with or without food.
- Verify patient name, dose, route, and time of administration.
- Assess patient's knowledge of medication and the reason for administration.
- Auscultate the abdomen for evidence of bowel sounds. Percuss and palpate the abdomen for tenderness and distention.
- Ascertain the time of the patient's last bowel movement and measure abdominal girth, if appropriate.

NURSING DIAGNOSES
- Deficient Knowledge
- Risk for Injury
- Impaired Swallowing

OUTCOME IDENTIFICATION AND PLANNING
Expected outcomes may include:
- Patient receives the medication via the tube and experiences the intended effect of the medication.
- Patient verbalizes knowledge of the medications given.
- Patient remains free from adverse effect and injury.
- Patient's gastrointestinal tube remains patent.

IMPLEMENTATION

ACTION	RATIONALE
1. Gather equipment. Check each medication order against the original in the medical record, according to	This comparison helps to identify errors that may have occurred when orders were transcribed. The primary care

ACTION	RATIONALE

facility policy. Clarify any inconsistencies. Check the patient's chart for allergies.

provider's order is the legal record of medication orders for each facility.

2. Know the actions, special nursing considerations, safe dose ranges, purpose of administration, and adverse effects of the medications to be administered. Consider the appropriateness of the medication for this patient.

This knowledge aids the nurse in evaluating the therapeutic effect of the medication in relation to the patient's disorder and can also be used to educate the patient about the medication.

3. Perform hand hygiene.

Hand hygiene prevents the spread of microorganisms.

4. Move the medication cart to the outside of the patient's room or prepare for administration in the medication area.

Organization facilitates error-free administration and saves time.

5. Unlock the medication cart or drawer. Enter pass code and scan employee identification, if required.

Locking the cart or drawer safeguards each patient's medication supply. Hospital accrediting organizations require medication carts to be locked when not in use. Entering pass code and scanning ID allow only authorized users into the system and identifies user for documentation by the computer.

6. **Prepare medications for one patient at a time.**

This prevents errors in medication administration.

7. Read the CMAR/MAR and select the proper medication from the patient's medication drawer or unit stock.

This is the *first* check of the label.

8. Compare the label with the CMAR/MAR. Check expiration dates and perform calculations, if necessary. Scan the bar code on the package, if required.

This is the *second* check of the label. Verify calculations with another nurse to ensure safety, if necessary.

ACTION	RATIONALE
9. Check to see if medications to be administered come in a liquid form. **If pills or capsules are to be given, check with pharmacy or drug reference to verify the ability to crush or open capsules.**	To prevent the tube from becoming clogged, all medications should be given in liquid form whenever possible. Medications in extended-release formulations should not be crushed before administration.
10. Prepare medication.	
Pills: Using a pill crusher, crush each pill one at a time. Dissolve the powder with water or other recommended liquid in a liquid medication cup, keeping each medication separate from the others. Keep the package label with the medication cup, for future comparison of information.	Some medications require dissolution in liquid other than water. The label is needed for an additional safety check. Some medications require preadministration assessments.
Liquid: When pouring liquid medications from a multi-dose bottle, hold the bottle with the label against the palm. Use the appropriate measuring device when pouring liquids, and read the amount of medication at the bottom of the meniscus at eye level. Wipe the lip of the bottle with a paper towel.	Liquid that may drip onto the label makes the label difficult to read. Accuracy is possible when the appropriate measuring device is used and then read accurately.
11. **When all medications for one patient have been prepared, recheck the label with the MAR before taking them to the patient.**	This is a *third* check to ensure accuracy and to prevent errors. Some facilities require the third check to occur at the bedside, after identifying the patient and before administration.
12. Lock the medication cart before leaving it.	Locking the cart or drawer safeguards the patient's medication supply. Hospital accrediting organizations require medication carts to be locked when not in use.
13. Transport medications to the patient's bedside carefully,	Careful handling and close observation prevent accidental or

ACTION	RATIONALE
and keep the medications in sight at all times.	deliberate disarrangement of medications.
14. **Ensure that the patient receives the medications at the correct time.**	Check agency policy, which may allow for administration within a period of 30 minutes before or 30 minutes after designated time.
15. Perform hand hygiene and put on PPE, if indicated.	Hand hygiene and PPE prevent the spread of microorganisms. PPE is required based on transmission precautions.
16. Identify the patient. Usually, the patient should be identified using two methods. Compare information with the CMAR or MAR.	Identifying the patient ensures the right patient receives the medications and helps prevent errors.
a. Check the name and identification number on the patient's identification band.	This is the most reliable method. Replace the identification band if it is missing or inaccurate in any way.
b. Ask the patient to state his or her name and birth date, based on facility policy.	This requires a response from the patient, but illness and strange surroundings often cause patients to be confused.
c. If the patient cannot identify himself or herself, verify the patient's identification with a staff member who knows the patient for the second source.	This is another way to double-check identity. Do not use the name on the door or over the bed, because these may be inaccurate.
17. Complete necessary assessments before administering medications. Check the patient's allergy bracelet or ask the patient about allergies. Explain what you are going to do, and the reason for doing it, to the patient.	Assessment is a prerequisite to administration of medications. Explanation relieves anxiety and facilitates cooperation.
18. Scan the patient's bar code on the identification band, if required.	This provides an additional check to ensure that th e medication is given to the right patient.

ACTION	RATIONALE
19. Assist the patient to the high Fowler's position, unless contraindicated.	This reduces the risk of aspiration.
20. Put on gloves.	Gloves prevent contact with mucous membranes and body fluids.
21. If the patient is receiving continuous tube feedings, pause the tube feeding pump.	If the pump is not stopped, tube feeding will flow out of the tube and onto the patient.
22. Pour the water into the irrigation container. Apply clamp on feeding tube, if present. Alternately, fold the gastric tube over on itself and pinch with fingers. Alternately, open port on gastric tube delegated to medication administration. If necessary, position stopcock to correct direction. Disconnect tubing for feeding or suction from gastric tube. Place cap on end of feeding tubing.	Fluid is ready for flushing of the tube. Applying clamp, folding the tube over and clamping, or correct positioning of stopcock prevents any backflow of gastric drainage. Covering the end of the feeding tubing prevents contamination.
23. **Check placement of tube, depending on type of tube and facility policy.**	Tube placement must be confirmed before administering anything through the tube to avoid inadvertent instillation in the respiratory tract.
24. Note the amount of any residual. Replace residual back into stomach, based on facility policy.	Research findings are inconclusive on the benefit of returning gastric volumes to the stomach or intestine to avoid fluid or electrolyte imbalance, which has been an accepted practice. Consult agency policy concerning this practice (Bourgault, et al., 2007; Keithley & Swanson, 2004; Metheny, 2008).
25. Fold gastric tube over and clamp with fingers. Remove 60-mL syringe. Remove the plunger of the syringe. Reinsert the syringe in the gastric	Folding the tube over and clamping it prevent any backflow of gastric drainage. Flushing the tube ensures all the residual is cleared from tube.

ACTION	RATIONALE
tube without the plunger. Pour 30 mL of water into the syringe. **Unclamp the tube and allow the water to enter the stomach via gravity infusion.**	
26. Administer the first dose of medication by pouring into the syringe. Follow with a 5- to 10-mL water flush between medication doses. Follow the last dose of medication with 30 to 60 mL of water flush.	Flushing between medications prevents any possible interactions between the medications. Flushing at the end maintains patency of the tube, prevents blockage by medication particles, and ensures all doses enter the stomach.
27. Clamp the tube, remove the syringe, and replace the feeding tubing. If a stopcock is used, position it to the correct direction. If a tube medication port was used, cap it. Unclamp the gastric tube and restart tube feeding, if appropriate for medications administered.	Some medications require the holding of the tube feeding for a certain period of time after administration. Consult a drug reference or a pharmacist.
28. Remove gloves. Assist the patient to a comfortable position. If receiving a tube feeding, the head of the bed must remain elevated at least 30 degrees.	Ensures patient comfort. Keeping the head of the bed elevated helps prevent aspiration.
29. Remove additional PPE, if used. Perform hand hygiene.	Removing PPE properly reduces the risk for infection transmission and contamination of other items. Hand hygiene prevents the spread of microorganisms.
30. Document the administration of the medication immediately after administration. See Documentation section below.	Timely documentation helps to ensure patient safety.
31. Evaluate the patient's response to medication within appropriate time frame.	The patient needs to be evaluated for therapeutic and adverse effects from the medication.

EVALUATION

- Patient receives the ordered medications and experiences the intended effects of the medications administered.
- Patient demonstrates a patent and functioning gastric tube.
- Patient verbalizes knowledge of the medications given, and remains free from adverse effect and injury.

DOCUMENTATION

- Document the administration of the medication immediately after administration, including date, time, dose, and route of administration on the CMAR/MAR or record using the required format. If using a bar-code system, medication administration is automatically recorded when it is scanned. PRN medications require documentation of the reason for administration. Prompt recording avoids the possibility of accidentally repeating the administration of the drug. Record the amount of gastric residual, if appropriate. Record the amount of liquid given on the intake and output record. If the drug was refused or omitted, record this in the appropriate area on the medication record and notify the primary care provider. This verifies the reason medication was omitted and ensures that the primary care provider is aware of the patient's condition.

GENERAL CONSIDERATIONS

- If medications are being administered via a nasogastric tube that is attached to suction, the tube should remain clamped, off suction, for a period of time after medication administration. This allows for medication absorption before returning to suction. Check facility policy and drug reference for specific drug requirements.
- If necessary to use a plunger in the irrigation syringe to administer medications, instill gently and slowly. Gravity administration is considered best to avoid excess pressure.
- Give medications separately and flush with water between each drug. Some medications may interact with each other or become less effective if mixed with other drugs.
- If the patient is receiving tube feedings, review information about the drugs to be administered. Absorption of some drugs (e.g., phenytoin [Dilantin]) is affected by tube feeding formulas. Discontinue a continuous tube feeding and leave the tube clamped for the required period of time before and after the medication has been given, according to the reference and facility protocol.
- Ongoing assessment is an important part of nursing care to evaluate patient response to administered medications and early detection of adverse effects. If an adverse effect is suspected, withhold further medication doses and notify the patient's primary healthcare provider. Additional intervention is based on type of reaction and patient assessment.

Skill · 99	Administering Medications by Intravenous Bolus or Push Through an Intravenous Infusion

A medication can be administered as an IV bolus or push. This involves a single injection of a concentrated solution directly into an IV line. Drugs given by IV push are used for intermittent dosing or to treat emergencies. The drug is administered very slowly over at least 1 minute. This can be done manually or a syringe pump may be used. Confirm exact administration times by consulting a pharmacist or drug reference.

EQUIPMENT

- Antimicrobial swab
- Watch with second hand, or stopwatch
- Clean gloves
- Additional PPE, as indicated
- Prescribed medication
- Syringe with a needleless device or 23- to 25-gauge,
- 1-inch needle (follow facility policy)
- Syringe pump if necessary
- Computer-generated Medication Administration Record (CMAR) or Medication Administration Record (MAR)

ASSESSMENT GUIDELINES

- Assess the patient for any allergies. Check the expiration date before administering medication.
- Assess the appropriateness of the drug for the patient. Assess the compatibility of the ordered medication and the IV fluid.
- Review assessment and laboratory data that may influence drug administration.
- Verify the patient's name, dose, route, and time of administration.
- Assess patient's IV site, noting any swelling, coolness, leakage of fluid from IV site, or pain.
- Assess the patient's knowledge of the medication. If the patient has a knowledge deficit about the medication, this may be the appropriate time to begin education about the medication.
- If the medication may affect the patient's vital signs, assess them before administration.
- If the medication is for pain relief, assess the patient's pain before and after administration.

NURSING DIAGNOSES

- Acute Pain
- Risk for Allergy Response
- Deficient Knowledge
- Risk for Infection
- Risk for Injury
- Anxiety

OUTCOME IDENTIFICATION AND PLANNING

Expected outcomes may include:
* Medication is given safely via the intravenous route.
* Patient experiences no adverse effect.
* Patient experiences no allergy response.
* Patient is knowledgeable about medication being added by bolus IV.
* Patient remains infection free.
* Patient has decreased anxiety.

IMPLEMENTATION

ACTION	RATIONALE
1. Gather equipment. Check medication order against the original order in the medical record, according to facility policy. Clarify any inconsistencies. Check the patient's chart for allergies. Verify the compatibility of the medication and IV fluid. Check a drug resource to clarify whether the medication needs to be diluted before administration. Check the infusion rate.	This comparison helps to identify errors that may have occurred when orders were transcribed. The primary care provider's order is the legal record of medication orders for each facility. Compatibility of medication and solution prevents complications. Delivers the correct dose of medication as prescribed.
2. Know the actions, special nursing considerations, safe dose ranges, purpose of administration, and adverse effects of the medications to be administered. Consider the appropriateness of the medication for this patient.	This knowledge aids the nurse in evaluating the therapeutic effect of the medication in relation to the patient's disorder and can also be used to educate the patient about the medication.
3. Perform hand hygiene.	Hand hygiene prevents the spread of microorganisms.
4. Move the medication cart to the outside of the patient's room or prepare for administration in the medication area.	Organization facilitates error-free administration and saves time.

ACTION	RATIONALE
5. Unlock the medication cart or drawer. Enter pass code and scan employee identification, if required.	Locking the cart or drawer safeguards each patient's medication supply. Hospital accrediting organizations require medication carts to be locked when not in use. Entering pass code and scanning ID allows only authorized users into the system and identifies user for documentation by the computer.
6. **Prepare medication for one patient at a time.**	This prevents errors in medication administration.
7. Read the CMAR/MAR and select the proper medication from the patient's medication drawer or unit stock.	This is the *first* check of the label.
8. Compare the label with the CMAR/MAR. Check expiration dates and perform calculations, if necessary. Scan the bar code on the package, if required.	This is the *second* check of the label. Verify calculations with another nurse to ensure safety, if necessary.
9. If necessary, withdraw medication from an ampule or vial as described in Skill 105 and Skill 106.	
10. **Recheck the label with the MAR before taking it to the patient.**	This is a *third* check to ensure accuracy and to prevent errors. Some facilities require the third check to occur at the bedside, after identifying the patient and before administration.
11. Lock the medication cart before leaving it.	Locking the cart or drawer safeguards the patient's medication supply. Hospital accrediting organizations require medication carts to be locked when not in use.
12. Transport medications and equipment to the patient's bedside carefully, and keep the medications in sight at all times.	Careful handling and close observation prevent accidental or deliberate disarrangement of medications. Having equipment available saves time and facilitates performance of the task.

ACTION	RATIONALE
13. **Ensure that the patient receives the medications at the correct time.**	Check agency policy, which may allow for administration within a period of 30 minutes before or 30 minutes after designated time.
14. Perform hand hygiene and put on PPE, if indicated.	Hand hygiene and PPE prevent the spread of microorganisms. PPE is required based on transmission precautions.
15. Identify the patient. Usually, the patient should be identified using two methods. Compare information with the CMAR/MAR.	Identifying the patient ensures the right patient receives the medications and helps prevent errors.
a. Check the name and identification number on the patient's identification band.	This is the most reliable method. Replace the identification band if it is missing or inaccurate in any way.
b. Ask the patient to state his or her name and birth date, based on facility policy.	This requires a response from the patient, but illness and strange surroundings often cause patients to be confused.
c. If the patient cannot identify himself or herself, verify the patient's identification with a staff member who knows the patient for the second source.	This is another way to double-check identity. Do not use the name on the door or over the bed, because these may be inaccurate.
16. Close curtains around bed and close the door to the room, if possible.	This provides patient privacy.
17. Complete necessary assessments before administering medications. Check the patient's allergy bracelet or ask the patient about allergies. Explain the purpose and action of the medication to the patient.	Assessment is a prerequisite to administration of medications. Explanation provides rationale, increases knowledge, and reduces anxiety.
18. Scan the patient's bar code on the identification band, if required.	Provides additional check to ensure that the medication is given to the right patient.

ACTION	RATIONALE
19. **Assess IV site for presence of inflammation or infiltration.**	IV medication must be given directly into a vein for safe administration.
20. If IV infusion is being administered via an infusion pump, pause the pump.	Pausing prevents infusion of fluid during bolus administration and activation of pump occlusion alarms.
21. Put on clean gloves.	Gloves prevent contact with blood and body fluids.
22. Select injection port on tubing that is closest to venipuncture site. Clean port with antimicrobial swab.	Using port closest to needle insertion site minimizes dilution of medication. Cleaning deters entry of microorganisms when port is punctured.
23. Uncap syringe. Steady port with your nondominant hand while inserting syringe into center of port.	This supports the injection port and lessens the risk for accidentally dislodging IV or entering the port incorrectly.
24. Move your nondominant hand to the section of IV tubing just above the injection port. Fold the tubing between your fingers.	This temporarily stops flow of gravity IV infusion and prevents medication from backing up tubing.
25. Pull back slightly on plunger just until blood appears in tubing.	This ensures injection of medication into the bloodstream.
26. **Inject the medication at the recommended rate.**	This delivers correct amount of medication at proper interval according to manufacturer's directions.
27. Release the tubing. Remove the syringe. Do not recap the used needle, if used. Engage the safety shield or needle guard, if present. Release the tubing and allow the IV fluid to flow. Discard the needle and syringe in the appropriate receptacle.	Proper disposal of the needle prevents injury.
28. Check IV fluid infusion rate. Restart infusion pump, if appropriate.	Injection of bolus may alter rate of fluid infusion, if infusing by gravity.

ACTION	RATIONALE
29. Remove gloves and additional PPE, if used. Perform hand hygiene.	Removing PPE properly reduces the risk for infection transmission and contamination of other items. Hand hygiene prevents the spread of microorganisms.
30. Document the administration of the medication immediately after administration. See Documentation section below.	Timely documentation helps to ensure patient safety.
31. Evaluate patient's response to medication within appropriate time frame.	The patient needs to be evaluated for therapeutic and adverse affects from the medication.

EVALUATION

- Medication is safely administered via IV bolus.
- Patient's anxiety is decreased.
- Patient does not experience adverse effects.
- Patient understands and complies with the medication regimen.

DOCUMENTATION

- Document the administration of the medication immediately after administration, including date, time, dose, route of administration, site of administration, and rate of administration on the CMAR/MAR or record using the required format. If using a bar-code system, medication administration is automatically recorded when it is scanned. PRN medications require documentation of the reason for administration. Prompt recording avoids the possibility of accidentally repeating the administration of the drug. If the drug was refused or omitted, record this in the appropriate area on the medication record and notify the primary care provider. This verifies the reason medication was omitted and ensures that the primary care provider is aware of the patient's condition.

GENERAL CONSIDERATIONS

- Facility policy may recommend the following variations when injecting a bolus IV medication:
  - Release folded tubing after each increment of the drug has been administered at prescribed rate to facilitate delivery of medication.
  - Use a syringe with 1 mL normal saline to flush tubing after an IV bolus is delivered to ensure that residual medication in tubing is not delivered too rapidly.

- Consider how fast IV fluid is flowing to determine whether a flush of normal saline is in order after administering medication. If IV fluid is flowing less than 50 mL per hour, it may take medication up to 30 minutes to reach patient. This depends on what type of tubing is being used in the agency.
- If the IV is a small gauge (22- to 24-gauge) placed in a small vein, a blood return may not occur even if IV is intact. Also, patient may complain of stinging and pain at site while medication is being administered due to irritation of vein. Placing a warm pack over the vein or slowing the rate may relieve discomfort.
- If the medication and IV solution are incompatible, a bolus may be given by flushing the tubing with normal saline before and after the medication bolus. Consult facility policy.
- Ongoing assessment is an important part of nursing care to evaluate patient response to administered medications and early detection of adverse effects. If an adverse effect is suspected, withhold further medication doses and notify the patient's primary healthcare provider. Additional intervention is based on type of reaction and patient assessment.

Skill · 100 — Administering a Piggyback Intermittent Intravenous Infusion of Medication

With intermittent IV infusion, the drug is mixed with a small amount of the IV solution, such as 50 to 100 mL, and administered over a short period at the prescribed interval (e.g., every 4 hours). The administration is most often performed using an intravenous infusion pump, which requires the nurse to program the infusion rate into the pump. 'Smart (computerized) pumps' are being used by many facilities for intravenous infusions, including intermittent infusions. Smart pumps also require programming of infusion rates by the nurse but also are able to identify dosing limits and practice guidelines to aid in safe administration. Administration may be achieved by gravity infusion, which requires the nurse to calculate the infusion rate in drops per minute. The best practice however, is to use an intravenous infusion pump.

The IV piggyback delivery system requires the intermittent or additive solution to be placed higher than the primary solution container. An extension hook provided by the manufacturer provides for easy lowering of the main IV container. The port on the primary IV line has a back-check valve that automatically stops the flow of the primary solution, allowing the secondary or piggyback solution to flow when connected. Because manufacturers' designs vary, it is important to check carefully the directions for the systems used in the facility. The nurse is responsible for calculating and regulating the infusion with an infusion pump or manually adjusting the flow rate of the IV intermittent infusion.

EQUIPMENT

- Medication prepared in labeled, small-volume bag
- Short secondary infusion tubing (microdrip or macrodrip)
- IV pump
- Needleless connector, if required, based on facility system
- Antimicrobial swab
- Metal or plastic hook
- IV pole
- Date label for tubing
- Computer-generated Medication Administration Record (CMAR) or Medication Administration Record (MAR)
- PPE, as indicated

ASSESSMENT GUIDELINES

- Assess the patient for any allergies.
- Check the expiration date before administering medication.
- Assess the appropriateness of the drug for the patient.
- Assess the compatibility of the ordered medication, diluent, and the infusing IV fluid.
- Review assessment and laboratory data that may influence drug administration.
- Verify patient name, dose, route, and time of administration.
- Assess the patient's knowledge of the medication. If the patient has a knowledge deficit about the medication, this may be the appropriate time to begin education about the medication.
- If the medication may affect the patient's vital signs, assess them before administration.
- Assess the IV insertion site, noting any swelling, coolness, leakage of fluid at site, redness, or pain.

NURSING DIAGNOSES

- Risk for Allergy Response
- Risk for Infection
- Deficient Knowledge
- Risk for Injury

OUTCOME IDENTIFICATION AND PLANNING

Expected outcomes may include:
- Medication is delivered via the intravenous route using sterile technique.
- Medication is delivered to the patient in a safe manner and at the appropriate infusion rate.
- Patient experiences no allergy response.
- Patient remains infection free.
- Patient understands and complies with the medication regimen.

IMPLEMENTATION

ACTION	RATIONALE
1. Gather equipment. Check each medication order against the original order in the medical record, according to facility policy. Clarify any inconsistencies. Check the patient's chart for allergies.	This comparison helps to identify errors that may have occurred when orders were transcribed. The primary care provider's order is the legal record of medication orders for each facility.
2. Know the actions, special nursing considerations, safe dose ranges, purpose of administration, and adverse effects of the medications to be administered. Consider the appropriateness of the medication for this patient.	This knowledge aids the nurse in evaluating the therapeutic effect of the medication in relation to the patient's disorder and can also be used to educate the patient about the medication.
3. Perform hand hygiene.	Hand hygiene prevents the spread of microorganisms.
4. Move the medication cart to the outside of the patient's room or prepare for administration in the medication area.	Organization facilitates error-free administration and saves time.
5. Unlock the medication cart or drawer. Enter pass code and scan employee identification, if required.	Locking of the cart or drawer safeguards each patient's medication supply. Hospital accrediting organizations require medication carts to be locked when not in use. Entering pass code and scanning ID allow only authorized users into the system and identify user for documentation by the computer.
6. **Prepare medications for one patient at a time.**	This prevents errors in medication administration.
7. Read the CMAR/MAR and select the proper medication from the patient's medication drawer or unit stock.	This is the *first* check of the label.

ACTION	**RATIONALE**
8. Compare the label with the CMAR/MAR. Check expiration dates. Confirm the prescribed or appropriate infusion rate. Calculate the drip rate if using a gravity system. Scan the bar code on the package, if required.	This is the *second* check of the label. Verify calculations with another nurse to ensure safety, if necessary. Infusing medication at appropriate rate prevents injury.
9. **When all medications for one patient have been prepared, recheck the label with the MAR before taking them to the patient.**	This is a *third* check to ensure accuracy and to prevent errors. Some facilities require the third check to occur at the bedside, after identifying the patient and before administration.
10. Lock the medication cart before leaving it.	Locking the cart or drawer safeguards the patient's medication supply. Hospital accrediting organizations require medication carts to be locked when not in use.
11. Transport medications to the patient's bedside carefully, and keep the medications in sight at all times.	Careful handling and close observation prevent accidental or deliberate disarrangement of medications.
12. **Ensure that the patient receives the medications at the correct time.**	Check agency policy, which may allow for administration within a period of 30 minutes before or 30 minutes after designated time.
13. Perform hand hygiene and put on PPE, if indicated.	Hand hygiene and PPE prevent the spread of microorganisms. PPE is required based on transmission precautions.
14. Identify the patient. Usually, the patient should be identified using two methods. Compare information with the CMAR/MAR.	Identifying the patient ensures the right patient receives the medications and helps prevent errors.
a. Check the name and identification number on the patient's identification band.	This is the most reliable method. Replace the identification band if it is missing or inaccurate in any way.

ACTION	RATIONALE
b. Ask the patient to state his or her name and birth date, based on facility policy.	This requires a response from the patient, but illness and strange surroundings often cause patients to be confused.
c. If the patient cannot identify himself or herself, verify the patient's identification with a staff member who knows the patient for the second source.	This is another way to double-check identity. Do not use the name on the door or over the bed, because these may be inaccurate.
15. Close the door to the room or pull the bedside curtain.	This provides patient privacy.
16. Complete necessary assessments before administering medications. Check the patient's allergy bracelet or ask the patient about allergies. Explain the purpose and action of the medication to the patient.	Assessment is a prerequisite to administration of medications. Explanation provides rationale, increases knowledge, and reduces anxiety.
17. Scan the patient's bar code on the identification band, if required.	Scanning provides an additional check to ensure that the medication is given to the right patient.
18. Assess the IV site for the presence of inflammation or infiltration.	IV medication must be given directly into a vein for safe administration.
19. Close the clamp on the short secondary infusion tubing. Using aseptic technique, remove the cap on the tubing spike and the cap on the port of the medication container, taking care to avoid contaminating either end.	Closing the clamp prevents fluid from entering the system until the nurse is ready. Maintaining sterility of tubing and medication port prevents contamination.
20. Attach infusion tubing to the medication container by inserting the tubing spike into the port with a firm push and twisting motion, taking care to avoid contaminating either end.	Maintaining sterility of tubing and medication port prevents contamination.

ACTION	RATIONALE
21. Hang piggyback container on IV pole, positioning it higher than the primary IV according to manufacturer's recommendations. Use metal or plastic hook to lower primary IV fluid container.	Position of containers influences the flow of IV fluid into the primary setup.
22. Place label on tubing with appropriate date.	Tubing for piggyback setup may be used for 48 to 96 hours, depending on agency policy. Label allows for tracking of the next date to change.
23. Squeeze drip chamber on tubing and release. Fill to the line or about half full. Open clamp and prime tubing. Close clamp. Place needleless connector on the end of the tubing, using sterile technique, if required.	This removes air from the tubing and preserves sterility of setup.
24. Use an antimicrobial swab to clean the access port or stopcock above the roller clamp on the primary IV infusion tubing.	This deters entry of microorganisms when the piggyback setup is connected to the port. Backflow valve in primary line secondary port stops flow of primary infusion while piggyback solution is infusing. Once completed, backflow valves open and flow of primary solution resumes.
25. Connect piggyback setup to the access port or stopcock. If using, turn the stopcock to the open position.	Needleless systems and stopcock setup eliminate the need for a needle and are recommended by the Centers for Disease Control and Prevention.
26. Open clamp on the secondary tubing. Set rate for secondary infusion on infusion pump and begin infusion. If using gravity infusion, use the roller clamp on the primary infusion tubing to regulate flow at prescribed delivery rate. Monitor medication infusion at periodic intervals.	Backflow valve in primary line secondary port stops flow of primary infusion while piggyback solution is infusing. Once completed, backflow valves open and flow of primary solution resumes. It is important to verify the safe administration rate for each drug to prevent effects.

ACTION	RATIONALE
27. Clamp tubing on piggyback set when solution is infused. Follow facility policy regarding disposal of equipment.	Most facilities allow the reuse of tubing for 48 to 96 hours. This reduces risk for contaminating primary IV setup.
28. Return primary IV fluid container to original height. **Check primary infusion rate on infusion pump. If using gravity infusion, readjust flow rate of primary IV.**	Most infusion pumps automatically restart primary infusion at previous rate after secondary infusion is completed. If using gravity infusion, piggyback medication administration may interrupt normal flow rate of primary IV. Rate readjustment may be necessary.
29. Remove PPE, if used. Perform hand hygiene.	Removing PPE properly reduces the risk for infection transmission and contamination of other items. Hand hygiene prevents the spread of microorganisms.
30. Document the administration of the medication immediately after administration. See Documentation section below.	Timely documentation helps to ensure patient safety.
31. Evaluate the patient's response to the medication within appropriate time frame. Monitor IV site at periodic intervals.	The patient needs to be evaluated for therapeutic and adverse effects from the medication.

EVALUATION

- Medication is delivered via the intravenous route using sterile technique.
- Medication is delivered to the patient in a safe manner and at the appropriate infusion rate.
- Patient experienced no allergy response.
- Patient remains infection free.
- Patient understands and complies with the medication regimen.

DOCUMENTATION

- Document the administration of the medication immediately after administration, including date, time, dose, route of administration, site of administration, and rate of administration on the CMAR/MAR or record using the required format. If using a bar-code system, medication administration is automatically recorded when scanned. PRN medications require documentation of the reason for administration. Prompt recording avoids the possibility of accidentally repeating the administration of the drug. If the drug was refused or omitted, record this in the appropriate area on the medication record and notify the primary care provider. This verifies the reason medication was omitted and ensures that the primary care provider is aware of the patient's condition. Document the volume of fluid administered on the intake and output record, if necessary.

GENERAL CONSIDERATIONS

• An alternate way to prime the secondary tubing, particularly if an administration set is in place from previous infusion, is to "backfill" the secondary tubing. Attach the medication bag to the secondary infusion tubing. Lower the medication bag below the main IV solution container and open the clamp on the secondary infusion tubing. This allows the primary IV solution to flow up the secondary tubing to the drip chamber, backfilling the tubing. Allow the solution to enter the drip chamber until the drip chamber is half full. Close the clamp on the secondary tubing and hang the medication container on the IV pole. Proceed with administration by lowering the primary IV container, as described above. This backfill method keeps the infusion system intact, preventing introduction of microorganisms and prevents loss of medication when the tubing is primed. Check facility policy regarding the use of backfilling.

• Ongoing assessment is an important part of nursing care to evaluate patient response to administered medications and early detection of adverse effects. If an adverse effect is suspected, withhold further medication doses and notify the patient's primary healthcare provider. Additional intervention is based on type of reaction and patient assessment.

Skill · 101   **Administering an Intermittent Intravenous Infusion of Medication via a Mini-Infusion Pump**

With intermittent IV infusion, the drug is mixed with a small amount of the IV solution, and administered over a short period at the prescribed interval (e.g., every 4 hours). The mini-infusion pump (syringe pump) for intermittent infusion is battery or electrical operated and allows medication mixed in a syringe to be connected to the primary line and delivered by mechanical pressure applied to the syringe plunger. "Smart (computerized) pumps" are being used by many facilities for IV infusions, including intermittent infusions. Smart pumps also require programming of infusion rates by the nurse, but also are able to identify dosing limits and practice guidelines to aid in safe administration.

EQUIPMENT
- Medication prepared in labeled syringe
- Mini-infusion pump and tubing
- Needleless connector, if required, based on facility system
- Antimicrobial swab
- Date label for tubing
- Computer-generated Medication Administration Record (CMAR) or Medication Administration Record (MAR)
- PPE, as indicated

ASSESSMENT GUIDELINES
- Assess the patient for any allergies. Check the expiration date before administering medication.
- Assess the appropriateness of the drug for the patient.
- Assess the compatibility of the ordered medication, diluent, and the infusing IV fluid.
- Review assessment and laboratory data that may influence drug administration.
- Verify patient name, dose, route, and time of administration. Assess the patient's knowledge of the medication. If the patient has a knowledge deficit about the medication, this may be the appropriate time to begin education about the medication.
- If the medication may affect the patient's vital signs, assess them before administration.
- Assess the IV insertion site, noting any swelling, coolness, leakage of fluid at site, redness, or pain.

NURSING DIAGNOSES
- Risk for Allergy Response
- Risk for Injury
- Deficient Knowledge
- Risk for Infection

OUTCOME IDENTIFICATION AND PLANNING
Expected outcomes may include:
- Medication is delivered via the intravenous route using sterile technique.
- Medication is delivered to the patient in a safe manner and at the appropriate infusion rate.
- Patient experiences no allergy response.
- Patient remains infection free.
- Patient understands and complies with the medication regimen.

IMPLEMENTATION

ACTION	RATIONALE
1. Gather equipment. Check each medication order against the original order in the medical record according to facility policy. Clarify any inconsistencies. Check the patient's chart for allergies.	This comparison helps to identify errors that may have occurred when orders were transcribed. The primary care provider order is the legal record of medication orders for each facility.
2. Know the actions, special nursing considerations, safe dose ranges, purpose of administration, and adverse effects of the medications to be administered. Consider the appropriateness of the medication for this patient.	This knowledge aids the nurse in evaluating the therapeutic effect of the medication in relation to the patient's disorder and can also be used to educate the patient about the medication.
3. Perform hand hygiene.	Hand hygiene prevents the spread of microorganisms.
4. Move the medication cart to the outside of the patient's room or prepare for administration in the medication area.	Organization facilitates error-free administration and saves time.
5. Unlock the medication cart or drawer. Enter pass code and scan employee identification, if required.	Locking the cart or drawer safeguards each patient's medication supply. Hospital accrediting organizations require medication carts to be locked when not in use. Entering pass code and scanning ID allows only authorized users into the system and identifies user for documentation by the computer.
6. **Prepare medications for one patient at a time.**	This prevents errors in medication administration.
7. Read the CMAR/MAR and select the proper medication from the patient's medication drawer or unit stock.	This is the *first* check of the label.

ACTION	RATIONALE
8. Compare the label with the CMAR/MAR. Check expiration dates. Confirm the prescribed or appropriate infusion rate. Scan the bar code on the package, if required.	This is the *second* check of the label. Verify calculations with another nurse to ensure safety, if necessary. Infusing medication at appropriate rate prevents injury.
9. **When all medications for one patient have been prepared, recheck the label with the MAR before taking them to the patient.**	This is the *third* check to ensure accuracy and to prevent errors. Some facilities require the third check to occur at the bedside, after identifying the patient and before administration.
10. Lock the medication cart before leaving it.	Locking the cart or drawer safeguards the patient's medication supply. Hospital accrediting organizations require medication carts to be locked when not in use.
11. Transport medications to the patient's bedside carefully, and keep the medications in sight at all times.	Careful handling and close observation prevent accidental or deliberate disarrangement of medications.
12. **Ensure that the patient receives the medications at the correct time.**	Check facility policy, which may allow for administration within a period of 30 minutes before or 30 minutes after designated time.
13. Perform hand hygiene and put on PPE, if indicated.	Hand hygiene and PPE prevent the spread of microorganisms. PPE is required based on transmission precautions.
14. Identify the patient. Usually, the patient should be identified using two methods. Compare information with the MAR/CMAR.	Identifying the patient ensures the right patient receives the medications and helps prevent errors.
a. Check the name and identification number on the patient's identification band.	This is the most reliable method. Replace the identification band if it is missing or inaccurate in any way.

ACTION	RATIONALE
b. Ask the patient to state his or her name and birth date, based on facility policy.	This requires a response from the patient, but illness and strange surroundings often cause patients to be confused.
c. If the patient cannot identify him or herself, verify the patient's identification with a staff member who knows the patient for the second source.	This is another way to double-check identity. Do not use the name on the door or over the bed, because these signs may be inaccurate.
15. Close the door to the room or pull the bedside curtain.	Provides patient privacy.
16. Complete necessary assessments before administering medications. Check the patient's allergy bracelet or ask the patient about allergies. Explain the purpose and action of the medication to the patient.	Assessment is a prerequisite to administration of medications. Explanation provides rationale, increases knowledge, and reduces anxiety.
17. Scan the patient's bar code on the identification band, if required.	Provides an additional check to ensure that the medication is given to the right patient.
18. Assess the IV site for the presence of inflammation or infiltration.	IV medication must be given directly into a vein for safe administration.
19. Using aseptic technique, remove the cap on the tubing and the cap on the syringe, taking care not to contaminate either end.	Maintaining sterility of tubing and syringe prevents contamination.
20. Attach infusion tubing to the syringe, taking care not to contaminate either end.	Maintaining sterility of tubing and medication port prevents contamination.
21. Place label on tubing with appropriate date.	Tubing for piggyback setup may be used for 48 to 96 hours, depending on facility policy. Label allows for tracking of the next date to change.
22. Fill tubing with medication by applying gentle pressure to syringe plunger. Place	This removes air from tubing and maintains sterility.

ACTION	RATIONALE
needleless connector on the end of the tubing, using sterile technique, if required.	
23. Insert syringe into mini-infusion pump according to manufacturer's directions.	Syringe must fit securely in pump apparatus for proper operation.
24. Use antimicrobial swab to clean the access port or stopcock below the roller clamp on the primary IV infusion tubing, usually the port closest to the IV insertion site.	This deters entry of microorganisms when the piggyback setup is connected to the port. Proper connection allows IV medication to flow into primary line.
25. Connect the secondary infusion to the primary infusion at the cleansed port.	Allows for delivery of medication.
26. Program pump to the appropriate rate and begin infusion. Set alarm if recommended by manufacturer.	Pump delivers medication at A controlled rate. Alarm is recommended for use with IV lock apparatus.
27. Clamp tubing on secondary set when solution is infused. Remove secondary tubing from access port and cap, or replace connector with a new, capped one, if reusing. Follow facility policy regarding disposal of equipment.	Many facilities allow reuse of tubing for 48 to 96 hours. Replacing connector or needle with a new, capped one maintains system sterility.
28. Check rate of primary infusion.	Administration of secondary infusion may interfere with primary infusion rate.
29. Remove PPE, if used. Perform hand hygiene.	Removing PPE properly reduces the risk for infection transmission and contamination of other items. Hand hygiene prevents the spread of microorganisms.
30. Document the administration of the medication immediately after administration. See Documentation section below.	Timely documentation helps to ensure patient safety.
31. Evaluate the patient's response to medication within appropriate time frame. Monitor IV site at periodic intervals.	The patient needs to be evaluated for therapeutic and adverse effects from the medication.

EVALUATION
• Medication is delivered via the intravenous route using sterile technique.
• Medication is delivered to the patient in a safe manner and at the appropriate infusion rate.
• Patient experiences no allergy response.
• Patient remains infection free.
• Patient understands and complies with the medication regimen.

DOCUMENTATION
• Document the administration of the medication immediately after administration, including date, time, dose, route of administration, site of administration, and rate of administration on the CMAR/MAR or record using the required format. If using a bar-code system, medication administration is automatically recorded when bar code is scanned. PRN medications require documentation of the reason for administration. Prompt recording avoids the possibility of accidentally repeating the administration of the drug. If the drug was refused or omitted, record this in the appropriate area on the medication record and notify the primary care provider. This verifies the reason medication was omitted and ensures that the primary care provider is aware of the patient's condition. Document the volume of fluid administered on the intake and output record, if necessary.

GENERAL CONSIDERATIONS
• Ongoing assessment is an important part of nursing care to evaluate patient response to administered medications and early detection of adverse effects. If an adverse effect is suspected, withhold further medication doses and notify the patient's primary healthcare provider. Additional intervention is based on type of reaction and patient assessment.

Skill • 102   **Administering an Intermittent Intravenous Infusion of Medication via a Volume-Control Administration Set**

With intermittent IV infusion, the drug is mixed with a small amount of the IV solution, such as 50 to 100 mL, and administered over a short period at the prescribed interval (e.g., every 4 hours). The administration is most often performed using an intravenous infusion pump, which requires the nurse to program the infusion rate into the pump. 'Smart (computerized) pumps' are being used by many facilities for intravenous infusions, including intermittent infusions. Smart pumps also require programming of infusion rates by the nurse, but also are able to identify dosing limits and practice guidelines to aid in safe administration. Administration may be achieved by gravity infusion, which requires the nurse to calculate the infusion rate in drops per minute. The best practice however, is to use an intravenous infusion pump.

This skill discusses using a volume-control administration set for intermittent IV infusion. The medication is diluted with a small amount of solution and administered through the patient's IV line. This type of equipment is commonly used for infusing solutions into children, critically ill patients, and older patients when the volume of fluid infused is a concern. Needleless devices (recommended by the Centers for Disease Control and Prevention and the Occupational Safety and Health Administration) prevent needlesticks and provide access to the primary venous line. Either a blunt-ended cannula or a recessed connection port may be used to connect intermittent IV infusions.

EQUIPMENT

- Prescribed medication
- Syringe with a needleless device or blunt needle, if required, based on facility system
- Volume-control set (Volutrol, Buretrol, Burette)
- Needleless connector or stopcock, if required
- Infusion pump, if needed
- Antimicrobial swab
- Date label for tubing
- Medication label
- Computer-generated Medication Administration Record (CMAR) or Medication Administration Record (MAR)
- PPE, as indicated

ASSESSMENT GUIDELINES

- Assess the patient for any allergies.
- Check the expiration date before administering medication.
- Assess the appropriateness of the drug for the patient.
- Assess the compatibility of the ordered medication, diluent, and the infusing IV fluid.
- Review assessment and laboratory data that may influence drug administration.
- Assess the patient's knowledge of the medication. If the patient has a knowledge deficit about the medication, this may be the appropriate time to begin education about the medication. If the medication may affect the patient's vital signs, assess them before administration.
- Assess the IV insertion site, noting any swelling, coolness, leakage of fluid at site, redness, or pain.

NURSING DIAGNOSES

- Risk for Allergy Response
- Risk for Injury
- Deficient Knowledge
- Risk for Infection

OUTCOME IDENTIFICATION AND PLANNING

Expected outcomes may include:
- Medication is delivered via the intravenous route using sterile technique.
- Medication is delivered to the patient in a safe manner and at the appropriate infusion rate.
- Patient experiences no allergy response.
- Patient remains infection free.
- Patient understands and complies with the medication regimen.

IMPLEMENTATION

ACTION	RATIONALE
1. Gather equipment. Check the medication order against the original order in the medical record, according to facility policy. Clarify any inconsistencies. Check the patient's chart for allergies. Verify the compatibility of the medication and IV fluid.	This comparison helps to identify errors that may have occurred when orders were transcribed. The primary care provider's order is the legal record of medication orders for each facility. Compatibility of medication and solution prevents complications.
2. Know the actions, special nursing considerations, safe dose ranges, purpose of administration, and adverse effects of the medications to be administered. Consider the appropriateness of the medication for this patient.	This knowledge aids the nurse in evaluating the therapeutic effect of the medication in relation to the patient's disorder and can also be used to educate the patient about the medication.
3. Perform hand hygiene.	Hand hygiene prevents the spread of microorganisms.
4. Move the medication cart to the outside of the patient's room or prepare for administration in the medication area.	Organization facilitates error-free administration and saves time.
5. Unlock the medication cart or drawer. Enter pass code and scan employee identification, if required.	Locking of the cart or drawer safeguards each patient's medication supply. Hospital accrediting organizations require medication carts to be locked

ACTION	RATIONALE
	when not in use. Entering pass code and scanning ID allows only authorized users into the system and identifies user for documentation by the computer.
6. **Prepare medication for one patient at a time.**	This prevents errors in medication administration.
7. Read the CMAR/MAR and select the proper medication from the patient's medication drawer or unit stock.	This is the *first* check of the label.
8. Compare the label with the CMAR/MAR. Check expiration dates and perform calculations, if necessary. Confirm the prescribed or appropriate infusion rate. Calculate the drip rate if using a gravity system. Scan the bar code on the package, if required. Check the infusion rate.	This is the *second* check of the label. Verify calculations with another nurse to ensure safety, if necessary. Delivers the correct dose of medication, as prescribed.
9. If necessary, withdraw medication from an ampule or vial as described in Skills 105 and 106. Attach needleless connector or blunt needle to the end of the syringe, if necessary.	Allows for entry into the volume-control administration set chamber.
10. **When all medications for one patient have been prepared, recheck their labels with the CMAR/MAR before taking them to the patient.**	This is the *third* check to ensure accuracy and to prevent errors. Some facilities require the third check to occur at the bedside, after identifying the patient and before administration.
11. Prepare medication label, including name of medication, dose, total volume, including diluent, and time of administration.	Allows for accurate identification of medication.
12. Lock the medication cart before leaving it.	Locking the cart or drawer safeguards the patient's medication supply. Hospital accrediting organizations require medication carts to be locked when not in use.

ACTION	RATIONALE
13. Transport medications and equipment to the patient's bedside carefully, and keep the medications in sight at all times.	Careful handling and close observation prevent accidental or deliberate disarrangement of medications. Having equipment available saves time and facilitates performance of the task.
14. **Ensure that the patient receives the medications at the correct time.**	Check facility policy, which may allow for administration within a period of 30 minutes before or 30 minutes after designated time.
15. Perform hand hygiene and put on PPE, if indicated.	Hand hygiene and PPE prevent the spread of microorganisms. PPE is required based on transmission precautions.
16. Identify the patient. Usually, the patient should be identified using two methods. Compare information with the CMAR/MAR.	Identifying the patient ensures the right patient receives the medications and helps prevent errors.
a. Check the name and identification number on the patient's identification band.	This is the most reliable method. Replace the identification band if it is missing or inaccurate in any way.
b. Ask the patient to state his or her name and birth date, based on facility policy.	This requires a response from the patient, but illness and strange surroundings often cause patients to be confused.
c. If the patient cannot identify himself or herself, verify the patient's identification with a staff member who knows the patient for the second source.	This is another way to double-check identity. Do not use the name on the door or over the bed, because these may be inaccurate.
17. Close the door to the room or pull the bedside curtain.	This provides patient privacy.
18. Complete necessary assessments before administering medications. Check the patient's allergy bracelet or ask the patient about	Assessment is a prerequisite to administration of medications. Explanation provides rationale, increases knowledge, and reduces anxiety.

ACTION	RATIONALE
allergies. Explain the purpose and action of the medication to the patient.	
19. Scan the patient's bar code on the identification band, if required.	Provides additional check to ensure that the medication is given to the right patient.
20. Assess IV site for presence of inflammation or infiltration.	IV medication must be given directly into a vein for safe administration.
21. Fill the volume-control administration set with the prescribed amount of IV fluid by opening the clamp between IV solution and the volume-control administration set. Follow manufacturer's instructions and fill with prescribed amount of IV solution. Close clamp.	This dilutes the medication in the minimal amount of solution. Reclamping prevents the continued addition of fluid to the volume to be mixed with the medication.
22. Check to make sure the air vent on the volume-control administration set chamber is open.	Air vent allows fluid in the chamber to flow at a regular rate.
23. Use antimicrobial swab to clean access port on volume-control administration set chamber.	This deters entry of microorganisms when the syringe enters the chamber.
24. Attach the syringe with a twisting motion into the access port while holding the syringe steady. Alternately, insert the needleless device or blunt needle into the port. Inject the medication into the chamber. Gently rotate the chamber.	This ensures that medication is evenly mixed with solution.
25. Attach the medication label to the volume-control device.	This identifies contents of the set and prevents medication error.
26. Use an antimicrobial swab to clean the access port or stopcock below the roller clamp on the primary IV infusion tubing, usually the port closest to the IV insertion site.	This deters entry of microorganisms when piggyback setup is connected to port. Proper connection allows IV medication to flow into primary line.

ACTION	RATIONALE
27. Connect the secondary infusion to the primary infusion at the cleansed port.	This allows for delivery of medication.
28. The volume-control administration set may be placed on an infusion pump with the appropriate dose programmed into the pump. Alternately, use the roller clamp on the volume-control administration set tubing to adjust the infusion to the prescribed rate.	Delivery over a 30- to 60-minute interval is a safe method of administering IV medication.
29. Discard the syringe in the appropriate receptacle.	Proper disposal prevents injury.
30. Clamp tubing on secondary set when solution is infused. Remove secondary tubing from the access port and cap or replace the connector with a new, capped one, if reusing. Follow facility policy regarding disposal of equipment.	Many facilities allow reuse of tubing for 48 to 96 hours. Replacing the connector or needle with a new, capped one maintains sterility of system.
31. Check rate of primary infusion.	Administration of secondary infusion may interfere with primary infusion rate.
32. Remove PPE, if used. Perform hand hygiene.	Removing PPE properly reduces the risk for infection transmission and contamination of other items. Hand hygiene prevents the spread of microorganisms.
33. Document the administration of the medication immediately after administration. See Documentation section below.	Timely documentation helps to ensure patient safety.
34. Evaluate the patient's response to medication within appropriate time frame. Monitor IV site at periodic intervals.	The patient needs to be evaluated for therapeutic and adverse effects from the medication. Visualization of the site also allows for assessment of any untoward effects.

EVALUATION

- Medication is delivered via the intravenous route using sterile technique.
- Medication is delivered to the patient in a safe manner and at the appropriate infusion rate.
- Patient experiences no allergy response.
- Patient remains infection free.
- Patient understands and complies with the medication regimen.

DOCUMENTATION

- Document the administration of the medication immediately after administration, including date, time, dose, route of administration, site of administration, and rate of administration on the CMAR/MAR or record using the required format. If using a bar-code system, medication administration is automatically recorded when scanned. PRN medications require documentation of the reason for administration. Prompt recording avoids the possibility of accidentally repeating the administration of the drug. If the drug was refused or omitted, record this in the appropriate area on the medication record and notify the primary care provider. This verifies the reason medication was omitted and ensures that the primary care provider is aware of the patient's condition. Document the volume of fluid administered on the intake and output record, if necessary.

GENERAL CONSIDERATIONS

- Ongoing assessment is an important part of nursing care to evaluate patient response to administered medications and early detection of adverse effects. If an adverse effect is suspected, withhold further medication doses and notify the patient's primary healthcare provider. Additional intervention is based on type of reaction and patient assessment.

Skill · 103 Mixing Medications From Two Vials in One Syringe

Preparation of medications in one syringe depends on how the medication is supplied. When using a single-dose vial and a multidose vial, air is injected into both vials and the medication in the multidose vial is drawn into the syringe first. This prevents the contents of the multidose vial from being contaminated with the medication in the single-dose vial. The CDC recommends that medications packaged as multiuse vials be assigned to a single patient whenever possible. In addition, it is recommended that the top of the vial be cleaned before each entry, as well as the use of a new sterile needle and syringe (CDC, 2008a; CDC, 2008b).

When considering mixing two medications in one syringe, ensure that the two drugs are compatible. Be aware of drug incompatibilities when preparing medications in one syringe. Certain medications, such as diazepam (Valium), are incompatible with other drugs in the same syringe. Other drugs have limited compatibility and should be administered within 15 minutes of preparation. Incompatible drugs may become cloudy or form a precipitate in the syringe. Such medications are discarded and prepared again in separate syringes. Mixing more than two drugs in one syringe is not recommended. If it must be done, contact the pharmacist to determine the compatibility of the three drugs, as well as the compatibility of their pH values and the preservatives that may be present in each drug. A drug-compatibility table should be available to nurses who are preparing medications.

Insulins, with many types available for use, are an example of medications that may be combined together in one syringe for injection. Insulins vary in their onset and duration of action and are classified as rapid acting, short acting, intermediate acting, and long acting. Before administering any insulin, be aware of the onset time, peak, and duration of effects, and ensure that proper food is available. Be aware that some insulins, such as Lantus and Levemir, cannot be mixed with other insulins. Refer to a drug reference for a listing of the different types of insulin and action specific to each type. Insulin dosages are calculated in units. The scale commonly used is U100, which is based on 100 units of insulin contained in 1 mL of solution.

The preparation of two types of insulin in one syringe is used as the example in the following procedure.

EQUIPMENT

- Two vials of medication (insulin in this example)
- Sterile syringe (insulin syringe in this example)
- Antimicrobial swabs
- Computer-generated Medication Administration Record (CMAR) or Medication Administration Record (MAR)

ASSESSMENT GUIDELINES

- Determine the compatibility of the two medications. Not all insulins can be mixed together. For example, Lantus and Levemir cannot be mixed with other insulins.
- Assess the contents of each vial of insulin. It is very important to be familiar with the particular drug's properties to be able to assess the quality of the medication in the vial before withdrawal. Unmodified preparations typically appear as clear substances, so they should be without particles or foreign matter. Modified preparations are typically suspensions, so they do not appear as clear substances. Keep in mind that it is no longer safe to use the terms "clear" and "cloudy" to designate types of insulin preparation. Insulin Glargine (Lantus) is a clear, long-acting insulin (24-hour duration).
- Check the expiration date before administering the medication.

- Assess the appropriateness of the drug for the patient.
- Review the assessment and laboratory data that may influence drug administration.
- Check the patient's blood glucose level, if appropriate, before administering the insulin.
- Verify patient name, dose, route, and time of administration.

NURSING DIAGNOSES
- Risk for Infection
- Risk for Injury
- Deficient Knowledge
- Anxiety

OUTCOME IDENTIFICATION AND PLANNING
Expected outcomes may include:
- Medication will be removed into a syringe in a sterile manner and the proper dose is prepared.

IMPLEMENTATION

ACTION	RATIONALE
1. Gather equipment. Check medication order against the original order in the medical record, according to facility policy.	This comparison helps to identify errors that may have occurred when orders were transcribed. The primary care provider's order is the legal record of medication orders for each facility.
2. Know the actions, special nursing considerations, safe dose ranges, purpose of administration, and adverse effects of the medication to be administered. Consider the appropriateness of the medication for this patient.	This knowledge aids the nurse in evaluating the therapeutic effect of the medication in relation to the patient's disorder and can also be used to educate the patient about the medication.
3. Perform hand hygiene.	Hand hygiene deters the spread of microorganisms.
4. Move the medication cart to the outside of the patient's room or prepare for administration in the medication area.	Organization facilitates error-free administration and saves time.

ACTION	RATIONALE
5. Unlock the medication cart or drawer. Enter pass code and scan employee identification, if required.	Locking the cart or drawer safeguards each patient's medication supply. Hospital accrediting organizations require medication carts to be locked when not in use. Entering pass code and scanning ID allows only authorized users into the system and identifies user for documentation by the computer.
6. **Prepare medications for one patient at a time.**	This prevents errors in medication administration.
7. Read the CMAR/MAR and select the proper medications from the patient's medication drawer or unit stock.	This is the *first* check of the labels.
8. Compare the labels with the CMAR/MAR. Check expiration dates and perform calculations, if necessary. Scan the bar code on the package, if required.	This is the *second* check of the labels. Verify calculations with another nurse to ensure safety, if necessary.
9. If necessary, remove the cap that protects the rubber stopper on each vial.	The cap protects the rubber top.
10. **If medication is a suspension (e.g., NPH insulin), roll and agitate the vial to mix it well.**	There is controversy regarding how to mix insulins in suspension. Some sources advise rolling the vial; others advise shaking the vial. Consult facility policy. Regardless of the method used, it is essential that the suspension be mixed well to avoid administering an inconsistent dose. Regular insulin, which is clear, does not need to be mixed before withdrawal.
11. Cleanse the rubber tops with antimicrobial swabs.	Antimicrobial swab removes surface contamination. Some sources question whether cleaning with alcohol actually disinfects or instead transfers resident bacteria from the hands to another surface.

ACTION	RATIONALE
12. Remove cap from needle by pulling it straight off. Touch the plunger at the knob only. Draw back an amount of air into the syringe that is equal to the dose of modified insulin to be withdrawn.	Pulling cap off in a straight manner prevents accidental needle-stick. Handling the plunger by the knob only ensures sterility of the shaft of the plunger. Before fluid is removed, injection of an equal amount of air is required to prevent the formation of a partial vacuum, because a vial is a sealed container. If not enough air is injected, the negative pressure makes it difficult to withdraw the medication.
13. Hold the modified vial on a flat surface. Pierce the rubber stopper in the center with the needle tip and inject the measured air into the space above the solution. Do not inject air into the solution. Withdraw the needle.	Unmodified insulin should never be contaminated with modified insulin. Placing air in the modified insulin first without allowing the needle to contact the insulin ensures that the second vial entered (unmodified) insulin is not contaminated by the medication in the other vial. Air bubbled through the solution could result in withdrawal of an inaccurate amount of medication.
14. Draw back an amount of air into the syringe that is equal to the dose of unmodified insulin to be withdrawn.	Before fluid is removed, injection of an equal amount of air is required to prevent the formation of a partial vacuum, because a vial is a sealed container. If not enough air is injected, the negative pressure makes it difficult to withdraw the medication.
15. Hold the unmodified vial on a flat surface. Pierce the rubber stopper in the center with the needle tip and inject the measured air into the space above the solution. Do not inject air into the solution. Keep the needle in the vial.	Air bubbled through the solution could result in withdrawal of an inaccurate amount of medication.
16. Invert vial of unmodified insulin. Hold the vial in one hand and use the other to withdraw	Holding the syringe at eye level facilitates accurate reading, and the vertical position makes

ACTION	RATIONALE

the medication. Touch the plunger at the knob only. **Draw up the prescribed amount of medication while holding the syringe at eye level and vertically.** Turn the vial over and then remove needle from vial.

removal of air bubbles from the syringe easy. First dose is prepared and is not contaminated by insulin that contains modifiers.

17. Check that there are no air bubbles in the syringe.

The presence of air in the syringe would result in an inaccurate dose of medication.

18. **Check the amount of medication in the syringe with the medication dose and discard any surplus.**

Careful measurement ensures that correct dose is withdrawn.

19. **Recheck the vial label with the CMAR/MAR.**

This is the *third* check to ensure accuracy and to prevent errors. Some facilities require the third check to occur at the bedside, after identifying the patient and before administration.

20. Calculate the endpoint on the syringe for the combined insulin amount by adding the number of units for each dose together.

Allows for accurate withdrawal of second dose.

21. Insert the needle into the modified vial and invert it, taking care not to push the plunger and inject medication from the syringe into the vial. Invert vial of modified insulin. Hold the vial in one hand and use the other to withdraw the medication. Touch the plunger at the knob only. **Draw up the prescribed amount of medication while holding the syringe at eye level and vertically. Take care to withdraw only the prescribed amount.** Turn the vial over and then remove needle from vial. Carefully recap the needle.

Previous addition of air eliminates need to create positive pressure. Holding the syringe at eye level facilitates accurate reading. Capping the needle prevents contamination and protects the nurse against accidental needlesticks. A one-handed recap method may be used as long as care is taken to ensure that the needle remains sterile.

ACTION	RATIONALE
Carefully replace the cap over the needle.	
22. **Check the amount of medication in the syringe with the medication dose.**	Careful measurement ensures that correct dose is withdrawn.
23. **Recheck the vial label with the CMAR/MAR.**	This is the *third* check to ensure accuracy and to prevent errors. Some facilities require the third check to occur at the bedside, after identifying the patient and before administration.
24. **Label the vials with the date and time opened, and store the vials containing the remaining medication according to facility policy.**	Because the vial is sealed, the medication inside remains sterile and can be used for future injections. Labeling the opened vials with a date and time limits its use after a specific time period. The CDC recommends that medications packaged as multiuse vials be assigned to a single patient whenever possible (CDC, 2008a; CDC, 2008b).
25. Lock medication cart before leaving it.	Locking the cart or drawer safeguards the patient's medication supply. Hospital accrediting organizations require medication carts to be locked when not in use.
26. Perform hand hygiene.	Hand hygiene deters the spread of microorganisms.
27. Proceed with administration, based on prescribed route.	See appropriate skill for prescribed route.

EVALUATION

- Medication is withdrawn into the syringe in a sterile manner and the proper dose is prepared.

DOCUMENTATION

- It is not necessary to record the removal of the medication from the vial. Record each medication administered on the CMAR/MAR or record using the required format immediately after it is administered, including date and time of administration. If using a bar-code system, medication administration is automatically recorded when the bar code is scanned. PRN medications require documentation of the reason for administration. Prompt recording avoids the possibility of accidentally repeating the administration of the drug. If the drug was refused or omitted, record this in the appropriate area on the medication record and notify the primary care provider. This verifies the reason medication was omitted and ensures that the primary care provider is aware of the patient's condition. Recording administration of a narcotic may require additional documentation on a narcotic record, stating drug count and other specific information. Record fluid intake if intake and output measurement is required.

GENERAL CONSIDERATIONS

• A patient with diabetes who is visually impaired may find it helpful to use a magnifying apparatus that fits around the syringe.
• Before attempting to explain or demonstrate devices that help low-vision diabetic patients to prepare their medication, attempt to use the device yourself under similar circumstances. To detect any difficulties the patient may experience, practice using the aid with your eyes closed or in a poorly lit room.
• School-age children are generally able to prepare and administer their own injections, such as insulin, with supervision (Kyle, 2008). Parents/significant others and the child should be involved in teaching.

Skill · 104 **Administering Oral Medications**

Drugs given orally are intended for absorption in the stomach and small intestine. The oral route is the most commonly used route of administration. It is usually the most convenient and comfortable route for the patient. After oral administration, drug action has a slower onset and a more prolonged, but less potent, effect than other routes.

EQUIPMENT

• Medication in disposable cup or oral syringe
• Liquid (e.g., water, juice) with straw, if not contraindicated
• Medication cart or tray
• Computer-generated Medication Administration Record (CMAR) or Medication Administration Record (MAR)
• PPE, as indicated

ASSESSMENT GUIDELINES

- Assess the appropriateness of the drug for the patient. Review medical history, allergy, assessment, and laboratory data that may influence drug administration.
- Assess the patient's ability to swallow medications. If the patient cannot swallow, is NPO, or is experiencing nausea or vomiting, withhold the medication, notify the primary care provider, and complete proper documentation.
- Assess the patient's knowledge of the medication. If the patient has a knowledge deficit about the medication, this may be the appropriate time to begin education about the medication.
- If the medication may affect the patient's vital signs, assess them before administration.
- If the medication is for pain relief, assess the patient's pain level before and after administration.
- Verify the patient name, dose, route, and time of administration.

NURSING DIAGNOSES

- Impaired Swallowing
- Risk for Aspiration
- Deficient Knowledge
- Anxiety
- Noncompliance

OUTCOME IDENTIFICATION AND PLANNING

Expected outcomes may include:
- Patient will swallow the medication.
- Patient will experience the desired effect from the medication.
- Patient will not aspirate.
- Patient experiences decreased anxiety.
- Patient does not experience adverse effects.
- Patient understands and complies with the medication regimen.

IMPLEMENTATION

ACTION	RATIONALE
1. Gather equipment. Check each medication order against the original in the medical record, according to facility policy. Clarify any inconsistencies. Check the patient's chart for allergies.	This comparison helps to identify errors that may have occurred when orders were transcribed. The primary care provider's order is the legal record of medication orders for each facility.

ACTION	RATIONALE

2. Know the actions, special nursing considerations, safe dose ranges, purpose of administration, and adverse effects of the medications to be administered. Consider the appropriateness of the medication for this patient.

This knowledge aids the nurse in evaluating the therapeutic effect of the medication in relation to the patient's disorder and can also be used to educate the patient about the medication.

3. Perform hand hygiene.

Hand hygiene prevents the spread of microorganisms.

4. Move the medication cart to the outside of the patient's room or prepare for administration in the medication area.

Organization facilitates error-free administration and saves time.

5. Unlock the medication cart or drawer. Enter pass code into the computer and scan employee identification, if required.

Locking the cart or drawer safeguards each patient's medication supply. Hospital accrediting organizations require medication carts to be locked when not in use. Entering pass code and scanning ID allows only authorized users into the computer system and identifies the user for documentation by the computer.

6. **Prepare medications for one patient at a time.**

This prevents errors in medication administration.

7. Read the CMAR/MAR and select the proper medication from the patient's medication drawer or unit stock.

This is the *first* check of the label.

8. Compare the label with the CMAR/MAR. Check expiration dates and perform calculations, if necessary. Scan the bar code on the package, if required.

This is the *second* check of the label. Verify calculations with another nurse to ensure safety, if necessary.

ACTION	RATIONALE

9. Prepare the required medications:

a. *Unit dose packages:* Place unit dose-packaged medications in a disposable cup. **Do not open the wrapper until at the bedside.** Keep narcotics and medications that require special nursing assessments in a separate container.

Wrapper is kept intact because the label is needed for an additional safety check. Special assessments may be required before giving certain medications. These may include assessing vital signs and checking laboratory test results.

b. *Multidose containers:* When removing tablets or capsules from a multidose bottle, pour the necessary number into the bottle cap and then place the tablets or capsules in a medication cup. Break only scored tablets, if necessary, to obtain the proper dosage. Do not touch tablets or capsules with hands.

Pouring medication into the cap allows for easy return of excess medication to the bottle. Pouring tablets or capsules into your hand is unsanitary.

c. *Liquid medication in multidose bottle:* When pouring liquid medications out of a multidose bottle, hold the bottle so the label is against the palm. Use the appropriate measuring device when pouring liquids, and read the amount of medication at the bottom of the meniscus at eye level. Wipe the lip of the bottle with a paper towel.

Liquid that may drip onto the label makes the label difficult to read. Accuracy is possible when the appropriate measuring device is used and then read accurately.

10. **When all medications for one patient have been prepared, recheck the labels with the CMAR/MAR before taking the medications to the patient. Replace**

This is a *third* check to ensure accuracy and to prevent errors. Locking the cart or drawer safeguards the patient's medication supply. Hospital accrediting organizations require medication

ACTION	RATIONALE
any multidose containers in the patient's drawer or unit stock. Lock the medication cart before leaving it.	carts to be locked when not in use. Some facilities require the third check to occur at the bedside, after identifying the patient and before administration.
11. Transport medications to the patient's bedside carefully, and keep the medications in sight at all times.	Careful handling and close observation prevent accidental or deliberate disarrangement of medications.
12. Ensure that the patient receives the medications at the correct time.	Check agency policy, which may allow for administration within a period of 30 minutes before or 30 minutes after the designated time.
13. Perform hand hygiene and put on PPE, if indicated.	Hand hygiene and PPE prevent the spread of microorganisms. PPE is required based on transmission precautions.
14. Identify the patient. Usually, the patient should be identified using two methods. Compare the information with the CMAR/MAR.	Identifying the patient ensures that the right patient receives the medications and helps prevent errors.
a. Check the name and identification number on the patient's identification band.	This is the most reliable method. Replace the identification band if it is missing or inaccurate in any way.
b. Ask the patient to state his or her name and birth date, based on facility policy.	This requires a response from the patient, but illness and strange surroundings often cause patients to be confused.
c. If the patient cannot identify him- or herself, verify the patient's identification with a staff member who knows the patient, for the second source.	This is another way to double check identity. Do not use the name on the door or over the bed, because these signs may be inaccurate.
15. Scan the patient's bar code on the identification band, if required.	The bar code provides an additional check to ensure that the medication is given to the right patient.

ACTION	RATIONALE
16. **Complete necessary assessments before administering medications. Check the patient's allergy bracelet or ask the patient about allergies. Explain the purpose and action of each medication to the patient.**	Assessment is a prerequisite to administration of medications.
17. Assist the patient to an upright or lateral position.	Swallowing is facilitated by proper positioning. An upright or side-lying position protects the patient from aspiration.
18. Administer medications:	
a. Offer water or other permitted fluids with pills, capsules, tablets, and some liquid medications.	Liquids facilitate swallowing of solid drugs. Some liquid drugs are intended to adhere to the pharyngeal area, in which case liquid is not offered with the medication.
b. Ask whether the patient prefers to take the medications by hand or in a cup.	This encourages the patient's participation in taking the medications.
19. **Remain with the patient until each medication is swallowed. Never leave medication at the patient's bedside.**	Unless you have seen the patient swallow the drug, the drug cannot be recorded as administered. The patient's chart is a legal record. Only with a physician's order can medications be left at the bedside.
20. Assist the patient to a comfortable position. Remove PPE, if used. Perform hand hygiene.	Promotes patient comfort. Proper removal of PPE prevents transmission of microorganisms. Hand hygiene deters the spread of microorganisms.
21. Document the administration of the medication immediately after administration. See Documentation section below.	Timely documentation helps to ensure patient safety.
22. Evaluate the patient's response to medication within an appropriate time frame.	The patient needs to be evaluated for therapeutic and adverse effects from the medication.

EVALUATION

• Patient swallows the medication, does not aspirate, verbalizes an understanding of the medication, experiences the desired effect from the medication, and does not experience adverse effects.

DOCUMENTATION

• Record each medication administered on the CMAR/MAR or record using the required format immediately after it is administered, including date and time of administration. If using a bar-code system, medication administration is automatically recorded when the bar code is scanned. PRN medications require documentation of the reason for administration. Prompt recording avoids the possibility of accidentally repeating the administration of the drug. If the drug was refused or omitted, record this in the appropriate area on the medication record and notify the primary care provider. This verifies the reason medication was omitted and ensures that the primary care provider is aware of the patient's condition. Recording the administration of a narcotic may require additional documentation on a narcotic record, stating drug count and other specific information. Record fluid intake if intake and output measurement is required.

GENERAL CONSIDERATIONS

• Some liquid medication preparations, such as suspensions, require agitation to ensure even distribution of medication in the solution. Be familiar with the specific requirements for medications you are administering.
• Place medications intended for sublingual absorption under the patient's tongue. Instruct the patient to allow the medication to dissolve completely. Reinforce the importance of not swallowing the medication tablet.
• Some oral medications are provided in powdered forms. Verify the correct liquid in which to dissolve the medication for administration. This information is usually included on the package; verify any unclear instructions with a pharmacist or medication reference. If there is more than one possible liquid in which to dissolve the medication, include the patient in the decision process; patients may find one choice more palatable than another.
• Ongoing assessment is an important part of nursing care to evaluate patient response to administered medications and early detection of adverse effects. If an adverse effect is suspected, withhold further medication doses and notify the patient's primary care provider. Additional intervention is based on type of reaction and patient assessment.
• If the patient questions a medication order or states the medication is different from the usual dose, always recheck and clarify with the original order and/or primary care provider before giving the medication.

- If the patient's level of consciousness is altered or his or her swallowing is impaired, check with the primary care provider to clarify the route of administration or alternative forms of medication. This may also be a solution for a pediatric or a confused patient who is refusing to take a medication.
- Patients with poor vision can request large-type labels on medication containers. A magnifying lens also may be helpful.
- Provide written medication information to reinforce discussion and education in the appropriate language, if the patient is literate. If the patient is unable to read, provide written information to family/significant other, if appropriate. Written information should be at a 5th-grade level to ensure ease of understanding.
- If the patient has difficulty swallowing tablets, it may be appropriate to crush the medication to facilitate administration. However, not all medications can be crushed or altered; long-acting and slow-release drugs are examples of medications that cannot be crushed. Therefore, it is important to consult a medication reference and/or pharmacist. If the medication can be crushed, use a pill-crusher or mortar and pestle to grind the tablet into a powder. Crush each pill one at a time. Dissolve the powder with water or other recommended liquid in a liquid medication cup, keeping each medication separate from the others. Keep the package label with the medication cup for future comparison of information. Combine the crushed medication with a small amount of soft food, such as applesauce or pudding, to facilitate administration.
- Elderly patients with arthritis may have difficulty opening childproof caps. On request, the pharmacist can substitute a cap that is easier to open. A rubber band twisted around the cap may provide a more secure grip for older patients.
- Consider large-print written information when appropriate.
- Physiologic changes associated with the aging process, including decreased gastric motility, muscle mass, acid production, and blood flow, can affect the patient's response to medication, including drug absorption and increased risk of adverse effects. Older adults are more likely to take multiple drugs, so drug interactions in the older adult are a very real and dangerous problem.

Skill · 105   Removing Medication From an Ampule

An ampule is a glass flask that contains a single dose of medication for parenteral administration. Because there is no way to prevent contamination of any unused portion of medication after the ampule is opened if not all the medication is used, discard any remaining medication. Remove medication from an ampule after its thin neck is broken.

EQUIPMENT

- Sterile syringe and filter needle
- Ampule of medication
- Small gauze pad

- Computer-generated Medication Administration Record (CMAR) or Medication Administration Record (MAR)

ASSESSMENT GUIDELINES

- Assess the medication in the ampule for any particles or discoloration.
- Assess the ampule for any cracks or chips. Check expiration date before administering the medication.
- Verify patient name, dose, route, and time of administration.
- Assess the appropriateness of the drug for the patient.
- Review assessment and laboratory data that may influence drug administration.

NURSING DIAGNOSES

- Risk for Infection
- Anxiety
- Deficient Knowledge
- Risk for Injury

OUTCOME IDENTIFICATION AND PLANNING

Expected outcomes may include:
- Medication will be removed in a sterile manner; it will be free from glass shards and the proper dose prepared.

IMPLEMENTATION

ACTION	RATIONALE
1. Gather equipment. Check the medication order against the original order in the medical record, according to facility policy. Clarify any inconsistencies. Check the patient's chart for allergies.	This comparison helps to identify errors that may have occurred when orders were transcribed. The primary care provider's order is the legal record of medication orders for each facility.
2. Know the actions, special nursing considerations, safe dose ranges, purpose of administration, and adverse effects of the medications to be administered. Consider the appropriateness of the medication for this patient.	This knowledge aids the nurse in evaluating the therapeutic effect of the medication in relation to the patient's disorder and can also be used to educate the patient about the medication.

ACTION	RATIONALE
3. Perform hand hygiene.	Hand hygiene deters the spread of microorganisms.
4. Move the medication cart to the outside of the patient's room or prepare for administration in the medication area.	Organization facilitates error-free administration and saves time.
5. Unlock the medication cart or drawer. Enter pass code and scan employee identification, if required.	Locking the cart or drawer safeguards each patient's medication supply. Hospital accrediting organizations require medication carts to be locked when not in use. Entering pass code and scanning ID allows only authorized users into the system and identifies user for documentation by the computer.
6. **Prepare medications for one patient at a time.**	This prevents errors in medication administration.
7. Read the CMAR/MAR and select the proper medication from the patient's medication drawer or unit stock.	This is the *first* check of the label.
8. Compare the label with the CMAR/MAR. Check expiration dates and perform calculations, if necessary. Scan the bar code on the package, if required.	This is the *second* check of the label. Verify calculations with another nurse to ensure safety, if necessary.
9. Tap the stem of the ampule or twist your wrist quickly while holding the ampule vertically.	This facilitates movement of medication in the stem to the body of the ampule.
10. Wrap a small gauze pad around the neck of the ampule.	This will protect your fingers from the glass as the ampule is broken.
11. Use a snapping motion to break off the top of the ampule along the scored line at its neck (FIGURE 1).	This protects your face and fingers from any shattered glass fragments.

ACTION	RATIONALE

Always break away from your body.

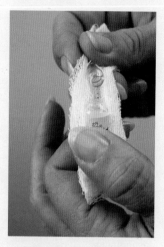

FIGURE 1 Using a snapping motion to break top of the ampule.

12. Attach filter needle to syringe. Remove the cap from the filter needle by pulling it straight off.	Use of a filter needle prevents the accidental withdrawing of small glass particles with the medication. Pulling the cap off in a straight manner prevents accidental needlestick.
13. Withdraw medication in the amount ordered plus a small amount more (approximately 30% more). **Do not inject air into the solution. Use either of the following methods. While inserting the filter needle into the ampule, be careful not to touch the rim.**	By withdrawing an additional small amount of medication, any air bubbles in the syringe can be displaced once the syringe is removed and there ample medication will still remain in the syringe. The contents of the ampule are not under pressure; therefore, air is unnecessary and will cause the contents to overflow. The rim of the ampule is considered contaminated.
a. Insert the tip of the needle into the ampule, which is upright on a flat surface, and withdraw fluid into	Handling the plunger at the knob only will keep the shaft of the plunger sterile.

ACTION	RATIONALE
the syringe. **Touch the plunger at the knob only.**	
b. Insert the tip of the needle into the ampule and invert the ampule. Keep the needle centered and not touching the sides of the ampule. Withdraw fluid into syringe. **Touch the plunger at the knob only.**	Surface tension holds the fluids in the ampule when inverted. If the needle touches the sides or is removed and then reinserted into the ampule, surface tension is broken, and fluid runs out. Handling the plunger at the knob only will keep the shaft of the plunger sterile.
14. Wait until the needle has been withdrawn to tap the syringe and expel the air carefully by pushing on the plunger. **Check the amount of medication in the syringe with the medication dose and discard any surplus, according to facility policy.**	Ejecting air into the solution increases pressure in the ampule and can force the medication to spill out over the ampule. Ampules may have overfill. Careful measurement ensures that the correct dose is withdrawn.
15. **Recheck the label with the CMAR/MAR.**	This is the *third* check to ensure accuracy and to prevent errors. Some facilities require the third check to occur at the bedside, after identifying the patient and before administration.
16. **Engage safety guard on filter needle and remove the needle. Discard the filter needle in a suitable container. Attach appropriate administration device to syringe.**	**The filter needle used to draw up medication should not be used to administer the medication, to prevent any glass shards from entering the patient.**
17. Discard the ampule in a suitable container.	Any medication that has not been removed from the ampule must be discarded because there is no way to maintain sterility of contents in an opened ampule.
18. Lock the medication cart before leaving it.	Locking the cart or drawer safeguards the patient's medication supply. Hospital accrediting organizations require medication carts to be locked when not in use.

ACTION	RATIONALE
19. Perform hand hygiene.	Hand hygiene deters the spread of microorganisms.
20. Proceed with administration, based on prescribed route.	See appropriate skill for prescribed route.

EVALUATION

• Medication is removed from the ampule in a sterile manner, free from glass shards, and the proper dose is prepared.

DOCUMENTATION

• It is not necessary to record the removal of the medication from the ampule. Record each medication administered on the CMAR/MAR or record using the required format immediately after it is administered, including date and time of administration. If using a bar-code system, medication administration is automatically recorded when the bar code scanned. PRN medications require documentation of the reason for administration. Prompt recording avoids the possibility of accidentally repeating the administration of the drug. If the drug was refused or omitted, record this in the appropriate area on the medication record and notify the primary care provider. This verifies the reason medication was omitted and ensures that the primary care provider is aware of the patient's condition. Recording administration of a narcotic may require additional documentation on a narcotic record, stating drug count and other specific information. Record fluid intake if intake and output measurement is required.

Skill · 106   Removing Medication From a Vial

A vial is a glass bottle with a self-sealing stopper through which medication is removed. For safety in transporting and storing, the vial top is usually covered with a soft metal cap that can be removed easily. The self-sealing stopper that is then exposed is the means of entrance into the vial. Single-dose vials are used once, then discarded, regardless of the amount of the drug that is used from the vial. Multidose vials contain several doses of medication and can be used multiple times. The Centers for Disease Control and Prevention (CDC) recommends that medications packaged as multiuse vials be assigned to a single patient whenever possible. In addition, it is recommended that the top of the vial be cleaned before each entry, as well as the use of a new sterile needle and syringe (CDC, 2008a; CDC, 2008b). The medication contained in a vial can be in liquid or powder form. Powdered forms must be dissolved in an appropriate diluent before administration. The following skill reviews removing liquid medication from a vial.

EQUIPMENT

- Sterile syringe and needle or blunt cannula (size depends on medication being administered and patient)
- Vial of medication
- Antimicrobial swab
- Second needle (optional)
- Filter needle (optional)
- Computer-generated Medication Administration Record (CMAR) or Medication Administration Record (MAR)

ASSESSMENT GUIDELINES

- Assess the medication in the vial for any discoloration or particles.
- Check expiration date before administering the medication.
- Verify patient name, dose, route, and time of administration.
- Assess the appropriateness of the drug for the patient.
- Review assessment and laboratory data that may influence drug administration.

NURSING DIAGNOSES

- Risk for Infection
- Risk for Injury
- Deficient Knowledge
- Anxiety

OUTCOME IDENTIFICATION AND PLANNING

Expected outcomes may include:
- Medication will be removed into a syringe in a sterile manner and that the proper dose is prepared.

IMPLEMENTATION

ACTION	RATIONALE
1. Gather equipment. Check the medication order against the original order in the medical record, according to facility policy.	This comparison helps to identify errors that may have occurred when orders were transcribed. The primary care provider's order

ACTION	RATIONALE
	is the legal record of medication orders for each facility.
2. Know the actions, special nursing considerations, safe dose ranges, purpose of administration, and adverse effects of the medication to be administered. Consider the appropriateness of the medication for this patient.	This knowledge aids the nurse in evaluating the therapeutic effect of the medication in relation to the patient's disorder and can also be used to educate the patient about the medication.
3. Perform hand hygiene.	Hand hygiene deters the spread of microorganisms.
4. Move the medication cart to the outside of the patient's room or prepare for administration in the medication area.	Organization facilitates error-free administration and saves time.
5. Unlock the medication cart or drawer. Enter pass code and scan employee identification, if required.	Locking the cart or drawer safeguards each patient's medication supply. Hospital accrediting organizations require medication carts to be locked when not in use. Entering pass code and scanning ID allows only authorized users into the system and identifies user for documentation by the computer.
6. **Prepare medications for one patient at a time.**	This prevents errors in medication administration.
7. Read the CMAR/MAR and select the proper medication from the patient's medication drawer or unit stock.	This is the *first* check of the label.
8. Compare the label with the CMAR/MAR. Check expiration dates and perform calculations, if necessary. Scan the bar code on the package, if required.	This is the *second* check of the label. Verify calculations with another nurse to ensure safety, if necessary.

ACTION	RATIONALE
9. Remove the metal or plastic cap on the vial that protects the rubber stopper.	Cap needs to be removed to access medication in vial.
10. **Swab the rubber top with the antimicrobial swab and allow to dry.**	Antimicrobial swab removes surface bacteria contamination. Allowing the alcohol to dry prevents it from entering the vial on the needle.
11. Remove the cap from the needle or blunt cannula by pulling it straight off. Touch the plunger at the knob only. Draw back an amount of air into the syringe that is equal to the specific dose of medication to be withdrawn. Some facilities require use of a filter needle when withdrawing premixed medication from multidose vials.	Pulling the cap off in a straight manner prevents accidental needlestick injury. Handling the plunger at the knob only will keep the shaft of the plunger sterile. Because a vial is a sealed container, before fluid is removed, injection of an equal amount of air is required to prevent the formation of a partial vacuum. If insufficient air is injected, the negative pressure makes it difficult to withdraw the medication. Using a filter needle prevents any solid material from being withdrawn through the needle.
12. Hold the vial on a flat surface. Pierce the rubber stopper in the center with the needle tip and inject the measured air into the space above the solution. Do not inject air into the solution.	Air bubbled through the solution could result in withdrawal of an inaccurate amount of medication.
13. **Invert the vial. Keep the tip of the needle or blunt cannula below the fluid level.**	This prevents air from being aspirated into the syringe.
14. Hold the vial in one hand and use the other to withdraw the medication. Touch the plunger at the knob only. **Draw up the prescribed amount of medication while holding the syringe vertically and at eye level.**	Handling the plunger at only the knob will keep the shaft of the plunger sterile. Holding the syringe at eye level facilitates accurate reading, and the vertical position makes removal of air bubbles from the syringe easy.

ACTION	RATIONALE
15. If any air bubbles accumulate in the syringe, tap the barrel of the syringe sharply and move the needle past the fluid into the air space to re-inject the air bubble into the vial. Return the needle tip to the solution and continue withdrawal of the medication.	Removal of air bubbles is necessary to ensure accurate dose of medication.
16. After the correct dose is withdrawn, remove the needle from the vial and carefully replace the cap over the needle. **If a filter needle has been used to draw up the medication, remove it and attach the appropriate administration device.** Some facilities require changing the needle, if one was used to withdraw the medication, before administering the medication.	This prevents contamination of the needle and protects against accidental needlesticks. A one-handed recap method may be used as long as care is taken not to contaminate the needle during the process. A filter needle used to draw up medication should not be used to administer the medication to prevent any solid material from entering the patient. Changing the needle may be necessary because passing the needle through the stopper on the vial may dull the needle.
17. **Check the amount of medication in the syringe with the medication dose and discard any surplus.**	Careful measurement ensures that correct dose is withdrawn.
18. **Recheck the label with the CMAR/MAR.**	This is the *third* check to ensure accuracy and to prevent errors. Some facilities require the third check to occur at the bedside, after identifying the patient and before administration.
19. **If a multidose vial is being used, label the vial with the date and time opened, and store the vial containing the remaining medication according to facility policy.**	Because the vial is sealed, the medication inside remains sterile and can be used for future injections. Labeling the opened vials with a date and time limits its use after a specific time period.

ACTION	RATIONALE
20. Lock the medication cart before leaving it.	Locking the cart or drawer safeguards the patient's medication supply. Hospital accrediting organizations require medication carts to be locked when not in use.
21. Perform hand hygiene.	Hand hygiene deters the spread of microorganisms.
22. Proceed with administration, based on prescribed route.	See appropriate skill for prescribed route.

EVALUATION

• Medication is withdrawn into the syringe in a sterile manner and the proper dose is prepared.

DOCUMENTATION

• It is not necessary to record the removal of the medication from the vial. Record each medication administered on the CMAR/MAR or record using the required format immediately after it is administered, including date and time of administration. If using a bar-code system, medication administration is automatically recorded when the bar code is scanned. PRN medications require documentation of the reason for administration. Prompt recording avoids the possibility of accidentally repeating the administration of the drug. If the drug was refused or omitted, record this in the appropriate area on the medication record and notify the primary care provider. This verifies the reason medication was omitted and ensures that the primary care provider is aware of the patient's condition. Recording administration of a narcotic may require additional documentation on a narcotic record, stating drug count and other specific information. Record fluid intake if intake and output measurement is required.

Skill · 107   **Applying a Transdermal Patch**

The transdermal route is being used more frequently to deliver medication. This involves applying to the patient's skin a disk or patch that contains medication intended for daily use or for longer intervals. Transdermal patches are commonly used to deliver hormones, narcotic analgesics, cardiac medications, and nicotine. Medication errors have occurred when patients apply multiple patches at once or fail to remove the overlay on the patch that exposes the skin to the medication. Narcotic analgesic patches are associated with the most adverse drug effects. Clear patches have a cosmetic advantage, but can be difficult to find on the patient's skin when they need to be removed or replaced.

EQUIPMENT
- Medication patch
- Gloves
- Scissors (optional)
- Washcloth, soap, and water
- Computer-generated Medication Administration Record

(CMAR) or Medication Administration Record (MAR)
- Additional PPE, as indicated

ASSESSMENT GUIDELINES
- Assess the patient for any allergies. Check the expiration date before administering medication. Assess the appropriateness of the drug for the patient.
- Review assessment and laboratory data that may influence drug administration.
- Verify patient name, dose, route, and time of administration.
- Assess the skin at the location where the patch will be applied. Many patches have different and specific instructions for where the patch is to be placed. For example, transdermal patches that contain estrogen can not be placed on breast tissue. The site should be clean, dry, and free of hair. Do not place transdermal patches on irritated or broken skin. Check the manufacturer's instructions for location of the patch.
- Assess the patient for any old patches. Do not place a new transdermal patch until old patches have been removed.
- Verify the application frequency for specific medication.
- Assess the patient's knowledge of the medication. If the patient has a knowledge deficit about the medication, this may be the appropriate time to begin education about the medication.
- If the medication may affect the patient's vital signs, assess them before administration.
- If the medication is for pain relief, assess the patient's pain before and after administration.

NURSING DIAGNOSES

• Risk for Allergy Response
• Deficient Knowledge
• Risk for Impaired Skin Integrity

OUTCOME IDENTIFICATION AND PLANNING

Expected outcomes may include:
• Medication is delivered via the transdermal route.
• Patient experiences no adverse effect.
• Patient's skin remains free from injury.
• Patient understands and complies with the medication regimen.

IMPLEMENTATION

ACTION

RATIONALE

1. Gather equipment. Check medication order against the original order in the medical record, according to facility policy. Clarify any inconsistencies. Check the patient's chart for allergies.

This comparison helps to identify errors that may have occurred when orders were transcribed. The primary care provider's order is the legal record of medication orders for each facility.

2. Know the actions, special nursing considerations, safe dose ranges, purpose of administration, and adverse effects of the medications to be administered. Consider the appropriateness of the medication for this patient.

This knowledge aids the nurse in evaluating the therapeutic effect of the medication in relation to the patient's disorder and can also be used to educate the patient about the medication.

3. Perform hand hygiene.

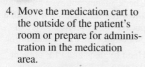

Hand hygiene prevents the spread of microorganisms.

4. Move the medication cart to the outside of the patient's room or prepare for administration in the medication area.

Organization facilitates error-free administration and saves time.

5. Unlock the medication cart or drawer. Enter pass code and scan employee identification, if required.

Locking of the cart or drawer safeguards each patient's medication supply. Hospital accrediting organizations require

ACTION	RATIONALE
	medication carts to be locked when not in use. Entering pass code and scanning ID allows only authorized users into the system and identifies user for documentation by the computer.
6. **Prepare medications for one patient at a time.**	This prevents errors in medication administration.
7. Read the CMAR/MAR and select the proper medication from the patient's medication drawer or unit stock.	This is the *first* check of the label.
8. Compare the label with the CMAR/MAR. Check expiration dates and perform calculations, if necessary. Scan the bar code on the package, if required.	This is the *second* check of the label. Verify calculations with another nurse to ensure safety, if necessary.
9. **When all medications for one patient have been prepared, recheck the label with the CMAR/MAR before taking them to the patient.**	This is a *third* check to ensure accuracy and to prevent errors. Some facilities require the third check to occur at the bedside, after identifying the patient and before administration.
10. Lock the medication cart before leaving it.	Locking the cart or drawer safeguards the patient's medication supply. Hospital accrediting organizations require medication carts to be locked when not in use.
11. Transport medications to the patient's bedside carefully, and keep the medications in sight at all times.	Careful handling and close observation prevent accidental or deliberate disarrangement of medications.
12. **Ensure that the patient receives the medications at the correct time.**	Check agency policy, which may allow for administration within a period of 30 minutes before or 30 minutes after designated time.
13. Perform hand hygiene and put on PPE, if indicated.	Hand hygiene and PPE prevent the spread of microorganisms. PPE is required based on transmission precautions.

ACTION	RATIONALE

14. Identify the patient. Usually, the patient should be identified using two methods. Compare information with the CMAR/MAR.

Identifying the patient ensures the right patient receives the medications and helps prevent errors.

   a. Check the name and identification number on the patient's identification band.

This is the most reliable method. Replace the identification band if it is missing or inaccurate in any way.

   b. Ask the patient to state his or her name and birth date, based on facility policy.

This requires a response from the patient, but illness and strange surroundings often cause patients to be confused.

   c. If the patient cannot identify him or herself, verify the patient's identification with a staff member who knows the patient for the second source.

This is another way to double-check identity. Do not use the name on the door or over the bed, because these signs may be inaccurate.

15. Complete necessary assessments before administering medications. Check the patient's allergy bracelet or ask the patient about allergies. Explain the purpose and action of each medication to the patient.

Assessment is a prerequisite to administration of medications.

16. Scan the patient's bar code on the identification band, if required.

This provides an additional check to ensure that the medication is given to the right patient.

17. Put on gloves.

Gloves protect the nurse when handling the medication on the transdermal patch.

18. Assess the patient's skin where patch is to be placed, looking for any signs of irritation or breakdown. Site should be clean, dry, and free of hair. Rotate application sites.

Transdermal patches should not be placed on skin that is irritated or broken down. Hair can prevent the patch from sticking to the skin. Rotating sites reduces risk for skin irritation.

19. **Remove any old transdermal patches from the patient's skin.** Fold the old

Leaving old patches on a patient while applying new ones may lead to delivery of a toxic level

ACTION	RATIONALE
patch in half with the adhesive sides sticking together and discard according to facility policy. Gently wash the area where the old patch was with soap and water.	of the drug. Folding sides together prevents accidental contact with remaining medication. Washing area with soap and water removes all traces of medication in that area.
20. Remove the patch from its protective covering. Initial and write the date and time of administration on the label side of the patch.	This allows for easy identification of application date and time.
21. Remove the covering on the patch without touching the medication surface. Apply the patch to the patient's skin. Use the palm of your hand to press firmly for about 10 seconds. Do not massage.	Touching the adhesive side may alter the amount of medication left on the patch. Pressing firmly for 10 seconds ensures that the patch stays on the patient's skin. Massaging site may increase absorption of medication.
22. Remove gloves and additional PPE, if used. Perform hand hygiene.	Removing PPE properly reduces the risk for infection transmission and contamination of other items. Hand hygiene prevents the spread of microorganisms.
23. Document the administration of the medication immediately after administration. See Documentation section below.	Timely documentation helps to ensure patient safety.
24. Evaluate the patient's response to medication within the appropriate time frame.	The patient needs to be evaluated for therapeutic and adverse effects from the medication.

EVALUATION

- Medication is delivered via the transdermal route.
- Patient experiences no adverse effect.
- Patient's skin remains intact and free from injury.
- Patient understands and complies with the medication regimen.

DOCUMENTATION

- Document the administration of the medication immediately after administration, including date, time, dose, route of administration, and site of administration on the CMAR/MAR or record using the required format. If using a bar-code system, medication administration is automatically recorded when the bar code is scanned. PRN medications require documentation of the reason for administration. Prompt recording avoids the possibility of accidentally repeating the administration of the drug. If the drug was refused or omitted, record this in the appropriate area on the medication record and notify the primary care provider. This verifies the reason medication was omitted and ensures that the primary care provider is aware of the patient's condition.

GENERAL CONSIDERATIONS

- Transdermal drug products have specific application sites, application intervals, and considerations. It is important to be knowledgeable about the specific drug administered. For example, fentanyl (Duragesic) may be applied to the chest, back, flank, and upper arm; is reapplied every three days; and patients may experience increased absorption with a temperature elevation higher than 102°F (Ball & Smith, 2008). Fentanyl iontophoretic transdermal system (Ionsys) may be applied to the chest or upper outer arm; it is reapplied every 24 hours or after 80 doses have been delivered, and contains metal parts, so should be removed before MRI, cardioversion, or defibrillation (Ball & Smith, 2008). Nitroglycerin (Minitran) may be placed on any hairless surface except on extremities below the knees or elbows, with the chest being the preferred site. It is reapplied every 12 to 14 hours, and patients should have a nitrate-free interval each day of 10 to 12 hours to ensure tolerance does not develop (Ball & Smith, 2008).
- Apply the patch at the same time of the day, according to the order and medication specifications.
- Check for dislodgement of the patch if the patient is active. Read information about the patch or consult with the pharmacist to determine reapplication schedule and procedure.
- Aluminum backing on a patch necessitates precautions if defibrillation is required. Burns and smoke may result.
- Assess for any skin irritation at application site. If necessary, remove the patch, wash the area carefully with soap and water, and allow skin to air dry. Apply a new patch at a different site. Assess the potential for adverse reaction.
- Ongoing assessment is an important part of nursing care to evaluate patient response to administered medications and early detection of adverse effects. If an adverse effect is suspected, withhold further medication doses and notify the patient's primary healthcare provider. Additional intervention is based on type of reaction and patient assessment.

Skill · 108   **Administering a Vaginal Cream**

Creams, foams, and tablets can be applied intravaginally using a narrow, tubular applicator with an attached plunger. Suppositories that melt when exposed to body heat are also administered by vaginal insertion. Suppositories should be refrigerated for storage. Time administration to allow the patient to lie down afterward to retain the medication.

EQUIPMENT

- Medication with applicator, if appropriate
- Water-soluble lubricant
- Perineal pad
- Washcloth, skin cleanser, and warm water
- Gloves
- Additional PPE, as indicated
- Computer-generated Medication Administration Record (CMAR) or Medication Administration Record (MAR)

ASSESSMENT GUIDELINES

- Assess the external genitalia and vaginal canal for redness, erythema, edema, drainage, or tenderness.
- Assess the patient for allergies.
- Verify patient name, dose, route, and time of administration.
- Assess the patient's knowledge of medication and procedure. If the patient has a knowledge deficit about the medication, this may be an appropriate time to begin education about the medication.
- Assess the patient's ability to cooperate with the procedure.

NURSING DIAGNOSES

- Deficient Knowledge
- Risk for Allergy Response
- Risk for Impaired Skin Integrity
- Acute Pain
- Anxiety

OUTCOME IDENTIFICATION AND PLANNING

Expected outcomes may include:
- Medication is administered successfully into the vagina.
- Patient understands the rationale for the vaginal instillation.
- Patient experiences no allergy response.
- Patient experiences no, or minimal, pain.
- Patient experiences minimal anxiety.

IMPLEMENTATION

ACTION	RATIONALE
1. Gather equipment. Check medication order against the original order in the medical record, according to facility policy. Clarify any inconsistencies. Check the patient's chart for allergies.	This comparison helps to identify errors that may have occurred when orders were transcribed. The primary care provider's order is the legal record of medication orders for each facility.
2. Know the actions, special nursing considerations, safe dose ranges, purpose of administration, and adverse effects of the medication to be administered. Consider the appropriateness of the medication for this patient.	This knowledge aids the nurse in evaluating the therapeutic effect of the medication in relation to the patient's disorder and can also be used to educate the patient about the medication.
3. Perform hand hygiene.	Hand hygiene prevents the spread of microorganisms.
4. Move the medication cart to the outside of the patient's room or prepare for administration in the medication area.	Organization facilitates error-free administration and saves time.
5. Unlock the medication cart or drawer. Enter pass code and scan employee identification, if required.	Locking of the cart or drawer safeguards each patient's medication supply. Hospital accrediting organizations require medication carts to be locked when not in use. Entering pass code and scanning ID allows only authorized users into the system and identifies user for documentation by the computer.
6. **Prepare medications for one patient at a time.**	This prevents errors in medication administration.
7. Read the CMAR/MAR and select the proper medication from the patient's medication drawer or unit stock.	This is the *first* check of the label.

ACTION	RATIONALE
8. Compare the label with the CMAR/MAR. Check expiration dates and perform calculations, if necessary. Scan the bar code on the package, if required.	This is the *second* check of the label. Verify calculations with another nurse to ensure safety, if necessary.
9. **When all medications for one patient have been prepared, recheck the label with the MAR before taking them to the patient.**	This is a *third* check to ensure accuracy and to prevent errors. Some facilities require the third check to occur at the bedside, after identifying the patient and before administration.
10. Lock the medication cart before leaving it.	Locking the cart or drawer safeguards the patient's medication supply. Hospital accrediting organizations require medication carts to be locked when not in use.
11. Transport medication to the patient's bedside carefully, and keep the medication in sight at all times.	Careful handling and close observation prevent accidental or deliberate disarrangement of medications.
12. **Ensure that the patient receives the medications at the correct time.**	Check agency policy, which may allow for administration within a period of 30 minutes before or 30 minutes after designated time.
13. Perform hand hygiene and put on PPE, if indicated.	Hand hygiene and PPE prevent the spread of microorganisms. PPE is required based on transmission precautions.
14. Identify the patient. Usually, the patient should be identified using two methods. Compare information with the CMAR/MAR.	Identifying the patient ensures the right patient receives the medications and helps prevent errors.
a. Check the name and identification number on the patient's identification band.	This is the most reliable method. Replace the identification band if it is missing or inaccurate in any way.
b. Ask the patient to state her name and birth date, based on facility policy.	This requires a response from the patient, but illness and strange surroundings often cause patients to be confused.

ACTION	RATIONALE
c. If the patient cannot identify herself, verify the patient's identification with a staff member who knows the patient for the second source.	This is another way to double-check identity. Do not use the name on the door or over the bed, because these signs may be inaccurate.
15. Complete necessary assessments before administering medications. Check the patient's allergy bracelet or ask the patient about allergies. Explain the purpose and action of the medication to the patient.	Assessment is a prerequisite to administration of medications.
16. Scan the patient's bar code on the identification band, if required.	Provides an additional check to ensure that the medication is given to the right patient.
17. Put on gloves.	Gloves protect the nurse from potential contact with contaminants and body fluids.
18. Ask the patient to void before inserting the medication.	Empties the bladder and helps to minimize pressure and discomfort during administration.
19. Position the patient so that she is lying on her back with the knees flexed. Maintain privacy with draping. Provide adequate light to visualize the vaginal opening.	Position provides access to vaginal canal and helps to retain medication in the canal. Draping limits exposure of the patient and promotes warmth and privacy. Adequate light facilitates ease of administration.
20. Spread labia with fingers, and cleanse area at vaginal orifice with washcloth and warm water, using a different corner of the washcloth with each stroke. Wipe from above the vaginal orifice downward toward the sacrum (front to back).	These techniques prevent contamination of vaginal orifice with debris surrounding the anus.
21. Remove gloves and put on new gloves.	Prevents spread of microorganisms.
22. Fill vaginal applicator with prescribed amount of cream.	This ensures the correct dosage of medication will be administered.

ACTION	RATIONALE
Alternately, remove the suppository from its wrapper and lubricate the round end with the water-soluble lubricant.	
23. Lubricate applicator with the lubricant, as necessary.	Ordinarily, lubrication is unnecessary, but it may be used to reduce friction while inserting the applicator.
24. Spread the labia with your nondominant hand and introduce applicator with your dominant hand gently, in a rolling manner, while directing it downward and backward.	This follows the normal contour of the vagina for its full length.
25. After applicator is properly positioned, labia may be allowed to fall in place if necessary to free the hand for manipulating the plunger. Push the plunger to its full length and then gently remove applicator with plunger depressed. Alternately, insert the rounded end of the suppository along the posterior wall of the canal. Insert to the length of the nurse's finger.	Pushing the plunger will gently deploy the cream into the vaginal orifice.
26. **Ask the patient to remain in the supine position for 5 to 10 minutes after insertion.** Offer the patient a perineal pad to collect drainage.	This gives the medication time to be absorbed in the vaginal cavity. As medication heats up, some medication may leak from vaginal orifice.
27. Dispose of applicator in appropriate receptacle or clean nondisposable applicator according to manufacturer's directions.	Disposal prevents transmission of microorganisms. Cleaning prepares the applicator for future use by patient.
28. Remove gloves and additional PPE, if used. Perform hand hygiene.	Removing PPE properly reduces the risk for infection transmission and contamination of other items. Hand hygiene prevents the spread of microorganisms.

ACTION	RATIONALE
29. Document the administration of the medication immediately after administration. See Documentation section below.	Timely documentation helps to ensure patient safety.
30. Evaluate the patient's response to medication within appropriate time frame.	The patient needs to be evaluated for therapeutic and adverse effects from the medication.

EVALUATION

- Patient receives the medication via the vagina.
- Patient understands the rationale for the medication administration.
- Patient experiences no allergy response.
- Patient experiences no or minimal discomfort.
- Patient experiences no or minimal anxiety.

DOCUMENTATION

- Document the administration of the medication immediately after administration, including date, time, dose, and route of administration on the CMAR/MAR or record using the required format. If using a bar-code system, medication administration is automatically recorded when the bar code is scanned. PRN medications require documentation of the reason for administration. Prompt recording avoids the possibility of accidentally repeating the administration of the drug. Document assessment, characteristics of any drainage, and the patient's response to the treatment, if appropriate. If the drug was refused or omitted, record this in the appropriate area on the medication record and notify the primary care provider. This verifies the reason medication was omitted and ensures that the primary care provider is aware of the patient's condition.

GENERAL CONSIDERATIONS

- Ongoing assessment is an important part of nursing care to evaluate patient response to administered treatments and early detection of adverse effects. If an adverse effect is suspected, notify the patient's primary healthcare provider. Additional intervention is based on type of reaction and patient assessment.

Skill · 109 Applying Montgomery Straps

Montgomery straps are prepared strips of nonallergenic tape with ties inserted through holes at one end. One set of straps is placed on either side of a wound, and the straps are tied like shoelaces to secure the dressings. When it is time to change the dressing, the straps are untied, the wound is treated, and then the straps are retied to hold the new dressing. Often a skin barrier is applied before the straps to protect the skin. The straps or ties need to be changed only if they become loose or soiled.

Montgomery straps are recommended to secure dressings on wounds that require frequent dressing changes, such as wounds with increased drainage. These straps allow the nurse to perform wound care without the need to remove adhesive strips, such as tape, with each dressing change, thus decreasing the risk of skin irritation and injury.

EQUIPMENT

- Clean disposable gloves
- Additional PPE, as indicated
- Dressings for wound care as ordered
- Commercially available Montgomery straps or 2- to 3-inch hypoallergenic tape and strings for ties
- Cleansing solution, usually normal saline
- Gauze pads
- Skin-protectant wipe
- Skin-barrier sheet (hydrocolloidal or nonhydrocolloidal)

ASSESSMENT GUIDELINES

- Assess the situation to determine the need for wound cleaning and a dressing change.
- Assess the integrity of any straps currently in use. Replace loose or soiled straps or ties.
- Confirm any medical orders relevant to wound care and any wound care included in the nursing plan of care.
- Assess the patient's level of comfort and the need for analgesics before wound care. Assess if the patient experienced any pain related to prior dressing changes and the effectiveness of interventions used to minimize the patient's pain.
- Assess the current dressing to determine if it is intact. Assess for excess drainage or bleeding or saturation of the dressing.
- Inspect the wound and the surrounding tissue. Assess the appearance of the wound for the approximation of wound edges, the color of the wound and surrounding area, and signs of dehiscence. Assess for the presence of sutures, staples, or adhesive closure strips. Note the stage of the healing process and characteristics of any drainage.
- Assess the surrounding skin for color, temperature, and edema, ecchymosis, or maceration.

NURSING DIAGNOSES

- Impaired Tissue Integrity
- Risk for Infection
- Risk for Injury
- Anxiety
- Acute Pain
- Disturbed Body Image
- Deficient Knowledge
- Impaired Skin Integrity
- Delayed Surgical Recovery

OUTCOME IDENTIFICATION AND PLANNING

Expected outcomes may include:

- Patient's skin is free from irritation and injury.
- Wound care is accomplished without contaminating the wound area, without causing trauma to the wound, and without causing the patient to experience pain or discomfort.
- Patient's wound continues to show signs of progression of healing.

IMPLEMENTATION

ACTION	RATIONALE
1. Review the medical orders for wound care or the nursing plan of care related to wound care.	Reviewing the order and plan of care validates the correct patient and correct procedure.
2. Gather the necessary supplies and bring to the bedside stand or overbed table.	Preparation promotes efficient time management and an organized approach to the task. Bringing everything to the bedside conserves time and energy. Arranging items nearby is convenient, saves time, and avoids unnecessary stretching and twisting of muscles on the part of the nurse.
3. Perform hand hygiene and put on PPE, if indicated.	Hand hygiene and PPE prevent the spread of microorganisms. PPE is required based on transmission precautions.
4. Identify the patient.	Identifying the patient ensures that the right patient receives the intervention and helps prevent errors.

ACTION	RATIONALE
5. Close curtains around bed and close door to room, if possible. Explain what you are going to do and why you are going to do it to the patient.	This ensures the patient's privacy. Explanation relieves anxiety and facilitates cooperation.
6. Assess the patient for possible need for nonpharmacologic pain-reducing interventions or analgesic medication before wound care dressing change. Administer appropriate prescribed analgesic. Allow sufficient time for analgesic to achieve its effectiveness before beginning the procedure.	Pain is a subjective experience influenced by past experience. Wound care and dressing changes can cause pain for some patients.
7. Place a waste receptacle at a convenient location for use during the procedure.	Having a waste container handy means that the soiled dressing may be discarded easily, without the spread of microorganisms.
8. Adjust bed to comfortable working height, usually elbow height of the caregiver (VISN 8 Patient Safety Center, 2009).	Having the bed at the proper height prevents back and muscle strain.
9. Assist the patient to a comfortable position that provides easy access to the wound area. Use a bath blanket to cover any exposed area other than the wound. Place a waterproof pad under the wound site.	Patient positioning and use of a bath blanket provide for comfort and warmth. Waterproof pad protects underlying surfaces.
10. Perform wound care and a dressing change as outlined in Skills 55, 56, 58 and 183, as ordered.	Wound care aids in healing and provides protection for the wound.
11. Put on clean gloves. Clean the skin on either side of the wound with the gauze, moistened with normal saline. Dry the skin.	Gloves prevent the spread of microorganisms. Cleaning and drying the skin prevents irritation and injury.

ACTION	RATIONALE
12. **Apply a skin protectant to the skin where the straps will be placed.**	Skin protectant minimizes the risk for skin breakdown and irritation.
13. Remove gloves.	Tape is easier to handle without gloves. Wound is covered with the dressing.
14. Cut the skin barrier to the size of the tape or strap. Apply the skin barrier to the patient's skin, near the dressing. Apply the sticky side of each tape or strap to the skin barrier sheet, so the openings for the strings are at the edge of the dressing (FIGURE 1). Repeat for the other side.	Skin barrier prevents skin irritation and breakdown.
15. Thread a separate string through each pair of holes in the straps. Tie one end of the string in the hole. Fasten the other end with the opposing tie, like a shoelace (FIGURE 2). **Do not secure too tightly.** Repeat according to the number of straps needed. If commercially prepared straps are used, tie strings like a shoelace. Note date and time of application on strap.	Ties hold the dressing in place. Tying the ties too tightly puts additional stress on the surrounding skin. Recording date and time provides a baseline for changing straps.

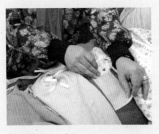

FIGURE 1 Applying Montgomery straps to the skin barrier on patient.

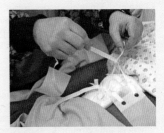

FIGURE 2 Tying Montgomery straps.

ACTION	RATIONALE
16. After securing the dressing, label dressing with date and time. Remove all remaining equipment; place the patient in a comfortable position, with side rails up and bed in the lowest position.	Recording date and time provides communication and demonstrates adherence to plan of care. Proper patient and bed positioning promotes safety and comfort.
17. Remove additional PPE, if used. Perform hand hygiene.	Removing PPE properly reduces the risk for infection transmission and contamination of other items. Hand hygiene prevents the spread of microorganisms.
18. Check all wound dressings every shift. More frequent checks may be needed if the wound is more complex or dressings become saturated quickly.	Checking dressings ensures the assessment of changes in patient condition and timely intervention to prevent complications.
19. Replace the ties and straps whenever they are soiled, or every 2 to 3 days. Straps can be reapplied onto skin barrier. Skin barrier can remain in place up to 7 days. Use a silicone-based adhesive remover to help remove the skin barrier.	Replacing soiled ties and straps prevents growth of pathogens. Minimizing removal of skin barrier prevents skin irritation and breakdown. A silicone-based adhesive remover allows for the easy, rapid, and painless removal without the associated problems of skin stripping (Rudoni, 2008; Stephen-Haynes, 2008).

EVALUATION

- Patient's skin is clean, dry, intact, and free from irritation and injury.
- Patient exhibits a clean wound area free of contamination and trauma.
- Patient verbalizes minimal to no pain or discomfort.
- Patient exhibits signs and symptoms indicative of progressive wound healing.

DOCUMENTATION

- Document the procedure, the patient's response, and your assessment of the area before and after application. Record a description of the wound, amount and character of the wound drainage, and an assessment of the surrounding skin. Note the type of dressing that was applied, including the application of skin protectant and a skin barrier. Document that Montgomery straps were applied to secure the dressings. Record the patient's response to the dressing care and associated pain assessment. Include any pertinent patient and family education.

GENERAL CONSIDERATIONS

- Guidelines from the Wound, Ostomy, Continence Nurses Society (WOCN) and National Pressure Ulcer Advisory Panel (NPUAP) recommend that clean gloves may be used to treat chronic wounds and pressure ulcers as long as the infection-control procedures are followed. The *no-touch technique* may be used within these guidelines. Clean gloves are used to handle dressing material. Irrigants and dressings are sterile. The wound is redressed by picking up dressing materials by the corner and placing the untouched side over the wound (NPUAP, 2007b; Wooten & Hawkins, 2005).

Skill · 110   **Moving a Patient Up in Bed With the Assistance of Another Nurse**

The patient is at risk for injuries from shearing forces while being moved. Evaluate the patient's condition, any activity restrictions, the patient's ability to assist with positioning and ability to understand directions, and the patient's body weight to decide how much additional assistance is needed. This is not a one-person task. Safe Patient Handling Algorithm 4 (in Skill 174) can assist in making decisions about patient handling and movement. Using assistance, appropriate lifting and repositioning devices, good body mechanics, and correct technique are important to avoid injuries to yourself and the patient. The procedure below describes moving a patient using a friction-reducing sheet.

EQUIPMENT

- Friction-reducing sheet or other friction-reducing device
- Nonsterile gloves, if indicated
- Additional caregivers to assist, based on assessment
- Full-body sling lift and cover sheet, if necessary, based on assessment and availability

ASSESSMENT GUIDELINES

- Review the medical record and nursing plan of care for conditions that may influence the patient's ability to move or to be positioned.
- Assess for tubes, IV lines, incisions, or equipment that may alter the positioning procedure.
- Assess the patient's level of consciousness, ability to understand and follow directions, and ability to assist with moving.
- Assess the patient's weight and your strength to determine the number of caregivers required to assist with the activity. Determine if there is a need for bariatric equipment.

- Assess the patient's skin for signs of irritation, redness, edema, or blanching.

NURSING DIAGNOSES

- Activity Intolerance
- Impaired Skin Integrity
- Risk for Injury
- Risk for Impaired Skin Integrity
- Acute Pain
- Impaired Bed Mobility
- Chronic Pain

OUTCOME IDENTIFICATION AND PLANNING

Expected outcomes may include:
- Patient remains free from injury and maintains proper body alignment during movement.
- Patient reports improved comfort.
- Patient's skin is clean, dry, and intact, without any redness, irritation, or breakdown.

IMPLEMENTATION

ACTION	RATIONALE
1. Review the medical record and nursing plan of care for conditions that may influence the patient's ability to move or to be positioned. Assess for tubes, IV lines, incisions, or equipment that may alter the positioning procedure. Identify any movement limitations. Consult patient handling algorithm, if available, to plan appropriate approach to moving the patient.	Reviewing the order and plan of care validates the correct patient and correct procedure. Identification of limitations and ability and use of an algorithm helps to prevent injury and aids in determining best plan for patient movement.
2. Perform hand hygiene and put on PPE, if indicated.	Hand hygiene and PPE prevent the spread of microorganisms. PPE is required based on transmission precautions.
3. Identify the patient. Explain the procedure to the patient.	Patient identification validates the correct patient and correct procedure. Discussion and explanation help allay anxiety and prepare the patient for what to expect.

ACTION	RATIONALE
4. Close curtains around bed or close the door to the room, if possible. Place the bed at an appropriate and comfortable working height, usually elbow height of the caregiver (VISN 8 Patient Safety Center, 2009). Adjust the head of the bed to a flat position or as low as the patient can tolerate. Placing the bed in slight Trendelenburg position aids movement, if the patient is able to tolerate it.	Closing the door or curtain provides for privacy. Proper bed height helps reduce back strain while you are performing the procedure. Flat positioning helps to decrease the gravitational pull of the upper body.
5. Remove all pillows from under the patient. Leave one at the head of the bed, leaning upright against the headboard.	Removing pillows from under the patient facilitates movement; placing a pillow at the head of the bed prevents accidental head injury against the top of the bed.
6. Position at least one nurse on either side of the bed, and lower both side rails.	Proper positioning and lowering the side rails facilitate moving the patient and minimize strain on the nurses.
7. If a friction-reducing sheet (or device) is not in place under the patient, place one under the patient's midsection.	A friction-reducing device supports the patient's weight and reduces friction during the repositioning.
8. Ask the patient (if able) to bend his or her legs and put his or her feet flat on the bed to assist with the movement.	Patient can use major muscle groups to push. Even if the patient is too weak to push on the bed, placing the legs in this fashion will assist with movement and prevent skin shearing on the heels.
9. Have the patient fold the arms across the chest. Have the patient (if able) lift the head with chin on chest.	Positioning in this manner provides assistance, reduces friction, and prevents hyperextension of the neck.
10. One nurse should be positioned on each side of the bed, at the patient's midsection, with feet spread shoulder width apart and one foot slightly in front of the other.	Doing so positions each nurse opposite the center of the body mass, lowers the center of gravity, and reduces the risk for injury.
11. If available on bed, engage mechanism to make the	Decreases friction and effort needed to move the patient.

ACTION	RATIONALE
bed surface firmer for repositioning.	
12. Grasp the friction-reducing sheet securely, close to the patient's body.	Having the sheet close to the body brings the patient's center of gravity closer to each nurse and provides for a secure hold.
13. Flex your knees and hips. Tighten your abdominal and gluteal muscles and keep your back straight.	Using the legs' large muscle groups and tightening muscles during transfer prevent back injury.
14. Shift your weight back and forth from your back leg to your front leg and count to three. On the count of three, move the patient up in bed. If possible, the patient can assist with the move by pushing with the legs. Repeat the process, if necessary, to get the patient to the right position.	The rocking motion uses the nurses' weight to counteract the patient's weight. Rocking develops momentum, which provides a smooth lift with minimal exertion by the nurses. If the patient assists, less effort is required by the nurses.
15. **Assist the patient to a comfortable position and readjust the pillows and supports, as needed. Return bed surface to normal position, if necessary. Raise the side rails. Place the bed in the lowest position. (FIGURE 1).**	Readjusting the bed with supports and side rails ensures patient safety and comfort.

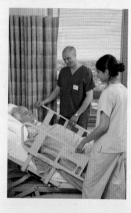

FIGURE 1 Adjusting bed to a safe and comfortable position.

ACTION	RATIONALE
16. Clean transfer aids per facility policy, if not indicated for single patient use. Remove gloves or other PPE, if used. Perform hand hygiene.	Proper cleaning of equipment between patient use prevents the spread of microorganisms. Removing PPE properly reduces the risk for infection transmission and contamination of other items. Hand hygiene prevents the spread of microorganisms.

EVALUATION

- Patient is moved up in bed without injury and maintains proper body alignment.
- Patient is comfortable.
- Patient demonstrates intact skin without evidence of any breakdown.

DOCUMENTATION

- Many facilities provide areas on the bedside flow sheet to document repositioning. Document the time of the patient's change of position, use of supports, and any pertinent observations, including skin assessment. Document the patient's tolerance of the position change. Document aids used to facilitate movement.

GENERAL CONSIDERATIONS

- When moving a patient with a leg or foot problem, such as a cast, wound, or fracture, one assistant should be assigned to lift and move that extremity.
- Calculate the Body Mass Index (BMI) for patients weighing over 300 pounds. If BMI exceeds 50, institute Bariatric Algorithms.

Skill · 111   Obtaining a Nasal Swab

A nasal swab provides a sample for culture to aid in the diagnosis of infection and detect the carrier state for certain organisms. A nasal swab may be used to diagnose infectious respiratory tract diseases, such as influenza. It is commonly used to detect the presence of organisms, such as *Staphylococcus aureus*, which may colonize on the skin in the nose, skin folds, hairline, perineum, and navel. These organisms often survive in these areas without causing infection, unless the organism invades the skin or deeper tissues (CDC, 2005). Some strains of *S. aureus* have developed resistance to antibiotics. A nasal swab can be part of the screening process to detect potential infection with drug-resistant microorganisms (Higgins, 2008e).

EQUIPMENT

- Nasal swab
- Sterile water (optional)
- Nonsterile gloves
- Additional PPE, as indicated
- Biohazard bag
- Appropriate label for specimen, based on facility policy and procedure

ASSESSMENT GUIDELINES

- Assess the patient's understanding of the collection procedure, reason for testing, and ability to cooperate.
- Inspect the patient's nares and for the presence of nasal symptoms, such as discharge, erythema, or congestion.
- Assess for conditions that would contraindicate obtaining a nasal swab, such as injury to the nares or nose, and surgery of nose.

NURSING DIAGNOSES

- Risk for Infection
- Acute Pain
- Deficient Knowledge

OUTCOME IDENTIFICATION AND PLANNING

Expected outcomes may include:

- An uncontaminated specimen is obtained without injury to the patient and sent to the laboratory promptly.
- Patient verbalizes an understanding of the rationale for the procedure.
- Patient verbalizes a decrease in anxiety related to specimen collection.

IMPLEMENTATION

ACTION	RATIONALE
1. Bring necessary equipment to the bedside stand or over-bed table. Check the expiration date on the swab package.	Bringing everything to the bedside conserves time and energy. Arranging items nearby is convenient, saves time, and avoids unnecessary stretching and twisting of muscles on the part of the nurse. Organization facilitates performance of tasks. Swab package is sterile and should not be used past expiration date.
2. Perform hand hygiene and put on PPE, if indicated.	Hand hygiene and PPE prevent the transmission of microorganisms. PPE is required based on transmission precautions.

ACTION	RATIONALE

3. Identify the patient. Discuss with the patient the need for a nasal swab. Explain to the patient the process by which the specimen will be collected.

Identifying the patient ensures the right patient receives the intervention and helps prevent errors. Discussion and explanation help to allay some of the patient's anxiety and prepare the patient for what to expect.

4. Check specimen label with patient identification bracelet. Label should include patient's name and identification number, time specimen was collected, route of collection, identification of the person obtaining the sample, and any other information required by agency policy.

Confirmation of patient identification information ensures the specimen is labeled correctly for the right patient.

5. Close curtains around bed or close the door to the room, if possible.

Closing the door or curtain provides for patient privacy.

6. Put on nonsterile gloves.

Gloves protect the nurse from exposure to blood or body fluids and prevent the transmission of microorganisms.

7. Ask the patient to tip his or her head back. Assist as necessary.

Tilting the head allows optimal access to the nares, which is where the swab will be inserted.

8. Peel open the swab packaging to expose the swab and collection tube. Remove the white plug from the collection tube and discard. Remove the swab from packaging by grasping the exposed end. Take care not to contaminate the swab by touching it to any other surface. Moisten with sterile water, depending on facility policy.

Swab must remain sterile to ensure the specimen is not contaminated. Moistening the end of the swab minimizes discomfort to the patient.

9. Insert swab 2 cm into one naris and rotate against the anterior nasal mucosa for 3 seconds or five rotations,

Contact with the mucosa is necessary to obtain potential pathogens.

ACTION	RATIONALE

depending on facility policy (FIGURE 1).

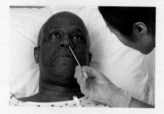

FIGURE 1 Inserting nasal swab into naris. (*Photo by B. Proud.*)

ACTION	RATIONALE
10. Remove the swab and repeat in the second naris, using the same swab.	Repeating in the second naris ensures accurate specimen.
11. Insert the swab fully into the collection tube, taking care not to touch any other surface. The handle end of the swab should fit snugly into the collection tube.	Swab must remain uncontaminated to ensure accurate results. Full insertion of the swab ensures it will remain in the collection tube.
12. Dispose of used equipment, per facility policy. Remove gloves. Perform hand hygiene.	Proper disposal of equipment reduces the transmission of microorganisms. Removing gloves properly reduces the risk for infection transmission and contamination of other items. Hand hygiene reduces the transmission of microorganisms.
13. Place label on the collection tube, per facility policy. Place container in plastic sealable biohazard bag.	Ensures specimen is labeled correctly for the right patient. Packaging the specimen in a biohazard bag prevents the person transporting the container from coming in contact with the specimen.
14. Remove other PPE, if used. Perform hand hygiene.	Removing PPE properly reduces the risk for infection transmission and contamination of other items. Hand hygiene reduces the transmission of microorganisms.

ACTION	RATIONALE
15. Transport specimen to laboratory immediately. If immediate transport is not possible, check with laboratory personnel or policy manual whether refrigeration is contraindicated.	Timely transport ensures accurate results.

EVALUATION

• The nasal swab is collected without contamination and sent to the laboratory as soon as possible.
• Patient does not experience injury.
• Patient verbalizes an understanding of the rationale for the specimen collection.
• Patient verbalizes a decrease in anxiety related to the procedure.

DOCUMENTATION

• Record the time the specimen was collected and sent to the laboratory. Document any pertinent assessments of the patient's nares and the presence of nasal symptoms, such as discharge, erythema, or congestion.

GENERAL CONSIDERATIONS

• If the patient has injury to the nares or nose or has had nose surgery, contact the physician or primary care provider to discuss the specimen collection. These conditions may prohibit collection.

Skill · 112   Obtaining a Nasopharyngeal Swab

A nasopharyngeal swab provides a sample for culture to aid in the diagnosis of infection and detect the carrier state for certain organisms. A swab on a flexible wire collects a specimen from the posterior nasopharynx. It is primarily used to detect viral infections. A nasopharyngeal swab is the optimal specimen for detection of *Bordetella pertussis* and *Corynebacterium diphtheriae*, as well as respiratory synctial virus, parainfluenza virus, and viruses causing rhinitis (Fischbach & Dunning, 2009).

EQUIPMENT

- Nasopharyngeal swab
- Penlight
- Tongue depressor
- Nonsterile gloves
- Additional PPE, as indicated
- Biohazard bag
- Appropriate label for specimen, based on facility policy and procedure

ASSESSMENT GUIDELINES

- Assess the patient's understanding of the collection procedure, reason for testing, and ability to cooperate.
- Assess the patient's nares and for the presence of nasal symptoms, such as discharge, erythema, or congestion.
- Inspect the patient's nasopharynx.
- Assess for conditions that would contraindicate obtaining a nasopharyngeal swab, such as injury to the nares or nose, and surgery of the nose or throat.

NURSING DIAGNOSES

- Risk for Infection
- Acute Pain
- Deficient Knowledge

OUTCOME IDENTIFICATION AND PLANNING

Expected outcomes may include:
- An uncontaminated specimen is obtained without injury to the patient and sent to the laboratory promptly.
- The patient verbalizes an understanding of the rationale for the procedure.
- The patient verbalizes a decrease in anxiety related to specimen collection.

IMPLEMENTATION

ACTION	RATIONALE
1. Bring necessary equipment to the bedside stand or overbed table. Check the expiration date on the swab package.	Bringing everything to the bedside conserves time and energy. Arranging items nearby is convenient, saves time, and avoids unnecessary stretching and twisting of muscles on the part of the nurse. Organization facilitates performance of tasks. Swab package is sterile and should not be used past expiration date.

ACTION	RATIONALE
2. Perform hand hygiene and put on PPE, if indicated.	Hand hygiene and PPE prevent the transmission of microorganisms. PPE is required based on transmission precautions.
3. Identify the patient. Discuss with patient the need for a nasopharyngeal swab. Explain to patient the process by which the specimen will be collected.	Identifying the patient ensures the right patient receives the intervention and helps prevent errors. Discussion and explanation help to allay some of the patient's anxiety and prepare the patient for what to expect.
4. Check the specimen label with the patient's identification bracelet. Label should include patient's name and identification number, time specimen was collected, route of collection, identification of person obtaining the sample, and any other information required by agency policy.	Confirmation of patient identification information ensures thespecimen is labeled correctly for the right patient.
5. Close curtains around bed or close the door to the room, if possible.	Closing the door or curtain provides for patient privacy.
6. Put on nonsterile gloves.	Gloves protect the nurse from exposure to blood or body fluids and prevent the transmission of microorganisms.
7. Ask the patient to cough tip back his or her head. Assist, as necessary.	Coughing clears the nasopharynx of material that may interfere with accurate sampling. Tilting the head allows optimal access to the nares, where the swab will be inserted.
8. Peel open the swab packaging to expose the swab and collection tube. Remove the cap from the collection tube and discard. Remove the swab from packaging by grasping the exposed end.	Swab must remain sterile to ensure specimen is not contaminated.

ACTION	RATIONALE
Take care not to contaminate the swab by touching it to any other surface.	
9. Ask the patient to open the mouth. Inspect the back of the patient's throat using the tongue depressor.	The swab must make contact with mucosa to ensure collection of potential pathogens.
10. Continue to observe the nasopharynx and insert the swab approximately 6 inches (adult) through one naris to the nasopharynx. Rotate the swab. Leave the swab in the nasopharynx for 15 to 30 seconds and remove. Take care not to touch the swab to the patient's tongue or sides of the nostrils.	Observation of nasopharynx during collection ensures an accurate specimen is collected. Swab must remain uncontaminated to ensure accurate results.
11. Insert the swab fully into the collection tube, taking care not to touch any other surface. The handle end of the swab should fit snugly into the collection tube.	Swab must remain uncontaminated to ensure accurate results. Full insertion of the swab ensures it will remain in the collection tube.
12. Dispose of used equipment per facility policy. Remove gloves. Perform hand hygiene.	Proper disposal of equipment reduces the transmission of microorganisms. Removing gloves properly reduces the risk for infection transmission and contamination of other items. Hand hygiene reduces the transmission of microorganisms.
13. Place label on the collection tube per facility policy. Place container in plastic sealable biohazard bag.	Ensures specimen is labeled correctly for the right patient. Packaging the specimen in a biohazard bag prevents the person transporting the container from coming in contact with the specimen.
14. Remove other PPE, if used. Perform hand hygiene.	Removing PPE properly reduces the risk for infection transmission and contamination of other items. Hand hygiene reduces the transmission of microorganisms.

ACTION	RATIONALE
15. Transport the specimen to the laboratory immediately. If immediate transport is not possible, check with laboratory personnel or policy manual whether refrigeration is contraindicated.	Timely transport ensures accurate results.

EVALUATION
- The nasopharyngeal swab is collected without contamination and sent to the laboratory as soon as possible.
- Patient does not experience injury.
- Patient verbalizes an understanding of the rationale for the specimen collection.
- Patient verbalizes a decrease in anxiety related to the procedure.

DOCUMENTATION
- Record the time the specimen was collected and sent. Document any pertinent assessments of the patient's nares and the presence of nasal symptoms, such as discharge, erythema, or congestion. Record significant assessments of the patient's oral cavity and throat.

GENERAL CONSIDERATIONS
- Warn the patient the procedure may cause slight discomfort.
- Caution the patient the procedure may cause gagging.

Skill · 113 **Inserting a Nasogastric (NG) Tube**

The nasogastric (NG) tube is passed through the nose and into the stomach. This type of tube permits the patient to receive nutrition through a tube feeding using the stomach as a natural reservoir for food. Another purpose of an NG tube may be to decompress or to drain unwanted fluid and air from the stomach. This application would be used, for example, to allow the intestinal tract to rest and promote healing after bowel surgery. The NG tube can also be used to monitor bleeding in the gastrointestinal (GI) tract, to remove undesirable substances (lavage), such as poisons, or to help treat an intestinal obstruction.

EQUIPMENT

- Nasogastric tube of appropriate size (8–18 French)
- Stethoscope
- Water-soluble lubricant
- Normal saline solution or sterile water, for irrigation, depending on facility policy
- Tongue blade
- Irrigations set, including a Toomey (20 to 50 mL)
- Flashlight
- Nonallergenic tape (1-inch wide)
- Tissues
- Glass of water with straw
- Topical anesthetic (lidocaine spray or gel) (optional)
- Clamp
- Suction apparatus (if ordered)
- Bath towel or disposable pad
- Emesis basin
- Safety pin and rubber band
- Nonsterile disposable gloves
- Additional PPE, as indicated
- Tape measure, or other measuring device
- Skin barrier
- pH paper

ASSESSMENT GUIDELINES

- Assess the patency of the patient's nares by asking the patient to occlude one nostril and breathe normally through the other. Select the nostril through which air passes more easily.
- Assess the patient's history for any recent facial trauma, polyps, blockages, or surgeries. Patients with facial fractures or facial surgeries present a higher risk for misplacement of the tube into the brain. Many institutions require a physician or advanced practice professional to place NG tubes in these patients.
- Inspect the abdomen for distention and firmness; auscultate for bowel sounds or peristalsis and palpate the abdomen for distention and tenderness. If the abdomen is distended, consider measuring the abdominal girth at the umbilicus to establish a baseline.

NURSING DIAGNOSES

- Imbalanced Nutrition, Less than Body Requirements
- Risk for Aspiration
- Deficient Knowledge
- Impaired Swallowing
- Risk for Disturbance in Body Image
- Acute Pain
- Nausea

OUTCOME IDENTIFICATION AND PLANNING

Expected outcomes may include:
- Nasogastric tube is passed into the patient's stomach without any complications.
- Patient demonstrates weight gain, indicating improved nutrition.
- Patient exhibits no signs and symptoms of aspiration.
- Patient rates pain as decreased from before insertion.
- Patient verbalizes an understanding of the reason for NG tube insertion.

IMPLEMENTATION

ACTION	RATIONALE

1. Verify the medical order for insertion of an NG tube.

Ensures the patient receives the correct treatment.

2. Perform hand hygiene and put on PPE, if indicated.

Hand hygiene and PPE prevent the spread of microorganisms. PPE is required based on transmission precautions.

3. Identify the patient.

Identifying the patient ensures the right patient receives the intervention and helps prevent errors.

4. Explain the procedure to the patient and explain the rationale why the tube is needed. Discuss the associated discomforts that may be experienced and possible interventions that may allay this discomfort. Answer any questions, as needed.

Explanation facilitates patient cooperation. Some patient surveys report that of all routine procedures, the insertion of an NG tube is considered the most painful. A lidocaine gel or spray is a possible option to decrease discomfort during NG tube insertion.

5. Gather equipment and select the appropriate NG tube.

This provides for an organized approach to task. NG tubes should be radioopaque, contain clearly visible markings for measurement, and may have multiple ports for aspiration.

6. Close the patient's beside curtain or door. Raise bed to a comfortable working position, usually elbow height of the caregiver (VISN 8 Patient Safety Center, 2009). Assist the patient to high Fowler's position or elevate the head of the bed 45 degrees if the patient is unable to maintain an upright position. Drape chest with bath towel or disposable pad. Have emesis basin and tissues handy.

Closing curtains or door provides for patient privacy. Having the bed at the proper height prevents back and muscle strain. Upright position is more natural for swallowing and protects against bronchial intubation aspiration, if the patient should vomit. Passage of tube may stimulate gagging and tearing of eyes.

ACTION	RATIONALE

7. **Measure the distance to insert tube by placing tip of tube at patient's nostril and extending to tip of earlobe and then to tip of xiphoid process (FIGURES 1 and 2). Mark tube with an indelible marker.**

Measurement ensures that tube will be long enough to enter patient's stomach.

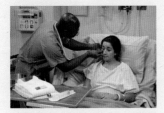

FIGURE 1 Measuring NG tube from nostril to tip of earlobe.

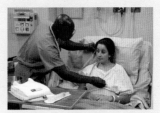

FIGURE 2 Measuring NG tube from tip of earlobe to xiphoid process.

8. Put on gloves. Lubricate tube tip (at least 2 to 4 inches) with water-soluble lubricant. Apply topical anesthetic to nostril and oropharynx, as appropriate.

Lubrication reduces friction and facilitates passage of the tube into the stomach. Water-soluble lubricant will not cause pneumonia if the tube accidentally enters the lungs. Topical anesthetics act as local anesthetics, reducing discomfort. Consult the primary care provider for an order for a topical anesthetic, such as lidocaine gel or spray, if needed.

9. After selecting the appropriate nostril, ask the patient to slightly flex head back against the pillow. Gently insert the tube into the nostril while directing the tube upward and backward along the floor of the nose. Patient may gag when tube reaches pharynx. Provide tissues for tearing or watering of eyes. Offer comfort and reassurance to the patient.

Following the normal contour of the nasal passage while inserting the tube reduces irritation and the likelihood of mucosal injury. The tube stimulates the gag reflex readily. Tears are a natural response as the tube passes into the nasopharynx. Many patients report that gagging and throat discomfort can be more painful than passing through the nostrils.

ACTION	RATIONALE

10. When pharynx is reached, instruct the patient to touch chin to chest. Encourage patient to sip water through a straw or swallow even if no fluids are permitted. Advance tube in downward and backward direction when patient swallows. Stop when patient breathes. **If gagging and coughing persist, stop advancing the tube and check placement of tube with tongue blade and flashlight.** If tube is curled, straighten it and attempt to advance it again. Keep advancing the tube until pen marking is reached. **Do not use force. Rotate tube if it meets resistance.**

Bringing the head forward helps close the trachea and open the esophagus. Swallowing helps advance the tube, causes the epiglottis to cover the opening of the trachea, and helps to eliminate gagging and coughing. Excessive coughing and gagging may occur if the tube has curled in the back of throat. Forcing the tube may injure mucous membranes.

11. **Discontinue procedure and remove tube if there are signs of distress, such as gasping, coughing, cyanosis, and inability to speak or hum.**

The tube is in the airway if the patient shows signs of distress and cannot speak or hum. If after three attempts, nasogastric insertion is unsuccessful, another nurse may try or the patient should be referred to another healthcare professional.

12. Secure the tube loosely to the nose or cheek until it is determined that the tube is in the patient's stomach:

Securing with tape stabilizes the tube while position is being determined.

   a. Attach syringe to end of tube and aspirate a small amount of stomach contents.

The tube is in the stomach if its contents can be aspirated: pH of aspirate can then be tested to determine gastric placement. If unable to obtain specimen, reposition the patient and flush the tube with 30 mL of air. This action may be necessary several times. Current literature recommends that the nurse ensures proper placement of the NG tube

ACTION	RATIONALE
	by relying on multiple methods and not on one method alone.
b. Measure the pH of aspirated fluid using pH paper or a meter. Place a drop of gastric secretions onto pH paper or place small amount in plastic cup and dip the pH paper into it. Within 30 seconds, compare the color on the paper with the chart supplied by the manufacturer.	Current research demonstrates that the use of pH is predictive of correct placement. The pH of gastric contents is acidic (less than 5.5). If the patient is taking an acid-inhibiting agent, the range may be 4.0 to 6.0. The pH of intestinal fluid is 7.0 or higher. The pH of respiratory fluid is 6.0 or higher. This method will not effectively differentiate between intestinal fluid and pleural fluid.
c. Visualize aspirated contents, checking for color and consistency.	Gastric fluid can be green with particles, off-white, or brown if old blood is present. Intestinal aspirate tends to look clear or straw-colored to a deep golden-yellow color. Also, intestinal aspirate may be greenish-brown if stained with bile. Respiratory or tracheobronchial fluid is usually off-white to tan and may be tinged with mucus. A small amount of blood-tinged fluid may be seen immediately after NG insertion.
d. Obtain radiograph (x-ray) of placement of tube, based on facility policy (and ordered by physician).	The x-ray is considered the most reliable method for identifying the position of the NG tube.
13. Apply skin barrier to tip and end of nose and allow to dry. Remove gloves and secure tube with a commercially prepared device (follow manufacturer's directions) or tape to patient's nose. To secure with tape:	Skin barrier improves adhesion and protects skin. Constant pressure of the tube against the skin and mucous membranes may cause tissue injury. Securing tube prevents migration of the tube inward and outward.
a. Cut a 4-inch piece of tape and split bottom 2 inches or use packaged nose tape for NG tubes.	

ACTION	RATIONALE

b. Place unsplit end over bridge of patient's nose.

c. Wrap split ends under tubing and up and over onto nose. **Be careful not to pull tube too tightly against nose.**

14. Put on gloves. Clamp tube and remove the syringe. Cap the tube or attach tube to suction, according to the medical orders.

Suction provides for decompression of stomach and drainage of gastric contents.

15. Measure length of exposed tube. Reinforce marking on tube at nostril with indelible ink. Ask the patient to turn the head to the side opposite the nostril in which the tube is inserted. Secure tube to patient's gown by using rubber band or tape and safety pin. For additional support, tube can be taped onto patient's cheek using a piece of tape. **If a double-lumen tube (e.g., Salem sump) is used, secure vent above stomach level.** Attach at shoulder level.

Tube length should be checked and compared with this initial measurement, in conjunction with pH measurement and visual assessment of aspirate. An increase in the length of the exposed tube may indicate dislodgement (Bourgault, et al., 2007; Smeltzer et al., 2010). The tube should be marked with an indelible marker at the nostril. This marking should be assessed each time the tube is used to ensure the tube has not become displaced. Securing prevents tension and tugging on the tube. Turning the head ensures adequate slack in the tubing to prevent tension when the patient turns the head. Securing the double-lumen tube above stomach level prevents seepage of gastric contents and keeps the lumen clear for venting air.

16. Assist with or provide oral hygiene at 2- to 4-hour intervals. Lubricate the lips generously and clean nares and lubricate, as needed. Offer analgesic throat lozenges or anesthetic spray for throat irritation, if needed.

Oral hygiene keeps mouth clean and moist, promotes comfort, and reduces thirst.

ACTION	RATIONALE
17. Remove equipment and return patient to a position of comfort. Remove gloves. Raise side rail and lower bed.	Promotes patient comfort and safety. Removing gloves properly reduces the risk for infection transmission and contamination of other items.
18. Remove additional PPE, if used. Perform hand hygiene.	Removing PPE properly reduces the risk for infection transmission and contamination of other items. Hand hygiene prevents transmission of microorganisms.

EVALUATION

- Patient exhibits a nasogastric tube placed into the stomach without any complications.
- Patient demonstrates weight gain, indicating improved nutrition.
- Patient remains free of any signs and symptoms of aspiration.
- Patient rates pain as decreased from before insertion.
- Patient verbalizes an understanding of the reason for NG tube insertion.

DOCUMENTATION

- Document the size and type of NG tube that was inserted and the measurement from the tip of the nose to the end of the exposed tube. Document the results of the x-ray that was taken to confirm the position of the tube, if applicable. Record a description of the gastric contents, including the pH of the contents. Document the naris where the tube is placed and the patient's response to the procedure. Include assessment data, both subjective and objective, related to the abdomen. Record the patient teaching that was discussed.

GENERAL CONSIDERATIONS

To promote patient safety when administering a tube feeding, be sure to do the following:

- Check tube placement before administering any fluids, medications, or feedings. Use multiple techniques: x-ray, external length marking/measurement, pH testing, and aspirate characteristics.
- Some patients require a nasointestinal tube. To insert a nasointestinal tube:
  - Measure tube from tip of nose to ear lobe and from ear lobe to xiphoid process. Add 8 to 10 inches for intestinal placement. Mark tubing at desired point.

- Place patient on his or her right side. Nasointestinal tube is usually placed in the stomach and allowed to advance through peristalsis through the pyloric sphincter (may take up to 24 hours).
- Administer medications to enhance GI motility, such as metoclopramide (Reglan), if ordered.
- Test pH of aspirate when tube has advanced to marked point to confirm placement in intestine. Confirm position by radiograph. Secure with tape once placement is confirmed.
- Monitoring for carbon dioxide to determine NG tube position and/or dislodgement has been investigated (May, 2007; Munera-Seeley, et al., 2008). This involves the use of a capnograph or a colorimetric end-tidal CO_2 detector to detect the presence of carbon dioxide, which would indicate tube positioning in the patient's airway instead of the stomach.

Skill · 114   Irrigating a Nasogastric Tube Connected to Suction

Nasogastric tubes can be used to decompress the stomach and to monitor for GI bleeding. The tube is usually attached to suction when used for these reasons or the tube may be clamped. The tube must be kept free from obstruction or clogging and is usually irrigated every 4 to 6 hours.

EQUIPMENT

- NG tube connected to continuous or intermittent suction
- Normal saline solution for irrigation
- Nonsterile gloves
- Additional PPE, as indicated
- Irrigation set (or a 60-mL catheter-tip syringe and cup for irrigating solution)
- Clamp
- Disposable pad or bath towel
- Emesis basin
- Tape measure, or other measuring device
- pH paper and measurement scale

ASSESSMENT GUIDELINES

- Assess abdomen by inspecting for presence of distention, auscultating for bowel sounds, and palpating the abdomen for firmness or tenderness. If the abdomen is distended, consider measuring the abdominal girth at the umbilicus.
- If the NG tube is attached to suction, assess suction to ensure that it is running at the prescribed pressure.
- Inspect drainage from NG tube, including color, consistency, and amount.

NURSING DIAGNOSES
• Imbalanced Nutrition: Less than Body Requirements
• Risk for Injury
• Risk for Deficient Fluid Volume Deficit

OUTCOME IDENTIFICATION AND PLANNING
Expected outcomes may include:
• Patency of the nasogastric tube will be maintained.
• Patient will not experience any trauma or injury.

IMPLEMENTATION

ACTION	RATIONALE
1. Assemble equipment. Verify the medical order or facility policy and procedure regarding frequency of irrigation, solution type, and amount of irrigant. Check expiration dates on irrigating solution and irrigation set.	Assembling equipment provides for organized approach to task. Verification ensures the patient receives correct intervention. Agency policy dictates safe interval for reuse of equipment.
2. Perform hand hygiene and put on PPE, if indicated.	Hand hygiene and PPE prevent the spread of microorganisms. PPE is required based on Transmission Precautions.
3. Identify the patient.	Identifying the patient ensures the right patient receives the intervention and helps prevent errors.
4. Explain the procedure to the patient and why this intervention is needed. Answer any questions, as needed. Perform key abdominal assessments as described above.	Explanation facilitates patient cooperation. Due to potential changes in patient's condition, assessment is vital before initiating intervention.
5. Pull the patient's bedside curtain. Raise bed to a comfortable working position, usually elbow height of the	Provides for privacy. Appropriate working height facilitates comfort and proper body mechanics for the nurse. This position

ACTION	RATIONALE
caregiver (VISN 8 Patient Safety Center, 2009). Assist patient to 30- to 45-degree position, unless this is contraindicated. Pour the irrigating solution into container.	minimizes risk for aspiration. Preparing the irrigation provides organized approach to the task.
6. Put on gloves. **Check placement of NG tube.** (Refer to Skill 113.)	Checking placement before the instillation of fluid is necessary to prevent accidental instillation into the respiratory tract if the tube has become dislodged.
7. Draw up 30 mL of saline solution (or amount indicated in the order or policy) into syringe.	This delivers measured amount of irrigant through tube. Saline solution (isotonic) compensates for electrolytes lost through nasogastric drainage.
8. Clamp suction tubing near connection site. If needed, disconnect tube from suction apparatus and lay on disposable pad or towel, or hold both tubes upright in nondominant hand.	Clamping protects patient from leakage of NG drainage.
9. Place tip of syringe in tube. **If Salem sump or doublelumen tube is used, make sure that syringe tip is placed in drainage port and not in blue air vent.** Hold syringe upright and gently insert the irrigant (or allow solution to flow in by gravity if agency policy or physician indicates). **Do not force solution into tube.**	Gentle insertion of saline solution (or gravity insertion) is less traumatic to gastric mucosa. The blue air vent acts to decrease pressure built up in the stomach when the Salem sump is attached to suction. It is not to be used for irrigation.
10. **If unable to irrigate tube, reposition patient and attempt irrigation again. Inject 10 to 20 mL of air and aspirate again. Check with primary care provider or follow agency policy, if repeated attempts to irrigate tube fail.**	Tube may be positioned against gastric mucosa, making it difficult to irrigate. Injection of air may reposition end of tube.

ACTION	RATIONALE
11. After irrigant has been instilled, hold end of NG tube over irrigation tray or emesis basin. Observe for return flow of NG drainage into available container. Alternately, you may reconnect the NG tube to suction and observe the return drainage as it drains into the suction container.	Return flow may be collected in an irrigating tray or other available container and measured. This amount will need to be subtracted from the irrigant to record the true NG drainage. A second method involves subtracting the total irrigant from the shift from the total NG drainage emptied over the entire shift, to find the true NG drainage. Check agency policy for guidelines. Observation determines patency of tube and correct operation of suction apparatus.
12. **If not already done, reconnect drainage port to suction, if ordered.**	Allows for continued removal of gastric contents as ordered.
13. **Inject air into blue air vent after irrigation is complete. Position the blue air vent above the patient's stomach.**	Following irrigation, the blue air vent is injected with air to keep it clear. Positioning the blue air vent above the stomach prevents the stomach contents from leaking from the NG tube.
14. Remove gloves. Lower the bed and raise side rails, as necessary. Assist the patient to a position of comfort. Perform hand hygiene.	Lowering bed and assisting the patient to a comfortable position promote safety and comfort.
15. Put on gloves. Measure returned solution, if collected outside of suction apparatus. Rinse equipment if it will be reused. Label with the date, patient's name, room number, and purpose (for NG tube/irrigation).	Gloves prevent contact with blood and body fluids. Irrigant placed in tube is considered intake; solution returned is recorded as output. Record on the intake and output record. Rinsing promotes cleanliness and infection control, and prepares equipment for next irrigation.
16. Remove gloves and additional PPE, if used. Perform hand hygiene.	Removing PPE properly reduces the risk for infection transmission and contamination of other items. Hand hygiene prevents transmission of microorganisms.

EVALUATION

• Patient demonstrates a patent and functioning NG tube.
• Patient reports no distress with irrigation.
• Patient remains free of any signs and symptoms of injury or trauma.

DOCUMENTATION

• Document assessment of the patient's abdomen. Record if the patient's NG tube is clamped or connected to suction, including the type of suction. Document the color and consistency of the NG drainage. Record the solution type and amount used to irrigate the NG tube, as well as ease of irrigation or if there was any difficulty related to the procedure. Record the amount of returned irrigant, if collected outside of the suction apparatus. Alternately, record irrigant amount so it can be subtracted from total NG drainage amount at the end of the shift. Record the patient's response to the procedure and any pertinent teaching points that were reviewed, such as instructions for the patient to contact the nurse for any feelings of nausea, bloating, or abdominal pain.

GENERAL CONSIDERATIONS

• A one-way antireflux valve may be used in the airflow lumen to prevent reflux of gastric contents through the airflow lumen. When pressure from gastric contents enters the airflow tubing, the valve closes to prevent secretions from exiting the tube. This valve is removed before flushing the lumen with air, and then replaced.

Skill · 115   Removing a Nasogastric Tube

When the NG tube is no longer necessary for treatment, the physician will order the tube to be removed. The NG tube is removed as carefully as it was inserted, to provide as much comfort as possible for the patient and to prevent complications. When the tube is removed, the patient must hold his or her breath to prevent aspiration of any secretions or fluid left in the tube as it is removed.

EQUIPMENT

• Tissues
• 50-mL syringe (optional)
• Nonsterile gloves
• Additional PPE, as indicated
• Stethoscope

• Disposable plastic bag
• Bath towel or disposable pad
• Normal saline solution for irrigation (optional)
• Emesis basin

ASSESSMENT GUIDELINES

• Perform an abdominal assessment by inspecting for the presence of distention; auscultating for bowel sounds; and palpating the abdomen for firmness or tenderness. If the abdomen is distended, consider measuring the abdominal girth at the umbilicus. If the patient reports any tenderness or nausea, exhibits any rigidity or firmness with distention, and if there is an absence of bowel sounds, confer with the primary care provider before discontinuing the NG tube.

• Assess any output from the NG tube, noting amount, color, and consistency.

NURSING DIAGNOSES

• Readiness for Enhanced Nutrition
• Risk for Aspiration

OUTCOME IDENTIFICATION AND PLANNING

Expected outcomes may include:
• Nasogastric tube is removed with minimal discomfort to the patient.
• Patient maintains an adequate nutritional intake.
• Patient's abdomen remains free from distention and tenderness.

IMPLEMENTATION

ACTION	RATIONALE
1. Check medical order for removal of NG tube.	This ensures correct implementation of physician's order.
2. Perform hand hygiene and put on PPE, if indicated.	Hand hygiene and PPE prevent the spread of microorganisms. PPE is required based on transmission precautions.
3. Identify the patient.	Identifying the patient ensures the right patient receives the intervention and helps prevent errors.
4. Explain the procedure to the patient and why this intervention is warranted. Describe that it will entail a quick few moments of discomfort. Perform key abdominal assessments as described above.	Patient cooperation is facilitated when explanations are provided. Due to changes in the patient's condition, assessment is vital before initiating an intervention.

ACTION	RATIONALE
5. Close curtains around bed and close the door to the room, if possible. Raise bed to a comfortable working position, usually elbow height of the caregiver (VISN 8 Patient Safety Center, 2009). Assist the patient into a 30- to 45-degree position. Place towel or disposable pad across patient's chest. Give tissues and emesis basin to patient.	Provides for privacy. Appropriate working height facilitates comfort and proper body mechanics for the nurse. Towel or pad protects patient from contact with gastric secretions. Emesis basin is helpful if patient vomits or gags. Tissues are necessary if patient wants to blow his or her nose when tube is removed.
6. Put on gloves. Discontinue suction and separate tube from suction. Unpin tube from patient's gown and carefully remove adhesive tape from patient's nose.	Gloves prevent contact with blood and body fluids. Disconnecting tube from suction and the patient allows for its unrestricted removal.
7. Check placement and attach syringe and flush with 10 mL of water or normal saline solution (optional) or clear with 30 to 50 mL of air.	Air or saline solution clears the tube of secretions, feeding, or debris.
8. Clamp tube with fingers by doubling tube on itself. Instruct patient to take a deep breath and hold it. Quickly and carefully remove tube while patient holds breath. Coil the tube in the disposable pad as you remove it from the patient.	Clamping prevents drainage of gastric contents into the pharynx and esophagus. The patient holds breath to prevent accidental aspiration of gastric secretions in tube. Careful removal minimizes trauma and discomfort for patient. Containing the tube in a towel while removing prevents leakage onto the patient.
9. Dispose of tube per agency policy. Remove gloves and place in bag. Perform hand hygiene.	This prevents contamination with microorganisms. Follow the biohazard policy of the institution.
10. Offer mouth care to patient and facial tissue to blow nose. Lower the bed and assist the patient to a position of comfort, as needed.	These interventions promote patient comfort.

ACTION	RATIONALE
11. Remove equipment and raise side rail and lower bed.	Promotes patient comfort and safety.
12. Put on gloves and measure the amount of nasogastric drainage in the collection device and record on output flow record, subtracting irrigant fluids, if necessary. Add solidifying agent to nasogastric drainage according to hospital policy.	Irrigation fluids are considered intake. To obtain the true nasogastric drainage, irrigant fluid amounts are subtracted from the total nasogastric drainage. Nasogastric drainage is recorded as part of the output of fluids from the patient. Solidifying agents added to liquid nasogastric drainage facilitate safe biohazard disposal.
13. Remove additional PPE, if used. Perform hand hygiene.	Removing PPE properly reduces the risk for infection transmission and contamination of other items. Hand hygiene prevents transmission of microorganisms.

EVALUATION

• Patient experiences minimal discomfort and pain on NG tube removal.
• Patient's abdomen remains free from distention and tenderness.
• Patient verbalizes measures to maintain an adequate nutritional intake.

DOCUMENTATION

• Document assessment of the abdomen. If an abdominal girth reading was obtained, record this measurement. Document the removal of the NG tube from the naris where it had been placed. Note if there is any irritation to the skin of the naris. Record the amount of NG drainage in the suction container on the patient's intake and output record as well as the color of the drainage. Record any pertinent teaching, such as instruction to patient to notify nurse if he or she experiences any nausea, abdominal pain, or bloating.

Skill · 116   Inserting a Nasopharyngeal Airway

Nasopharyngeal airways, frequently referred to as nasal trumpets, are curved soft rubber or plastic tubes inserted into the back of the pharynx through the nose in patients who are breathing spontaneously. The nasal trumpet provides a route from the nares to the pharynx to help maintain a patent airway. These airways may be indicated if the teeth are clenched, the tongue is enlarged, or the patient needs frequent nasopharyngeal suctioning.

EQUIPMENT
- Nasal airway of appropriate size (size range for adolescent to adult is 24 Fr–36 Fr)
- Disposable gloves
- Water-soluble lubricant
- Suction equipment
- Mask (if necessary)
- Goggles (if necessary)
- Additional PPE, as indicated

ASSESSMENT GUIDELINES
- Assess patient's lung sounds. If lung sounds are diminished, patient may need nasal airway to keep airway patent. If lung sounds are coarse or wheezing is noted, patient may need the nasal airway to help with suctioning.
- Assess patient's respiratory rate and effort. If patient is not getting enough air or if patient needs to be suctioned, the respiratory rate will generally increase and the patient may have retractions, nasal flaring, and grunting.
- Assess the oxygen saturation level. If the patient is not getting enough air or if the patient needs to be suctioned, the oxygen saturation level will generally decrease.
- Assess for the presence of nasal conditions, such as a deviated septum or recent nasal or oral surgery, and increased risk for bleeding, such as anticoagulant therapy, which would contraindicate the use of a nasopharyngeal airway.

NURSING DIAGNOSES
- Risk for Aspiration
- Risk for Activity Intolerance
- Risk for Injury
- Ineffective Airway Clearance
- Risk for Impaired Skin Integrity
- Risk for Infection

OUTCOME IDENTIFICATION AND PLANNING
Expected outcomes may include:
- Patient will sustain and maintain a patent airway.
- Patient demonstrates a respiratory rate and depth within normal limits and equal, clear lung sounds bilaterally.

IMPLEMENTATION

ACTION

RATIONALE

1. Bring necessary equipment to the bedside stand or over-bed table.

Bringing everything to the bedside conserves time and energy. Arranging items nearby is convenient, saves time, and avoids unnecessary stretching and twisting of muscles on the part of the nurse

2. Perform hand hygiene and put on PPE, if indicated.

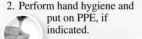

Hand hygiene and PPE prevent the spread of microorganisms. PPE is required based on transmission precautions.

3. Identify the patient.

Identifying the patient ensures the right patient receives the intervention and helps prevent errors.

4. Close curtains around bed and close door to room if possible.

This ensures the patient's privacy.

5. Explain what you are going to do and the reason to the patient, even if the patient does not appear to be alert.

Explanation alleviates fears. Even if patient appears unconscious, the nurse should explain what is happening.

6. Put on disposable gloves. If patient is coughing or has copious secretions, a mask and goggles should also be worn.

Gloves and personal protective equipment prevent contact with contaminants.

7. **Measure the nasopharyngeal airway for correct size.** The nasopharyngeal airway length is measured by holding the airway on the side of the patient's face. The airway should reach from the tragus of the ear to the nostril plus 1″. The diameter should be slightly smaller than the diameter of the nostril.

Correct size ensures correct insertion and fit, allowing for conformation of the airway to the curvature of the nasopharynx.

ACTION	RATIONALE
8. Adjust bed to a comfortable working level, usually elbow height of the care giver (VISN 8, 2006). Lower side rail closer to you. **If patient is awake and alert, position patient supine in semi-Fowler's position. If patient is not conscious or alert, position patient in a side-lying position.**	Having the bed at the proper height prevents back and muscle strain. By raising the head of the bed or placing patient in the side-lying position, the nurse is helping to protect the airway if the patient should vomit during the placement of the nasopharyngeal airway.
9. Suction patient if necessary.	Suctioning removes excess secretions and helps maintain patent airway.
10. Lubricate the nasopharyngeal airway generously with the water-soluble lubricant, covering the airway from the tip to the guard rim.	The water-soluble lubricant helps prevent injury to the mucosa as the airway is inserted.
11. Gently insert the airway into the naris, narrow end first, until the rim is touching the naris (FIGURE 1). If resistance is met, stop and try other naris.	To prevent injury, the airway should not be forced into the naris.

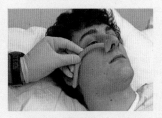

FIGURE 1 Inserting nasopharyngeal airway.

12. Check placement by closing the patient's mouth and place your fingers in front of the tube opening to check for air movement. Assess the pharynx to visualize the tip of the airway behind the uvula. Assess the nose for blanching or stretching of the skin.	This ensures correct placement and prevents injury. The skin should not be blanched or appear stretched due to the nasopharyngeal airway. If this occurs, a smaller size airway is needed.

ACTION	RATIONALE
13. Remove gloves and raise the 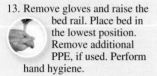 bed rail. Place bed in the lowest position. Remove additional PPE, if used. Perform hand hygiene.	Raising side rails and proper bed height provides for patient comfort and safety. Removing PPE properly reduces the risk for infection transmission and contamination of other items. Hand hygiene prevents the spread of microorganisms.
14. **Remove the airway, clean in warm soapy water, and place in other naris at least every 8 hours, or according to facility policy.**	The nasopharyngeal airway may cause tissue trauma and skin breakdown if left in place for too long. Secretions can accumulate on surface and contribute to irritation and tissue trauma.

EVALUATION

• Patient maintains a clear, patent airway with minimal to no secretions.
• Patient exhibits an oxygen saturation level >95% and respiratory rate remains in the normal range.

DOCUMENTATION

• Document the placement of the nasopharyngeal airway, including size of airway, nares used for placement, assessment pre- and post-intervention, and removal/cleaning.

GENERAL CONSIDERATIONS

• If the patient coughs or gags on insertion, the nasal trumpet may be too long. Assess the pharynx. The tip of the airway should be visualized behind the uvula.
• The skin, mucous membranes, and tissues of older adults are more fragile and prone to injury and breakdown. Extra care on insertion to prevent injury and extra vigilance to provide oral hygiene and assessment of the area is necessary.

Skill · 117   Administering Medication via a Small-Volume Nebulizer

Many medications to help with respiratory problems may be delivered via the respiratory system using a small-volume nebulizer. Nebulizers disperse fine particles of liquid medication into the deeper passages of the respiratory tract, where absorption occurs. The treatment continues until all the medication in the nebulizer cup has been inhaled.

EQUIPMENT
- Stethoscope
- Medication
- Nebulizer tubing and chamber
- Air compressor or oxygen hookup
- Sterile saline (if not premeasured)
- Computerized-generated Medication Administration Record (CMAR) or Medication Administration Record (MAR)
- PPE, as indicated

ASSESSMENT GUIDELINES
- Assess lung sounds before and after use to establish a baseline and determine the effectiveness of the medication. Frequently, patients will have wheezes or coarse lung sounds before medication administration.
- If ordered, assess oxygen saturation level before medication administration. The oxygenation level will usually increase after the medication is administered.
- Verify patient name, dose, route, and time of administration.
- Assess the patient's knowledge and understanding of the medication's purpose and action.

NURSING DIAGNOSES
- Ineffective Airway Clearance
- Ineffective Breathing Pattern
- Impaired Gas Exchange
- Deficient Knowledge
- Risk for Activity Intolerance

OUTCOME IDENTIFICATION AND PLANNING
Expected outcomes may include:
- Patient receives the medication.
- Patient exhibits improved lung sound and respiratory effort.
- Patient's demonstrates steps for use of nebulizer.
- Patient verbalizes an understanding of medication purpose and action.

IMPLEMENTATION

ACTION

RATIONALE

1. Gather equipment. Check each medication order against the original order in the medical record, according to facility policy. Clarify any inconsistencies. Check the patient's chart for allergies.

   This comparison helps to identify errors that may have occurred when orders were transcribed. The primary care provider's order is the legal record of medication orders for each facility.

2. Know the actions, special nursing considerations, safe dose ranges, purpose of administration, and adverse effects of the medications to be administered. Consider the appropriateness of the medication for this patient.

   This knowledge aids the nurse in evaluating the therapeutic effect of the medication in relation to the patient's disorder and can also be used to educate the patient about the medication.

3. Perform hand hygiene.

   Hand hygiene prevents the spread of microorganisms.

4. Move the medication cart to the outside of the patient's room or prepare for administration in the medication area.

   Organization facilitates error-free administration and saves time.

5. Unlock the medication cart or drawer. Enter pass code and scan employee identification, if required.

   Locking the cart or drawer safeguards each patient's medication supply. Hospital accrediting organizations require medication carts to be locked when not in use. Entering pass code and scanning ID allows only authorized users into the system and identifies user for documentation by the computer.

6. **Prepare medications for one patient at a time.**

   This prevents errors in medication administration.

ACTION	RATIONALE
7. Read the CMAR/MAR and select the proper medication from the patient's medication drawer or unit stock.	This is the *first* check of the label.
8. Compare the label with the CMAR/MAR. Check expiration dates and perform calculations, if necessary. Scan the bar code on the package, if required.	This is the *second* check of the label. Verify calculations with another nurse to ensure safety, if necessary.
9. **When all medications for one patient have been prepared, recheck the label with the MAR before taking them to the patient.**	This is a *third* check to ensure accuracy and to prevent errors. Some facilities require the third check to occur at the bedside, after identifying the patient and before administration.
10. Lock the medication cart before leaving it.	Locking the cart or drawer safeguards the patient's medication supply. Hospital accrediting organizations require medication carts to be locked when not in use.
11. Transport medications to the patient's bedside carefully, and keep the medications in sight at all times.	Careful handling and close observation prevent accidental or deliberate disarrangement of medications.
12. **Ensure that the patient receives the medications at the correct time.**	Check agency policy, which may allow for administration within a period of 30 minutes before or 30 minutes after designated time.
13. Perform hand hygiene and put on PPE, if indicated.	Hand hygiene and PPE prevent the spread of microorganisms. PPE is required based on transmission precautions.
14. Identify the patient. Usually, the patient should be identified using two methods. Compare information with the CMAR/MAR.	Identifying the patient ensures the right patient receives the medications and helps prevent errors.
a. Check the name and identification number on the	This is the most reliable method. Replace the identification band if

ACTION	RATIONALE
patient's identification band.	it is missing or inaccurate in any way.
b. Ask the patient to state his or her name and birth date, based on facility policy.	This requires a response from the patient, but illness and strange surroundings often cause patients to be confused.
c. If the patient cannot identify him- or herself, verify the patient's identification with a staff member who knows the patient for the second source.	This is another way to double-check identity. Do not use the name on the door or over the bed, because these signs may be inaccurate.
15. Complete necessary assessments before administering medications. Check the patient's allergy bracelet or ask the patient about allergies. Explain what you are going to do, and the reason for doing it, to the patient.	Assessment is a prerequisite to administration of medications. Explanation relieves anxiety and facilitates cooperation.
16. Scan the patient's bar code on the identification band, if required.	Provides an additional check to ensure that the medication is given to the right patient.
17. Remove the nebulizer cup from the device and open it. Place premeasured unit-dose medication in the bottom section of the cup or use a dropper to place a concentrated dose of medication in cup and add prescribed diluent, if required.	To get enough volume to make a fine mist, normal saline may need to be added to the concentrated medication.
18. Screw the top portion of the nebulizer cup back in place and attach the cup to the nebulizer. Attach one end of tubing to the stem on the bottom of the nebulizer cuff and the other end to the air compressor or oxygen source.	Air or oxygen must be forced through the nebulizer to form a fine mist.

ACTION	RATIONALE
19. Turn on the air compressor or oxygen. Check that a fine medication mist is produced by opening the valve. Have patient place mouthpiece into mouth and grasp securely with teeth and lips.	If there is no fine mist, make sure that medication has been added to the cup and that the tubing is connected to the air compressor or oxygen outlet. Adjust flow meter if necessary.
20. **Instruct patient to inhale slowly and deeply through the mouth. A nose clip may be necessary if the patient is also breathing through the nose. Hold each breath for a slight pause, before exhaling.**	While the patient inhales and holds the breath, the medication comes in contact with the respiratory tissue and is absorbed. The longer the breath is held, the more medication can be absorbed.
21. Continue this inhalation technique until all medication in the nebulizer cup has been aerosolized (usually about 15 minutes). Once the fine mist decreases in amount, gently flick the sides of the nebulizer cup.	Once the fine mist stops, the medication is no longer being aerosolized. By gently flicking the cup sides, any medication that is stuck to the sides is knocked into the bottom of the cup, where it can become aerosolized.
22. Have the patient gargle and rinse with tap water after using the nebulizer, as necessary. Clean the nebulizer according to the manufacturer's directions.	Rinsing is necessary when using inhaled steroids, because oral fungal infections can occur. Rinsing removes medication residue from the mouth. The buildup of medication in the device can affect how the medication is delivered, as well as attract bacteria.
23. Remove gloves and additional PPE, if used. Perform hand hygiene.	Removing PPE properly reduces the risk for infection transmission and contamination of other items. Hand hygiene prevents the spread of microorganisms.
24. Document the administration of the medication immediately after administration. See Documentation section below.	Timely documentation helps to ensure patient safety.

ACTION	RATIONALE
25. Evaluate patient's response to medication within appropriate time frame. **Reassess lung sounds, oxygenation saturation if ordered, and respirations.**	The patient needs to be evaluated for therapeutic and adverse effects from the medication. Lung sounds and oxygenation saturation may improve after nebulizer use. Respirations may decrease after nebulizer use.

EVALUATION

- Patient receives the medication.
- Patient exhibits improved lung sounds and respiratory effort.
- Patient demonstrates correct steps for use and verbalizes an understanding of the need of the medication. Information about medication theraphy associated with MDI use.

DOCUMENTATION

- Document the administration of the medication immediately after administration, including date, time, dose, and route of administration on the CMAR/MAR or record using the required format. If using a bar-code system, medication administration is recorded automatically when scanned. PRN medications require documentation of the reason for administration. Prompt recording avoids the possibility of accidentally repeating the administration of the drug. Document respiratory rate, oxygen saturation, if applicable, lung assessment, and the patient's response to the treatment, if appropriate. If the drug was refused or omitted, record this in the appropriate area on the medication record and notify the primary care provider. This verifies the reason medication was omitted and ensures that the primary care provider is aware of the patient's condition.

GENERAL CONSIDERATIONS

- Ongoing assessment is an important part of nursing care to evaluate patient response to administered medications and early detection of adverse effects. If an adverse effect is suspected, withhold further medication doses and notify the patient's primary healthcare provider. Additional intervention is based on type of reaction and patient assessment.

Skill • 118   Applying Negative Pressure Wound Therapy

Negative-pressure wound therapy (NPWT) (or topical negative pressure [TNP]) promotes wound healing and wound closure through the application of uniform negative pressure on the wound bed. NPWT results in a reduction in bacteria in the wound and the removal of excess wound fluid, while providing a moist wound healing environment. The negative pressure results in mechanical tension on the wound tissues, stimulating cell proliferation, blood flow to wounds, and the growth of new blood vessels. An open-cell foam dressing is applied in the wound. A fenestrated tube is connected to the foam, allowing the application of the negative pressure. The dressing and distal tubing are covered by a transparent, occlusive, air-permeable dressing that provides a seal, allowing the application of the negative pressure. Excess wound fluid is removed through tubing, and it also acts to pull the wound edges together.

Negative-pressure wound therapy is used to treat a variety of acute or chronic wounds, wounds with heavy drainage, wounds failing to heal, or wounds healing slowly. Examples of such wounds include pressure ulcers; arterial, venous, and diabetic ulcers; dehisced surgical wounds, infected wounds, skin graft sites, and burns. NPWT is not considered for use in the presence of active bleeding; wounds with exposed blood vessels, organs, or nerves; malignancy in wound tissue; presence of dry/necrotic tissue; or with fistulas of unknown origin (Hess, 2008; Preston, 2008; Thompson, 2008). Cautious use is indicated in the presence of unrelieved pressure, anticoagulant therapy, poor nutritional status, and immunosuppressant therapy (Preston, 2008). Candidates must be assessed for preexisting bleeding disorders, use of anticoagulants and other medications, or use of supplements that prolong bleeding times, such as aspirin or ginkgo biloba (Malli, 2005; Preston, 2008). NPWT dressings are changed every 48 to 72 hours, depending on the manufacturer's specifications and medical orders. Infected wounds may require dressing changes every 12 to 24 hours.

The following is an outline of the procedure for V.A.C. Therapy (KCl), as an example of NPWT. There are many manufacturers of NPWT systems. The nurse should be familiar with the components of, and procedures related to, the particular system in use.

EQUIPMENT
- Negative pressure unit (V.A.C. ATS unit)
- Evacuation/collection canister
- V.A.C. Foam dressing
- V.A.C. Drape
- T.R.A.C. pad
- Skin-protectant wipes
- Sterile gauze sponge
- A sterile irrigation set, including a basin, irrigant container, and irrigation syringe
- Sterile irrigation solution, as ordered by the physician, warmed to body temperature
- Waste receptacle to dispose of contaminated materials

* Sterile gloves (2 pairs)
* Sterile scissors
* Clean disposable gloves
* Gown, mask, eye protection

* Additional PPE, as indicated
* Sterile scissors
* Waterproof pad and bath blanket

ASSESSMENT GUIDELINES

* Confirm the medical order for the application of NPWT. Check the patient's chart and question the patient about current treatments and medications that may contraindicate the application.
* Assess the situation to determine the need for a dressing change. Confirm any medical orders relevant to wound care and any wound care included in the nursing plan of care.
* Assess the patient's level of comfort and the need for analgesics before wound care. Assess if the patient experienced any pain related to prior dressing changes and the effectiveness of interventions used to minimize the patient's pain.
* Assess the current dressing to determine if it is intact. Assess for excess drainage, bleeding, or saturation of the dressing.
* Inspect the wound and the surrounding tissue. Assess the location, appearance of the wound, stage (if appropriate), drainage, and types of tissue present in the wound. Measure the wound. Note the stage of the healing process and characteristics of any drainage.
* Assess the surrounding skin for color, temperature, edema, ecchymosis, or maceration.

NURSING DIAGNOSES

* Anxiety
* Disturbed Body Image
* Acute Pain
* Risk for Infection
* Risk for Injury
* Deficient Knowledge
* Impaired Tissue Integrity

OUTCOME IDENTIFICATION AND PLANNING

Expected outcomes may include:
* Negative-pressure wound therapy is accomplished without contaminating the wound area or causing trauma to the wound, and without causing the patient to experience pain or discomfort.
* Negative-pressure device functions correctly and the appropriate and ordered pressure is maintained throughout therapy.
* Patient's wound exhibits progression in healing.

IMPLEMENTATION

ACTION	RATIONALE
1. Review the medical order for the application of negative-pressure wound therapy, including the ordered pressure setting for the device.	Reviewing the order validates the correct patient and correct procedure.
2. Gather the necessary supplies and bring them to the bedside stand or overbed table.	Preparation promotes efficient time management and an organized approach to the task. Bringing everything to the bedside conserves time and energy. Arranging items nearby is convenient, saves time, and avoids unnecessary stretching and twisting of muscles on the part of the nurse.
3. Perform hand hygiene and put on PPE, if indicated.	Hand hygiene and PPE prevent the spread of microorganisms. PPE is required based on transmission precautions.
4. Identify the patient.	Identifying the patient ensures that the right patient receives the intervention and helps prevent errors.
5. Close curtains around bed and close door to room, if possible. Explain what you are going to do and why you are going to do it to the patient.	This ensures the patient's privacy. Explanation relieves anxiety and facilitates cooperation.
6. Assess the patient for possible need for nonpharmacologic pain-reducing interventions or analgesic medication before wound care dressing change. Administer appropriate prescribed analgesic. Allow sufficient time for analgesic to achieve its effectiveness before beginning the procedure.	Pain is a subjective experience influenced by past experience. Wound care and dressing changes may cause pain for some patients.

ACTION	RATIONALE
7. Adjust bed to comfortable working height, usually elbow height of the caregiver (VISN 8 Patient Safety Center, 2009).	Having the bed at the proper height prevents back and muscle strain.
8. Assist the patient to a comfortable position that provides easy access to the wound area. Position the patient so the irrigation solution will flow from the clean end of the wound toward the dirty end. Expose the area and drape the patient with a bath blanket if needed. Put a waterproof pad under the wound area.	Patient positioning and draping provide for comfort and warmth. Gravity directs the flow of liquid from the least contaminated to the most contaminated area. Waterproof pad protects the patient and the bed linens.
9. Have the disposal bag or waste receptacle within easy reach for use during the procedure.	Having the waste container handy means that soiled dressings and supplies can be discarded easily, without the spread of microorganisms.
10. Using sterile technique, prepare a sterile field and add all the sterile supplies needed for the procedure to the field. Pour warmed sterile irrigating solution into the sterile container.	Proper preparation ensures that supplies are within easy reach and sterility is maintained. Warmed solution may result in less discomfort.
11. Put on a gown, mask, and eye protection.	Use of PPE is part of Standard Precautions. A gown protects your clothes from contamination if splashing should occur. Goggles protect mucous membranes of your eyes from contact with irrigant fluid.
12. Put on clean gloves. Carefully and gently remove the dressing. If there is resistance, use a silicone-based adhesive remover to help remove the drape. **Note the number of pieces of foam removed from the wound.**	Gloves protect the nurse from handling contaminated dressings. A silicone-based adhesive remover allows for the easy, rapid, and painless removal without the associated problems of skin stripping (Rudoni, 2008; Stephen-Haynes, 2008). Counting

ACTION	RATIONALE
Compare with the documented number from the previous dressing change.	the number of pieces of foam assures the removal of all foam that was placed during the previous dressing change.
13. Discard the dressings in the receptacle. Remove your gloves and put them in the receptacle.	Proper disposal of dressings and used gloves prevents the spread of microorganisms.
14. Put on sterile gloves. Using sterile technique, irrigate the wound (see Skill 183).	Irrigation removes exudate and debris.
15. Clean the area around the skin with normal saline. Dry the surrounding skin with a sterile gauze sponge.	Moisture provides a medium for growth of microorganisms.
16. Assess the wound for appearance, stage, or the presence of eschar, granulation tissue, epithelialization, undermining, tunneling, necrosis, sinus tract, and drainage. Assess the appearance of the surrounding tissue. Measure the wound.	This information provides evidence about the wound healing process and/or the presence of infection.
17. Wipe intact skin around the wound with a skin-protectant wipe and allow it to dry well.	Skin protectant provides a barrier against irritation and breakdown.
18. Remove gloves if they become contaminated and discard them into the receptacle.	Proper disposal of gloves prevents spread of microorganisms.
19. Put on a new pair of sterile gloves, if necessary. Using sterile scissors, cut the foam to the shape and measurement of the wound. Do not cut foam over the wound. More than one piece of foam may be necessary if the first piece is cut too small. Carefully place the foam in the wound. Ensure foam-to-foam	Aseptic technique maintains sterility of items to come in contact with wound. Foam should fill the wound but not cover intact surrounding skin. Foam fragments may fall into wound if cutting is performed over the wound. Foam-to-foam contact allows for even distribution of negative pressure. Recording the number of pieces of foam aids in assuring

ACTION	RATIONALE
contact if more than one piece is required. Note the number of pieces of foam placed in the wound.	the removal of all foam with next dressing change.
20. Trim and place the V.A.C. Drape to cover the foam dressing and an additional 3- to 5-cm border of intact periwound tissue. V.A.C. Drape may be cut into multiple pieces for easier handling.	The occlusive air-permeable V.A.C. drape provides a seal, allowing the application of the negative pressure.
21. Choose an appropriate site to apply the T.R.A.C. Pad.	T.R.A.C. Pad should be placed in the area where the greatest fluid flow and optimal drainage is anticipated. Avoid placing over bony prominences or within creases in the tissue.
22. Pinch the drape and cut a 2-cm hole through it. Apply the T.R.A.C. Pad (FIGURE 1). Remove the V.A.C. Canister from the package and insert it into the V.A.C. Therapy Unit until it locks into place. Connect T.R.A.C. Pad tubing to canister tubing and check that the clamps on each tube are open. Turn on the power to the V.A.C. Therapy Unit and select the prescribed therapy setting.	A hole in the drape allows for removal of fluid and/or exudate. The canister provides a collection chamber for drainage.

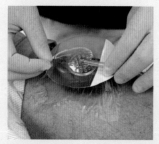

FIGURE 1 Applying the T.R.A.C. Pad.

ACTION	RATIONALE
23. Assess the dressing to ensure seal integrity. The dressing should be collapsed, shrinking to the foam and skin.	Shrinkage confirms good seal, allowing for accurate application of pressure and treatment.
24. Remove and discard gloves. Apply tape, Montgomery straps, or roller gauze to secure the dressings. Alternately, many commercial wound products are self-adhesive and do not require additional tape.	Tape or other securing products are easier to apply after gloves have been removed. Proper disposal of gloves prevents the spread of microorganisms.
25. Label dressing with date and time. Remove all remaining equipment; place the patient in a comfortable position, with side rails up and bed in the lowest position.	Recording date and time provides communication and demonstrates adherence to plan of care. Proper patient and bed positioning promotes safety and comfort.
26. Remove PPE, if used. Perform hand hygiene.	Removing PPE properly reduces the risk for infection transmission and contamination of other items. Hand hygiene prevents the spread of microorganisms.
27. Check all wound dressings every shift. More frequent checks may be needed if the wound is more complex or dressings become saturated quickly.	Checking dressings ensures the assessment of changes in patient condition and timely intervention to prevent complications.

EVALUATION

• Negative-pressure wound therapy is applied without contaminating the wound area, causing trauma to the wound, and without causing the patient to experience pain or discomfort.
• Negative-pressure device functions correctly and the appropriate, ordered pressure is maintained throughout therapy.
• Patient's wound exhibits progression in healing.

DOCUMENTATION

• Record your assessment of the wound, including evidence of granulation tissue, presence of necrotic tissue, stage (if appropriate), and characteristics of drainage. Include the appearance of the surrounding skin. Document the cleansing or irrigation of the wound and solution used. Document the application of the NPWT, noting the pressure setting, patency, and seal of the dressing. Describe the color and characteristics of the drainage in the collection chamber. Record pertinent patient and family education and any patient reaction from this procedure, including the presence of pain and effectiveness or ineffectiveness of pain interventions.

GENERAL CONSIDERATIONS

- Change the wound dressing every 48 hours for noninfected wounds, or every 12 to 24 hours for infected wounds. Time dressing changes to allow for wound assessment by the other members of the healthcare team.
- Measure and record the amount of drainage each shift as part of the intake and output record.
- Be alert for audible and visual alarms on the vacuum device to alert you to problems, such as tipping of the device greater than 45 degrees, a full collection canister, an air leak in the dressing, or dislodgment of the canister.
- NPWT should operate for 24 hours. It should not be shut off for more than 2 hours in a 24-hour period. When NPWT is restarted, irrigate the wound per medical order or facility policy, and apply a new NPWT dressing.
- When maceration of the surrounding skin beneath the occlusive dressing occurs, this may be treated by placing a barrier or wafer dressing beneath the transparent dressing to protect the skin. Verify with facility policy as needed.

Skill · 119 **Instilling Nose Drops**

Nasal instillations are used to treat allergies, sinus infections, and nasal congestion. Medications with a systemic effect, such as vasopressin, may also be prepared as a nasal instillation. The nose is normally not a sterile cavity, but because of its connection with the sinuses, observe medical asepsis carefully when using nasal instillations.

EQUIPMENT

- Medication
- Dropper, if not part of medication container
- Gloves
- Additional PPE, as indicated
- Tissue
- Computer-generated Medication Administration Record (CMAR) or Medication Administration Record (MAR)

ASSESSMENT GUIDELINES

- Assess the nares for redness, erythema, edema, drainage, or tenderness.
- Assess the patient for allergies.
- Verify patient name, dose, route, and time of administration.
- Assess the patient's knowledge of medication and procedure. If the patient has a knowledge deficit about the medication, this may be an appropriate time to begin education about the procedure.
- Assess the patient's ability to cooperate with the procedure.

NURSING DIAGNOSES

- Deficient Knowledge
- Risk for Allergy Response

OUTCOME IDENTIFICATION AND PLANNING

Expected outcomes may include:
- Medication is administered successfully into the nose.
- Patient understands the rationale for the nose-drop instillation.
- Patient experiences no allergy response.
- Patient's skin remains intact.
- Patient experiences no, or minimal, pain.

IMPLEMENTATION

ACTION	RATIONALE
1. Gather equipment. Check medication order against the original order in the medical record, according to facility policy. Clarify any inconsistencies. Check the patient's chart for allergies.	This comparison helps to identify errors that may have occurred when orders were transcribed. The primary care provider's order is the legal record of medication orders for each facility.
2. Know the actions, special nursing considerations, safe dose ranges, purpose of administration, and adverse effects of the medication to be administered. Consider the appropriateness of the medication for this patient.	This knowledge aids the nurse in evaluating the therapeutic effect of the medication in relation to the patient's disorder and can also be used to educate the patient about the medication.
3. Perform hand hygiene.	Hand hygiene prevents the spread of microorganisms.

ACTION	RATIONALE
4. Move the medication cart to the outside of the patient's room or prepare for administration in the medication area.	Organization facilitates error-free administration and saves time.
5. Unlock the medication cart or drawer. Enter pass code and scan employee identification, if required.	Locking the cart or drawer safeguards each patient's medication supply. Hospital accrediting organizations require medication carts to be locked when not in use. Entering pass code and scanning ID allows only authorized users into the system and identifies user for documentation by the computer.
6. **Prepare medications for one patient at a time.**	This prevents errors in medication administration.
7. Read the CMAR/MAR and select the proper medication from the patient's medication drawer or unit stock.	This is the *first* check of the label.
8. Compare the label with the CMAR/MAR. Check expiration dates and perform calculations, if necessary. Scan the bar code on the package, if required.	This is the *second* check of the label. Verify calculations with another nurse to ensure safety, if necessary.
9. **When all medications for one patient have been prepared, recheck the label with the CMAR/MAR before taking them to the patient.**	This is a *third* check to ensure accuracy and to prevent errors. Some facilities require the third check to occur at the bedside, after identifying the patient and before administration.
10. Lock the medication cart before leaving it.	Locking the cart or drawer safeguards the patient's medication supply. Hospital accrediting organizations require medication carts to be locked when not in use.
11. Transport medications to the patient's bedside carefully, and keep the medications in sight at all times.	Careful handling and close observation prevent accidental or deliberate disarrangement of medications.

ACTION	RATIONALE
12. **Ensure that the patient receives the medications at the correct time.**	Check agency policy, which may allow for administration within a period of 30 minutes before or 30 minutes after designated time.
13. Perform hand hygiene and put on PPE, if indicated.	Hand hygiene and PPE prevent the spread of microorganisms. PPE is required based on transmission precautions.
14. Identify the patient. Usually, the patient should be identified using two methods. Compare information with the CMAR/MAR.	Identifying the patient ensures the right patient receives the medications and helps prevent errors.
a. Check the name and identification number on the patient's identification band.	This is the most reliable method. Replace the identification band if it is missing or inaccurate in any way.
b. Ask the patient to state his or her name and birth date, based on facility policy.	This requires a response from the patient, but illness and strange surroundings often cause patients to be confused.
c. If the patient cannot identify him or herself, verify the patient's identification with a staff member who knows the patient for the second source.	This is another way to double-check identity. Do not use the name on the door or over the bed, because these signs may be inaccurate.
15. Complete necessary assessments before administering medications. Check the patient's allergy bracelet or ask the patient about allergies. Explain the purpose and action of each medication to the patient.	Assessment is a prerequisite to administration of medications.
16. Scan the patient's bar code on the identification band, if required.	Provides an additional check to ensure that the medication is given to the right patient.
17. Put on gloves.	Gloves protect the nurse from potential contact with contaminants and body fluids.

ACTION	RATIONALE
18. Provide patient with paper tissues and ask patient to blow his or her nose.	Blowing the nose clears the nasal mucosa prior to medication administration.
19. Have patient sit up with head tilted well back. If patient is lying down, tilt head back over a pillow.	These positions allow the solution to flow well back into the nares. Do not tilt the head if patient has a cervical spine injury.
20. Draw sufficient solution into dropper for both nares. Do not return excess solution to a stock bottle.	Returning solution to a stock bottle increases the risk for contamination of the stock bottle.
21. Ask the patient to breathe through the mouth. Hold tip of nose up and place dropper just above naris, about 1/3 inch. Instill the prescribed number of drops in one naris and then into the other. Protect dropper with a piece of soft tubing if patient is an infant or young child. Avoid touching naris with dropper.	Breathing through the mouth helps prevent aspiration of solution. The soft tubing will protect the patient's nares from injury during administration of medication. Touching the naris may cause the patient to sneeze and will contaminate the dropper.
22. Have patient remain in position with head tilted back for a few minutes.	Tilting the head back prevents the escape of the medication.
23. Remove gloves. Assist the patient to a comfortable position.	This ensures patient comfort.
24. 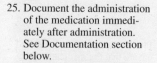 Remove additional PPE, if used. Perform hand hygiene.	Removing PPE properly reduces the risk for infection transmission and contamination of other items. Hand hygiene prevents the spread of microorganisms.
25. Document the administration of the medication immediately after administration. See Documentation section below.	Timely documentation helps to ensure patient safety.
26. Evaluate the patient's response to the procedure and medication within appropriate time frame.	The patient needs to be evaluated for therapeutic and adverse effects from the medication.

EVALUATION

- Patient receives the nose drops successfully.
- Patient understands the rationale for nose-drop instillation.
- Patient experiences no allergy response.
- Patient experiences no, or minimal, pain or discomfort.

DOCUMENTATION

- Document the administration of the medication, including date, time, dose, route of administration, and site of administration, specifically right, left, or both nares, on the CMAR/MAR or record using the required format. If using a bar-code system, medication administration is automatically recorded when the bar code is scanned. PRN medications require documentation of the reason for administration. Prompt recording avoids the possibility of accidentally repeating the administration of the drug. Document pre- and postadministration assessments, characteristics of any drainage, and the patient's response to the treatment, if appropriate. If the drug was refused or omitted, record this in the appropriate area on the medication record and notify the primary care provider. This verifies the reason medication was omitted and ensures that the primary care provider is aware of the patient's condition.

GENERAL CONSIDERATIONS

- Ongoing assessment is an important part of nursing care to evaluate patient response to administered treatments and early detection of adverse effects. If an adverse effect is suspected, notify the patient's primary healthcare provider. Additional intervention is based on type of reaction and patient assessment.

Skill · 120   Assisting the Patient with Oral Care

Poor oral hygiene is reported to lead to the colonization of the oropharyngeal secretions by respiratory pathogens. Diligent oral hygiene care can improve oral health and limit the growth of pathogens in the oropharyngeal secretions, decreasing the incidence of aspiration pneumonia and other systemic diseases (Yoon & Steele, 2007; AACN, 2006). The mouth requires care even during illness, but sometimes care must be modified to meet a patient's needs. If the patient can assist with mouth care, provide the necessary materials. Oral care is important not only to prevent dental caries but also to improve the patient's self-image. Oral care should be done at least twice a day for ambulatory patients.

EQUIPMENT

- Toothbrush
- Toothpaste
- Emesis basin
- Glass with cool water
- Disposable gloves
- Additional PPE, as indicated

- Towel
- Mouthwash (optional)
- Washcloth or paper towel
- Lip lubricant (optional)
- Dental floss

ASSESSMENT GUIDELINES

- Assess the patient's oral hygiene preferences: frequency, time of day, and type of hygiene products.
- Assess for any physical activity limitations.
- Assess patient's oral cavity and dentition. Look for any inflammation or bleeding of the gums. Look for ulcers, lesions, and yellow or white patches. The yellow or white patches may indicate a fungal infection called thrush. Assess for signs of dehydration (dry mucosa) and dental decay. Look at the lips for dryness or cracking. Ask the patient if he or she is having pain, dryness, soreness, or difficulty chewing or swallowing.
- Assess patient's ability to perform own care.

NURSING DIAGNOSES

- Risk for Aspiration
- Ineffective Health Maintenance
- Impaired Oral Mucous Membrane
- Disturbed Body Image
- Deficient Knowledge

OUTCOME IDENTIFICATION AND PLANNING

Expected outcomes may include:
- The patient's mouth and teeth will be clean.
- The patient verbalizes positive body image.
- The patient will verbalize the importance of oral care.

IMPLEMENTATION

ACTION	RATIONALE
1. Perform hand hygiene and put on gloves if assisting with oral care, and/or other PPE, if indicated.	Hand hygiene and PPE prevent the spread of microorganisms. PPE is required based on transmission precautions.
2. Identify the patient. Explain the procedure to the patient.	Identifying the patient ensures the right patient receives the intervention and helps prevent errors. Explanation facilitates cooperation.

ACTION	RATIONALE
3. Assemble equipment on overbed table within patient's reach.	Organization facilitates performance of task.
4. Close the room door or curtains. Place the bed at an appropriate and comfortable working height; usually elbow height of the caregiver (VISN 8 Patient Safety Center, 2009).	Closing the door or curtains provides privacy. Proper bed height helps reduce back strain while performing the procedure.
5. Lower side rail and assist the patient to a sitting position if permitted, or turn patient onto side. Place towel across patient's chest. Raise bed to a comfortable working position.	The sitting or side-lying position prevents aspiration of fluids into the lungs. The towel protects the patient from dampness.
6. Encourage the patient to brush own teeth, or assist if necessary.	
a. Moisten toothbrush and apply toothpaste to bristles.	Water softens the bristles.
b. Place brush at a 45-degree angle to gum line and brush from gum line to crown of each tooth (FIGURE 1). Brush outer and inner surfaces. Brush back and forth across biting surface of each tooth.	Facilitates removal of plaque and tartar. The 45-degree angle of brushing permits cleansing of all tooth surface areas.

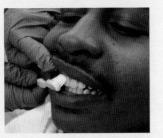

FIGURE 1 Brushing from the gum line to the crown of each tooth.

ACTION	RATIONALE
c. Brush tongue gently with toothbrush (FIGURE 2).	Removes coating on the tongue. Gentle motion does not stimulate gag reflex.

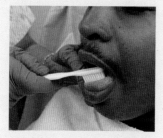

FIGURE 2 Brushing the tongue.

ACTION	RATIONALE
d. Have patient rinse vigorously with water and spit into emesis basin. Repeat until clear. Suction may be used as an alternative for removal of fluid and secretions from the mouth.	The vigorous swishing motion helps to remove debris. Suction is appropriate if patient is unable to expectorate well.
7. Assist patient to floss teeth, if appropriate:	Flossing aids in removal of plaque and promotes healthy gum tissue.
a. Remove approximately 6 inches of dental floss from container or use a plastic floss holder. Wrap the floss around the index fingers, keeping about 1 to 1½ inches of floss taut between the fingers.	The floss must be held taut to get between the teeth.
b. Insert floss gently between teeth, moving it back and forth downward to the gums.	Trauma to the gums can occur if floss is forced between teeth.
c. Move the floss up and down, first on one side of a tooth and then on the side of the other tooth, until the surfaces are clean. Repeat in the spaces between all teeth.	This ensures that the sides of both teeth are cleaned.

ACTION	RATIONALE
d. Instruct patient to rinse mouth well with water after flossing.	Vigorous rinsing helps to remove food particles and plaque that have been loosened by flossing.
8. Offer mouthwash if patient prefers.	Mouthwash leaves a pleasant taste in the mouth.
9. Offer lip balm or petroleum jelly.	Lip balm lubricates lips and prevents drying.
10. Remove equipment. Remove gloves and discard. Raise side rail and lower bed. Assist patient to a position of comfort.	Removing gloves properly reduces the risk for infection transmission and contamination of other items. These actions promote patient comfort and safety.
11. Remove any other PPE, if used. Perform hand hygiene.	Removing PPE properly reduces the risk for infection transmission and contamination of other items. Hand hygiene prevents the spread of microorganisms.

EVALUATION

- The patient receives oral care and experiences little to no discomfort.
- The patient states mouth feels refreshed.
- The patient verbalizes an understanding of reasons for proper oral care.

DOCUMENTATION

- Record oral assessment, significant observations and unusual findings, such as bleeding or inflammation. Document any teaching done. Document procedure and patient response.

GENERAL CONSIDERATIONS

- A soft bristled toothbrush with a small head should be used even when the patient has no or few teeth. It is the only effective way to remove plaque and debris from the teeth, gums, and tongue (Holman, et al., 2005).
- When meeting the oral hygiene needs of patients with cognitive impairments, maintain a relaxed demeanor. Use calming language. Try to determine phrases and terms the patient understands in relation to hygiene and make use of them. Offer frequent reassurance.
- A patient receiving chemotherapy medication may have bleeding gums and extremely sensitive mucous membranes. Use a soft sponge toothette for cleaning, and a saltwater rinse (half teaspoon salt in 1 cup of warm water) (Polovich, et al., 2009).

| Skill · 121 | **Providing Oral Care for the Dependent Patient** |

Adequate oral hygiene care is imperative to promote the patient's sense of well-being and prevent deterioration of the oral cavity. Poor oral hygiene is reported to lead to the colonization of the oropharyngeal secretions by respiratory pathogens. Diligent oral hygiene care can improve oral health and limit the growth of pathogens in the oropharyngeal secretions, decreasing the incidence of aspiration pneumonia and other systemic diseases (Yoon & Steele, 2007; AACN, 2006). Physical limitations, such as those associated with aging, often lead to less than adequate oral hygiene. The dexterity required for adequate brushing and flossing may decrease with age or illness. Older patients may be dependent on caregivers for oral hygiene. Patients with cognitive impairment, such as dementia, are also at risk for inadequate oral hygiene (Bailey, et al., 2005). If the patient is unable to perform oral hygiene, make certain that the mouth receives care as often as necessary to keep it clean and moist, as often as every 1 or 2 hours if necessary. This is especially important for patients who cannot drink or are not permitted fluids by mouth. Moisten the mouth with water, if allowed, and lubricate the lips often enough to keep the membranes well moistened.

EQUIPMENT

- Toothbrush
- Toothpaste
- Emesis basin
- Glass with cool water
- Disposable gloves
- Additional PPE, as indicated
- Towel
- Mouthwash (optional)
- Dental floss (optional)
- Denture-cleaning equipment (if necessary)
- Denture cup
- Denture cleaner
- 4 × 4 gauze
- Washcloth or paper towel
- Lip lubricant (optional)
- Sponge toothette
- Irrigating syringe with rubber tip (optional)
- Suction catheter with suction apparatus (optional)

ASSESSMENT GUIDELINES

- Assess the patient's oral hygiene preferences, if possible: frequency, time of day, and type of hygiene products.
- Assess for any physical activity limitations.
- Assess the patient's level of consciousness and overall ability to assist with oral care and respond to directions. Alterations in cognitive function and/or consciousness increase the risk for alterations in oral tissue and structure integrity.
- Assess the patient's risk for oral hygiene problems.
- Assess the patient's gag reflex. Decreased or absent gag reflex increases the risk for aspiration.

- Assess patient's oral cavity and dentition. Look for any inflammation or bleeding of the gums. Look for ulcers, lesions, and yellow or white patches. The yellow or white patches may indicate a fungal infection called thrush.
- Assess for signs of dehydration (dry mucosa) and dental decay. Look at the lips for dryness or cracking.
- If possible, ask the patient if he or she is having pain, dryness, soreness, or difficulty chewing or swallowing.

NURSING DIAGNOSES
- Ineffective Health Maintenance
- Impaired Oral Mucous Membrane
- Disturbed Body Image
- Deficient Knowledge
- Risk for Aspiration

OUTCOME IDENTIFICATION AND PLANNING
Expected outcomes may include:
- Patient's mouth and teeth will be clean.
- Patient will not experience impaired oral mucous membranes.
- Patient will participate as much as possible with oral care.
- Patient will demonstrate improvement in body image.
- Patient will verbalize an understanding about the importance of oral care.

IMPLEMENTATION

ACTION	RATIONALE
1. Perform hand hygiene and put on PPE, if indicated.	Hand hygiene and PPE prevent the spread of microorganisms. PPE is required based on transmission precautions.
2. Identify the patient. Explain procedure to patient.	Identifying the patient ensures the right patient receives the intervention and helps prevent errors. Explanation facilitates cooperation.
3. Assemble equipment on overbed table within reach.	Organization facilitates performance of task.
4. Close the room door or curtains. Place the bed at an appropriate and comfortable working height, usually elbow height of the caregiver	Cleaning another person's mouth is invasive and may be embarrassing (Holman, et al., 2005). Closing the door or curtains provides privacy. Proper bed height

ACTION	RATIONALE

(VISN 8 Patient Safety Center, 2009). Lower one side rail and position patient on the side, with head tilted forward. Place towel across patient's chest and emesis basin in position under chin. Put on gloves.

5. Gently open the patient's mouth by applying pressure to lower jaw at the front of the mouth. Remove dentures, if present (see Skill 49). Brush the teeth and gums carefully with toothbrush and paste (FIGURE 1). Lightly brush the tongue.

helps reduce back strain while performing the procedure. The side-lying position with head forward prevents aspiration of fluid into lungs. Towel and emesis basin protect patient from dampness. Gloves prevent the spread of microorganisms.

Toothbrush provides friction necessary to clean areas where plaque and tartar accumulate.

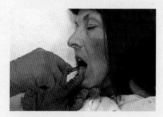

FIGURE 1 Carefully brushing patient's teeth.

6. Use toothette dipped in water to rinse the oral cavity. If desired, insert the rubber tip of the irrigating syringe into patient's mouth and rinse gently with a small amount of water (FIGURE 2). **Position patient's head to allow for return of water or use suction apparatus to remove the water from the oral cavity (FIGURE 3).**

Rinsing helps clean debris from the mouth. Forceful irrigation may cause aspiration.

ACTION	RATIONALE

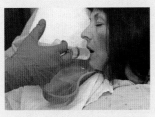

FIGURE 2 Using irrigating syringe and a small amount of water to rinse mouth.

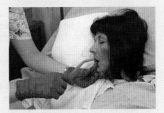

FIGURE 3 Using suction to remove excess fluid.

ACTION	RATIONALE
7. Clean the dentures before replacing (see Skill 49).	Cleaning maintains dentures and oral hygiene. Plaque can accumulate on dentures and can promote oropharyngeal colonization of pathogens (Yoon & Steele, 2007).
8. Apply lubricant to patient's lips.	This prevents drying and cracking of lips.
9. Remove equipment and return patient to a position of comfort. Remove your gloves. Raise side rail and lower bed.	Promotes patient comfort and safety. Removing gloves properly reduces the risk for infection transmission and contamination of other items.
10. Remove additional PPE, if used. Perform hand hygiene.	Removing PPE properly reduces the risk for infection transmission and contamination of other items. Hand hygiene prevents the spread of microorganisms.

EVALUATION

- Patient's oral cavity is clean and free from complications.
- Patient states or demonstrates improved body image.
- If able, the patient verbalizes a basic understanding of the need for oral care.

DOCUMENTATION

- Record oral assessment, significant observations, and unusual findings, such as bleeding or inflammation. Document any teaching done. Document procedure and patient response.

SPECIAL CONSIDERATIONS

* Suction toothbrushes may be used with patients with dysphagia, including those on enteral feedings (Yoon & Steele, 2007).
* A soft bristled toothbrush with a small head should be used even when the patient has no or few teeth. It is the only effective way to remove plaque and debris from the teeth, gums, and tongue (Holman, et al., 2005).
* When meeting the oral hygiene needs of patients with cognitive impairments, maintain a relaxed demeanor. Use calming language. Try to determine phrases and terms the patient understands in relation to hygiene and make use of them. Offer frequent reassurance.
* A patient receiving chemotherapy medication may have bleeding gums and extremely sensitive mucous membranes. Use a soft sponge toothette for cleaning, and a salt water rinse (half teaspoon salt in 1 cup of warm water) (Polovich, et al., 2005).

Skill · 122   Inserting an Oropharyngeal Airway

An oropharyngeal airway is a semicircular tube of plastic or rubber inserted into the back of the pharynx through the mouth in a patient who is breathing spontaneously. The oropharyngeal airway can help protect the airway of an unconscious patient by preventing the tongue from falling back against the posterior pharynx and blocking it. Once the patient regains consciousness, the oropharyngeal airway is removed. Tape is not used to hold the airway in place because the patient should be able to expel the airway once he or she becomes alert. The nurse can insert this device at the bedside with little to no trauma to the unconscious patient. Oropharyngeal airways may also be used to aid in ventilation during a code situation and to facilitate suctioning an unconscious or semiconscious patient. Alternately, airway support may be provided with a nasopharyngeal airway. Nasopharyngeal airways, frequently referred to as nasal trumpets, are curved soft rubber or plastic tubes inserted into the back of the pharynx through the nose in patients who are breathing spontaneously.

EQUIPMENT

* Oropharyngeal airway of appropriate size
* Disposable gloves
* Suction equipment
* Goggles or face shield (optional)
* Flashlight (optional)
* Additional PPE, as indicated

ASSESSMENT GUIDELINES

- Assess patient's level of consciousness and ability to protect the airway.
- Assess amount and consistency of oral secretions.
- Auscultate lung sounds. If the tongue is occluding the airway, lung sounds may be diminished.
- Assess for loose teeth or recent oral surgery, which may contraindicate the use of an oropharyngeal airway.

NURSING DIAGNOSES

- Risk for Aspiration
- Ineffective Airway Clearance
- Risk for Injury

OUTCOME IDENTIFICATION AND PLANNING

Expected outcomes may include:
- Patient will sustain a patent airway.
- Patient remains free of aspiration and injury.

IMPLEMENTATION

ACTION	RATIONALE
1. Bring necessary equipment to the bedside stand or over-bed table.	Bringing everything to the bed-side conserves time and energy. Arranging items nearby is convenient, saves time, and avoids unnecessary stretching and twisting of muscles on the part of the nurse.
2. Perform hand hygiene and put on PPE, if indicated.	Hand hygiene and PPE prevent the spread of microorganisms. PPE is required based on transmission precautions.
3. Identify the patient.	Identifying the patient ensures the right patient receives the intervention and helps prevent errors.
4. Close curtains around bed and close the door to the room, if possible.	This ensures the patient's privacy.

ACTION	RATIONALE
5. Explain to the patient what you are going to do and the reason for doing it, even though the patient does not appear to be alert.	Explanation alleviates fears. Even though a patient appears unconscious, the nurse should explain what is happening.
6. Put on disposable gloves; put on goggles or face shield, as indicated.	Gloves and other PPE prevent contact with contaminants and body fluids.
7. Measure the oropharyngeal airway for correct size. Measure the oropharyngeal airway by holding the airway on the side of the patient's face. The airway should reach from the opening of the mouth to the back angle of the jaw.	Correct size ensures correct insertion and fit, allowing for conformation of the airway to the curvature of the palate.
8. **Check mouth for any loose teeth, dentures, or other foreign material. Remove dentures or material if present.**	Prevents aspiration or swallowing of objects. During insertion, the airway may push any foreign objects in the mouth to the back of the throat.
9. Position patient in semi-Fowler's position.	This position facilitates airway insertion and helps prevent the tongue from moving back against the posterior pharynx.
10. Suction patient if necessary.	This removes excess secretions and helps maintain patent airway.
11. Open patient's mouth by using your thumb and index finger to gently pry teeth apart. **Insert the airway with the curved tip pointing up toward the roof of the mouth (FIGURE 1).**	This is done to advance the tip of the airway past the tongue, toward the back of the throat.

FIGURE 1 Sliding in the airway.

ACTION	RATIONALE
12. Slide the airway across the tongue to the back of the mouth. Rotate the airway 180 degrees as it passes the uvula. The tip should point down and the curvature should follow the contour of the roof of the mouth. A flashlight can be used to confirm the position of the airway with the curve fitting over the tongue.	This is done to shift the tongue anteriorly, thereby allowing the patient to breathe through and around the airway.
13. Ensure accurate placement and adequate ventilation by auscultating breath sounds.	If the airway is placed correctly, lung sounds should be audible and equal in all lobes.
14. Position patient on his or her side when airway is in place.	This position helps keep the tongue out of the posterior pharynx area and helps to prevent aspiration if the unconscious patient should vomit.
15. Remove gloves and additional PPE, if used. Perform hand hygiene.	Removing PPE properly reduces the risk for infection transmission and contamination of other items. Hand hygiene prevents the spread of microorganisms.
16. Remove the airway for a brief period every 4 hours, or according to facility policy. Assess mouth, provide mouth care, and clean the airway according to facility policy before reinserting it.	Tissue irritation and ulceration can result from prolonged use of an airway. Mouth care provides moisture to mucous membranes and helps maintain tissue integrity.

EVALUATION

• Patient exhibits a patent airway with oxygen saturation levels >95%.
• Patient remains free of injury and aspiration.

DOCUMENTATION

• Document airway placement, airway size, removal/cleaning, assessment before and after intervention, and oxygen saturation level.

GENERAL CONSIDERATIONS

- Wearing gloves, remove the airway briefly every 4 hours to provide mouth care. Assess the mouth and tongue for tissue irritation, tooth damage, bleeding, and ulceration. Ensure that the lips and tongue are not between the teeth and the airway to prevent injury.
- When reinserting the oropharyngeal airway, attempt to insert it on the other side of the mouth. This helps to prevent tongue and mouth irritation.
- Suction secretions, as needed, by manipulating around and through the oropharyngeal airway.

Skill · 123   Changing and Emptying an Ostomy Appliance

The word *ostomy* is a term for a surgically formed opening from the inside of an organ to the outside. The intestinal mucosa is brought out to the abdominal wall and a *stoma*, the part of the ostomy that is attached to the skin, is formed by suturing the mucosa to the skin. An *ileostomy* allows liquid fecal content from the ileum of the small intestine to be eliminated through the stoma. A *colostomy* permits formed feces in the colon to exit through the stoma. Colostomies are further classified by the part of the colon from which they originate. Ostomy appliances or pouches are applied to the opening to collect stool. They should be emptied promptly, usually when they are one-third to one-half full. If they are allowed to fill up, they may leak or become detached from the skin. Ostomy appliances are available in a one-piece (barrier backing already attached to the pouch) or two-piece (separate pouch that fastens to the barrier backing) system; they are usually changed every 3 to 7 days, although they could be changed more often. Proper application minimizes the risk for skin breakdown around the stoma. This skill addresses changing a one-piece appliance. A one-piece appliance consists of a pouch with an integral adhesive section that adheres to the patient's skin. The adhesive flange is generally made from hydrocolloid. The accompanying Skill Variation addresses changing a two-piece appliance.

EQUIPMENT

- Basin with warm water
- Skin cleanser, towel, washcloth
- Silicone-based adhesive remover
- Gauze squares
- Washcloth or cotton balls
- Skin protectant, such as SkinPrep
- One-piece ostomy appliance
- Closure clamp, if required for appliance
- Stoma measuring guide
- Graduated container, toilet, or bedpan
- Ostomy belt (optional)
- Disposable gloves
- Additional PPE, as indicated
- Small plastic trash bag
- Waterproof disposable pad

ASSESSMENT GUIDELINES

- Assess current ostomy appliance, looking at product style, condition of appliance, and stoma (if bag is clear). Note length of time the appliance has been in place.
- Determine the patient's knowledge of ostomy care.
- Assess the skin surrounding the stoma.
- Assess any abdominal scars, if surgery was recent.
- Assess the amount, color, consistency, and odor of stool from the ostomy.

NURSING DIAGNOSES

- Risk for Impaired Skin Integrity
- Deficient Knowledge
- Disturbed Body Image
- Ineffective Coping
- Constipation
- Diarrhea

OUTCOME IDENTIFICATION AND PLANNING

Expected outcomes may include:
- Stoma appliance is applied correctly to the skin to allow stool to drain freely.
- Patient exhibits a moist red stoma with intact skin surrounding the stoma.
- Patient demonstrates knowledge of how to apply the appliance.
- Patient demonstrates positive coping skills.
- Patient expels stool that is appropriate in consistency and amount for the ostomy location.
- Patient verbalizes a positive self-image.

IMPLEMENTATION

ACTION	RATIONALE
1. Bring necessary equipment to the bedside stand or over-bed table.	Bringing everything to the bedside conserves time and energy. Arranging items nearby is convenient, saves time, and avoids unnecessary stretching and twisting of muscles on the part of the nurse.
2. Perform hand hygiene and put on PPE, if indicated.	Hand hygiene and PPE prevent the spread of microorganisms. PPE is required based on transmission precautions.

ACTION	RATIONALE
3. Identify the patient.	Identifying the patient ensures the right patient receives the intervention and helps prevent errors.
4. Close curtains around bed and close the door to the room, if possible. Explain what you are going to do and why you are going to do it to the patient. Encourage the patient to observe or participate if possible.	This ensures the patient's privacy. Explanation relieves anxiety and facilitates cooperation. Discussion promotes cooperation and helps to minimize anxiety. Having the patient observe or assist encourages self-acceptance.
5. Assist the patient to a comfortable sitting or lying position in bed or a standing or sitting position in the bathroom.	Either position should allow the patient to view the procedure in preparation to learn to perform it independently. Lying flat or sitting upright facilitates smooth application of the appliance.

Emptying an Appliance

ACTION	RATIONALE
6. Put on disposable gloves. Remove clamp and fold end of pouch upward like a cuff.	Gloves prevent contact with blood, body fluids, and microorganisms. Creating a cuff before emptying prevents additional soiling and odor.
7. Empty contents into bedpan, toilet, or measuring device.	Appliances do not need rinsing because rinsing may reduce appliance's odor barrier.
8. Wipe the lower 2 inches of the appliance or pouch with toilet tissue.	Drying the lower section removes any additional fecal material, thus decreasing odor problems.
9. Uncuff edge of appliance or pouch and apply clip or clamp, or secure Velcro closure. Ensure the curve of the clamp follows the curve of the patient's body. Remove gloves. Assist patient to a comfortable position.	The edge of the appliance or pouch should remain clean. The clamp secures closure. Hand hygiene deters spread of microorganisms. Ensures patient comfort.

ACTION	RATIONALE

10. If appliance is not to be changed, remove additional PPE, if used. Perform hand hygiene.

Removing PPE properly reduces the risk for infection transmission and contamination of other items. Hand hygiene prevents the spread of microorganisms.

Changing an Appliance

11. Place a disposable pad on the work surface. Set up the wash basin with warm water and the rest of the supplies. Place a trash bag within reach.

Protects surface. Organization facilitates performance of procedure.

12. Put on clean gloves. Place waterproof pad under the patient at the stoma site. Empty the appliance as described previously.

Protects linens and patient from moisture. Emptying the contents before removal prevents accidental spillage of fecal material.

13. Gently remove pouch faceplate from skin by pushing skin from appliance rather than pulling appliance from skin. Start at the top of the appliance, while keeping the abdominal skin taut. Apply a silicone-based adhesive remover by spraying or wiping with the remover wipe.

The seal between the surface of the faceplate and the skin must be broken before the faceplate can be removed. Harsh handling of the appliance can damage the skin and impair the development of a secure seal in the future. Silicone-based adhesive remover allows for the rapid and painless removal of adhesives and prevents skin stripping (Rudoni, 2008; Stephen-Haynes, 2008).

14. Place the appliance in the trash bag, if disposable. If reusable, set aside to wash in lukewarm soap and water and allow to air dry after the new appliance is in place.

Thorough cleaning and airing of the appliance reduce odor and deterioration of the appliance. For esthetic and infection-control purposes, discard used appliances appropriately.

15. Use toilet tissue to remove any excess stool from stoma. Cover stoma with gauze pad. Clean skin around stoma with mild soap and water or a cleansing agent and a washcloth. Remove all old adhesive

Toilet tissue, used gently, will not damage the stoma. The gauze absorbs any drainage from the stoma while the skin is being prepared. Cleaning the skin removes excretions and old adhesive and skin protectant.

ACTION	RATIONALE

from skin; use an adhesive remover, as necessary.
Do not apply lotion to peristomal area.

Excretions or a buildup of other substances can irritate and damage the skin. Lotion will prevent a tight adhesive seal.

16. Gently pat area dry. Make sure skin around the stoma is thoroughly dry. Assess stoma and condition of surrounding skin.

Careful drying prevents trauma to skin and stoma. An intact, properly applied urinary collection device protects skin integrity. Any change in color and size of the stoma may indicate circulatory problems.

17. Apply skin protectant to a 2-inch (5-cm) radius around the stoma, and allow it to dry completely, which takes about 30 seconds.

The skin needs protection from the excoriating effect of the excretion and appliance adhesive. The skin must be perfectly dry before the appliance is placed to get good adherence and to prevent leaks.

18. Lift the gauze squares for a moment and measure the stoma opening, using the measurement guide. Replace the gauze. Trace the same-size opening on the back center of the appliance. Cut the opening 1/8 inch larger than the stoma size.

The appliance should fit snugly around the stoma, with only 1/8 inch of skin visible around the opening. A faceplate opening that is too small can cause trauma to the stoma. If the opening is too large, exposed skin will be irritated by stool.

19. Remove the backing from the appliance. Quickly remove the gauze squares and ease the appliance over the stoma. Gently press onto the skin while smoothing over the surface. Apply gentle pressure to the appliance for 5 minutes.

The appliance is effective only if it is properly positioned and adhered securely.

20. Close bottom of appliance or pouch by folding the end upward and using the clamp or clip that comes with the product, or secure Velcro closure. Ensure the curve of the clamp follows the curve of the patient's body.

A tightly sealed appliance will not leak and cause embarrassment and discomfort for the patient.

ACTION	RATIONALE
21. Remove gloves. Assist the patient to a comfortable position. Cover the patient with bed linens. Place the bed in the lowest position.	Provides warmth and promotes comfort and safety.
22. Put on clean gloves. Remove or discard equipment and assess patient's response to the procedure.	Gloves prevent contact with blood, body fluids, and microorganisms that contaminate the used equipment. The patient's response may indicate acceptance of the ostomy as well as the need for health teaching.
23. Remove gloves and additional PPE, if used. Perform hand hygiene.	Removing PPE properly reduces the risk for infection transmission and contamination of other items. Hand hygiene prevents the spread of microorganisms.

EVALUATION

• Patient tolerates the procedure without pain and the peristomal skin remains intact without excoriation.
• Odor is contained within the closed system.
• Patient participates in ostomy appliance care, demonstrates positive coping skills, and expels stool that is appropriate in consistency and amount for the location of the ostomy.

DOCUMENTATION

• Document appearance of stoma, condition of peristomal skin, characteristics of drainage (amount, color, consistency, unusual odor), and patient's reaction to procedure.

Skill Variation   Applying a Two-Piece Appliance

A two-piece colostomy appliance is composed of a pouch and a separate adhesive faceplate. The faceplate is left in place for a period of time, usually 2 to 5 days. During this period, when the colostomy appliance requires changing, only the bag needs to be replaced. There are two main types of two-piece appliance: those that 'click' together and those that 'adhere' together. The clicking Tupperware-type joining action provides extra security as there is a sensation when the appliance is secured,

(continued on page 670)

Applying a Two-Piece Appliance *continued*

which the patient can feel. One problem with this type of system is that those with reduced manual dexterity may find it difficult to secure. Another disadvantage is that it is less discreet because the parts of the appliance that click together are more bulky than the one-piece system. Two-piece appliances with an adhesive system have the advantage that they are more discreet than conventional two-piece systems. They may also be simpler to use for those with poor manual dexterity. A potential disadvantage is that if the adhesive is not joined correctly and forms a crease, then feces or flatus may leak out, causing odor and embarrassment (Burch & Sica, 2007). Regardless of the type of two-piece appliance in use, the procedure to change is basically the same.

1. Bring necessary equipment to the bedside stand or overbed table.

2. Perform hand hygiene and put on PPE, if indicated.

3. Identify the patient.

4. Close curtains around the bed and close door to room, if possible. Explain what you are going to do and why you are going to

do it to the patient. Encourage patient to observe or participate if possible.

5. Assist the patient to a comfortable sitting or lying position in bed or a standing or sitting position in the bathroom.

6. Place a disposable pad on the work surface. Set up the wash basin with warm water and the rest of the supplies. Place a trash bag within reach.

7. Put on clean gloves. Place waterproof pad under the patient at the stoma site. Empty the appliance as described previously in Skill 123.

8. Gently remove pouch faceplate from skin by pushing skin from appliance rather than pulling appliance from skin. Start at the top of the appliance, while keeping the abdominal skin taut. Apply a silicone-based adhesive remover by spraying or wiping with the remover wipe.

9. Place the appliance in the trash bag, if disposable. If reusable, set aside to wash in lukewarm soap and water and allow to air dry after the new appliance is in place.

10. Use toilet tissue to remove any excess stool from stoma. Cover stoma with gauze pad. Clean skin around stoma with mild soap and water or a

Applying a Two-Piece Appliance *continued*

cleansing agent and a washcloth. Remove all old adhesive from skin; use an adhesive remover as necessary. Do not apply lotion to peristomal area.

11. Gently pat area dry. Make sure skin around stoma is thoroughly dry. Assess stoma and condition of surrounding skin.

12. Apply skin protectant to a 2-inch (5-cm) radius around the stoma, and allow it to dry completely, which takes about 30 seconds.

13. Lift the gauze squares for a moment and measure the stoma opening, using the measurement guide. Replace the gauze. Trace the same-size opening on the back center of the appliance faceplate. Cut the opening 1/8 inch larger than the stoma size.

14. Remove the backing from the faceplate. Quickly remove the gauze squares and ease the faceplate over the stoma. Gently press onto the skin while smoothing over the surface. Apply gentle pressure to faceplate for 5 minutes.

15. Apply the appliance pouch to the faceplate following manufacturer's directions. If using a 'click' system, lay the ring on the pouch over the ring on the faceplate. Ask the patient to tighten stomach muscles,

if possible. Beginning at one edge of the ring, push the pouch ring onto the faceplate ring (FIGURE 1). A 'click' should be heard when the pouch is secured onto the faceplate.

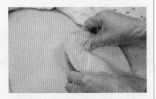

FIGURE 1 Securing appliance pouch to the faceplate.

16. If using an 'adhere' system, remove the paper backing from the faceplate and pouch. Starting at one edge, carefully match the pouch adhesive with the faceplate adhesive. Press firmly and smooth the pouch onto the faceplate, taking care to avoid creases.

17. Close bottom of pouch by folding the end upward and using clamp or clip that comes with product, or secure Velcro closure. Ensure the curve of the clamp follows the curve of the patient's body.

18. Remove gloves. Assist the patient to a comfortable position. Cover the patient with bed linens. Place the bed in the lowest position.

(continued on page 672)

Applying a Two-Piece Appliance *continued*

19. Put on clean gloves. Remove or discard equipment and assess patient's response to the procedure.

20. Remove gloves and additional PPE, if used. Perform hand hygiene.

Skill · 124   **Emptying and Changing a Stoma Appliance on an Ileal Conduit**

An ileal conduit is a cutaneous urinary diversion. An ileal conduit involves a surgical resection of the small intestine, with transplantation of the ureters to the isolated segment of small bowel. This separated section of the small intestine is then brought to the abdominal wall, where urine is excreted through a stoma, a surgically created opening on the body surface. Such diversions are usually permanent, and the patient wears an external appliance to collect the urine because elimination of the urine from the stoma cannot be controlled voluntarily. The frequency of changing the appliance depends on the type being used. The usual wear time is 5 days. The appliance usually is changed after a time of low fluid intake, such as in the early morning. Urine production is less at this time, making changing the appliance easier. Proper application minimizes the risk for skin breakdown around the stoma.

EQUIPMENT

- Basin with warm water
- Skin cleanser, towel, washcloth
- Silicone-based adhesive remover
- Gauze squares
- Washcloth or cotton balls
- Skin protectant
- Ostomy appliance
- Stoma measuring guide
- Graduated container
- Ostomy belt (optional)
- Disposable gloves
- Additional PPE, as indicated
- Waterproof disposable pad
- Small plastic trash bag

ASSESSMENT GUIDELINES

- Assess current ileal conduit appliance, observing product style, condition of appliance, and stoma (if bag is clear). Note length of time the appliance has been in place.
- Determine the patient's knowledge of care of the ileal conduit, including level of self-care and ability to manipulate equipment.
- After the appliance is removed, assess the skin surrounding the ileal conduit.

- Assess the condition of any abdominal scars or incisional areas, if surgery to create the urinary diversion was recent.

NURSING DIAGNOSES
- Impaired Urinary Elimination
- Risk for Impaired Skin Integrity
- Disturbed Body Image
- Deficient Knowledge

OUTCOME IDENTIFICATION AND PLANNING
Expected outcomes may include:
- Stoma appliance is applied correctly to the skin to allow urine to drain freely.
- Patient exhibits a moist red stoma with intact skin surrounding the stoma.
- Patient demonstrates knowledge of how to apply the appliance.
- Patient verbalizes positive self-image.

IMPLEMENTATION

ACTION

1. Bring necessary equipment to the bedside stand or over-bed table.

2. Perform hand hygiene and put on PPE, if indicated.

3. Identify the patient.

4. Close curtains around bed and close the door to the room, if possible. Explain what you are going to do and why you are going to do it to the patient. Encourage the

RATIONALE

Bringing everything to the bedside conserves time and energy. Arranging items nearby is convenient, saves time, and avoids unnecessary stretching and twisting of muscles on the part of the nurse.

Hand hygiene and PPE prevent the spread of microorganisms. PPE is required based on transmission precautions.

Identifying the patient ensures the right patient receives the intervention and helps prevent errors.

This ensures the patient's privacy. Explanation relieves anxiety and facilitates cooperation. Discussion promotes cooperation and helps to minimize anxiety. Having the patient observe or

ACTION	RATIONALE
patient to observe or partici-pate if possible.	assist encourages self-acceptance.
5. Assist the patient to a com-fortable sitting or lying posi-tion in bed or a standing or sitting position in the bath-room. If the patient is in bed, adjust the bed to a comfort-able working height, usually elbow height of the caregiver (VISN 8 Patient Safety Cen-ter, 2009). Place waterproof pad under the patient at the stoma site.	Either position should allow the patient to view the procedure in preparation for learning to per-form it independently. Lying flat or sitting upright facilitates smooth application of the appli-ance. Having the bed at the proper height prevents back and muscle strain. A waterproof pad protects linens and patient from moisture.

Emptying the Appliance

ACTION	RATIONALE
6. Put on gloves. Hold end of appliance over a bedpan, toi-let, or measuring device. Remove the end cap from the spout. Open spout and empty contents into the bedpan, toi-let, or measuring device.	Gloves protect the nurse from exposure to blood and body flu-ids. Emptying the pouch before handling it reduces the likelihood of spilling the excretions.
7. Close the spout. Wipe the spout with toilet tissue. Replace the cap.	Drying the spout removes any urine.
8. Remove equipment. Remove gloves. Assist the patient to a comfortable position.	Proper removal of PPE prevents the transmission of microorgan-isms. Ensures patient comfort.
9. If appliance is not to be changed, place bed in lowest position. Remove additional PPE, if used. Perform hand hygiene.	Lowering the bed promotes patient safety. Removing PPE properly reduces the risk for infection transmission and con-tamination of other items. Hand hygiene prevents the spread of microorganisms.

Changing the Appliance

ACTION	RATIONALE
10. Place a disposable water-proof pad on the overbed table or other work area. Set up the wash basin with warm water and the rest of the sup-plies. Place a trash bag within reach.	The pad protects the surface. Organization facilitates perfor-mance of procedure.

ACTION	RATIONALE
11. Put on clean gloves. Place waterproof pad under the patient at the stoma site. Empty the appliance as necessary as described in steps 6–8.	Waterproof pad protects linens and patient from moisture. Emptying the contents before removal prevents accidental spillage of fecal material.
12. Gently remove appliance faceplate from skin by pushing skin from the appliance rather than pulling the appliance from skin. Start at the top of the appliance, while keeping the skin taut. Apply a silicone-based adhesive remover by spraying or wiping with the remover wipe.	The seal between the surface of the faceplate and the skin must be broken before the faceplate can be removed. Harsh handling of the appliance can damage the skin and impair the development of a secure seal in the future. Silicone-based adhesive remover allows for the rapid and painless removal of adhesives and prevents skin stripping (Rudoni, 2008; Stephen-Haynes, 2008).
13. Place the appliance in the trash bag, if disposable. If reusable, set aside to wash in lukewarm soap and water and allow to air dry after the new appliance is in place.	Thorough cleaning and airing of the appliance reduce odor and deterioration of the appliance. For aesthetic and infection-control purposes, used appliances should be discarded appropriately.
14. Clean skin around the stoma with mild soap and water or a cleansing agent and a washcloth. Remove all old adhesive from skin; additional adhesive remover may be used. Do not apply lotion to peristomal area.	Cleaning the skin removes excretions and old adhesive and skin protectant. Excretions or a buildup of other substances can irritate and damage the skin. Lotion will prevent a tight adhesive seal.
15. Gently pat area dry. **Make sure skin around stoma is thoroughly dry.** Assess stoma and condition of surrounding skin.	Careful drying prevents trauma to skin and stoma. An intact, properly applied urinary collection device protects skin integrity. Any change in color and size of the stoma may indicate circulatory problems.
16. Place one or two gauze squares over stoma opening.	Continuous drainage must be absorbed to keep skin dry during appliance change.

ACTION	RATIONALE
17. Apply skin protectant to a 2-inch (5-cm) radius around the stoma, and allow it to dry completely, which takes about 30 seconds.	
18. Lift the gauze squares for a moment and measure the stoma opening, using the measurement guide. Replace the gauze. Trace the same size opening on the back center of the appliance. Cut the opening 1/8 inch larger than the stoma size (FIGURE 1). Check that the spout is closed and the end cap is in place.	The appliance should fit snugly around the stoma, with only 1/8 inch of skin visible around the opening. A faceplate opening that is too small can cause trauma to the stoma. If the opening is too large, exposed skin will be irritated by urine. A closed spout and secured end cap prevent urine from leaking from the appliance.

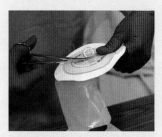

FIGURE 1 Cutting the faceplate opening 1/8 inch larger than stoma size.

ACTION	RATIONALE
19. Remove the backing from the appliance. Quickly remove the gauze squares and discard appropriately; ease the appliance over the stoma. **Gently press onto the skin while smoothing over the surface. Apply gentle pressure to the appliance for a few minutes.**	The appliance is effective only if it is properly positioned and adhered securely.
20. Secure optional belt to the appliance and around the patient.	An elasticized belt helps support the appliance for some people.

ACTION	RATIONALE
21. Remove gloves. Assist the patient to a comfortable position. Cover the patient with bed linens. Place the bed in the lowest position.	Removing gloves reduces risk of transmission of microorganisms. Positioning and covering provide warmth and promote comfort. Bed in lowest position promotes patient safety.
22. Put on clean gloves. Remove or discard any remaining equipment and assess patient's response to procedure.	The patient's response may indicate acceptance of the ostomy as well as the need for health teaching.
23. Remove gloves and additional PPE, if used. Perform hand hygiene.	Removing PPE properly reduces the risk of infection transmission and contamination of other items. Hand hygiene prevents the spread of microorganisms.

EVALUATION

- Ileal conduit appliance is changed without trauma to stoma or peristomal skin, or leaking.
- Urine is draining freely into the appliance.
- Patient's skin surrounding the stoma is clean, dry, and intact.
- Patient shows an interest in learning to perform the appliance change and verbalizes positive self-image.

DOCUMENTATION

- Document the procedure, including the appearance of the stoma, condition of the peristomal skin, characteristics of the urine, and the patient's response to the procedure.

GENERAL CONSIDERATIONS

- If using a two-piece appliance, after applying the faceplate, snap the appliance pouch in place. Lay the pouch flange over the flange on the faceplate. Start at the bottom and push as you run your fingers around the flange, snapping the pouch onto the flange.

Skill · 125 **Using an Oxygen Hood**

Oxygen hoods are generally used to deliver oxygen to infants. They can supply an oxygen concentration up to 80% to 90%. Use of oxygen hoods enable the oxygen percentage to be measured more accurately and make appropriate humidification possible (Pease, 2006). The oxygen hood is placed over the infant's head and shoulders, and allows easy access to the chest and lower body. The hoods are made of hard plastic or vinyl with a metal frame.

EQUIPMENT
- Oxygen source
- Oxygen hood (head box)
- Oxygen analyzer
- Humidification device
- PPE, as indicated

ASSESSMENT GUIDELINES
- Assess the patient's lung sounds. Many respiratory conditions may cause the patient's oxygen demand to increase.
- Assess the oxygen saturation level. The primary care provider will usually order a baseline for the pulse oximeter (i.e., deliver oxygen to keep pulse ox greater than 95%).
- Assess skin color. A pale or cyanotic patient may not be receiving enough oxygen.
- Assess patient for any signs of respiratory distress, such as nasal flaring, grunting, or retractions; oxygen-depleted patients often exhibit these signs.

NURSING DIAGNOSES
- Impaired Gas Exchange
- Ineffective Breathing Pattern
- Ineffective Airway Clearance

OUTCOME IDENTIFICATION AND PLANNING
Expected outcomes may include:
- Patient exhibits an oxygen saturation level within acceptable parameters.
- Patient will remain free of signs and symptoms of respiratory distress.
- Patient's respiratory status, including respiratory rate and depth, will be in the normal range for the patient's age group.
- Patient's skin will be dry, and without evidence of breakdown.

IMPLEMENTATION

ACTION	RATIONALE
1. Bring necessary equipment to the bedside stand or over-bed table.	Bringing everything to the bed-side conserves time and energy. Arranging items nearby is convenient, saves time, and avoids unnecessary stretching and twisting of muscles on the part of the nurse.
2. Perform hand hygiene and put on PPE, if indicated.	Hand hygiene and PPE prevent the spread of microorganisms. PPE is required based on transmission precautions.
3. Identify the patient.	Identifying the patient ensures the right patient receives the intervention and helps prevent errors.
4. Close curtains around bed and close the door to the room, if possible.	This ensures the patient's privacy.
5. Explain what you are going to do and the reason for doing it to the patient and parents/guardians. Review safety precautions necessary when oxygen is in use.	Explanation relieves anxiety and facilitates cooperation. Oxygen supports combustion.
6. Calibrate the oxygen analyzer according to manufacturer's directions.	This ensures accurate readings and appropriate adjustments to therapy.
7. Place hood on crib. Connect humidifier to oxygen source in the wall. Connect the oxygen tubing to the hood. Adjust flow rate as ordered by physician. Check that oxygen is flowing into the hood.	Oxygen forced through a water reservoir is humidified before it is delivered to the patient, thus preventing dehydration of the mucous membranes.
8. Turn analyzer on. **Place oxygen analyzer probe in hood.**	The analyzer will give an accurate reading of the concentration of oxygen in the hood or bed.

ACTION	RATIONALE
9. Adjust oxygen flow as necessary, based on sensor readings. Once oxygen levels reach the prescribed amount, place hood over the patient's head (FIGURE 1). The hood should not rub against the infant's neck, chin, or shoulder.	Patient will receive oxygen once placed under the hood. Pressure and irritation could result in alterations in the infant's skin integrity.

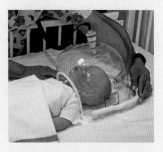

FIGURE 1 Placing oxygen hood over infant.

10. If using the soft vinyl hood, roll small blankets or towels and place around edges where hood meets crib (if needed) to keep oxygen concentration at desired level.	The blankets help keep the edges of the hood sealed and prevent oxygen from escaping.
Do not block hole in top of hood if present. If using a vinyl hood, the vent hole covering may need to be removed.	This hole allows for the escape of carbon dioxide; blocking it may cause a buildup of carbon dioxide in the hood.
11. Instruct family members not to raise edges of the hood.	Every time the hood is raised, oxygen is released.
12. Reassess patient's respiratory status, including respiratory rate, effort, oxygen saturation, and lung sounds. Note any signs of respiratory distress, such as tachypnea,	This assesses the effectiveness of oxygen therapy.

ACTION	RATIONALE

nasal flaring, grunting, retractions, or dyspnea.

13. Remove PPE, if used. Perform hand hygiene.

Removing PPE properly reduces the risk for infection transmission and contamination of other items. Hand hygiene prevents the spread of microorganisms.

14. Frequently check bedding and patient's head for moisture. Change linen and dry skin as needed to keep the patient dry.

The humidification delivered in an oxygen hood makes cloth moist, which would be uncomfortable for the patient and possibly lower body temperature.

15. Monitor the patient's body temperature at regular intervals.

Hypothermia can result from administering cool oxygen.

EVALUATION

• Patient exhibits an oxygen saturation level within acceptable parameters.
• Patient remains free of dyspnea, nasal flaring, grunting, or use of accessory muscles when breathing, and respirations remain in normal range for age.

DOCUMENTATION

• Document amount of oxygen applied, respiratory rate, oxygen saturation level, and assessment before and after intervention.

Skill · 126   Administering Oxygen by Mask

When a patient requires a higher concentration of oxygen than a nasal cannula can deliver (6 L or 44% oxygen concentration), use an oxygen mask. Fit the mask carefully to the patient's face to avoid leakage of oxygen. The mask should be comfortably snug, but not tight against the face. Disposable and reusable face masks are available. The most commonly used types of masks are the simple facemask, the partial rebreather mask, the nonrebreather mask, and the Venturi mask.

EQUIPMENT

- Flow meter connected to oxygen supply
- Humidifier with sterile distilled water, if necessary, for the type of mask prescribed
- Face mask, specified by primary care provider
- Gauze to pad elastic band (optional)
- PPE, as indicated

ASSESSMENT GUIDELINES

- Assess patient's oxygen saturation level before starting oxygen therapy to provide a baseline for evaluating the effectiveness of oxygen therapy.
- Assess patient's respiratory status, including respiratory rate, effort, and lung sounds. Note any signs of respiratory distress, such as tachypnea, nasal flaring, use of accessory muscles, or dyspnea.

NURSING DIAGNOSES

- Impaired Gas Exchange
- Ineffective Breathing Pattern
- Ineffective Airway Clearance
- Risk for Activity Intolerance
- Excess Fluid Volume
- Decreased Cardiac Output

OUTCOME IDENTIFICATION AND PLANNING

Expected outcomes may include:
- Patient will exhibit an oxygen saturation level within acceptable parameters.
- Patient will not experience dyspnea.
- Patient will demonstrate effortless respirations in the normal range for age group, without evidence of nasal flaring or use of accessory muscles.

IMPLEMENTATION

ACTION	RATIONALE
1. Bring necessary equipment to the bedside stand or overbed table.	Bringing everything to the bedside conserves time and energy. Arranging items nearby is convenient, saves time, and avoids unnecessary stretching and twisting of muscles on the part of the nurse
2. Perform hand hygiene and put on PPE, if indicated.	Hand hygiene and PPE prevent the spread of microorganisms. PPE is required based on transmission precautions.

ACTION	RATIONALE
3. Identify the patient.	Identifying the patient ensures the right patient receives the intervention and helps prevent errors.
4. Close curtains around bed and close the door to the room, if possible.	This ensures the patient's privacy.
5. Explain what you are going to do and the reason for doing it to the patient. Review safety precautions necessary when oxygen is in use. Place "No Smoking" signs in appropriate areas.	Explanation relieves anxiety and facilitates cooperation. Oxygen supports combustion; a small spark could cause a fire.
6. Attach face mask to oxygen source (with humidification, if appropriate, for the specific mask). Start the flow of oxygen at the specified rate. For a mask with a reservoir, be sure to allow oxygen to fill the bag before proceeding to the next step.	Oxygen forced through a water reservoir is humidified before it is delivered to the patient, thus preventing dehydration of the mucous membranes. A reservoir bag must be inflated with oxygen because the bag is the oxygen supply source for the patient.
7. Position face mask over the patient's nose and mouth (FIGURE 1). Adjust the elastic strap so that the mask fits snugly but comfortably on the face. Adjust the flow rate to the prescribed rate.	A loose or poorly fitting mask will result in oxygen loss and decreased therapeutic value. Masks may cause a feeling of suffocation, and the patient needs frequent attention and reassurance.

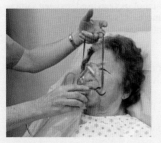

FIGURE 1 Applying face mask over the patient's nose and mouth.

ACTION	RATIONALE
8. If the patient reports irritation or redness is noted, use gauze pads under the elastic strap at pressure points to reduce irritation to ears and scalp.	Pads reduce irritation and pressure and protect the skin.
9. Reassess patient's respiratory status, including respiratory rate, effort, and lung sounds. Note any signs of respiratory distress, such as tachypnea, nasal flaring, use of accessory muscles, or dyspnea.	This helps assess the effectiveness of oxygen therapy.
10. Remove PPE, if used. Perform hand hygiene.	Removing PPE properly reduces the risk for infection transmission and contamination of other items. Hand hygiene prevents the spread of microorganisms.
11. **Remove the mask and dry the skin every 2 to 3 hours if the oxygen is running continuously. Do not use powder around the mask.**	The tight-fitting mask and moisture from condensation can irritate the skin on the face. There is a danger of inhaling powder if it is placed on the mask.

EVALUATION

- Patient exhibits an oxygen saturation level within acceptable parameters.
- Patient demonstrates an absence of respiratory distress and accessory muscle use and exhibits respiratory rate and depth within normal parameters for age group.

DOCUMENTATION

- Document type of mask used, amount of oxygen used, oxygen saturation level, lung sounds, and rate/pattern of respirations. Document your assessment before and after intervention.

GENERAL CONSIDERATIONS

- It is important to ensure the mask fits snugly around the patient's face. If it is loose, it will not effectively deliver the right amount of oxygen.
- The mask must be removed for the patient to eat, drink, and take medications. Obtain an order for oxygen via nasal cannula for use during meal times and limit the amount of times the mask is removed to maintain adequate oxygenation.

Skill · 127   Administering Oxygen by Nasal Cannula

A nasal cannula, also called nasal prongs, is the most commonly used oxygen delivery device. The cannula is a disposable plastic device with two protruding prongs for insertion into the nostrils. The cannula connects to an oxygen source with a flow meter and, many times, a humidifier. It is commonly used because the cannula does not impede eating or speaking and is used easily in the home. Disadvantages of this system are that it can be dislodged easily and can cause dryness of the nasal mucosa. A nasal cannula is used to deliver from 1 L/minute to 6 L/minute of oxygen.

EQUIPMENT

- Flow meter connected to oxygen supply
- Humidifier with sterile distilled water (optional for low-flow system)
- Nasal cannula and tubing
- Gauze to pad tubing over ears (optional)
- PPE, as indicated

ASSESSMENT GUIDELINES

- Assess the patient's oxygen saturation level before starting oxygen therapy to provide a baseline for evaluating the effectiveness of oxygen therapy.
- Assess the patient's respiratory status, including respiratory rate, effort, and lung sounds. Note any signs of respiratory distress, such as tachypnea, nasal flaring, use of accessory muscles, or dyspnea.

NURSING DIAGNOSES

- Impaired Gas Exchange
- Ineffective Breathing Pattern
- Ineffective Airway Clearance
- Risk for Activity Intolerance
- Excess Fluid Volume
- Decreased Cardiac Output

OUTCOME IDENTIFICATION AND PLANNING

Expected outcomes may include:
- Patient will exhibit an oxygen saturation level within acceptable parameters.
- Patient will not experience dyspnea.
- Patient will demonstrate effortless respirations in the normal range for age group, without evidence of nasal flaring or use of accessory muscles.

IMPLEMENTATION

ACTION	RATIONALE
1. Bring necessary equipment to the bedside stand or over-bed table.	Bringing everything to the bedside conserves time and energy. Arranging items nearby is convenient, saves time, and avoids unnecessary stretching and twisting of muscles on the part of the nurse.
2. Perform hand hygiene and put on PPE, if indicated.	Hand hygiene and PPE prevent the spread of microorganisms. PPE is required based on transmission precautions.
3. Identify the patient. 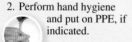	Identifying the patient ensures the right patient receives the intervention and helps prevent errors.
4. Close curtains around bed and close the door to the room, if possible.	This ensures the patient's privacy.
5. Explain what you are going to do and the reason for doing it to the patient. Review safety precautions necessary when oxygen is in use. Place "No Smoking" signs in appropriate areas.	Explanation relieves anxiety and facilitates cooperation. Oxygen supports combustion; a small spark could cause a fire.
6. Connect nasal cannula to oxygen setup with humidification, if one is in use. Adjust flow rate as ordered. Check that oxygen is flowing out of prongs.	Oxygen forced through a water reservoir is humidified before it is delivered to the patient, thus preventing dehydration of the mucous membranes. Low-flow oxygen does not require humidification.
7. Place prongs in patient's nostrils (FIGURE 1). Place tubing over and behind each ear with adjuster comfortably under chin. Alternately, the tubing may be placed around the patient's head, with the adjuster at the back or base	Correct placement of the prongs and fastener facilitates oxygen administration and patient comfort. Pads reduce irritation and pressure and protect the skin.

ACTION

RATIONALE

of the head. Place gauze pads at ear beneath the tubing, as necessary.

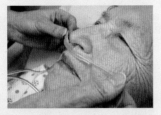

FIGURE 1 Applying cannula to nares.

8. Adjust the fit of the cannula as necessary. Tubing should be snug but not tight against the skin.

Proper adjustment maintains the prongs in the patient's nose. Excessive pressure from tubing could cause irritation and pressure to the skin.

9. **Encourage patient to breathe through the nose, with the mouth closed.**

Nose breathing provides for optimal delivery of oxygen to the patient. The percentage of oxygen delivered can be reduced in patients who breathe through the mouth.

10. Reassess patient's respiratory status, including respiratory rate, effort, and lung sounds. Note any signs of respiratory distress, such as tachypnea, nasal flaring, use of accessory muscles, or dyspnea.

These assess the effectiveness of oxygen therapy.

11. Remove PPE, if used. Perform hand hygiene.

Removing PPE properly reduces the risk for infection transmission and contamination of other items. Hand hygiene prevents the spread of microorganisms.

12. Put on clean gloves. Remove and clean the cannula and assess nares at least every 8 hours, or according to agency recommendations. Check nares for evidence of irritation or bleeding.

The continued presence of the cannula causes irritation and dryness of the mucous membranes.

EVALUATION

- Patient demonstrates an oxygen saturation level within acceptable parameters.
- Patient remains free of dyspnea, nasal flaring, or accessory muscle use and demonstrates respiratory rate and depth within normal ranges.

DOCUMENTATION

- Document your assessment before and after intervention. Document the amount of oxygen applied, the patient's respiratory rate, oxygen saturation, and lung sounds.

Skill · 128   Using an Oxygen Tent

Oxygen tents are often used in children who will not leave a facemask or nasal cannula in place. The oxygen tent gives the patient freedom to move in the bed or crib while humidified oxygen is being delivered; however, it is difficult to keep the tent closed, because the child may want contact with his or her parents. It is also difficult to maintain a consistent level of oxygen and to deliver oxygen at a rate higher than 30% to 50%. Frequent assessment of the child's pajamas and bedding is necessary because the humidification quickly creates moisture, leading to damp clothing and linens, and, possibly, hypothermia.

EQUIPMENT

- Oxygen source
- Oxygen tent
- Humidifier compatible with tent
- Oxygen analyzer
- Small blankets for blanket rolls
- PPE, as indicated

ASSESSMENT GUIDELINES

- Assess the patient's lung sounds. Secretions may cause the patient's oxygen demand to increase.
- Assess the oxygen saturation level. The primary care provider will usually order a baseline for the pulse oximeter (i.e., deliver oxygen to keep pulse oximetry greater than 95%).
- Assess skin color. A pale or cyanotic patient may not be receiving sufficient oxygen.
- Assess patient for any signs of respiratory distress, such as nasal flaring, grunting, or retractions; oxygen-depleted patients often exhibit these signs.

NURSING DIAGNOSES
- Impaired Gas Exchange
- Ineffective Airway Clearance
- Ineffective Breathing Pattern
- Risk for Activity Intolerance
- Decreased Cardiac Output
- Excess Fluid Volume
- Risk for Impaired Skin Integrity

OUTCOME IDENTIFICATION AND PLANNING
Expected outcomes may include:
- Patient exhibits an oxygen saturation level within acceptable parameters.
- Patient will remain free of signs and symptoms of respiratory distress.
- Patient's respiratory status, including respiratory rate and depth, will be in the normal range for the patient's age group.
- Patient's skin will be dry, without evidence of breakdown.

IMPLEMENTATION

ACTION	RATIONALE
1. Bring necessary equipment to the bedside stand or over-bed table.	Bringing everything to the bed-side conserves time and energy. Arranging items nearby is convenient, saves time, and avoids unnecessary stretching and twisting of muscles on the part of the nurse.
2. Perform hand hygiene and put on PPE, if indicated.	Hand hygiene and PPE prevent the spread of microorganisms. PPE is required based on transmission precautions.
3. Identify the patient.	Identifying the patient ensures the right patient receives the intervention and helps prevent errors.
4. Close curtains around bed and close the door to the room, if possible.	This ensures the patient's privacy.

ACTION	RATIONALE
5. Explain what you are going to do and the reason for doing it to the patient and parents/guardians. Review safety precautions necessary when oxygen is in use.	Explanation relieves anxiety and facilitates cooperation. Oxygen supports combustion; a small spark could cause a fire.
6. Calibrate the oxygen analyzer according to manufacturer's directions.	Ensures accurate readings and appropriate adjustments to therapy.
7. Place tent over crib or bed. Connect the humidifier to the oxygen source in the wall and connect the tent tubing to the humidifier. Adjust flow rate as ordered by physician. Check that oxygen is flowing into tent.	Oxygen forced through a water reservoir is humidified before it is delivered to the patient, thus preventing dehydration of the mucous membranes.
8. Turn analyzer on. Place oxygen analyzer probe in tent, out of patient's reach.	The analyzer will give an accurate reading of the concentration of oxygen in the crib or bed.
9. Adjust oxygen as necessary, based on sensor readings. Once oxygen levels reach the prescribed amount, place patient in the tent (FIGURE 1).	Patient will receive oxygen once placed in the tent.
10. Roll small blankets like a jelly roll and tuck tent edges under blanket rolls, as necessary (FIGURE 2).	The blanket helps keep the edges of the tent flap from coming up and letting oxygen out.

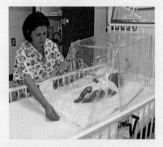

FIGURE 1 Placing patient in the tent.

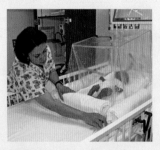

FIGURE 2 Tucking edges under blanket rolls.

ACTION	RATIONALE
11. **Encourage patient and family members to keep tent flap closed.**	Every time the tent flap is opened, oxygen is released.
12. Reassess patient's respiratory status, including respiratory rate, effort, and lung sounds. Note any signs of respiratory distress, such as tachypnea, nasal flaring, use of accessory muscles, grunting, retractions, or dyspnea.	This assesses the effectiveness of oxygen therapy.
13. Remove PPE, if used. Perform hand hygiene.	Removing PPE properly reduces the risk for infection transmission and contamination of other items. Hand hygiene prevents the spread of microorganisms.
14. Frequently check bedding and patient's pajamas for moisture. Change as needed to keep the patient dry.	The large amount of humidification delivered in an oxygen tent quickly makes cloth moist, which would be uncomfortable for the patient and may affect temperature regulation.

EVALUATION

- Patient exhibits an oxygen saturation level within acceptable parameters.
- Patient remains free of dyspnea, nasal flaring, grunting, or use of accessory muscles when breathing.
- Patient's respirations remain in normal range for age group.

DOCUMENTATION

- Document amount of oxygen applied, respiratory rate, oxygen saturation level, and assessment before and after intervention.

Skill · 129   **Using an External (Transcutaneous) Pacemaker**

Electrical therapy is used to terminate or control potentially lethal dysrhythmias quickly. A temporary pacemaker consists of an external, battery-powered pulse generator and a lead or electrode system to electrically stimulate heartbeat. Transcutaneous pacing can temporarily supply an electrical current in the heart when electrical conduction is abnormal. In a life-threatening situation, when time is critical, a transcutaneous pacemaker is the best choice. This device works by sending an electrical impulse from the pulse generator to the patient's heart by way of two electrodes, which are placed on the front and back of the patient's chest. This stimulates the contraction of cardiac muscle fibers through electrical stimulation (depolarization) of the myocardium. Transcutaneous pacing is quick and effective, but is usually used as short-term therapy until the situation resolves or transvenous pacing can be initiated. Transcutaneous pacing is contraindicated in patients with severe hypothermia and prolonged brady-asystolic cardiac arrest (Craig, 2005).

EQUIPMENT

- Transcutaneous pacing generator
- Transcutaneous pacing electrodes
- Cardiac monitor

ASSESSMENT GUIDELINES

- Review the patient's medical record and plan of care for information about the patient's need for pacing. Transcutaneous pacing is generally an emergency measure.
- Assess the patient's initial cardiac rhythm, including a rhythm strip and 12-lead ECG.
- Monitor heart rate, respiratory rate, level of consciousness, and skin color.
- If pulselessness occurs, initiate CPR.

NURSING DIAGNOSES

- Decreased Cardiac Output
- Anxiety
- Deficient Knowledge
- Risk for Injury

OUTCOME IDENTIFICATION AND PLANNING

Expected outcomes may include:
- External transcutaneous pacemaker is applied correctly without adverse effect to the patient.
- Patient regains signs of circulation, including the capture of at least the minimal set heart rate.

• Patient's heart and lungs maintain adequate function to sustain life.
• Patient does not experience injury.

IMPLEMENTATION

ACTION

RATIONALE

1. Bring necessary equipment to the bedside stand or over-bed table.

Bringing everything to the bedside conserves time and energy. Arranging items nearby is convenient, saves time, and avoids unnecessary stretching and twisting of muscles on the part of the nurse. Organization facilitates performance of tasks.

2. Perform hand hygiene and put on PPE, if indicated.

Hand hygiene and PPE prevent the transmission of microorganisms. PPE is required based on transmission precautions.

3. Identify the patient.

Verification of the patient's identity validates that the correct procedure is being done on the correct patient.

4. If the patient is responsive, explain the procedure to the patient. Explain that it involves some discomfort and that you will administer medication to keep him or her comfortable and help him or her relax. Administer analgesia and sedation, as ordered, if not an emergency situation.

External pacemakers are typically used with unconscious patients because most alert patients cannot tolerate the uncomfortable sensations produced by the high energy levels needed to pace externally. If responsive, the patient will most likely be sedated.

5. Close curtains around bed and close the door to the room, if possible.

This provides for patient privacy.

6. If necessary, clip the hair over the areas of electrode placement. **Do not shave the area.**

Shaving can cause tiny nicks in the skin, causing skin irritation. Also, the current from the pulse generator could cause discomfort.

ACTION	RATIONALE
7. Attach cardiac monitoring electrodes to the patient in the lead I, II, and III positions. Do this even if the patient is already on telemetry monitoring. If you select the lead II position, adjust the LL (left leg) electrode placement to accommodate the anterior pacing electrode and the patient's anatomy.	Connecting the telemetry electrodes to the pacemaker is required.
8. Attach the patient monitoring electrodes to the ECG cable and into the ECG input connection on the front of the pacing generator. Set the selector switch to the 'Monitor on' position.	These actions ensure that the equipment is functioning properly.
9. Note the ECG waveform on the monitor. Adjust the R-wave beeper volume to a suitable level and activate the alarm by pressing the "Alarm on" button. Set the alarm for 10 to 20 beats lower and 20 to 30 beats higher than the intrinsic rate.	These actions ensure that the equipment is functioning properly.
10. Press the "Start/Stop" button for a printout of the waveform.	A printout provides objective data.
11. Apply the two pacing electrodes. Make sure the patient's skin is clean and dry to ensure good skin contact. Pull the protective strip from the posterior electrode (marked "Back") and apply the electrode on the left side of the thoracic spinal column, just below the scapula (FIGURE 1).	This placement ensures that the electrical stimulus must travel only a short distance to the heart.
12. Apply the anterior pacing electrode (marked "Front"), which has two protective	This placement ensures that the electrical stimulus must travel only a short distance to the heart.

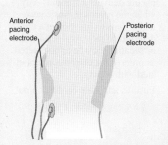

FIGURE 1 Transcutaneous pace-maker pads in place.

strips—one covering the gelled area and one covering the outer rim. Expose the gelled area and apply it to the skin in the anterior position, to the left side of the sternum in the usual V_2 to V_5 position, centered close to the point of maximal cardiac impulse (see FIGURE 1). Move this electrode around to get the best waveform. Then, expose the electrode's outer rim and firmly press it to the skin.

13. Prepare to pace the heart. After making sure the energy output in milliamperes (mA) is on 0, connect the electrode cable to the monitor output cable.

This sets the pacing threshold.

14. Check the waveform, looking for a tall QRS complex in lead II.

15. Check the selector switch to "Pacer on." Select synchronous (demand) or asynchronous (fixed-rate or

Asynchronous pacing delivers a stimulus at a set (fixed) rate regardless of the occurrence of spontaneous myocardial

ACTION	RATIONALE

nondemand) mode, per medical orders. **Tell the patient he or she may feel a thumping or twitching sensation. Reassure the patient you will provide medication if the discomfort is intolerable.**

16. Set the pacing rate dial to 10 to 20 beats higher than the intrinsic rhythm. Look for pacer artifact or spikes, which will appear as you increase the rate. If the patient does not have an intrinsic rhythm, set the rate at 80 beats/minute (Craig, 2005).

17. Set the pacing current output (in milliamperes [mA]). For patients with bradycardia, start with the minimal setting and **slowly increase the amount of energy delivered to the heart by adjusting the "Output" mA dial. Do this until electrical capture is achieved: you will see a pacer spike followed by a widened QRS complex and a tall broad T wave that resembles a premature ventricular contraction.**

18. Increase output by 2 mA or 10%. **Do not go higher because of the increased risk of discomfort to the patient.**

depolarizations. Synchronous pacing delivers a stimulus only when the heart's intrinsic pacemaker fails to function at a predetermined rate. Analgesia and/or sedation may be administered as ordered for discomfort associated with pacing.

Ensures adequate cardiac output.

Ensures adequate cardiac output.

Increasing the output ensures consistent capture. With full capture, the patient's heart rate should be approximately the same as the pacemaker rate set on the machine. The usual pacing threshold is 40 to 80 mA. Thresholds may vary due to recent cardiothoracic surgery, pericardial effusions, cardiac tamponade, acidosis, and

ACTION	RATIONALE
	hypoxia. These conditions may require higher thresholds.
19. Assess for mechanical capture: Presence of a pulse and signs of improved cardiac output (increased blood pressure, improved level of consciousness, improved body temperature).	Both electrical and mechanical capture must occur to benefit the patient (Del Monte, 2006).
20. For patients with asystole, start with the full output. If capture occurs, slowly decrease the output until capture is lost, then add 2 mA or 10% more.	Increasing the output ensures consistent capture. With full capture, the patient's heart rate should be approximately the same as the pacemaker rate set on the machine. The usual pacing threshold is 40 to 80 mA.
21. Secure the pacing leads and cable to the patient's body.	This prevents accidental displacement of the electrode, resulting in failure to pace or sense.
22. Monitor the patient's heart rate and rhythm to assess ventricular response to pacing. Assess the patient's vital signs, skin color, level of consciousness, and peripheral pulses. Take blood pressure in both arms.	Assessment helps determine the effectiveness of the paced rhythm. If the blood pressure reading is significantly higher in one arm, use that arm for measurements.
23. Assess the patient's pain and administer analgesia/sedation, as ordered, to ease the discomfort of chest wall muscle contractions (Craig, 2005).	Analgesia and sedation promote patient comfort.
24. Perform a 12-lead ECG and additional ECGs daily or with clinical changes.	ECG monitoring provides a baseline for further evaluation.
25. Continually monitor the ECG readings, noting capture, sensing, rate, intrinsic beats, and competition of paced and intrinsic rhythms. If the pacemaker is sensing correctly,	Continuous monitoring helps evaluate the patient's condition and determine the effectiveness of therapy.

ACTION	RATIONALE
the sense indicator on the pulse generator should flash with each beat.	
26. Remove PPE, if used. Perform hand hygiene.	Removing PPE properly reduces the risk for infection transmission and contamination of other items. Hand hygiene and proper disposal of equipment reduces the transmission of microorganisms.

EVALUATION

- External transcutaneous pacemaker is applied correctly without adverse effect to the patient.
- Patient regains signs of circulation, including the capture of at least the minimal set heart rate.
- Patient's heart and lungs maintain adequate function to sustain life.
- Patient does not experience injury.

DOCUMENTATION

- Document the reason for pacemaker use, time that pacing began, electrode locations, pacemaker settings, patient's response to the procedure and to temporary pacing, complications, and nursing actions taken. Document the patient's pain-intensity rating, analgesia or sedation administered, and the patient's response. If possible, record a rhythm strip before, during, and after pacemaker placement; any time that pacemaker settings are changed; and whenever the patient receives treatment because of a complication due to the pacemaker.

GENERAL CONSIDERATIONS

- Do not leave patients unattended during noninvasive pacing. It is safe to touch the patient and perform procedures during pacing (e.g., CPR). Gloves should be worn.
- Monitor for changes in the patient's underlying rhythm. Ventricular fibrillation requires immediate defibrillation.
- Check the skin where the electrodes are placed for skin burns or tissue damage. Reposition as needed.
- Avoid using the carotid pulse to confirm mechanical capture. Electrical stimulation can cause jerky muscle contractions that may be interpreted as carotid pulsations. Assess the femoral pulse.

- If the patient needs emergency defibrillation, make sure the pacemaker can withstand the procedure. If you are unsure, disconnect the pulse generator to avoid damage.
- Do not place the electrodes over a bony area, because bone conducts current poorly.
- With a female patient, place the anterior electrodes under the patient's breast but not over her diaphragm.
- Do not use electrical equipment that is not grounded, such as telephones, electric shaver, television, or lamps; otherwise, the patient may experience microshock.
- If defibrillation is indicated, position defibrillator electrode pads at least 1 inch away from pacing electrodes to avoid arching of electricity. Turn transcutaneous pacemaker off during CPR (Jevon, 2007c).

Skill · 130 Caring for a Patient Receiving Patient Controlled Analgesia

Patient-controlled analgesia (PCA) allows patients to control the administration of their own medication within predetermined safety limits. This approach can be used with oral analgesic agents as well as with infusions of opioid analgesic agents by intravenous, subcutaneous, epidural, and perineural routes (D'Arcy, 2008a; Pasero, 2004; Smeltzer, Bare, et al., 2010). PCA provides effective, individualized analgesia and comfort. This drug delivery system may be used to manage acute and chronic pain in a healthcare facility or the home.

The PCA pump permits the patient to self-administer medication (bolus doses) with episodes of increased pain or painful activities. A PCA pump is electronically controlled by a timing device. The PCA system consists of a portable infusion pump containing a reservoir or chamber for a syringe that is prefilled with the prescribed medication, usually an opioid, or dilute anesthetic solutions in the case of epidural administration (D'Arcy, 2008a; Roman & Cabaj, 2005; Smeltzer, Bare, et al., 2010). When pain occurs, the patient pushes a button that activates the PCA device to deliver a small, preset bolus dose of the analgesic. A lockout interval that is programmed into the PCA unit prevents reactivation of the pump and administration of another dose during that period of time. The pump mechanism can also be programmed to deliver only a specified amount of analgesic within a given time interval (basal rate; most commonly every hour or, occasionally, every 4 hours). These safeguards limit the risk for overmedication and allow the patient to evaluate the effect of the previous dose. PCA pumps also have a locked safety system that prohibits tampering with the device.

Nursing responsibilities for patients receiving medications via a PCA pump include patient/family teaching, initial setup of the device, monitoring the device to ensure proper functioning, and frequent assessment of the patient's response, including pain/discomfort control and presence of adverse effects. Additional information related to epidural infusions is discussed in Skill 69.

EQUIPMENT

- PCA system
- Syringe filled with medication
- PCA system tubing
- Antimicrobial swabs
- Appropriate label for syringe and tubing, based on facility policy and procedure
- Second nurse to verify medication and programmed pump
- information, if necessary, according to facility policy
- Pain assessment tool and/or scale
- Computerized medication administration record (CMAR) or medication administration record (MAR)
- Nonsterile gloves
- Additional PPE, as indicated

ASSESSMENT GUIDELINES

- Review the patient's medical record and plan of care for specific instructions related to PCA therapy, including the primary care provider's orders and conditions indicating the need for therapy. Check the medical order for the prescribed drug, initial loading dose, dose for self-administration, and lockout interval.
- Check to ensure proper functioning of the unit.
- Assess the patient's level of consciousness and understanding of PCA therapy and the rationale for its use.
- Review the patient's history for conditions that might contraindicate therapy, such as respiratory limitations, history of substance abuse, or psychiatric disorder. Review the patient's medical record and assess for factors contributing to an increased risk for respiratory depression, such as the use of a basal infusion, the patient's age, obesity, upper abdominal surgery, sleep apnea, concurrent CNS depressants, and impaired organ functioning (Hagle et al., 2004).
- Determine the prescribed route for administration. Inspect the site to be used for the infusion for signs of infiltration or infection. If the route is via an intravenous infusion, ensure that the line is patent and the current solution is compatible with the drug ordered.
- Assess the patient's pain and level of discomfort using an appropriate assessment tool. Assess the characteristics of any pain, and for other symptoms that often occur with the pain, such as headache or restlessness. Ask the patient what interventions have and have not been successful in the past to promote comfort and relieve pain.
- Assess the patient's vital signs. Assess the patient's respiratory status, including rate, depth, and rhythm, and oxygen saturation level using pulse oximetry.
- Also, assess the patient's sedation score. Determine the patient's response to the intervention to evaluate effectiveness and for the presence of adverse effects.

NURSING DIAGNOSES

- Acute Pain
- Deficient Knowledge
- Chronic Pain
- Fear
- Anxiety
- Ineffective Coping
- Risk for Injury

OUTCOME IDENTIFICATION AND PLANNING

Expected outcomes may include:
- Patient reports increased comfort and/or decreased pain, without adverse effects, oversedation, and respiratory depression.
- Patient displays decreased anxiety, improved coping skills, and an understanding of the therapy and the reason for its use.

IMPLEMENTATION

ACTION	RATIONALE
1. Gather equipment. Check the medication order against the original physician's order according to agency policy. Clarify any inconsistencies. Check the patient's chart for allergies.	This comparison helps to identify errors that may have occurred when orders were transcribed. The physician's order is the legal record of medication orders for each agency.
2. Know the actions, special nursing considerations, safe dose ranges, purpose of administration, and adverse effects of the medications to be administered. Consider the appropriateness of the medication for this patient.	This knowledge aids the nurse in evaluating the therapeutic effect of the medication in relation to the patient's disorder and can also be used to educate the patient about the medication.
3. Prepare the medication syringe or other container, based on facility policy, for administration.	Proper preparation and administration procedure prevent errors.
4. Perform hand hygiene and put on PPE, if indicated.	Hand hygiene and PPE prevent the spread of microorganisms. PPE is required based on transmission precautions.

ACTION	RATIONALE
5. Identify the patient. 	Identifying the patient ensures the right patient receives the intervention and helps prevent errors.
6. Show the patient the device, and explain the function of the device and the reason for its use. Explain the purpose and action of the medication to the patient.	Explanation encourages patient understanding and cooperation and reduces apprehension.
7. Plug the PCA device into the electrical outlet, if necessary. Check status of battery power, if appropriate.	The PCA device requires a power source (electricity or battery) to run. Most units will alarm to acknowledge a low battery state.
8. Close curtains around bed and close the door to the room.	Closing the door or pulling the curtain provides patient privacy.
9. Complete necessary assessments before administering medication. Check allergy bracelet or ask patient about allergies. Assess the patient's pain, using an appropriate assessment tool and measurement scale.	Assessment is a prerequisite to administration of medications. Accurate assessment is necessary to guide treatment/relief interventions and evaluate the effectiveness of pain control measures.
10. **Check the label on the pre-filled drug syringe with the medication record and patient identification.** Obtain verification of information from a second nurse, according to facility policy. If using a barcode administration system, scan the barcode on the medication label, if required.	This action verifies that the correct drug and dosage will be administered to the correct patient. Confirmation of information by a second nurse helps prevent errors (D'Arcy, 2008a). Scanning the barcode provides an additional check to ensure that the medication is given to the right patient.
11. If using a barcode administration system, scan the patient's barcode on the identification band, if required.	This provides an additional check to ensure that the medication is given to the right patient.

ACTION	RATIONALE
12. Connect tubing to prefilled syringe and place the syringe into the PCA device. **Prime the tubing.**	Doing so prepares the device to deliver the drug. Priming the tubing purges air from the tubing and reduces the risk for air embolism.
13. Set the PCA device to administer the loading dose, if ordered, and then program the device based on the medical order for medication dosage, dose interval, and lockout interval. Obtain verification of information from a second nurse, according to facility policy.	These actions ensure that the appropriate drug dosage will be administered. Confirmation of information by a second nurse helps prevent errors.
14. Put on gloves. Using antimicrobial swab, clean connection port on intravenous infusion line or other site access, based on route of administration. Connect the PCA tubing to the patient's intravenous infusion line or appropriate access site, based on the specific site used. Secure the site per facility policy and procedure. Remove gloves. Initiate the therapy by activating the appropriate button on the pump.	Gloves prevent contact with blood and body fluids. Cleaning the connection port reduces the risk of infection. Connection and initiation are necessary to allow drug delivery to the patient.
15. Remind the patient to press the button each time he or she needs relief from pain.	Instruction promotes correct use of the device.
16. Assess the patient's pain at least every 4 hours or more often, as needed. Monitor vital signs, especially respiratory status, including oxygen saturation at least every 4 hours or more often as needed.	Continued assessment at frequent intervals helps evaluate the effectiveness of the drug and reduces the risk for complications (D'Arcy, 2008a; D'Arcy, 2007a).
17. Assess the patient's sedation score and end-tidal carbon	Sedation occurs before clinically significant respiratory depression

ACTION	RATIONALE
dioxide level (capnography) at least every 4 hours or more often, as needed.	(D'Arcy, 2008a). Respiratory depression may occur with the use of narcotic analgesics. Capnography is a more reliable indicator of respiratory depression (D'Arcy, 2007a).
18. Assess the infusion site periodically, according to facility policy and nursing judgment. Assess the patient's use of the medication, noting number of attempts and number of doses delivered. Replace the drug syringe when it is empty.	Continued assessment of the infusion site is necessary for early detection of problems. Continued assessment of the patient's use of medication and its effect is necessary to ensure adequate pain control without adverse effect. Replacing the syringe ensures continued drug delivery.
19. Make sure the control (dosing button) is within the patient's reach.	Easy access to the control is essential for the patient's use of the device.
20. Remove gloves and additional PPE, if used. Perform hand hygiene.	Removing PPE properly reduces the risk for infection transmission and contamination of other items. Hand hygiene prevents transmission of microorganisms.

EVALUATION

• Patient reports increased comfort and/or decreased pain, without adverse effects, oversedation, and respiratory depression.
• Patient displays decreased anxiety and improved coping skills.
• Patient verbalizes an understanding of the therapy and the reason for its use.

DOCUMENTATION

• Document the date and time PCA therapy was initiated, initial pain assessment, drug and loading dose administered, if appropriate, and individual dosing and time interval. Document continued pain, sedation level, capnography results, vital sign assessments, and patient's response to therapy.

GENERAL CONSIDERATIONS

• A wide variety of PCA devices are available on the market. Check the manufacturer's instructions before using the device.

- Adults and children who are cognitively and physically able to use the PCA equipment and are able to understand that pressing a button can result in pain relief are appropriate candidates for PCA therapy (D'Arcy, 2008; Pasero & McCaffery, 2005).
- PCA is considered safe because the analgesic administered most often is an opioid, which causes sedation before respiratory depression. A sedated patient cannot self-administer a dose, reducing the risk of an overdose (D'Arcy, 2008; Hagle et al., 2004; Marders, 2004; Pasero & McCaffery, 2005a).
- Family members and nurses may need to remind the patient to push the button. If someone other than the patient delivers a dose, the risk for oversedation is increased (D'Arcy, 2008; Hagle et al., 2004; Pasero & McCaffery, 2005; Wuhrman, et al., 2007).
- Some facilities have developed clinical practice guidelines for authorized agent controlled analgesia (AACA). In these cases, one family member (caregiver-controlled analgesia [CCA]) or primary nurse (nurse-controlled analgesia [NCA]) is designated as the primary pain manager and only that person can press the PCA button for the patient. In the case of family members, the primary pain manager must be chosen carefully and taught to asses for pain and the adverse effect of the medication. Additionally, nursing staff must be vigilant in assessing the patient's need for, and response to, the medication, following the same assessment guidelines previously discussed. It is very important to follow facility guidelines to ensure safe administration (D'Arcy, 2007a; Hagle, et al., 2004; Pasero & McCaffery, 2005; Wuhrman, et al., 2007).
- If using a device that provides continuous and bolus doses, the cumulative doses per hour should not exceed the total hourly dose ordered by the physician.
- Vital-sign monitoring is crucial, especially when initiating therapy. Encourage the patient to practice coughing and deep breathing to promote ventilation and prevent pooling of secretions.
- A narcotic antagonist, such as naloxone (Narcan), must be readily available in case the patient develops respiratory complications related to drug therapy.
- A fentanyl patient-controlled transdermal system (PCTS) is another patient-controlled delivery technique for pain medication. The small device contains the medication in a reservoir in the patch and attaches to the patient's upper arm or chest with adhesive. When the patient pushes the button on the device, the medication is delivered by iontophoresis, an electrical current that introduces the medication into the tissues. The device is preprogrammed to deliver fixed 40-μg doses of fentanyl. Each patch holds 80 doses, with minimal time between doses of 10 minutes. The device will deliver the maximum 80 doses or will operate for 24 hours from the first dose, whichever occurs first. The patch then shuts off. If continued use is required, it is replaced with a new device, in another location. It is not for use with patients with implanted devices, such as pacemakers, that are sensitive to electricity (D'Arcy, 2005a; D'Arcy, 2005b; Koo, 2005; Layzell, 2008).

Skill · 131   Caring for a Peritoneal Dialysis Catheter

Peritoneal dialysis is a method of removing fluid and wastes from the body of a patient with kidney failure. A catheter inserted through the abdominal wall into the peritoneal cavity allows a special fluid (dialysate) to be infused and then drained from the body, removing waste products and excess fluid. The exit site is not disturbed initially after insertion, to allow for healing. Generally, this time frame is 7 to 10 days post-insertion (Redmond & Doherty, 2005). Once the exit site has healed, exit site care is an important part of patient care. The catheter insertion site is a site for potential infection, possibly leading to catheter tunnel infection and peritonitis (inflammation of the peritoneal membrane). Therefore, meticulous care is needed. The incidence of exit site infections can be reduced through a daily cleansing regimen by the patient or caregiver (Bernardini et al., 2005; Redmond & Doherty, 2005). Often, in the acute care setting, catheter care is performed using aseptic technique, to reduce the risk for a hospital-acquired infection. At home, clean technique can be used by the patient and caregivers.

EQUIPMENT

- Face masks (2)
- Sterile gloves
- Nonsterile gloves
- Additional PPE, as indicated
- Antimicrobial cleansing agent, per facility policy
- Sterile gauze squares (4)
- Sterile basin
- Sterile drain sponge
- Topical antibiotic, such as mupirocin or gentamicin, depending on order and policy
- Sterile applicator
- Plastic trash bag
- Bath blanket

ASSESSMENT GUIDELINES

- Inspect peritoneal dialysis catheter exit site for any erythema, drainage, bleeding, tenderness, swelling, skin irritation or breakdown, or leakage. These signs could indicate exit site or tunnel infection.
- Assess abdomen for tenderness, pain, and guarding.
- Assess the patient for nausea, vomiting, and fever, which could indicate peritonitis.
- Assess the patient's knowledge about measures to care for the exit site.

NURSING DIAGNOSES

- Risk for Impaired Skin Integrity
- Risk for Infection
- Deficient Knowledge

OUTCOME IDENTIFICATION AND PLANNING

Expected outcomes may include:
- Peritoneal dialysis catheter dressing change is completed using aseptic technique without trauma to the site or patient.
- Patient's catheter site is clean, dry, and intact, without evidence of inflammation or infection.
- Patient participates in care, as appropriate.

IMPLEMENTATION

ACTION	RATIONALE
1. Bring necessary equipment to the bedside stand or overbed table.	Bringing everything to the bedside conserves time and energy. Arranging items nearby is convenient, saves time, and avoids unnecessary stretching and twisting of muscles on the part of the nurse.
2. Perform hand hygiene and put on PPE, if indicated.	Hand hygiene and PPE prevent the spread of microorganisms. PPE is required based on transmission precautions.
3. Identify the patient.	Identifying the patient ensures the right patient receives the intervention and helps prevent errors.
4. Close curtains around bed and close the door to the room, if possible. Explain what you are going to do and why you are going to do it to the patient. Encourage the patient to observe or participate, if possible.	This ensures the patient's privacy. Explanation relieves anxiety and facilitates cooperation. Discussion promotes cooperation and helps to minimize anxiety. Having the patient observe or assist encourages self-acceptance.
5. Adjust bed to comfortable working height, usually elbow height of the caregiver (VISN 8 Patient Safety Center, 2009). Assist the patient to a supine position. Expose the abdomen, draping the patient's chest with the bath blanket, exposing only the catheter site.	Having the bed at the proper height prevents back and muscle strain. The supine position is usually the best way to gain access to the peritoneal dialysis catheter. Use of bath blanket provides patient warmth and avoids unnecessary exposure.

ACTION	RATIONALE
6. Put on unsterile gloves. Put on one of the facemasks; have patient put on the other mask.	Gloves protect the nurse from contact with blood and bodily fluids. Use of facemasks deters the spread of microorganisms.
7. Gently remove old dressing, noting odor, amount and color of drainage, leakage, and condition of skin around the catheter. Discard dressing in appropriate container.	Drainage, leakage, and skin condition can indicate problems with the catheter, such as infection.
8. Remove gloves and discard. Set up sterile field. Open packages. Using aseptic technique, place two sterile gauze squares in basin with antimicrobial agent. Leave two sterile gauze squares opened on sterile field. Alternately (based on facility's policy), place sterile antimicrobial swabs on the sterile field. Place sterile applicator on field. Squeeze a small amount of the topical antibiotic on one of the gauze squares on the sterile field.	Until the catheter site has healed, aseptic technique is necessary for site care to prevent infection.
9. Put on sterile gloves. Pick up dialysis catheter with nondominant hand. With the antimicrobial-soaked gauze/swab, cleanse the skin around the exit site using a circular motion, starting at the exit site and then slowly going outward 3 to 4 inches. Gently remove crusted scabs if necessary.	Aseptic technique is necessary to prevent infection. The antimicrobial agent cleanses the skin and removes any drainage or crust from the wound, reducing the risk for infection.
10. Continue to hold catheter with your nondominant hand. After skin has dried, clean the catheter with an antimicrobial-soaked gauze, beginning at exit	Antimicrobial agents cleanse the catheter and remove any drainage or crust from the tube, reducing the risk for infection.

ACTION	RATIONALE
site, going around catheter, and then moving up to end of catheter. Gently remove crusted secretions on the tube, if necessary.	
11. Using the sterile applicator, apply the topical antibiotic to the catheter exit site, if prescribed.	Application of mupirocin and gentamicin at the catheter exit site prevents exit site infection and peritonitis (Bernardini et al., 2005; The Joanna Briggs Institute, 2004).
12. Place sterile drain sponge around exit site. Then place a 4 × 4 gauze over exit site. Remove your gloves and secure edges of gauze pad with tape. Some institutions recommend placing a transparent dressing over the gauze pads instead of tape. Remove masks.	The drain sponge and 4 × 4 gauze pad are used to absorb any drainage from the exit site. Occlusion of the site with a dressing deters contamination of site. Once the site is covered, masks are no longer necessary.
13. Coil the exposed length of tubing and secure to the dressing or the patient's abdomen with tape.	Anchoring the catheter absorbs any tugging, preventing tension on, and irritation to, the skin or abdomen.
14. Assist the patient to a comfortable position. Cover the patient with bed linens. Place the bed in the lowest position.	Positioning and covering provide warmth and promote comfort. A bed in the low position promotes patient safety.
15. Put on clean gloves. Remove or discard equipment and assess the patient's response to the procedure.	These actions deter the spread of microorganisms. The patient's response may indicate acceptance of the catheter or the need for health teaching.
16. Remove gloves and additional PPE, if used. Perform hand hygiene.	Removing PPE properly reduces the risk for infection transmission and contamination of other items. Hand hygiene prevents the spread of microorganisms.

EVALUATION
• Peritoneal dialysis catheter dressing change is completed using aseptic technique without trauma to the site or patient.
• Patient's catheter site is clean, dry, and intact, without evidence of redness, irritation, or excoriation.
• Patient verbalizes appropriate measures to care for the site.

DOCUMENTATION
• Document the dressing change, including condition of skin surrounding the exit site, drainage, or odor, as well as the patient's reaction to procedure, and any patient teaching provided.

GENERAL CONSIDERATIONS
• Patients with a peritoneal dialysis catheter should avoid baths and public pools.
• Patients performing own site care should be reminded of the importance of good handwashing before self-care.
• Once the site is healed, some primary care providers do not require patients to wear a dressing unless the site is leaking. The patient may shower with an occlusive dressing over the exit site. The catheter exit site should be cleansed after showering.
• Often, clean technique, instead of sterile technique, is used by the patient and caregivers in the home.

Skill · 132 | **Using Personal Protective Equipment**

Personal protective equipment (PPE) refers to specialized clothing or equipment worn by an employee for protection against infectious materials. PPE is used in healthcare settings to improve personnel safety in the healthcare environment through the appropriate use of PPE (CDC, 2004a). This equipment includes clean (unsterile) and sterile gloves, impervious gowns/aprons, surgical and high-efficiency particulate air (HEPA) masks, N95 disposable masks, face shields, and protective eyewear/goggles.

Understanding the potential contamination hazards related to the patient's diagnosis and condition and the institutional policies governing PPE is very important. The type of PPE used will vary based on the type of exposure anticipated and category precautions: Standard Precautions and Transmission-Based Precautions, including Contact, Droplet, or Airborne Precautions. It is the nurse's responsibility to enforce the proper wearing of PPE during patient care for members of the healthcare team.

EQUIPMENT

- Gloves
- Mask (surgical or particulate respirator)
- Impervious gown
- Protective eyewear (does not include eyeglasses)

ASSESSMENT GUIDELINES

- Assess the situation to determine the necessity for PPE.
- Check the patient's chart for information about a suspected or diagnosed infection or communicable disease.
- Determine the possibility of exposure to blood and body fluids, and identify the necessary equipment to prevent exposure.
- Refer to the infection control manual provided by your facility.

NURSING DIAGNOSES

- Risk for Infection
- Deficient Knowledge
- Ineffective Protection
- Bowel Incontinence
- Diarrhea
- Impaired Skin Integrity

OUTCOME IDENTIFICATION AND PLANNING

Expected outcomes may include:
- Transmission of microorganisms is prevented.
- Patient and staff remain free of exposure to potentially infectious microorganisms.
- Patient verbalizes information about the rationale for PPE use.

IMPLEMENTATION

ACTION	RATIONALE
1. Check medical record and nursing plan of care for type of precautions and review precautions in infection control manual.	Mode of transmission of organism determines type of precautions required.
2. Plan nursing activities before entering patient's room.	Organization facilitates performance of task and adherence to precautions.
3. Perform hand hygiene.	Hand hygiene prevents the spread of microorganisms.

ACTION	RATIONALE
4. Provide instruction about precautions to patient, family members, and visitors.	Explanation encourages cooperation of patient and family and reduces apprehension about precaution procedures.
5. Put on gown, gloves, mask, and protective eyewear, based on the type of exposure anticipated and category of isolation precautions.	Use of PPE interrupts chain of infection and protects patient and nurse. Gown should protect entire uniform. Gloves protect hands and wrists from microorganisms. Masks protect nurse or patient from droplet nuclei and large-particle aerosols. Eyewear protects mucous membranes in the eye from splashes.
a. Put on the gown, with the opening in the back. Tie gown securely at neck and waist.	Gown should fully cover the torso from the neck to knees, arms to the end of wrists, and wrap around the back.
b. Put on the mask or respirator over your nose, mouth, and chin. Secure ties or elastic bands at the middle of the head and neck. If respirator is used, perform a fit check. Inhale; the respirator should collapse. Exhale; air should not leak out.	Masks protect nurse or patient from droplet nuclei and large-particle aerosols. A mask must fit securely to provide protection.
c. Put on goggles. Place over eyes and adjust to fit. Alternately, a face shield could be used to take the place of the mask and goggles.	Eyewear protects mucous membranes in the eye from splashes. Must fit securely to provide protection.
d. Put on clean disposable gloves. Extend gloves to cover the cuffs of the gown.	Gloves protect hands and wrists from microorganisms.
6. Identify the patient. Explain the procedure to the patient. Continue with patient care as appropriate.	Patient identification validates the correct patient and correct procedure. Discussion and explanation help allay anxiety and prepare the patient for what to expect.

ACTION	RATIONALE

Remove PPE

7. Remove PPE: Except for respirator, remove PPE at the doorway or in an anteroom. Remove respirator after leaving the patient's room and closing door.

Proper removal prevents contact with, and the spread of, microorganisms. Outside front of equipment is considered contaminated. The inside, outside back, and ties on head and back are considered clean, which are areas of PPE that are not likely to have been in contact with infectious organisms.

a. If impervious gown has been tied in front of the body at the waistline, untie waist strings before removing gloves.

Front of gown, including waist strings, are contaminated. If tied in front of body, the ties must be untied before removing gloves.

b. Grasp the outside of one glove with the opposite gloved hand and peel off, turning the glove inside out as you pull it off. Hold the removed glove in the remaining gloved hand.

Outside of gloves are contaminated.

c. Slide fingers of ungloved hand under the remaining glove at the wrist, taking care not to touch the outer surface of the glove.

Ungloved hand is clean and should not touch contaminated areas.

d. Peel off the glove over the first glove, containing the one glove inside the other. Discard in appropriate container.

Proper disposal prevents transmission of microorganisms.

e. To remove the goggles or face shield: Handle by the headband or earpieces. Lift away from the face. Place in designated receptacle for reprocessing or in an appropriate waste container.

Outside of goggles or face shield is contaminated. Handling by headband or earpieces and lifting away from face prevents transmission of microorganisms. Proper disposal prevents transmission of microorganisms.

f. To remove gown: Unfasten ties, if at the neck and back. Allow the gown to

Gown front and sleeves are contaminated. Touching only the inside of the gown and pulling

ACTION	RATIONALE
fall away from shoulders. Touching only the inside of the gown, pull away from the torso. Keeping hands on the inner surface of the gown, pull from arms. Turn gown inside out. Fold or roll into a bundle and discard.	it away from the torso prevents transmission of microorganisms. Proper disposal prevents transmission of microorganisms.
g. To remove mask or respirator: Grasp the neck ties or elastic, then top ties or elastic and remove. Take care to avoid touching front of mask or respirator. Discard in waste container. If using a respirator, save for future use in the designated area.	Front of mask or respirator is contaminated; **Do Not Touch.** Not touching the front and proper disposal prevent transmission of microorganisms.
8. Perform hand hygiene immediately after removing all PPE.	Hand hygiene prevents spread of microorganisms.

EVALUATION

• Transmission of microorganisms is prevented.
• Patient and staff remain free from exposure to potentially infectious microorganisms.
• Patient verbalizes an understanding about the rationale for use of PPE.

DOCUMENTATION

• It is not usually necessary to document the use of specific articles of PPE or each application of PPE. However, document the implementation and continuation of specific transmission-based precautions as part of the patient's care.

Skill · 133   Applying Pneumatic Compression Devices

Pneumatic compression devices (PCDs) consist of fabric sleeves containing air bladders that apply brief pressure to the legs. Intermittent compression pushes blood from the smaller blood vessels into the deeper vessels and into the femoral veins. This action enhances blood flow and venous return and promotes fibrinolysis, deterring venous thrombosis. The sleeves are attached by tubing to an air pump. The sleeve may cover the entire leg or may extend from the foot to the knee.

Pneumatic compression devices may be used in combination with antiembolism stockings (graduated compression stockings) and anticoagulant therapy to prevent thrombosis formation. They can be used preoperatively and postoperatively with patients at risk for blood clot formation. They are also prescribed for patients with other risk factors for clot formation, including inactivity or immobilization, chronic venous disease, and malignancies.

EQUIPMENT

- Compression sleeves of appropriate size based on the manufacturer's guidelines
- Inflation pump with connection tubing
- Nonsterile gloves and/or other PPE, as indicated

ASSESSMENT GUIDELINES

- Assess the patient's history, medical record, and current condition and status to identify risk for development of deep-vein thrombosis.
- Assess the skin integrity of the lower extremities. Identify any leg conditions that would be exacerbated by the use of the compression device or would contraindicate its use.
- Review the patient's record and nursing plan of care to verify the order from the primary care provider for use.

NURSING DIAGNOSES

- Delayed Surgical Recovery
- Impaired Physical Mobility
- Risk for Injury
- Risk for Peripheral Neurovascular Dysfunction
- Fatigue

OUTCOME IDENTIFICATION AND PLANNING

Expected outcomes may include:
- Patient maintains adequate circulation in extremities.
- Patient is free from symptoms of neurovascular compromise.

IMPLEMENTATION

ACTION	RATIONALE
1. Review the medical record and nursing plan of care for conditions that may contraindicate the use of the PCD.	Reviewing the medical record and plan of care validates the correct patient and correct procedure and minimizes the risk for injury.
2. Perform hand hygiene. Put on PPE, as indicated.	Hand hygiene and PPE prevent the spread of microorganisms. PPE is required based on transmission precautions.
3. Identify the patient. Explain the procedure to the patient.	Patient identification validates the correct patient and correct procedure. Discussion and explanation help allay anxiety and prepare the patient for what to expect.
4. Close curtains around bed or close the door to the room, if possible. Place the bed at an appropriate and comfortable working height, usually elbow height of the caregiver (VISN 8 Patient Safety Center, 2009).	Closing the door or curtains provides privacy. Proper bed height helps reduce back strain.
5. Hang the compression pump on the foot of the bed and plug it into an electrical outlet. Attach the connecting tubing to the pump.	Equipment preparation promotes efficient time management and provides an organized approach to the task.
6. Remove the compression sleeves from the package and unfold them. Lay the unfolded sleeves on the bed with the cotton lining facing up. Note of the markings indicating the correct placement for the ankle and popliteal areas.	Proper placement of the sleeves prevents injury.
7. Apply antiembolism stockings, if ordered. Place a sleeve under the patient's leg with the tubing toward the	Proper placement prevents injury.

ACTION

RATIONALE

heel (FIGURE 1). Each one fits either leg. For total leg sleeves, place the behind-the-knee opening at the popliteal space to prevent pressure there. For knee-high sleeves, make sure the back of the ankle is over the ankle marking.

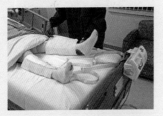

FIGURE 1 Placing PCD sleeves under the patient's legs with the tubing toward the heel.

8. Wrap the sleeve snugly around the patient's leg so that two fingers fit between the leg and the sleeve. Secure the sleeve with the Velcro fasteners. Repeat for the second leg, if bilateral therapy is ordered. Connect each sleeve to the tubing, following manufacturer's recommendations.

Correct placement ensures appropriate, but not excessive, compression of the extremity.

9. Set the pump to the prescribed maximal pressure (usually 35 to 55 mm Hg). Make sure the tubing is free from kinks. Check that the patient can move about without interrupting the airflow. Turn on the pump. Initiate cooling setting, if available.

Proper pressure setting ensures patient safety and prevents injury. Some devices have a cooling setting available to increase patient comfort.

10. Observe the patient and the device during the first cycle. Check the audible alarms. Check the sleeves and pump at least once per shift or per facility policy.

Observation and frequent checking ensure proper fit and inflation and reduce the risk for injury from the device.

ACTION	RATIONALE
11. Place the bed in the lowest position. Make sure the call bell and other necessary items are within easy reach.	Returning the bed to the lowest position and having the call bell and other items readily available promote patient safety.
12. Remove PPE, if used. Perform hand hygiene.	Removing PPE properly reduces the risk for infection transmission and contamination of other items. Hand hygiene prevents the spread of microorganisms.
13. Assess the extremities for peripheral pulses, edema, changes in sensation, and movement. Remove the sleeves and assess and document skin integrity every 8 hours.	Assessment provides for early detection and prompt intervention for possible complications, including skin irritation.

EVALUATION

• Patient exhibits adequate circulation in extremities without symptoms of neurovascular compromise.

DOCUMENTATION

• Document the time and date of application of the PCD, the patient's response to therapy, and understanding of the therapy. Document the status of the alarms and pressure settings. Note the use of the cooling setting, if appropriate.

GENERAL CONSIDERATIONS

• PCDs are contraindicated in patients with suspected or existing deep-vein thrombosis. They should not be used for patients with arterial occlusive disease, severe edema, cellulitis, phlebitis, a skin graft, or an infection of the extremity.
• Use the cooling setting, if the unit has one. The skin under the sleeve can become wet with diaphoresis, which can increase the risk for impaired skin integrity.
• Generally, the PCDs should be worn continuously. They may be removed for bathing, walking, and physical therapy. Use is usually discontinued when the patient is ambulating consistently.
• The risk for deep-vein thrombosis formation and injury is greater if the sleeves are not applied correctly.

Skill · 134	**Providing Postoperative Care When Patient Returns to Room**

Postoperative care facilitates recovery from surgery and supports the patient in coping with physical changes or alterations. Nursing interventions promote physical and psychological health, prevent complications, and teach self-care skills for the patient to use after the hospital stay. After surgery, patients spend time on the postanesthesia care unit (PACU). From the PACU, they are transferred back to their rooms. At this time, nursing care focuses on accurate assessments and associated interventions. Ongoing assessments are crucial for early identification of postoperative complications.

EQUIPMENT (VARIES DEPENDING ON THE SURGERY)

- Electronic blood pressure machine
- Blood pressure cuff
- Electronic thermometer
- Pulse oximeter
- Stethoscope
- IV pump, IV solutions
- Antiembolism stockings
- Pneumatic compression devices
- Tubes, drains, vascular access tubing
- Incentive spirometer
- PPE, as indicated
- Blankets, as needed

ASSESSMENT GUIDELINES

- Assess the patient's mental status, positioning, and vital signs.
- Assess the patient's oxygen saturation level, skin color, respiratory status, and cardiovascular status.
- Assess the patient's neurovascular status, depending on the type of surgery.
- Assess the operative site, drains/tubes, and intravenous site(s).
- Perform a pain assessment.
- A wide variety of factors increase the risk for postoperative complications. Ongoing postoperative assessments and interventions are used to decrease the risk for postoperative complications.
- Assessment of the patient's and family's learning needs is also important.

NURSING DIAGNOSES

- Anxiety
- Hypothermia
- Risk for Infection
- Impaired Skin Integrity
- Acute Pain
- Risk for Aspiration
- Risk for Imbalanced Body Temperature
- Risk for Perioperative Positioning Injury
- Risk for Imbalanced Fluid Volume

- Impaired Physical Mobility
- Ineffective Airway Clearance
- Risk for Spiritual Distress
- Impaired Gas Exchange
- Disturbed Body Image
- Impaired Urinary Elimination

OUTCOME IDENTIFICATION AND PLANNING

Expected outcomes may include:
- Patient will recover from the surgery.
- Patient is free from anxiety.
- Patient's temperature remains between 97.7°F and 99.5°F.
- Patient's vital signs remain stable.
- Patient will remain free from infection.
- Patient will not experience any skin breakdown.
- Patient will regain mobility.
- Patient will have pain managed appropriately.
- Patient is comfortable with body image.
- Specific expected outcomes are individualized based on risk factors, the surgical procedure, and the patient's unique needs.

IMPLEMENTATION

ACTION	RATIONALE
Immediate Care	
1. When patient returns from the PACU, obtain a report from the PACU nurse and review the operating room and PACU data.	Obtaining this report ensures accurate communication and promotes continuity of care.
2. Perform hand hygiene and put on PPE, if indicated.	Hand hygiene and PPE prevent the spread of microorganisms. PPE is required based on transmission precautions.
3. Identify the patient.	Identifying the patient ensures the right patient receives the intervention and helps prevent errors.
4. Close curtains around bed and close the door to the room, if possible. Explain what you are going to do and why you are going to do it to the patient.	This ensures the patient's privacy. Explanation relieves anxiety and facilitates cooperation.

ACTION	RATIONALE
5. **Place patient in a safe position (semi- or high Fowler's or side-lying). Note level of consciousness.**	A sitting position facilitates deep breathing; the side-lying position with neck slightly extended prevents aspiration and airway obstruction. Alternate positions may be appropriate based on the type of surgery.
6. **Obtain vital signs. Monitor and record vital signs frequently.** Assessment order may vary, but usual frequency includes taking vital signs every 15 minutes the first hour, every 30 minutes the next 2 hours, every hour for 4 hours, and finally every 4 hours.	Comparison with baseline preoperative vital signs may indicate impending shock or hemorrhage. Some institutions use a paper or computer flow sheet to record initial postoperative data.
7. Assess the patient's respiratory status. Measure the patient's oxygen saturation level.	Comparison with baseline preoperative respiratory assessment may indicate impending respiratory complications.
8. Assess the patient's cardiovascular status.	Comparison with baseline preoperative cardiovascular assessment may indicate impending cardiovascular complications.
9. Assess the patient's neurovascular status, based on the type of surgery performed.	Comparison with baseline preoperative neurovascular assessment may indicate impending neurovascular complications.
10. Provide for warmth, using heated or extra blankets, as necessary. Assess skin color and condition.	The operating room is a cold environment. Hypothermia is uncomfortable and may lead to cardiac arrhythmias and impaired wound healing.
11. Check dressings for color, odor, presence of drains, and amount of drainage. Mark the drainage on the dressing by circling the amount, and include the time. Turn the patient to assess visually under the patient for bleeding from the surgical site.	Hemorrhage and shock are life-threatening complications of surgery and early recognition is essential.

ACTION	RATIONALE
12. Verify that all tubes and drains are patent and equipment is operative; note amount of drainage in collection device. If an indwelling urinary (Foley) catheter is in place, note urinary output.	This ensures maintenance of vital functions.
13. Verify and maintain IV infusion at correct rate.	This replaces fluid loss and prevents dehydration and electrolyte imbalances.
14. Assess for pain and relieve it by administering medications ordered by the physician. If the patient has been instructed in use of PCA for pain management, review its use. Check record to verify if analgesic medication was administered in the PACU.	Observe for nonverbal behavior that may indicate pain, such as grimacing, crying, and restlessness. Analgesics and other non-pharmacologic pain strategies are used for relief of postoperative pain.
15. Provide for a safe environment. Keep bed in low position with side rails up, based on facility policy. Have call bell within patient's reach.	This prevents accidental injury. Easy access to call bell permits patient to call for nurse when necessary.
16. Remove PPE, if used. Perform hand hygiene.	Removing PPE properly reduces the risk for infection transmission and contamination of other items. Hand hygiene prevents transmission of microorganisms.

Ongoing Care

17. Promote optimal respiratory function.	Anesthetic agents may depress respiratory function. Patients who have existing respiratory or cardiovascular disease, have abdominal or chest incisions, who are obese, elderly, or in a poor state of nutrition are at greater risk for respiratory complications.
a. Assess respiratory rate, depth, quality, color, and capillary refill. Ask if the patient is experiencing any difficulty breathing.	Postoperative analgesic medication can reduce the rate and quality of the respiratory effort.

ACTION	RATIONALE
b. Assist with coughing and deep-breathing exercises (see Skill 46).	
c. Assist with incentive spirometry (see Skill 85).	
d. Assist with early ambulation.	
e. Provide frequent position change.	
f. Administer oxygen, as ordered.	
g. Monitor pulse oximetry (see Skill 138).	
18. Promote optimal cardiovascular function:	Preventive measures can improve venous return and circulatory status.
a. Assess apical rate, rhythm, and quality and compare with peripheral pulses, color, and blood pressure. Ask if the patient has any chest pains or shortness of breath.	
b. Provide frequent position changes.	
c. Assist with early ambulation.	
d. Apply antiembolism stockings or pneumatic compression devices, if ordered and not in place. If in place, assess for integrity.	
e. Provide leg and range-of-motion exercises if not contraindicated (see Skills 96 and 140).	
19. Promote optimal neurologic function:	
a. Assess level of consciousness, motor and sensation.	Anesthetic and pain management agents can alter neurologic function.

ACTION	RATIONALE
b. Determine the level of orientation to person, place, and time.	Older patients may take longer to return to their level of orientation before surgery. Drug and anesthetics will delay this return.
c. Test motor ability by asking the patient to move each extremity.	Anesthesia alters motor and sensory function.
d. Evaluate sensation by asking the patient if he or she can feel your touch on an extremity.	
20. Promote optimal renal and urinary function and fluid and electrolyte status. Assess intake and output, evaluate for urinary retention and monitor serum electrolyte levels.	Anesthetic agents and surgical manipulation in the area may temporarily depress bladder tone and response causing urinary retention.
a. Promote voiding by offering bedpan at regular intervals, noting the frequency, amount, and if any burning or urgency symptoms.	Frequency, burning, or urgency may indicate possible urinary tract abnormality.
b. Monitor urinary catheter drainage if present.	The primary care provider needs to be notified if the urinary output is less than 30 mL/hour or 240 mL/8-hour period.
c. Measure intake and output.	Intake and output are good indicators of fluid balance.
21. Promote optimal gastrointestinal function and meet nutritional needs:	
a. Assess abdomen for distention and firmness. Ask if patient feels nauseated, any vomiting, and if passing flatus.	Anesthetic agents and narcotics depress peristalsis and normal functioning of the gastrointestinal tract. Flatus indicates return of peristalsis.
b. Auscultate for bowel sounds.	Presence of bowel sounds indicates return of peristalsis.
c. Assist with diet progression; encourage fluid intake; monitor intake.	Patients may experience nausea after surgery and are encouraged to resume diet slowly, starting with clear liquids and advancing as tolerated.

ACTION	RATIONALE
d. Medicate for nausea and vomiting as ordered by physician.	Antiemetics are frequently ordered to alleviate postoperative nausea.
22. Promote optimal wound healing.	Alterations in nutritional, circulatory, and metabolic status may predispose patient to infection and delayed healing.
a. Assess condition of wound for presence of drains and any drainage.	
b. Use surgical asepsis for dressing changes.	Surgical asepsis reduces the risk of infection.
c. Inspect all skin surfaces for beginning signs of pressure ulcer development and use pressure-relieving supports to minimize potential skin breakdown.	Lying on the operating room table in the same position can predispose some patients to pressure ulcer formation, especially in patients who have undergone surgery lasting more than 4 hours.
23. Promote optimal comfort and relief from pain.	This shortens recovery period and facilitates return to normal function.
a. Assess for pain (location and intensity using scale).	Control of postoperative pain promotes patient comfort and recovery.
b. Provide for rest and comfort; provide extra blankets, as needed, for warmth.	Patients may experience chilling in the postoperative period.
c. Administer pain medications or other nonpharmacologic methods, as needed.	
24. Promote optimal meeting of psychosocial needs:	This facilitates individualized care and patient's return to normal health.
a. Provide emotional support to patient and family, as needed.	
b. Explain procedures and offer explanations regarding postoperative recovery, as needed, to both patient and family members.	

EVALUATION

- Patient recovers from surgery.
- Patient is free from anxiety.
- Patient's temperature remains between 97.7°F and 99.5°F.
- Patient's vital signs remain stable.
- Patient remains free from infection.
- Patient does not experience skin breakdown.
- Patient regains mobility.
- Patient experiences adequate pain control.
- Patient is comfortable with body image.
- Specific expected outcomes are individualized based on risk factors, the surgical procedure, and the patient's unique needs.

DOCUMENTATION

- Document the time that the patient returns from PACU to the surgical unit. Record the patient's level of consciousness, vital signs, all assessments, and condition of dressing. If patient has oxygen running, an IV, or any other equipment, record this information. Document the pain assessment and interventions that were instituted to alleviate this pain, as well as the patient's response to the interventions. Document any patient teaching that is reviewed with the patient, such as use of incentive spirometer.

GENERAL CONSIDERATIONS

- Be aware of baseline sensory deficits. Ensure appropriate aids are in place, such as glasses or hearing aids. Lack of appropriate aids may impact postoperative assessments, such as level of consciousness.
- For patients undergoing throat surgery, such as a tonsillectomy, evaluate swallowing pattern. A patient who has had throat surgery and swallows frequently may be bleeding from the incision site.
- In the obese patient, medications may not perform as expected related to the lack of serum proteins that are needed to bind with drugs to support their effectiveness. Additionally, due to the larger kidney mass of the obese patient, renal elimination rates of certain drugs are increased, reducing the effectiveness of these drugs.
- Check to make sure that the mattress for the obese patient is of high quality, because this patient is at greater risk for skin breakdown due to the poor vascular supply of adipose tissue.
- Ensure that written postoperative instructions specific to the patient and follow-up appointments with the surgeon or other healthcare professionals are provided to each patient upon discharge from the hospital or outpatient center. Information, such as signs and symptoms to report to the primary care provider, as well as restrictions in activity and diet need to be addressed. In addition, patients discharged the same day as their surgery are required to have a responsible individual accompany them home, and a contact telephone number is to be provided in case of emergency. The patient should be alert and

oriented, or mental status should be at the patient's baseline. The vital signs of the patient should be stable.

- In the elderly patient, postoperative pneumonia can be a very serious complication resulting in death. Therefore, it is especially important to encourage and assist the patient in using the incentive spirometer and with deep-breathing exercises.
- Older patients may take longer to return to their level of orientation before surgery. Drug and anesthetics will delay this return.

Skill · 135   Assessing the Apical Pulse by Auscultation

An apical pulse is auscultated (listened to) over the apex of the heart, as the heart beats. The cardiovascular system is composed of the heart and the blood vessels. The heart is a cone-shaped, muscular pump, divided into four hollow chambers. The upper chambers, the atria (singular, atrium), receive blood from the veins (the superior and inferior vena cava and the left and right pulmonary veins). The lower chambers, the ventricles, force blood out of the heart through the arteries (the left and right pulmonary arteries and the aorta). One-way valves that direct blood flow through the heart are located at the entrance (tricuspid and mitral valves) and exit (pulmonic and aortic valves) of each ventricle. Heart sounds, which are produced by closure of the valves of the heart, are characterized as "lub-dub." The apical pulse is the result of closure of the mitral and tricuspid valves ("lub") and the aortic and pulmonic valves ("dub"). The combination of the two sounds is counted as one beat. Pulse rates are measured in beats per minute. The normal pulse rate for adolescents and adults ranges from 60 to 100 beats per minute. Pulse rhythm is also assessed. Pulse rhythm is the pattern of the beats and the pauses between them. Pulse rhythm is normally regular; the beats and the pauses between occur at regular intervals. An irregular pulse rhythm occurs when the beats and pauses between beats occur at unequal intervals.

An apical pulse is assessed when giving medications that alter heart rate and rhythm. In addition, if a peripheral pulse is difficult to assess accurately because it is irregular, feeble, or extremely rapid, assess the apical rate. In adults, the apical rate is counted for 1 full minute by listening with a stethoscope over the apex of the heart. Apical pulse measurement is also the preferred method of pulse assessment for infants and children less than 2 years of age (Kyle, 2008).

EQUIPMENT

- Watch with second hand or digital readout
- Stethoscope
- Alcohol swab
- Pencil or pen, paper or flow sheet, computerized record
- Nonsterile gloves, if appropriate; additional PPE, as indicated

ASSESSMENT GUIDELINES

- Assess for factors that could affect apical pulse rate and rhythm, such as the patient's age, amount of exercise, fluid balance, and medications.
- Note baseline or previous apical pulse measurements.

NURSING DIAGNOSES

- Decreased Cardiac Output
- Risk for Decreased Cardiac Tissue Perfusion
- Deficient Fluid Volume
- Acute Pain

OUTCOME IDENTIFICATION AND PLANNING

Expected outcomes may include:
- Patient's pulse is assessed accurately without injury and the patient experiences minimal discomfort.

IMPLEMENTATION

ACTION	RATIONALE
1. Check medical order or nursing care plan for frequency of pulse assessment. More frequent pulse measurement may be appropriate based on nursing judgment. Identify the need to obtain an apical pulse measurement.	Provides for patient safety and appropriate care.
2. Perform hand hygiene and put on PPE, if indicated.	Hand hygiene and PPE prevent the spread of microorganisms. PPE is required based on transmission precautions.
3. Identify the patient.	Identifying the patient ensures the right patient receives the intervention and helps prevent errors.

ACTION	RATIONALE
4. Close curtains around bed and close the door to the room, if possible. Discuss procedure with patient and assess patient's ability to assist with the procedure.	This ensures the patient's privacy. Explanation relieves anxiety and facilitates cooperation.
5. Put on gloves as appropriate.	Gloves are not usually worn to obtain a pulse measurement unless contact with blood or body fluids is anticipated. Gloves prevent contact with blood and body fluids.
6. Use alcohol swab to clean the diaphragm of the stethoscope. Use another swab to clean the earpieces, if necessary.	Cleaning with alcohol deters transmission of microorganisms.
7. Assist patient to a sitting or reclining position and expose chest area.	This position facilitates identification of the site for stethoscope placement.
8. Move the patient's clothing to expose only the apical site.	The site must be exposed for pulse assessment. Exposing only the apical site keeps the patient warm and maintains his or her dignity.
9. Hold the stethoscope diaphragm against the palm of your hand for a few seconds.	Warming the diaphragm promotes patient comfort.
10. **Palpate the space between the fifth and sixth ribs (fifth intercostal space), and move to the left midclavicular line.** Place the diaphragm over the apex of the heart (FIGURE 1 and FIGURE 2).	Positions the stethoscope over the apex of the heart, where the heartbeat is best heard.

ACTION

RATIONALE

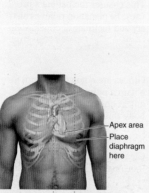

Midsternum   Midclavicular line

FIGURE 1 Locating the apical pulse: apex area.

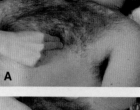

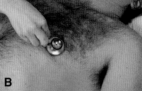

FIGURE 2 The apical pulse is usually found at (**A**) the fifth intercostal space just inside the midclavicular line and can be heard (**B**) over the apex of the heart.

ACTION	RATIONALE
11. Listen for heart sounds ("lub-dub"). Each "lub-dub" counts as one beat.	These sounds occur as the heart valves close.
12. Using a watch with a second hand, count the heartbeat for 1 minute.	Counting for a full minute increases the accuracy of assessment.
13. When measurement is completed, remove gloves, if worn. Cover the patient and help him or her to a position of comfort.	Removing PPE properly reduces the risk for infection transmission and contamination of other items. Ensures patient comfort.
14. Clean the diaphragm of the stethoscope with an alcohol swab.	Cleaning with alcohol deters transmission of microorganisms.
15. Remove additional PPE, if used. Perform hand hygiene	Removing PPE properly reduces the risk for infection transmission and contamination of other items. Hand hygiene prevents the spread of microorganisms.

EVALUATION

• Patient's pulse is assessed accurately without injury and the patient experiences minimal discomfort.

DOCUMENTATION

• Record pulse rate and rhythm on paper, flow sheet, or computerized record. Report abnormal findings to the appropriate person. Identify site of assessment.

GENERAL CONSIDERATIONS

• If a peripheral pulse is difficult to assess accurately because it is irregular, feeble, or extremely rapid, assess the apical rate.

Skill • 136   **Assessing a Peripheral Pulse by Palpation**

The pulse is a throbbing sensation that can be palpated over a peripheral artery, such as the radial artery or the carotid artery. Peripheral pulses result from a wave of blood being pumped into the arterial circulation by the contraction of the left ventricle. Each time the left ventricle contracts to eject blood into an already full aorta, the arterial walls in the cardiovascular system expand to compensate for the increase in pressure of the blood. Characteristics of the pulse, including rate, quality, or amplitude, and rhythm, provide information about the effectiveness of the heart as a pump and the adequacy of peripheral blood flow.

Pulse rates are measured in beats per minute. The normal pulse rate for adolescents and adults ranges from 60 to 100 beats per minute. Pulse quality (amplitude) describes the quality of the pulse in terms of its fullness—strong or weak. It is assessed by the feel of the blood flow through the vessel. Pulse rhythm is the pattern of the pulsations and the pauses between them. Pulse rhythm is normally regular; the pulsations and the pauses between occur at regular intervals. An irregular pulse rhythm occurs when the pulsations and pauses between beats occur at unequal intervals.

Assess the pulse by palpating peripheral arteries, by auscultating the apical pulse with a stethoscope, or by using a portable Doppler ultrasound. To assess the pulse accurately, you need to know which site to choose and what method is most appropriate for the patient. Place your fingers over the artery so that the ends of your fingers are flat against the patient's skin when palpating peripheral pulses. Do not press with the tip of the fingers only.

EQUIPMENT

- Watch with second hand or digital readout
- Pencil or pen, paper or flow sheet, computerized record
- Nonsterile gloves, if appropriate; additional PPE, as indicated

ASSESSMENT GUIDELINES

- Choose a site to assess the pulse. For an adult patient, the most common site for obtaining a peripheral pulse is the radial pulse. For a child older than 2 years, palpate the radial pulse. For children younger than 2 years of age, auscultate the apical pulse.
- Assess for factors that could affect pulse characteristics, such as the patient's age, amount of exercise, fluid balance, and medications. Note baseline or previous pulse measurements.

NURSING DIAGNOSES

- Decreased Cardiac Output
- Ineffective Peripheral Tissue Perfusion
- Acute Pain
- Deficient Fluid Volume

OUTCOME IDENTIFICATION AND PLANNING

Expected outcomes may include:
- Patient's pulse is assessed accurately without injury.
- Patient experiences minimal discomfort.

IMPLEMENTATION

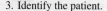 ACTION	RATIONALE
1. Check medical order or nursing care plan for frequency of pulse assessment. More frequent pulse measurement may be appropriate based on nursing judgment.	Assessment and measurement of vital signs at appropriate intervals provides important data about the patient's health status.
2. Perform hand hygiene and put on PPE, if indicated.	Hand hygiene and PPE prevent the spread of microorganisms. PPE is required based on transmission precautions.
3. Identify the patient.	Identifying the patient ensures the right patient receives the intervention and helps prevent errors.

ACTION	RATIONALE
4. Close curtains around bed and close the door to the room, if possible. Discuss the procedure with the patient and assess the patient's ability to assist with the procedure.	This ensures the patient's privacy. Explanation relieves anxiety and facilitates cooperation.
5. Put on gloves as appropriate.	Gloves are not usually worn to obtain a pulse measurement unless contact with blood or body fluids is anticipated. Gloves prevent contact with blood and body fluids.
6. Select the appropriate peripheral site based on assessment data.	Ensures safety and accuracy of measurement.
7. Move the patient's clothing to expose only the site chosen.	The site must be exposed for pulse assessment. Exposing only the site keeps the patient warm and maintains his or her dignity.
8. Place your first, second, and third fingers over the artery (FIGURE 1). **Lightly compress the artery so pulsations can be felt and counted.**	The sensitive fingertips can feel the pulsation of the artery.

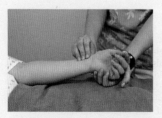

FIGURE 1 Palpating the radial pulse.

9. Using a watch with a second hand, count the number of pulsations felt for 30 seconds. Multiply this number by 2 to calculate the rate for 1 minute. **If the rate, rhythm, or amplitude of the pulse is**	Ensures accuracy of measurement and assessment.

ACTION	RATIONALE
abnormal in any way, palpate and count the pulse for 1 minute.	
10. Note the rhythm and amplitude of the pulse.	Provides additional assessment data regarding the patient's cardiovascular status.
11. When measurement is completed, remove gloves, if worn. Cover the patient and help him or her to a position of comfort.	Removing PPE properly reduces the risk for infection transmission and contamination of other items. Ensures patient comfort.
12. Remove additional PPE, if used. Perform hand hygiene.	Removing PPE properly reduces the risk for infection transmission and contamination of other items. Hand hygiene prevents the spread of microorganisms.

EVALUATION

• Patient's pulse is assessed accurately without injury and the patient experiences minimal discomfort.

DOCUMENTATION

• Record pulse rate, amplitude, and rhythm on paper flow sheet, or computerized record. Identify site of assessment. Report abnormal findings to the appropriate person.

GENERAL CONSIDERATIONS

• The normal heart rate varies by age.
• When palpating a carotid pulse, lightly press only one side of the neck at a time. Never attempt to palpate both carotid arteries at the same time. Bilateral palpation could result in reduced cerebral blood flow (Weber & Kelly, 2007).
• If a peripheral pulse is difficult to assess accurately because it is irregular, feeble, or extremely rapid, assess the apical rate.

Skill • 137   Assessing Peripheral Pulse Using a Portable Doppler Ultrasound Device

The pulse is a throbbing sensation that can be palpated over a peripheral artery, such as the radial artery or the carotid artery. Peripheral pulses result from a wave of blood being pumped into the arterial circulation by the contraction of the left ventricle. Each time the left ventricle contracts to eject blood into an already full aorta, the arterial walls in the cardiovascular system expand to compensate for the increase in pressure of the blood. Characteristics of the pulse, including rate, quality, or amplitude, and rhythm, provide information about the effectiveness of the heart as a pump and the adequacy of peripheral blood flow.

Pulse rates are measured in beats per minute. The normal pulse rate for adolescents and adults ranges from 60 to 100 beats per minute. Pulse rhythm is the pattern of the pulsations and the pauses between them. Pulse rhythm is normally regular; the pulsations and the pauses between occur at regular intervals. An irregular pulse rhythm occurs when the pulsations and pauses between beats occur at unequal intervals.

Assess the pulse by palpating peripheral arteries, by auscultating the apical pulse with a stethoscope, or by using a portable Doppler ultrasound. An ultrasound or Doppler device amplifies sound. It is especially useful if the pulse is weak, or to assess the circulatory status of a surgical or injury site. Doppler ultrasound is used to assess peripheral pulses. To assess the pulse accurately, you need to know which site to choose and what method is most appropriate for the patient.

EQUIPMENT
- Watch with second hand or digital readout
- Portable Doppler ultrasound
- Conducting gel
- Pencil or pen, paper or flow sheet, computerized record
- Nonsterile gloves, if appropriate; additional PPE, as indicated

ASSESSMENT GUIDELINES
- Choose a site to assess the pulse. For an adult patient, the most common site for obtaining a peripheral pulse is the radial pulse. For a child older than 2 years, palpate the radial pulse. For children younger than 2 years of age, auscultate the apical pulse. The site may be determined by other patient health problems, such as recent arteriovenous surgery, or injury.
- Assess for factors that could affect pulse characteristics, such as the patient's age, amount of exercise, fluid balance, and medications. Note baseline or previous pulse measurements.

NURSING DIAGNOSES
- Decreased Cardiac Output
- Ineffective Peripheral Tissue Perfusion

• Acute Pain
• Deficient Fluid Volume

OUTCOME IDENTIFICATION AND PLANNING

Expected outcomes may include:
• Patient's pulse is assessed accurately without injury.
• Patient experiences minimal discomfort.

IMPLEMENTATION

ACTION	RATIONALE
1. Check physician's order or nursing care plan for frequency of pulse assessment. More frequent pulse measurement may be appropriate based on nursing judgment. Determine the need to use a Doppler ultrasound device for pulse assessment.	Assessment and measurement of vital signs at appropriate intervals provides important data about the patient's health status.
2. Perform hand hygiene and put on PPE, if indicated.	Hand hygiene and PPE prevent the spread of microorganisms. PPE is required based on transmission precautions.
3. Identify the patient.	Identifying the patient ensures the right patient receives the intervention and helps prevent errors.
4. Close curtains around bed and close the door to the room, if possible. Discuss the procedure with patient and assess the patient's ability to assist with the procedure.	This ensures the patient's privacy. Explanation relieves anxiety and facilitates cooperation.
5. Put on gloves, as appropriate.	Gloves are not usually worn to obtain a pulse measurement unless contact with blood or body fluids is anticipated. Gloves prevent contact with blood and body fluids.
6. Select the appropriate peripheral site based on assessment data.	Ensures safety and accuracy of measurement.

ACTION	RATIONALE
7. Move the patient's clothing to expose only the site chosen.	The site must be exposed for pulse assessment. Exposing only the site keeps the patient warm and maintains his or her dignity.
8. Remove Doppler from charger and turn it on. Make sure that volume is set at low. Apply conducting gel to the site where you are auscultating the pulse.	Removing from charger and turning on prepare the device for use. Conduction gel is necessary to provide conduction of sound from artery to Doppler.
9. Hold the Doppler base in your nondominant hand. With your dominant hand, place the Doppler probe tip in the gel. Adjust the volume as needed. Move the Doppler tip around until the pulse is heard (FIGURE 1). **Using a watch with a second hand, count the heartbeat for 1 minute.**	Locates arterial pulse for reading. Ensures accuracy of measurement and assessment.

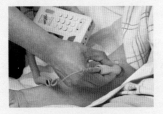

FIGURE 1 Moving the Doppler tip until pulse is heard.

10. Note the rhythm of the pulse.	Provides additional assessment data regarding patient's cardiovascular status.
11. Remove the Doppler tip and turn the Doppler off. Wipe excess gel off of the patient's skin with a tissue. Place a small X over the spot where the pulse is located with an indelible pen, depending on facility policy.	Removing gel from patient's skin promotes patient comfort. Marking the site allows for easier future assessment. It can also make palpating the pulse easier since the exact location of the pulse is known.

ACTION	RATIONALE
12. Wipe any gel remaining on the Doppler probe off with a tissue. Clean the Doppler probe per facility policy or manufacturer's recommendations.	Appropriate cleaning deters the spread of microorganisms. Equipment should be left ready for use.
13. Remove gloves. Cover the patient and help him or her to a position of comfort.	Removing PPE properly reduces the risk for infection transmission and contamination of other items. Ensures patient comfort.
14. Remove PPE, if used. Perform hand hygiene.	Removing PPE properly reduces the risk for infection transmission and contamination of other items. Hand hygiene deters the spread of microorganisms.
15. Return the Doppler ultrasound device to the charge base.	Equipment should be left ready for use.

EVALUATION
- Patient's pulse is assessed accurately without injury and the patient experiences minimal discomfort.

DOCUMENTATION
- Record pulse rate and rhythm on paper, flow sheet, or computerized record. Identify site of assessment and that it was obtained with a Doppler. Report abnormal findings to the appropriate person.

GENERAL CONSIDERATIONS
- The normal heart rate varies by age.

Skill · 138 Using a Pulse Oximeter

Pulse oximetry is a noninvasive technique that measures the arterial oxyhemoglobin saturation (SaO_2 or SpO_2) of arterial blood. A sensor, or probe, uses a beam of red and infrared light that travels through tissue and blood vessels. One part of the sensor emits the light and another part receives the light. The oximeter then calculates the amount of light that has been absorbed by arterial blood. Oxygen saturation is determined by the amount of each light absorbed; unoxygenated hemoglobin absorbs more red light and oxygenated hemoglobin absorbs more infrared light. Sensors are available for use on a finger, a toe, a foot (infants), an earlobe, forehead, and the bridge of the nose. It is important to use the appropriate sensor for the intended site; use of a sensor on a site other than that for what it is intended can result in inaccurate or unreliable readings (Haynes, 2007). Circulation to the sensor site must be adequate to ensure accurate readings. Pulse oximeters also display a measured pulse rate.

It is important to know the patient's hemoglobin level before evaluating oxygen saturation because the test measures only the percentage of oxygen carried by the available hemoglobin. Thus, even a patient with low hemoglobin level could appear to have a normal SpO_2 because most of that hemoglobin is saturated. However, the patient may not have enough oxygen to meet body needs. Also, take into consideration the presence of preexisting health conditions, such as COPD. Parameters for acceptable oxygen saturation readings may be different for these patients. Be aware of any medical orders regarding acceptable ranges and/or check with the patient's physician. A range of 95% to 100% is considered normal SpO_2; values less than or equal to 90% are abnormal, indicate that oxygenation to the tissues is inadequate, and should be investigated for potential hypoxia or technical error (Booker, 2008a; DeMeulenaere, 2007).

Pulse oximetry is useful for monitoring patients receiving oxygen therapy, titrating oxygen therapy, monitoring those at risk for hypoxia, and postoperative patients. Pulse oximetry does not replace arterial blood gas analysis. Desaturation indicates gas exchange abnormalities.

EQUIPMENT

- Pulse oximeter with an appropriate sensor or probe
- Alcohol wipe(s) or disposable cleansing cloth
- Nail polish remover (if necessary)
- PPE, as indicated

ASSESSMENT GUIDELINES

- Assess the patient's skin temperature and color, including the color of the nail beds. Temperature is a good indicator of blood flow. Warm skin indicates adequate circulation. In a well-oxygenated patient, the skin and nail beds are usually pink. Skin that is bluish or dusky indicates hypoxia (inadequate amount of oxygen available to the cells).
- Check capillary refill; prolonged capillary refill indicates a reduction in blood flow.
- Assess the quality of the pulse proximal to the sensor application site.
- Auscultate the lungs.
- Note the amount of oxygen and delivery method if the patient is receiving supplemental oxygen.

NURSING DIAGNOSES

• Risk for Decreased Cardiac Tissue Perfusion
• Risk for Ineffective Cerebral Tissue Perfusion
• Impaired Gas Exchange
• Ineffective Airway Clearance
• Activity Intolerance

OUTCOME IDENTIFICATION AND PLANNING

Expected outcomes may include:
• Patient will exhibit arterial blood oxygen saturation within acceptable
  parameters, or greater than 95%.

IMPLEMENTATION

ACTION	RATIONALE
1. Review chart for any health problems that would affect the patient's oxygenation status.	Identifying influencing factors aids in interpretation of results.
2. Bring necessary equipment to the bedside stand or over-bed table.	Bringing everything to the bedside conserves time and energy. Arranging items nearby is convenient, saves time, and avoids unnecessary stretching and twisting of muscles on the part of the nurse.
3. Perform hand hygiene and put on PPE, if indicated.	Hand hygiene and PPE prevent the spread of microorganisms. PPE is required based on transmission precautions.
4. Identify the patient.	Identifying the patient ensures the right patient receives the intervention and helps prevent errors.
5. Close curtains around bed and close the door to the room, if possible. Explain what you are going to do and why you are going to do it to the patient.	This ensures the patient's privacy. Explanation relieves anxiety and facilitates cooperation.
6. Select an adequate site for application of the sensor.	Inadequate circulation can interfere with the oxygen saturation (SpO$_2$) reading.

ACTION	RATIONALE
a. Use the patient's index, middle, or ring finger.	Fingers are easily accessible.
b. Check the proximal pulse and capillary refill at the pulse closest to the site.	Brisk capillary refill and a strong pulse indicate that circulation to the site is adequate.
c. If circulation at the site is inadequate, consider using the earlobe, forehead, or bridge of nose.	These alternate sites are highly vascular alternatives.
d. Use a toe only if lower extremity circulation is not compromised.	Peripheral vascular disease is common in lower extremities.
7. Select proper equipment:	
a. If one finger is too large for the probe, use a smaller one. A pediatric probe may be used for a small adult.	Inaccurate readings can result if the probe or sensor is not attached correctly.
b. Use probes appropriate for patient's age and size.	Probes come in adult, pediatric, and infant sizes.
c. Check if patient is allergic to adhesive. A nonadhesive finger clip or reflectance sensor is available.	A reaction may occur if the patient is allergic to adhesive substance.
8. Prepare the monitoring site. Cleanse the selected area with the alcohol wipe or disposable cleansing cloth. Allow the area to dry. If necessary, remove nail polish and artificial nails after checking pulse oximeter's manufacturer instructions.	Skin oils, dirt, or grime on the site can interfere with the passage of light waves. Research is conflicting regarding the effect of dark color nail polish and artificial nails; refer to facility policy and pulse oximeter's manufacturer instructions (Collins & Andersen, 2007; DeMeulenaere, 2007).
9. **Apply probe securely to skin (FIGURE 1). Make sure that the light-emitting sensor and the light-receiving sensor are aligned opposite each other (not necessary to check if placed on forehead or bridge of nose).**	Secure attachment and proper alignment promote satisfactory operation of the equipment and accurate recording of the SpO_2.

ACTION	RATIONALE

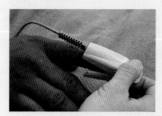

FIGURE 1 Attaching probe to patient's finger.

10. Connect the sensor probe to the pulse oximeter, turn the oximeter on, and check operation of the equipment (audible beep, fluctuation of bar of light or waveform on face of oximeter) (FIGURE 2).

Audible beep represents the arterial pulse, and fluctuating waveform or light bar indicates the strength of the pulse. A weak signal will produce an inaccurate recording of the SpO$_2$. Tone of beep reflects SpO$_2$ reading. If SpO$_2$ drops, tone becomes lower in pitch.

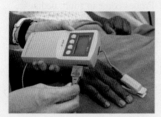

FIGURE 2 Connecting sensor probe to unit.

11. Set alarms on pulse oximeter. Check manufacturer's alarm limits for high and low pulse rate settings.

Alarm provides an additional safeguard and signals when high or low limits have been surpassed.

12. Check oxygen saturation at regular intervals, as ordered by primary care provider, nursing assessment, and signaled by alarms. Monitor hemoglobin level.

Monitoring SpO$_2$ provides ongoing assessment of the patient's condition. A low hemoglobin level may be satisfactorily saturated yet inadequate to meet a patient's oxygen needs.

13. Remove sensor on a regular basis and check for skin irritation or signs of pressure (every 2 hours for spring-tension sensor or every 4 hours for adhesive finger or toe sensor).

Prolonged pressure may lead to tissue necrosis. Adhesive sensor may cause skin irritation.

ACTION	RATIONALE
14. Clean nondisposable sensors according to the manufacturer's directions. Remove PPE, if used. Perform hand hygiene.	Cleaning equipment between patient use reduces the spread of microorganisms. Removing PPE properly reduces the risk for infection transmission and contamination of other items. Hand hygiene prevents the spread of microorganisms.

EVALUATION

• Patient exhibits an oxygen saturation level within acceptable parameters, or greater than 95%, and a heart rate that correlates with the pulse measurement.

DOCUMENTATION

• Document the type of sensor and location used, the assessment of the proximal pulse and capillary refill, pulse oximeter reading, the amount of oxygen and delivery method if the patient is receiving supplemental oxygen; lung assessment, if relevant; and any other relevant interventions required as a result of the reading.

GENERAL CONSIDERATIONS

• Accuracy of readings can be influenced by conditions that decrease arterial blood flow, such as peripheral edema, hypotension, and peripheral vascular disease.
• Correlate the pulse reading on the pulse oximeter with the patient's heart rate. Variation between pulse and heart rate may indicate that not all pulsations are being detected and another sensor site may be required (Moore, 2007).
• Excessive motion of sensor probe site, such as with extremity tremors or shivering, can also interfere with obtaining an accurate reading.
• Bradycardia and irregular cardiac rhythms may also cause inaccurate readings.
• In patients with low cardiac index (cardiac output in liters per minute divided by body surface area in square meters), the forehead sensor may be better than the digit sensor for pulse oximetry (Fernandez, et al., 2007).

Skill · 139   Monitoring Temperature Using an Overhead Radiant Warmer

Neonates, infants who are exposed to stressors or chilling (e.g., from undergoing numerous procedures), and infants who have an underlying condition that interferes with thermoregulation (e.g., prematurity) are highly susceptible to heat loss. Therefore, radiant warmers are used for infants who have trouble maintaining body temperature. In addition, use of a radiant warmer minimizes the oxygen and calories that the infant would expend to maintain body temperature, thereby minimizing the effects of body temperature changes on metabolic activity.

An overhead radiant warmer warms the air to provide a neutral thermal environment, one that is neither too warm nor too cool for the patient. The incubator temperature is adjusted to maintain an anterior abdominal skin temperature of 36.5°C (97.7°F), but at least 36°C (96.8°F), using servo-control (automatic thermostat) (Sinclair, 2002).

EQUIPMENT
- Overhead warmer
- Temperature probe
- Aluminum foil probe cover
- Axillary or rectal thermometer, based on facility policy
- PPE, as indicated

ASSESSMENT GUIDELINES
- Assess the patient's temperature using the axillary or rectal route, based on facility policy, and assess the patient's fluid intake and output.

NURSING DIAGNOSES
- Hyperthermia
- Hypothermia
- Risk for Imbalanced Body Temperature
- Ineffective Thermoregulation

OUTCOME IDENTIFICATION AND PLANNING
Expected outcomes may include:
- Infant's temperature is maintained within normal limits without injury.

IMPLEMENTATION

ACTION	RATIONALE
1. Check medical order or nursing care plan for the use of a radiant warmer.	Provides for patient safety and appropriate care.

ACTION	RATIONALE

2. Perform hand hygiene and put on PPE, if indicated.

Hand hygiene and PPE prevent the spread of microorganisms. PPE is required based on transmission precautions.

3. Identify the patient.

Identifying the patient ensures the right patient receives the intervention and helps prevent errors.

4. Close curtains around bed and close the door to the room, if possible. Discuss procedure with patient's family.

This ensures the patient's privacy. Explanation reduces the family's apprehension and encourages family cooperation.

5. Plug in the warmer. Turn the warmer to the manual setting. Allow the blankets to warm before placing the infant under the warmer.

By allowing the blankets to warm before placing the infant under the warmer, you are preventing heat loss through conduction. By placing the warmer on the manual setting, you are keeping the warmer at a set temperature no matter how warm the blankets become.

6. **Switch the warmer setting to automatic. Set the warmer to the desired abdominal skin temperature, usually 36.5°C.**

The automatic setting ensures that the warmer will regulate the amount of radiant heat depending on the temperature of the infant's skin. The temperature should be adjusted so that the infant does not become too warm or too cold.

7. Place the infant under the warmer. Attach the probe to the infant's abdominal skin at mid-epigastrium, halfway between the xiphoid and the umbilicus. Cover with a foil patch.

The foil patch prevents direct warming of the probe, allowing the probe to read only the infant's temperature.

8. When the abdominal skin temperature reaches the desired set point, check the patient's axillary or rectal temperature, based on facility

By monitoring the infant's temperature, you are watching for signs of hyperthermia or hypothermia.

ACTION	RATIONALE
policy, to be sure it is within the normal range.	
9. Adjust the warmer's set point slightly, as needed, if the axillary or rectal temperature is abnormal. Do not change the set point if the axillary or rectal temperature is normal.	By monitoring the infant's temperature, you are watching for signs of hyperthermia or hypothermia. This prevents the infant from becoming too warm or too cool.
10. Remove additional PPE, if used. Perform hand hygiene.	Removing PPE properly reduces the risk for infection transmission and contamination of other items. Hand hygiene deters the spread of microorganisms.
11. Check frequently to be sure the probe maintains contact with the patient's skin. Continue to monitor temperature and other vital signs.	Poor contact will cause overheating. Entrapment of the probe under the arm or between the infant and mattress will cause underheating. Monitoring of vital signs assesses patient status.

EVALUATION

• Infant is placed under a radiant warmer, the temperature is well controlled, and the infant experiences no injury.

DOCUMENTATION

• Document initial assessment of the infant, including body temperature; the placement of the infant under the radiant warmer; and the settings of the radiant warmer. Document incubator air temperatures, as well as subsequent skin and axillary or rectal temperatures, and other vital signs measurements.

GENERAL CONSIDERATIONS

• Radiant warmers increase insensible water loss in low-birthweight babies in the newborn period. This water loss needs to be taken into account when daily fluid requirements are calculated.
• Plastic surgeons may order overhead radiant warmers to be used for patients who have undergone extremity or digit reattachment surgery. In this case, judge the heat by the probe's reading of the skin temperature.

Skill · 140   Providing Range-of-Motion Exercises

Range of motion (ROM) is the complete extent of movement of which a joint is normally capable. Taking part in routine activities of daily living helps to use muscle groups that keep many joints in an effective range of motion. When all or some of the normal activities are impossible, attention is given to the joints not being used or to those that have limited use. When the patient does the exercise for himself or herself, it is referred to as active range of motion. Exercises performed by the nurse without participation by the patient are referred to as passive range of motion. Exercises should be as active as the patient's physical condition permits. Allow the patient to do as much individual activity as his or her condition permits. Range-of-motion exercises should be initiated as soon as possible because body changes can occur after only 3 days of impaired mobility.

EQUIPMENT
- Gloves, as indicated
- Additional PPE, as indicated

ASSESSMENT GUIDELINES
- Review the medical record and nursing plan of care for any conditions or orders that will limit mobility.
- Perform a pain assessment before the time for the exercises. If the patient reports pain, administer the prescribed medication in sufficient time to allow for the full effect of the analgesic.
- Assess the patient's ability to perform ROM exercises. Inspect and palpate joints for redness, tenderness, pain, swelling, or deformities.

NURSING DIAGNOSES
- Impaired Physical Mobility
- Deficient Knowledge
- Impaired Bed Mobility
- Acute Pain
- Activity Intolerance
- Chronic Pain
- Fatigue
- Impaired Skin Integrity

OUTCOME IDENTIFICATION AND PLANNING
Expected outcomes may include:
- Patient maintains joint mobility.
- Patient improves or maintains muscle strength.
- Muscle atrophy and contractures are prevented.

IMPLEMENTATION

ACTION	RATIONALE
1. Review the physician's orders and nursing plan of care for patient activity. Identify any movement limitations.	Reviewing the order and plan of care validates the correct patient and correct procedure. Identification of limitations prevents injury.
2. Perform hand hygiene and put on PPE, if indicated.	Hand hygiene and PPE prevent the spread of microorganisms. PPE is required based on transmission precautions.
3. Identify the patient. Explain the procedure to the patient.	Patient identification validates the correct patient and correct procedure. Discussion and explanation help allay anxiety and prepare the patient for what to expect.
4. Close curtain around bed and close the door to the room, if possible. Place the bed at an appropriate and comfortable working height, usually elbow height of the caregiver (VISN 8 Patient Safety Center, 2009). Adjust the head of the bed to a flat position or as low as the patient can tolerate.	Closing the door or curtains provides privacy. Proper bed height helps reduce back strain while performing the procedure.
5. Stand on the side of the bed where the joints are to be exercised. Lower side rail on that side, if in place. Uncover only the limb to be used during the exercise.	Standing on the side to be exercised and lowering the side rail prevent strain on the nurse's back. Proper draping provides for privacy and warmth.
6. Perform the exercises slowly and gently, providing support by holding the areas proximal and distal to the joint. Repeat each exercise two to five times, moving each joint in a smooth and rhythmic manner. **Stop movement if the patient complains of pain or if you meet resistance.**	Slow, gentle movements with support prevent discomfort and muscle spasms resulting from jerky movements. Repeated movement of muscles and joints improves flexibility and increases circulation to the body part. Pain may indicate the exercises are causing damage.

ACTION	RATIONALE
7. While performing the exercises, begin at the head and move down one side of the body at a time. **Encourage the patient to do as many of these exercises by him- or herself as possible.**	Proceeding from head to toe one side at a time promotes efficient time management and an organized approach to the task. Both active and passive exercises improve joint mobility and increase circulation to the affected part, but only active exercise increases muscle mass, tone, and strength and improves cardiac and respiratory functioning.
8. Move the chin down to rest on the chest. Return the head to a normal upright position. Tilt the head as far as possible toward each shoulder.	These movements provide for flexion, extension, and lateral flexion of the head and neck.
9. Move the head from side to side, bringing the chin toward each shoulder.	These movements provide for rotation of neck.
10. Start with the arm at the patient's side and lift the arm forward to above the head. Return the arm to the starting position at the side of the body.	These movements provide for flexion and extension of the shoulder.
11. With the arm back at the patient's side, move the arm laterally to an upright position above the head, and then return it to the original position. Move the arm across the body as far as possible.	These movements provide for abduction and adduction of the shoulder.
12. Raise the arm at the side until the upper arm is in line with the shoulder. Bend the elbow at a 90-degree angle and move the forearm upward and downward, then return the arm to the side.	These movements provide for internal and external rotation of the shoulder.
13. Bend the elbow and move the lower arm and hand upward toward the shoulder	These movements provide for flexion and extension of the elbow.

ACTION

RATIONALE

(FIGURE 1). Return the lower arm and hand to the original position while straightening the elbow.

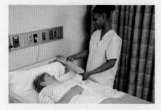

FIGURE 1 Bending the patient's elbow, lower arm, and hand upward toward the shoulder.

14. Rotate the lower arm and hand so the palm is up. Rotate the lower arm and hand so the palm of the hand is down.

These movements provide for supination and pronation of the forearm.

15. Move the hand downward toward the inner aspect of the forearm. Return the hand to a neutral position even with the forearm. Then move the dorsal portion of the hand backward as far as possible.

These movements provide for flexion, extension, and hyperextension of the wrist.

16. Bend the fingers to make a fist, and then straighten them out. Spread the fingers apart and return them back together. Touch the thumb to each finger on the hand.

These movements provide for flexion, extension, abduction, and adduction of the fingers.

17. Extend the leg and lift it upward. Return the leg to the original position beside the other leg.

These movements provide for flexion and extension of the hip.

18. Lift the leg laterally away from the patient's body. Return the leg back toward the other leg and try to extend it beyond the midline (FIGURE 2).

These movements provide for abduction and adduction of the hip.

ACTION

RATIONALE

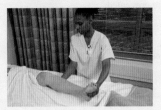

FIGURE 2 Returning the leg back toward the other leg and trying to extend it beyond the midline if possible.

ACTION	RATIONALE
19. Turn the foot and leg toward the other leg to rotate it internally. Turn the foot and leg outward away from the other leg to rotate it externally.	These movements provide for internal and external rotation of the hip.
20. Bend the leg and bring the heel toward the back of the leg. Return the leg to a straight position.	These movements provide for flexion and extension of the knee.
21. At the ankle, move the foot up and back until the toes are upright. Move the foot with the toes pointing downward.	These movements provide for dorsiflexion and plantar flexion of the ankle.
22. Turn the sole of the foot toward the midline. Turn the sole of the foot outward.	These movements provide for inversion and eversion of the ankle.
23. Curl the toes downward, and then straighten them out. Spread the toes apart and bring them together.	These movements provide for flexion, extension, abduction, and adduction of the toes.
24. Repeat these exercises on the other side of the body. Encourage the patient to do as many of these exercises by himself or herself as possible.	Repeating motions on the other side provides exercise for the entire body.
25. **When finished, make sure the patient is comfortable, with the side rails up and the bed in the lowest position.**	Proper positioning with raised side rails and proper bed height provide for patient comfort and safety.
26. Remove gloves and any other PPE, if used. Perform hand hygiene.	Removing PPE properly reduces the risk for infection transmission and contamination of other items. Hand hygiene prevents the spread of microorganisms.

EVALUATION

- Patient maintains or improves joint mobility and muscle strength.
- Muscle atrophy and contractures are prevented.

DOCUMENTATION

- Document the exercises performed, any significant observations, and the patient's reaction to the activities.

GENERAL CONSIDERATIONS

- Many of these exercises can be incorporated into daily activities, such as during bathing.
- An order from the primary care provider and specific instructions should be obtained to perform ROM exercises for patients with acute arthritis, fractures, torn ligaments, joint dislocation, acute myocardial infarction, and bone tumors or metastases.

Skill · 141   Administering a Rectal Suppository

Rectal suppositories are used primarily for their local action, such as laxatives and fecal softeners. Systemic effects are also achieved with rectal suppositories. It is important to ensure the suppository is placed past the internal anal sphincter and against the rectal mucosa.

EQUIPMENT

- Suppository
- Water-soluble lubricant
- Clean gloves
- Computer-generated Medication Administration Record (CMAR)
- or Medication Administration Record (MAR)
- Additional PPE, as indicated

ASSESSMENT GUIDELINES

- Assess the rectal area for any alterations in integrity. Suppository should not be administered to patients who have had recent rectal or prostate surgery.
- Assess recent laboratory values, particularly the patient's white blood cell and platelet counts. Patients who are thrombocytopenic or neutropenic should not receive rectal suppositories. Rectal suppositories should not be administered to patients at risk for cardiac arrhythmias.
- Assess relevant body systems for the particular medication being administered.
- Assess the patient for allergies.
- Verify patient name, dose, route, and time of administration.

• Assess the patient's knowledge of medication and procedure. If the patient has a knowledge deficit about the medication, this may be an appropriate time to begin education about the medication.
• Assess the patient's ability to cooperate with the procedure.

NURSING DIAGNOSES

• Deficient Knowledge
• Risk for Injury
• Anxiety
• Constipation

OUTCOME IDENTIFICATION AND PLANNING

Expected outcomes may include:
• Medication is administered successfully into the rectum.
• Patient understands the rationale for the rectal instillation.
• Patient experiences no allergy response.
• Patient's skin remains intact.
• Patient experiences no, or minimal, pain.
• Patient experiences minimal anxiety.

IMPLEMENTATION

ACTION	RATIONALE
1. Gather equipment. Check medication order against the original order in the medical record, according to facility policy. Clarify any inconsistencies. Check the patient's chart for allergies.	This comparison helps to identify errors that may have occurred when orders were transcribed. The primary care provider's order is the legal record of medication orders for each facility.
2. Know the actions, special nursing considerations, safe dose ranges, purpose of administration, and adverse effects of the medication to be administered. Consider the appropriateness of the medication for this patient.	This knowledge aids the nurse in evaluating the therapeutic effect of the medication in relation to the patient's disorder and can also be used to educate the patient about the medication.
3. Perform hand hygiene.	Hand hygiene prevents the spread of microorganisms.
4. Move the medication cart to the outside of the patient's	Organization facilitates error-free administration and saves time.

ACTION	RATIONALE
room or prepare for administration in the medication area.	
5. Unlock the medication cart or drawer. Enter pass code and scan employee identification, if required.	Locking the cart or drawer safeguards each patient's medication supply. Hospital accrediting organizations require medication carts to be locked when not in use. Entering pass code and scanning ID allows only authorized users into the system and identifies user for documentation by the computer.
6. **Prepare medications for one patient at a time.**	This prevents errors in medication administration.
7. Read the CMAR/MAR and select the proper medication from the patient's medication drawer or unit stock.	This is the *first* check of the label.
8. Compare the label with the CMAR/MAR. Check expiration dates and perform calculations, if necessary. Scan the bar code on the package, if required.	This is the *second* check of the label. Verify calculations with another nurse to ensure safety, if necessary.
9. **When all medications for one patient have been prepared, recheck the label with the CMAR/MAR before taking them to the patient.**	This is a *third* check to ensure accuracy and to prevent errors. Some facilities require the third check to occur at the bedside, after identifying the patient and before administration.
10. Lock the medication cart before leaving it.	Locking the cart or drawer safeguards the patient's medication supply. Hospital accrediting organizations require medication carts to be locked when not in use.
11. Transport medications to the patient's bedside carefully, and keep the medications in sight at all times.	Careful handling and close observation prevent accidental or deliberate disarrangement of medications.
12. **Ensure that the patient receives the medications at the correct time.**	Check agency policy, which may allow for administration within a period of 30 minutes before or 30 minutes after designated time.

ACTION	RATIONALE

13. Perform hand hygiene and put on PPE, if indicated.

Hand hygiene and PPE prevent the spread of microorganisms. PPE is required based on transmission precautions.

14. Identify the patient. Usually, the patient should be identified using two methods. Compare information with the MAR/CMAR.

Identifying the patient ensures the right patient receives the medications and helps prevent errors.

   a. Check the name and identification number on the patient's identification band.

This is the most reliable method. Replace the identification band if it is missing or inaccurate in any way.

   b. Ask the patient to state his or her name and birth date, based on facility policy.

This requires a response from the patient, but illness and strange surroundings often cause patients to be confused.

   c. If the patient cannot identify him- or herself, verify the patient's identification with a staff member who knows the patient for the second source.

This is another way to double-check identity. Do not use the name on the door or over the bed, because these signs may be inaccurate.

15. Complete necessary assessments before administering medications. Check the patient's allergy bracelet or ask the patient about allergies. Explain the purpose and action of each medication to the patient.

Assessment is a prerequisite to administration of medications.

16. Scan the patient's bar code on the identification band, if required.

Provides an additional check to ensure that the medication is given to the right patient.

17. Put on gloves.

Gloves protect the nurse from potential contact with contaminants, mucous membranes, and body fluids.

18. Assist the patient to his or her left side in a Sims' position. Drape accordingly to only expose the buttocks.

Positioning allows for easy access to anal area. Left side decreases chance of expulsion of the suppository. Proper draping maintains privacy.

ACTION	RATIONALE
19. Remove the suppository from its wrapper. Apply lubricant to the rounded end. Lubricate the index finger of your dominant hand.	Lubricant reduces friction on administration and increases patient comfort.
20. Separate the buttocks with your nondominant hand and instruct the patient to breathe slowly and deeply through his or her mouth while the suppository is being inserted.	Slow, deep breaths help to relax the anal sphincter and reduce discomfort.
21. Using your index finger, insert the suppository, round end first, along the rectal wall. Insert about 3 to 4 inches.	Suppository must make contact with the rectal mucosa for absorption to occur.
22. Use toilet tissue to clean any stool or lubricant from around the anus. Release the buttocks. Encourage the patient to remain on his or her side for at least 5 minutes and retain the suppository for the appropriate amount of time for the specific medication.	Prevents skin irritation. Prevents accidental expulsion of suppository and ensures absorption of medication.
23. Remove additional PPE, if used. Perform hand hygiene.	Removing PPE properly reduces the risk for infection transmission and contamination of other items. Hand hygiene prevents the spread of microorganisms.
24. Document the administration of the medication immediately after administration. See Documentation section below.	Timely documentation helps to ensure patient safety.
25. Evaluate patient's response to the medication within appropriate time frame.	The patient needs to be evaluated for therapeutic and adverse effects from the medication.

EVALUATION

• Medication is administered successfully into the rectum.
• Patient understood the rationale for the rectal instillation.
• Patient did not experience adverse effect.

- Patient's skin remains intact.
- Patient experiences minimal anxiety.

DOCUMENTATION

- Document the administration of the medication immediately after administration, including date, time, dose, and route of administration on the CMAR/MAR or record using the required format. If using a bar-code system, medication administration is automatically recorded when the bar code is scanned. PRN medications require documentation of the reason for administration. Prompt recording avoids the possibility of accidentally repeating the administration of the drug. Document your assessments, and the patient's response to the treatment, if appropriate. If the drug was refused or omitted, record this in the appropriate area on the medication record and notify the physician. This verifies the reason medication was omitted and ensures that the physician is aware of the patient's condition.

GENERAL CONSIDERATIONS

- If the suppository is for laxative purposes, it must remain in position for 35 to 45 minutes, or until the patient feels the urge to defecate.
- Ongoing assessment is an important part of nursing care to evaluate patient response to administered medications and early detection of adverse effects. If an adverse effect is suspected, withhold further medication doses and notify the patient's primary healthcare provider. Additional intervention is based on type of reaction and patient assessment.

Skill · 142   Assessing Respiration

Under normal conditions, healthy adults breathe about 12 to 20 times per minute. Infants and children breathe more rapidly. The depth of respirations varies normally from shallow to deep. The rhythm of respirations is normally regular, with each inhalation/exhalation and the pauses between occurring at regular intervals. An irregular respiratory rhythm occurs when the inhalation/exhalation cycle and the pauses between occur at unequal intervals.

Assess respiratory rate, depth, and rhythm by inspection (observing and listening) or by listening with the stethoscope. Determine the rate by counting the number of breaths per minute. If respirations are very shallow and difficult to detect, observe the sternal notch, where respiration is more apparent. With an infant or young child, assess respirations before taking the temperature so that the child is not crying, which would alter the respiratory status.

Move immediately from the pulse assessment to counting the respiratory rate to avoid letting the patient know you are counting respirations. Patients should be unaware of the respiratory assessment because, if they are conscious of the procedure, they might alter their breathing patterns or rate.

EQUIPMENT
- Watch with second hand or digital readout
- Pencil or pen, paper or flow sheet, computerized record
- PPE, as indicated

ASSESSMENT GUIDELINES
- Assess the patient for factors that could affect respirations, such as exercise, medications, smoking, chronic illness or conditions, neurologic injury, pain, and anxiety.
- Note baseline or previous respiratory measurements.
- Assess patient for any signs of respiratory distress, which include retractions, nasal flaring, grunting, orthopnea (breathing more easily in an upright position), or tachypnea (rapid respirations).

NURSING DIAGNOSES
- Ineffective Breathing Pattern
- Ineffective Airway Clearance
- Impaired Gas Exchange
- Risk for Decreased Cardiac Tissue Perfusion
- Risk for Activity Intolerance
- Excess Fluid Volume

OUTCOME IDENTIFICATION AND PLANNING
Expected outcomes may include:
- Patient's respirations are assessed accurately without injury and the patient experiences minimal discomfort.

IMPLEMENTATION

ACTION	RATIONALE
1. While your fingers are still in place for the pulse measurement, after counting the pulse rate, observe the patient's respirations.	The patient may alter the rate of respirations if he or she is aware they are being counted.
2. Note the rise and fall of the patient's chest.	A complete cycle of an inspiration and an expiration composes one respiration.

ACTION	RATIONALE
3. Using a watch with a second hand, count the number of respirations for 30 seconds. Multiply this number by 2 to calculate the respiratory rate per minute.	Sufficient time is necessary to observe the rate, depth, and other characteristics.
4. If respirations are abnormal in any way, count the respirations for at least 1 full minute.	Increased time allows the detection of unequal timing between respirations.
5. Note the depth and rhythm of the respirations.	Provides additional assessment data regarding patient's respiratory status.
6. When measurement is completed, remove gloves, if worn. Cover the patient and help him or her to a position of comfort.	Removing PPE properly reduces the risk for infection transmission and contamination of other items. Ensures patient comfort.
7. Remove additional PPE, if used. Perform hand hygiene.	Removing PPE properly reduces the risk for infection transmission and contamination of other items. Hand hygiene deters the spread of microorganisms.

EVALUATION
• Patient's respirations are assessed without the patient altering the rate, rhythm, or depth of respirations.

DOCUMENTATION
• Document respiratory rate, depth, and rhythm on paper, flow sheet, or computerized record. Report any abnormal findings to the appropriate person.

GENERAL CONSIDERATIONS
• If respiratory rate is irregular, count respirations for 1 minute.

Implementing Alternatives to the Use of Restraints

There is growing concern regarding the use of physical restraint in healthcare institutions and a move toward minimizing and eliminating the use of restraints. The goal of evidence-based practice related to the use of restraints is to avoid using restraints rather than to apply them with any clinical justification (Park & Tang, 2007). The use of physical restraints is associated with patient injury and even death (Joanna Briggs, 2002a). Restraint minimization programs and alternatives to physical restraints require education for healthcare providers and are multiple activity programs (Joanna Briggs, 2002b; Park & Tang, 2007). The following skill outlines possible alternatives to restraint use.

EQUIPMENT
- Personal Protective Equipment (PPE), as indicated
- Additional intervention tools, as appropriate (refer to sample intervention equipment in this skill)

ASSESSMENT GUIDELINES
- Assess the patient's status. Determine whether a pattern of behavior (wandering, fall risk, interfering with medical devices, resistive to care, danger to self or others) exists that increases the risk for use of restraints. Assess to determine the meaning and cause of the behavior.
- Assess for pain. Assess respiratory status, vital signs, blood glucose level, fluid and electrolyte issues, and medications.
- Assess the patient's functional, mental, and psychological status.
- Evaluate the patient's environment, including noise level, lighting, floor surfaces, design/suitability of equipment and furniture, visual cues, barriers to mobility, space for privacy, and clothing.
- Assess and evaluate the effectiveness of restraint alternatives.

NURSING DIAGNOSES
- Acute Confusion
- Anxiety
- Risk for Injury
- Self-Mutilation
- Risk for Self-Mutilation
- Disturbed Sensory Perception
- Risk for Suicide
- Risk for Self-Directed Violence
- Risk for Other-Directed Violence

OUTCOME IDENTIFICATION AND PLANNING

Expected outcomes may include:
• The use of restraints is avoided.
• Patient and others remain free from harm.

IMPLEMENTATION

ACTION	RATIONALE
1. Perform hand hygiene and put on PPE, if indicated.	Hand hygiene and PPE prevent the spread of microorganisms. PPE is required based on transmission precautions.
2. Identify the patient.	Identifying the patient ensures the right patient receives the intervention and helps prevent errors.
3. Explain the rationale for interventions to the patient and family/significant others.	Explanation helps reduce anxiety and promotes compliance and understanding.
4. Include the patient's family and/or significant others in the plan of care.	This promotes continuity of care and cooperation.
5. Identify behavior(s) that place the patient at risk for restraint use. Assess the patient's status and environment, as outlined above.	Behaviors, such as interference with therapy or treatment, risk for falls, agitation, restlessness, resistance to care, wandering, and/or cognitive impairment put the patient at risk for restraint use.
	Assessment and interpretation of patient behavior identifies unmet physiologic or psychosocial needs, acute changes in mental or physical status; provides for appropriate environments and individualized care; and respects patient's needs and rights (Evans & Cotter, 2008; Joanna Briggs, 2002a; Park & Tang, 2007).
6. Identify triggers or contributing factors to patient behaviors. Evaluate medication usage for medications that	Removal of contributing factors and/or triggers can decrease the need for restraint use. Possible changes in prescribed medications

ACTION	RATIONALE
could contribute to cognitive and movement dysfunction and an increased risk for falls	can be addressed to decrease adverse effects and decrease need for restraint use.
7. Assess the patient's functional, mental, and psychological status and the environment, as outlined above.	Assessment provides a better understanding of the reason for the behavior, leading to individualized interventions that can eliminate restraint use and provide for patient safety.
8. Provide adequate lighting. Use a night light during sleeping hours.	Appropriate lighting can reduce disruptive behavior related to fear in an unfamiliar environment.
9. Consult with primary care provider and other appropriate healthcare providers regarding the continued need for treatments/therapies and the use of the least invasive method to deliver care.	Exploring the possibility of administering treatment in a less intrusive manner or discontinuing treatment no longer needed can remove stimulus for behavior that increases the risk for restraint use.
10. Assess the patient for pain and discomfort. Provide appropriate pharmacologic and nonpharmacologic interventions.	Unrelieved pain can contribute to behaviors that increase the risk for restraint use.
11. Ask a family member or significant other to stay with the patient.	Having someone stay with the patient provides companionship and familiarity.
12. Reduce unnecessary environmental stimulation and noise.	Increased stimulation can contribute to behaviors that increase risk for restraint use.
13. Provide simple, clear, and direct explanations for treatments and care. Repeat to reinforce, as needed.	Explanation helps reduce anxiety and promotes compliance and understanding.
14. Distract and redirect using a calm voice.	Distraction and redirection can reduce or remove behaviors that increase the risk for restraint use.
15. Increase the frequency of patient observation and surveillance: 1-hour or 2-hour nursing rounds, including pain assessment, toileting	Patient care rounds/nursing rounds improve identification of unmet needs, which can decrease behaviors that increase risk for restraint use (Joanna Briggs,

ACTION	RATIONALE
assistance, patient comfort, personal items in reach, and patient needs.	2002a; Meade et al., 2006; Weisgram & Raymond, 2008).
16. Implement fall precaution interventions.	Behaviors that increase risk for use of restraints also increase risk for falls.
17. Camouflage tube and other treatment sites with clothing, elastic sleeves, or bandaging.	Camouflaging tubes and other treatment sites removes stimulus that can trigger behaviors that increase risk for restraint use.
18. Ensure the use of glasses and hearing aids, if necessary.	Glasses and hearing aids allow for correct interpretation of the environment and activities to reduce confusion.
19. Consider relocation to a room close to the nursing station.	Relocation close to the nursing station provides for the opportunity for increased frequency of observation.
20. Encourage daily exercise/ provide exercise and activities or relaxation techniques.	Activity provides an outlet for energy and stimulation, decreasing behaviors associated with increased risk for restraint use.
21. Make the environment as homelike as possible; provide familiar objects.	Familiarity provides reassurance and comfort, decreasing apprehension and reducing behaviors associated with increased risk for restraint use.
22. Allow restless patient to walk after ensuring that environment is safe. Use a large plant or piece of furniture as a barrier to limit wandering from designated area.	Activity provides outlet for energy and stimulation, decreasing behaviors associated with increased risk for restraint use.
23. Consider the use of patient attendant or sitter.	An attendant or sitter provides companionship and supervision.
24. Remove PPE, if used. Perform hand hygiene.	Removing PPE properly reduces the risk for infection transmission and contamination of other items. Hand hygiene prevents transmission of microorganisms.

EVALUATION

- Use of restraints is avoided.
- Patient and others remain free from harm.

DOCUMENTATION

- Document patient assessment. Include appropriate interventions to reduce need for restraints in nursing plan of care. Document patient and family teaching relative to use of interventions. Document interventions included in care.

Skill · 144   **Applying an Elbow Restraint**

Elbow restraints are generally used on infants and children, but may be used with adults. They prevent the patient from bending the elbows and reaching incisions or therapeutic devices. The patient can move all joints and extremities except the elbow. **Restraints should be used only after less restrictive methods have failed.** Ensure compliance with ordering, assessment, and maintenance procedures.

EQUIPMENT

- Elbow restraint
- Padding, as necessary
- PPE, as indicated

ASSESSMENT GUIDELINES

- Assess the patient's physical condition and the potential for injury to self or others. A confused patient who might remove devices needed to sustain life is considered at risk for injury to self and may require the use of restraints.
- Assess the patient's behavior, including the presence of confusion, agitation, combativeness, and ability to understand and follow directions.
- Evaluate the appropriateness of the least restrictive restraint device.
- Inspect the arm where the restraint will be applied. Baseline skin condition should be established for comparison at future assessments while the restraint is in place. Consider using another form of restraint if the restraint may cause further injury at the site.
- Assess capillary refill and proximal pulses in the arm to which the restraint is to be applied. This helps to determine the circulation in the extremity before applying the restraint. The restraint should not interfere with circulation.
- Measure the distance from the patient's shoulder to wrist to determine which size of elbow restraint to apply.

NURSING DIAGNOSES

* Risk for Injury
* Risk for Impaired Skin Integrity
* Anxiety

OUTCOME IDENTIFICATION AND PLANNING

Expected outcomes may include:

* Patient is constrained by the restraint, remains free from injury, and the restraint does not interfere with therapeutic devices.
* Patient does not experience impaired skin integrity.
* Patient does not injure himself or herself due to the restraints.
* Patient's family will demonstrate an understanding about the use of the restraint and their role in the patient's care.

IMPLEMENTATION

ACTION	RATIONALE
1. Determine need for restraints. Assess the patient's physical condition, behavior, and mental status. Refer to review material in the chapter introduction.	Restraints should be used only as a last resort when alternative measures have failed and the patient is at increased risk for harming self or others.
2. Confirm agency policy for application of restraints. **Secure an order from the primary care provider or validate that the order has been obtained within the past 24 hours.**	Policy protects the patient and the nurse and specifies guidelines for application as well as type of restraint and duration. **The Joint Commission (TJC) standards require that a new order for restraints must be written every 24 hours.**
3. Perform hand hygiene and put on PPE, if indicated.	Hand hygiene and PPE prevent the spread of microorganisms. PPE is required based on transmission precautions.
4. Identify the patient.	Identifying the patient ensures the right patient receives the intervention and helps prevent errors.

ACTION	RATIONALE
5. Explain reason for use to patient and family. Clarify how care will be given and how needs will be met. Explain that restraint is a temporary measure.	Explanation to patient and family may lessen confusion and anger and provide reassurance. A clearly stated agency policy on application of restraints should be available for patient and family to read. In a long-term care facility, the family must give consent before a restraint is applied.
6. Apply restraint according to manufacturer's directions:	Proper application prevents injury. Proper application ensures that there is no interference with patient's circulation.
a. Choose the correct size of the least restrictive type of device that allows the greatest possible degree of mobility.	This provides minimal restriction.
b. Pad bony prominences that may be affected by the restraint.	Padding helps prevent injury.
c. Spread elbow restraint out flat. Place middle of elbow restraint behind patient's elbow. The restraint should not extend below the wrist or place pressure on the axilla.	Elbow restraint should be placed in middle of arm to ensure that patient cannot bend the elbow. Patient should be able to move wrist. Pressure on the axilla may lead to skin impairment.
d. Wrap restraint snugly around the patient's arm, but make sure that two fingers can easily fit under restraint.	Wrapping snugly ensures that patient will not be able to remove the device. Being able to insert two fingers helps to prevent impaired circulation and potential alterations in neurovascular status.
e. Secure Velcro straps around the restraint.	Velcro straps will hold the restraint in place and prevent its removal.
f. Apply the restraint to the opposite arm if patient can move arm.	Bilateral elbow restraints are needed if a patient can move both arms.
g. Thread Velcro strap from one elbow restraint across the back and into the loop	Strap across the back prevents patient from wiggling out of elbow restraints.

ACTION	RATIONALE
on the opposite elbow restraint.	
7. **Assess circulation to fingers and hand.**	Circulation should not be impaired from elbow restraint.
8. Remove PPE, if used. Perform hand hygiene.	Removing PPE properly reduces the risk for infection transmission and contamination of other items. Hand hygiene prevents transmission of microorganisms.
9. Assess the patient at least every hour or according to facility policy, which is required. An assessment should include the following: the placement of the restraint, neurovascular assessment, and skin integrity. Assess for signs of sensory deprivation, such as increased sleeping, daydreaming, anxiety, inconsolable crying, and panic.	Improperly applied restraints may cause alterations in circulation, skin tears, abrasions, or bruises. Decreased circulation may result in impaired skin integrity. Use of restraints may decrease environmental stimulation and result in sensory deprivation.
10. **Remove restraint at least every 2 hours or according to agency policy and patient need. Remove restraint at least every 2 hours for children ages 9 to 17 years and at least every 1 hour for children under age 9, or according to agency policy and patient need.** Perform range-of-motion exercises.	Removal allows the nurse to assess the patient and reevaluate need for restraint. Allows interventions for toileting, provision of nutrition and liquids, exercise, and change of position. Exercise increases circulation in restrained extremity.
11. Evaluate patient for continued need of restraint. Reapply restraint only if continued need is evident.	Continued need must be documented for reapplication.
12. Reassure patient at regular intervals. **Keep call bell within easy reach.**	Reassurance demonstrates caring and provides an opportunity for sensory situation as well as ongoing assessment and evaluation. Parent or child old enough to use call bell can use it to summon assistance quickly.

EVALUATION

- Patient is constrained by the restraint, remains free from injury, and the restraint does not interfere with therapeutic devices.
- Patient does not experience impaired skin integrity.
- Patient does not injure himself or herself due to the restraints.
- Patient's family will demonstrate an understanding about the use of restraints and their role in the patient's care.

DOCUMENTATION

- Document alternative measures attempted before applying restraint. Document patient assessment before application. Record patient and family education regarding restraint use and their understanding. Document family consent, if necessary, according to facility policy. Document reason for restraining patient, date and time of application, type of restraint, times when removed, and result and frequency of nursing assessment. Obtain a new order after 24 hours if restraints are still necessary.

Skill · 145   Applying an Extremity Restraint

Cloth extremity restraints immobilize one or more extremities. They may be indicated after other measures have failed to prevent a patient from removing therapeutic devices, such as intravenous access devices, endotracheal tubes, oxygen, or other treatment interventions. Restraints can be applied to the hands, wrists, or ankles. **Restraints should be used only after less restrictive methods have failed. Ensure compliance with ordering, assessment, and maintenance procedures.**

EQUIPMENT

- Appropriate cloth restraint for the extremity that is to be immobilized
- Padding, if necessary, for bony prominences
- PPE, as indicated

ASSESSMENT GUIDELINES

- Assess the patient's physical condition and the potential for injury to self or others. A confused patient who might remove devices needed to sustain life is considered at risk for injury to self and may require the use of restraints.
- Assess the patient's behavior, including the presence of confusion, agitation, combativeness, and ability to understand and follow directions.

- Evaluate the appropriateness of the least restrictive restraint device. For example, if the patient has had a stroke and cannot move the left arm, a restraint may be needed only on the right arm.
- Inspect the extremity where the restraint will be applied. Establish baseline skin condition for comparison at future assessments while the restraint is in place. Consider using another form of restraint if the restraint may cause further injury at the site.
- Assess for adequate circulation in the extremity to which the restraint is to be applied, including capillary refill and proximal pulses.

NURSING DIAGNOSES

- Risk for Injury
- Acute Confusion
- Risk for Impaired Skin Integrity
- Anxiety

OUTCOME IDENTIFICATION AND PLANNING

- Patient is constrained by the restraint, remains free from injury, and the restraint does not interfere with therapeutic devices.
- Patient does not experience impaired skin integrity.
- Patient does not injure himself or herself due to the restraints.
- Patient's family will demonstrate an understanding about the use of the restraint and their role in the patient's care.

IMPLEMENTATION

ACTION	RATIONALE
1. Determine need for restraints. Assess patient's physical condition, behavior, and mental status.	Restraints should be used only as a last resort when alternative measures have failed and the patient is at increased risk for harming self or others.
2. Confirm agency policy for application of restraints. **Secure an order from the primary care provider, or validate that the order has been obtained within the past 24 hours.**	Policy protects the patient and the nurse and specifies guidelines for application as well as type of restraint and duration. **The Joint Commission (TJC) standards require that a new order for restraints must be written every 24 hours.**
3. Perform hand hygiene and put on PPE, if indicated.	Hand hygiene and PPE prevent the spread of microorganisms. PPE is required based on transmission precautions.

ACTION	RATIONALE

4. Identify the patient.

Identifying the patient ensures the right patient receives the intervention and helps prevent errors.

5. Explain the reason for restraint use to patient and family. Clarify how care will be given and how needs will be met. Explain that the restraint is a temporary measure.

Explanation to patient and family may lessen confusion and anger and provide reassurance. A clearly stated agency policy on application of restraints should be available for patient and family to read. In a long-term care facility, the family must give consent before a restraint is applied.

6. Include the patient's family and/or significant others in the plan of care.

This promotes continuity of care and cooperation.

7. Apply restraint according to manufacturer's directions:

Proper application prevents injury.

a. Choose the least restrictive type of device that allows the greatest possible degree of mobility.

This provides minimal restriction.

b. Pad bony prominences.

Padding helps prevent skin injury.

c. Wrap the restraint around the extremity with the soft part in contact with the skin. If a hand mitt is being used, pull it over the hand with the cushion to the palmar aspect of hand. Secure in place with the Velcro straps.

This prevents excess pressure on extremity.

8. **Ensure that two fingers can be inserted between the restraint and the patient's wrist or ankle.**

Proper application ensures that there is no interference with the patient's circulation and potential alteration in neurovascular status.

9. Maintain restrained extremity in normal anatomic position. Use a **quick-release knot** to tie the restraint to the bed

Maintaining a normal position lessens possibility of injury. A quick-release knot ensures that restraint will not tighten when

ACTION	RATIONALE

frame, not side rail. The restraint may also be attached to a chair frame. The site should not be readily accessible to the patient.

pulled and can be removed quickly in an emergency. Securing the restraint to a side rail may injure the patient when the side rail is lowered. Tying restraint out of patient's reach promotes security.

10. Remove PPE, if used. Perform hand hygiene.

Removing PPE properly reduces the risk for infection transmission and contamination of other items. Hand hygiene prevents transmission of microorganisms.

11. Assess the patient at least every hour or according to facility policy. Assessment should include the following: the placement of the restraint, neurovascular assessment of the affected extremity, and skin integrity. In addition, assess for signs of sensory deprivation, such as increased sleeping, daydreaming, anxiety, panic, and hallucinations.

Improperly applied restraints may cause skin tears, abrasions, or bruises. Decreased circulation may result in paleness, coolness, decreased sensation, tingling, numbness, or pain in the extremity. Use of restraints may decrease environmental stimulation and result in sensory deprivation.

12. **Remove restraint at least every 2 hours, or according to agency policy and patient need.** Perform range-of-motion exercises.

Removal allows the nurse to assess the patient and reevaluate the need for restraint. It also allows interventions for toileting, provision of nutrition and liquids, exercise, and change of position. Exercise increases circulation in the restrained extremity.

13. Evaluate patient for continued need of restraint. Reapply restraint only if continued need is evident and order is still valid.

Continued need must be documented for reapplication.

14. Reassure patient at regular intervals. Provide continued explanation of rationale for interventions, reorientation if necessary, and plan of care. **Keep call bell within easy reach.**

Reassurance demonstrates caring and provides an opportunity for sensory situation as well as ongoing assessment and evaluation. Patient can use call bell to summon assistance quickly.

EVALUATION

- Patient remains free of injury to self or others; circulation to extremity remains adequate; and skin integrity is not impaired under the restraint.
- Patient and family are aware of rationale for restraints.

DOCUMENTATION

- Document alternative measures attempted before applying restraint. Document patient assessment before application. Record patient and family education and understanding regarding restraint use. Document family consent, if necessary, according to facility policy. Document reason for restraining patient, date and time of application, type of restraint, times when removed, and result and frequency of nursing assessment. Obtain a new order after 24 hours if restraints are still necessary.

GENERAL CONSIDERATIONS

- Do not position patient flat in a supine position with wrist restraints. If patient vomits, aspiration may occur.
- Check restraint for correct size before applying. Extremity restraints are available in different sizes. If restraint is too large, patient may free the extremity. If restraint is too small, circulation may be affected.
- Consider keeping a pair of scissors with emergency supplies in case the restraints cannot be untied quickly.

Skill · 146   **Applying a Mummy Restraint**

A mummy restraint is appropriate for short-term restraint of an infant or small child to control the child's movements during examination or to provide care for the head and neck. **Restraints should be used only after less restrictive methods have failed.** Ensure compliance with ordering, assessment, and maintenance procedures.

EQUIPMENT

- Small blanket or sheet
- PPE, as indicated

ASSESSMENT GUIDELINES

- Assess patient's behavior and need for restraint. Assess for wounds or therapeutic devices that may be affected by the restraint. Another form of restraint may be more appropriate to prevent injury.

NURSING DIAGNOSES

• Risk for Injury
• Anxiety
• Impaired Physical Mobility

OUTCOME IDENTIFICATION AND PLANNING

Expected outcomes may include:
• Patient is contained by the restraint, remains free from injury, and the restraint does not interfere with therapeutic devices.
• Examination and/or treatment is provided without incident.
• Patient's family will demonstrate an understanding about the use of the restraint and their role in the patient's care.

IMPLEMENTATION

ACTION	RATIONALE
1. Determine need for restraints. Assess the patient's physical condition, behavior, and mental status. Refer to review material in the chapter introduction.	Restraints should be used only as a last resort when alternative measures have failed, and the patient is at increased risk for harming self or others.
2. Confirm agency policy for application of restraints. **Secure an order from the primary care provider or validate that the order has been obtained within the past 24 hours.**	Policy protects the patient and the nurse and specifies guidelines for application as well as type of restraint and duration. **The Joint Commission (TJC) standards require that a new order for restraints must be written every 24 hours.**
3. Perform hand hygiene and put on PPE, if indicated.	Hand hygiene and PPE prevent the spread of microorganisms. PPE is required based on transmission precautions.
4. Identify the patient.	Identifying the patient ensures the right patient receives the intervention and helps prevent errors.
5. Explain reason for restraint use to patient and family. Clarify how care will be	Explanation to patient and family may lessen confusion and anger and provide reassurance. A

ACTION	RATIONALE
given and needs will be met. Explain that restraint is a temporary measure.	clearly stated agency policy on application of restraints should be available for patient and family to read. In a long-term care facility, the family must give consent before a restraint is applied.
6. Open the blanket or sheet. Place the child on the blanket, with edge of blanket at or above neck level.	This positions child correctly on the blanket.
7. Position the child's right arm alongside his or her body. Left arm should not be constrained at this time. Pull the right side of the blanket tightly over the child's right shoulder and chest. Secure under the left side of the child's body (FIGURE 1).	Wrapping snugly ensures that child will not be able to wiggle out.
8. Position the left arm alongside the child's body. Pull the left side of the blanket tightly over the child's left shoulder and chest. Secure under the right side of his or her body (FIGURE 2).	Wrapping snugly ensures that child will not be able to wiggle out.

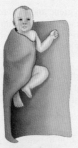

FIGURE 1 Pulling blanket over right shoulder and chest and securing under patient's left side.

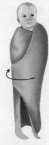

FIGURE 2 Securing blanket under right side of body.

ACTION	RATIONALE
9. Fold the lower part of blanket up and pull over the child's body. Secure under the child's body on each side or with safety pins (Figure 3).	This ensures that child will not be able to wiggle out.

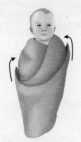

FIGURE 3 Securing lower corner of blanket under each side of the patient's body.

ACTION	RATIONALE
10. Stay with child while the mummy wrap is in place. Reassure the child and parents at regular intervals. Once examination or treatment is completed, unwrap the child.	Remaining with the child prevents injury. Reassurance demonstrates caring and provides an opportunity for ongoing assessment and evaluation.
11. Remove PPE, if used. Perform hand hygiene.	Removing PPE properly reduces the risk for infection transmission and contamination of other items. Hand hygiene prevents transmission of microorganisms.

EVALUATION

• Patient is constrained by the restraint, remains free from injury, and the restraint does not interfere with therapeutic devices.
• Examination or treatment is provided without incident.
• Patient's family demonstrates an understanding of the rationale for the mummy restraint.

DOCUMENTATION

• Document alternative measures attempted before applying restraint. Document patient assessment before application. Record patient and family education and understanding regarding restraint use. Document family consent, if necessary, according to facility policy. Document reason for restraining patient, date and time of application, type of restraint, times when removed, and result and frequency of nursing assessment.

Skill · 147   Applying a Waist Restraint

Waist restraints are a form of restraint that is applied to the patient's torso. It is applied over the patient's clothes, gown, or pajamas. When using a waist restraint, patients can move their extremities but cannot get out of the chair or bed. **Restraints should be used only after less restrictive methods have failed.** Ensure compliance with ordering, assessment, and maintenance procedures. **Historically, vest or jacket restraints were used to prevent similar patient movement, but their use has significantly decreased due to concerns for the potential risk for asphyxiation with the device. Research suggests that waist restraints pose the same potential risk for asphyxial death as vest restraints (Capezuti et al., 2008). Healthcare providers need to be aware of this potential outcome and weigh it against possible benefit from use of the device.**

EQUIPMENT
- Waist restraint
- Additional padding as needed
- PPE, as indicated

ASSESSMENT GUIDELINES
- Assess the patient's physical condition and the potential for injury to self or others. A confused patient who is being treated with devices needed to sustain life, such as pulmonary intubation, might attempt to ambulate and is considered at risk for injury to self, and may require the use of restraints.
- Assess the patient's behavior, including the presence of confusion, agitation, combativeness, and ability to understand and follow directions.
- Evaluate the appropriateness of the least restrictive restraint device.
- Inspect the patient's torso for any wounds or therapeutic devices that may be affected by the waist restraint. Consider using another form of restraint if the restraint may cause further injury at the site.
- Assess the patient's respiratory effort. If applied incorrectly, the waist restraint can restrict the patient's ability to breathe.

NURSING DIAGNOSES

• Risk for Injury
• Risk for Impaired Skin Integrity
• Anxiety
• Acute Confusion
• Wandering
• Impaired Physical Mobility

OUTCOME IDENTIFICATION AND PLANNING

Expected outcomes may include:
• Patient is constrained by the restraint, remains free from injury, and the restraint does not interfere with therapeutic devices.
• Patient does not experience impaired skin integrity.
• Patient does not injure himself or herself due to the restraints.
• Patient's family will demonstrate an understanding about the use of the restraint and their role in the patient's care.

IMPLEMENTATION

ACTION	RATIONALE
1. Determine need for restraints. Assess patient's physical condition, behavior, and mental status.	Restraints should be used only as a last resort when alternative measures have failed and the patient is at increased risk for harming self or others.
2. Confirm agency policy for application of restraints. **Secure an order from the primary care provider or validate that the order has been obtained within the past 24 hours.**	Policy protects the patient and the nurse and specifies guidelines for application as well as type of restraint and duration. **The Joint Commission (TJC) standards require that a new order for restraints must be written every 24 hours.**
3. Perform hand hygiene and put on PPE, if indicated.	Hand hygiene and PPE prevent the spread of microorganisms. PPE is required based on transmission precautions.
4. Identify the patient.	Identifying the patient ensures the right patient receives the intervention and helps prevent errors.
5. Explain the reason for restraint use to the patient	Explanation to patient and family may lessen confusion and anger and provide reassurance. A

ACTION	RATIONALE
and family. Clarify how care will be given and how needs will be met. Explain that restraint is a temporary measure.	clearly stated agency policy on application of restraints should be available for patient and family to read. In a long-term care facility, the family must give consent before a restraint is applied.
6. Include the patient's family and/or significant others in the plan of care.	This promotes continuity of care and cooperation.
7. Apply restraint according to manufacturer's directions:	Proper application prevents injury. Proper application ensures that there is no interference with patient's respiration.
a. Choose the correct size of the least restrictive type of device that allows the greatest possible degree of mobility.	This provides minimal restriction.
b. Pad bony prominences that may be affected by the waist restraint.	Padding helps prevent injury.
c. Assist patient to a sitting position, if not contraindicated.	This will assist the nurse in helping the patient into the waist restraint.
d. Place waist restraint on the patient over gown. Bring ties through slots in restraint. Position slots at patient's back.	Placing the waist restrain over the gown protects the patient's skin. Positioning the slots with the ties at the back keeps them out of the patient's vision.
e. Pull the ties secure. Ensure that it is not too tight and there are no wrinkles in the waist restraint.	Securing too tightly could impede breathing. Wrinkles in the restraint may lead to skin impairment.
f. Insert fist between restraint and patient to ensure that breathing is not constricted. Assess respirations after restraint is applied.	This prevents impaired respirations.
8. Use a quick-release knot to tie the restraint to the bed frame, not side rail. If patient is in a wheelchair,	A quick-release knot ensures that restraint will not tighten when pulled and can be removed quickly in an emergency. Securing the

ACTION	RATIONALE

lock the wheels and place the ties under the armrests and tie behind the chair. Site should not be readily accessible to the patient.

restraint to a side rail may injure the patient when the side rail is lowered. Tying the restraint out of the patient's reach promotes security.

9. Remove PPE, if used. Perform hand hygiene.

Removing PPE properly reduces the risk for infection transmission and contamination of other items. Hand hygiene prevents transmission of microorganisms.

10. Assess the patient at least every hour or according to facility policy, which is required. An assessment should include the following: the placement of the restraint, respiratory assessment, and skin integrity. Assess for signs of sensory deprivation, such as increased sleeping, daydreaming, anxiety, panic, and hallucinations.

Improperly applied restraints may cause difficulty breathing, skin tears, abrasions, or bruises. Decreased circulation may result in impaired skin integrity. Use of restraints may decrease environmental stimulation and result in sensory deprivation.

11. **Remove restraint at least every 2 hours or according to agency policy and patient need.** Perform range-of-motion exercises.

Removal allows the nurse to assess the patient and reevaluate need for restraint. Allows interventions for toileting, provision of nutrition and liquids, exercise, and change of position. Exercise increases circulation in restrained extremity.

12. Evaluate patient for continued need of restraint. Reapply restraint only if continued need is evident and order is still valid.

Continued need must be documented for reapplication.

13. Reassure patient at regular intervals. Provide continued explanation of rationale for interventions, reorientation, if necessary, and plan of care. **Keep call bell within easy reach.**

Reassurance demonstrates caring and provides an opportunity for sensory situation as well as ongoing assessment and evaluation. Patient can use call bell to summon assistance quickly.

14. Perform hand hygiene.

Hand hygiene deters the spread of microorganisms.

EVALUATION
- Patient remains free of injury.
- Patient's respirations are easy and effortless.
- Integrity of patient's skin under the restraint is maintained.
- Patient and family demonstrate understanding of the rationale for using the restraints.

DOCUMENTATION
- Document alternative measures attempted before applying the restraint. Document patient assessment before application. Record patient and family education and understanding regarding restraint use. Document family consent, if necessary, according to facility policy. Document reason for restraining patient, date and time of application, type of restraint, times when removed, and result and frequency of nursing assessment. Obtain a new order after 24 hours if restraints are still necessary.

GENERAL CONSIDERATIONS
- Consider keeping a pair of scissors with emergency supplies in case the restraints cannot be untied quickly.

Skill · 148 · **Using a Handheld Resuscitation Bag and Mask**

If the patient is not breathing with an adequate rate and depth, or if the patient has lost the respiratory drive, a bag and mask may be used to deliver oxygen until the patient is resuscitated or can be intubated with an endotracheal tube. Bag and mask devices are frequently referred to as Ambu bags ("air mask bag unit") or BVMs ("bag-valve-mask" device). The bags come in infant, pediatric, and adult size. The bag consists of an oxygen reservoir (commonly referred to as the tail), oxygen tubing, the bag itself, a one-way valve to prevent secretions from entering the bag, an exhalation port, an elbow so that the bag can lie across the patient's chest, and a mask.

EQUIPMENT
- Handheld resuscitation device with a mask
- Oxygen source
- Disposable gloves
- Face shield or goggles and mask
- Additional PPE, as indicated

ASSESSMENT GUIDELINES

- Assess the patient's respiratory effort and drive. If the patient is breathing less than 10 breaths per minute, is breathing too shallowly, or is not breathing at all, assistance with a BVM may be needed.
- Assess the oxygen saturation level. Patients who have decreased respiratory effort and drive may also have a decreased oxygen saturation level.
- Assess the heart rate and rhythm. Bradycardia may occur with a decreased oxygen saturation level, leading to a cardiac dysrhythmia.
- Many times, a BVM is used in a crisis situation. Manual ventilation is also used during airway suctioning.

NURSING DIAGNOSES

- Ineffective Breathing Pattern
- Impaired Gas Exchange
- Risk for Aspiration
- Decreased Cardiac Output

OUTCOME IDENTIFICATION AND PLANNING

Expected outcomes may include:
- Patient will exhibit signs and symptoms of adequate oxygen saturation.
- Patient will receive adequate volume of respirations with BVM.
- Patient will maintain normal sinus rhythm.

IMPLEMENTATION

ACTION	RATIONALE
1. If not a crisis situation, perform hand hygiene.	Hand hygiene prevents the spread of microorganisms.
2. Put on PPE, as indicated.	PPE prevents the spread of microorganisms. PPE is required based on transmission precautions.
3. If not an emergency, identify the patient.	Identifying the patient ensures the right patient receives the intervention and helps prevent errors.

ACTION	RATIONALE
4. Explain what you are going to do and the reason for doing it to the patient, even if the patient does not appear to be alert.	Explanation alleviates fears. Even if the patient appears unconscious, the nurse should explain what is happening.
5. Put on disposable gloves. Put on face shield or goggles and mask.	Using gloves deters the spread of microorganisms. Personal protective equipment protects the nurse from pathogens.
6. **Ensure that the mask is connected to the bag device, the oxygen tubing is connected to the oxygen source, and the oxygen is turned on, at a flow rate of 10 to 15 L per minute. This may be done through visualization or by listening to the open end of the reservoir or tail: if air is heard flowing, the oxygen is attached and on.**	Expected results might not be accomplished if the oxygen is not attached and on.
7. If possible, get behind head of bed and remove headboard. **Slightly hyperextend patient's neck (unless contraindicated). If unable to hyperextend, use jaw thrust maneuver to open airway.**	Standing at head of bed makes positioning easier when obtaining seal of mask to face. Hyperextending the neck opens the airway.
8. Place mask over patient's face with opening over oral cavity. If mask is teardrop-shaped, the narrow portion should be placed over the bridge of the nose.	This helps ensure an adequate seal so that oxygen may be forced into the lungs.
9. **With dominant hand, place three fingers on the mandible, keeping head slightly hyperextended. Place thumb and one finger in C position around the mask, pressing hard enough to form a seal around the patient's face (FIGURE 1).**	This helps ensure that an adequate seal is formed so that oxygen may be forced into the lungs.

ACTION	RATIONALE

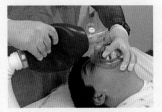

FIGURE 1 Creating a seal between mask and patient's face.

10. **Using nondominant hand, gently and slowly (over 2 to 3 seconds) squeeze the bag, watching the chest for symmetric rise.** If two people are available, one person should maintain a seal on the mask with two hands while the other squeezes the bag to deliver the ventilation and oxygenation.

Volume of air needed is based on patient's size. Enough has been delivered if chest is rising. If air is introduced rapidly, it may enter the stomach.

11. Deliver the breaths with the patient's own inspiratory effort, if present. Avoid delivering breaths when the patient exhales. Deliver one breath every 5 seconds, if patient's own respiratory drive is absent. Continue delivering breaths until patient's drive returns or until patient is intubated and attached to mechanical ventilation.

Once patient's airway has been stabilized or patient is breathing on own, bag-mask delivery can be stopped.

12. Dispose of equipment appropriately.

Reduces the risk for transmission of microorganisms and contamination of other items.

13. Remove face shield or goggles and mask. Remove gloves and additional PPE, if used. Perform hand hygiene.

Removing PPE properly reduces the risk for infection transmission and contamination of other items. Hand hygiene prevents the spread of microorganisms.

EVALUATION

- Patient demonstrates improved skin color and nail beds without evidence of cyanosis.
- Patient's oxygen saturation level is above 95%, and heart rate is in normal sinus rhythm.
- Patient maintains a patent airway and exhibits spontaneous respirations.

DOCUMENTATION

- Document the incident, including patient's respiratory effort before initiation of bag-mask breaths, lung sounds, oxygen saturation, chest symmetry, and resolution of incident (i.e., intubation or patient's respiratory drive returns).

GENERAL CONSIDERATIONS

- Air can be forced into the stomach during manual ventilation with a mask, causing abdominal distention. This distension can cause vomiting and possible aspiration. Be alert for vomiting; watch through the mask. If the patient starts to vomit, stop ventilating immediately, remove the mask, wipe and suction vomitus as needed, then resume ventilation.

Skill · 149 | **Employing Seizure Precautions and Seizure Management**

Seizures occur when the electrical system of the brain malfunctions. Sudden excessive discharge from cerebral neurons results in episodes of abnormal motor, sensory, autonomic, or psychic activity, or a combination of these (Hickey, 2009; Smeltzer et al., 2010). During a seizure, patients are at risk for hypoxia, vomiting, and pulmonary aspiration. All patients with seizures presenting to the hospital must be placed under seizure precautions to minimize the risk of physical injury (Bhanushali & Helmers, 2008). Seizure management includes interventions by the nurse to prevent aspiration, protect the patient from injury, provide care after the seizure, and document the details of the event (Bhanushali & Helmers, 2008; Hickey, 2009).

EQUIPMENT

- PPE, as indicated
- Portable or wall suction unit with tubing
- A commercially prepared suction kit with an appropriate size catheter or
- Sterile suction catheter with Y-port in the appropriate size (Adult: 10 Fr–16 Fr)
- Sterile disposable container
- Sterile gloves
- Oral airway

- Bed rail padding
- Oxygen apparatus
- Nasal cannula or mask to deliver oxygen
- Handheld bag valve/resuscitation bag

ASSESSMENT GUIDELINES

- Assess for preexisting conditions that increase the patient's risk for seizure activity; for example, history of seizure disorder or epilepsy, cerebrovascular disease, hypoxemia, head injury, hypertension, central nervous system infections, metabolic conditions (e.g., renal failure, hypocalcemia, hypoglycemia), brain tumor, drug/alcohol withdrawal, or allergies.
- Assess circumstances before the seizure, such as visual, auditory, or olfactory stimuli, tactile stimuli, emotional or psychological disturbances, sleep, or hyperventilation.
- Assess for the occurrence of an aura; note where the movements or stiffness begin; and gaze position and position of the head when the seizure begins.
- Assess the body part(s) and the type of movement(s) involved in the seizure. Assess pupil sizes; if eyes remained open during seizure; whether eyes or head turned to one side.
- Assess for the presence or absence of repeated involuntary motor activity (e.g., repeated swallowing); incontinence of urine or stool; duration of seizure; presence of unconsciousness and duration; obvious paralysis or weakness of arms or legs after seizure; and inability to speak, movements, sleeping, and/or confusion after seizure.
- Assess the patient for injury after the seizure is over.

NURSING DIAGNOSES

- Fear
- Ineffective Coping
- Deficient Knowledge

OUTCOME IDENTIFICATION AND PLANNING

Expected outcomes may include:
- Patient remains free from injury.
- Other specific outcomes will be formulated depending on the identified nursing diagnosis.

IMPLEMENTATION

ACTION	RATIONALE
1. Review the medical record and nursing plan of care for conditions that would place the patient at risk for seizures. Review the medical orders and the nursing plan of care for orders for seizure precautions.	Reviewing the order and plan of care validates the correct patient and correct procedure.

Seizure Precautions

ACTION	RATIONALE
2. Gather the necessary supplies and bring to the bedside stand or overbed table.	Preparation promotes efficient time management and organized approach to the task. Bringing everything to the bedside conserves time and energy. Arranging items nearby is convenient, saves time, and avoids unnecessary stretching and twisting of muscles on the part of the nurse.
3. Perform hand hygiene and put on PPE, if indicated.	Hand hygiene and PPE prevent the spread of microorganisms. PPE is required based on transmission precautions.
4. Identify the patient.	Identifying the patient ensures the right patient receives the intervention and helps prevent errors.
5. Close curtains around bed and close the door to the room, if possible. Explain what you are going to do and why you are going to do it to the patient.	This ensures the patient's privacy. Explanation relieves anxiety and facilitates cooperation.
6. Place the bed in the lowest position with two to three side rails elevated. Apply padding to side rails.	Bed in lowest position promotes safety and decreases risk of injury. Rail padding also decreases risk of injury.
7. Attach oxygen apparatus to oxygen access in the wall at the head of the bed. Place nasal cannula or mask equipment in a location where it is easily reached if needed.	During a seizure, patients are at risk for hypoxia, vomiting, and pulmonary aspiration. Ready access ensures availability of oxygen in the event of a seizure.

ACTION	RATIONALE
8. Attach suction apparatus to vacuum access in the wall at the head of the bed. Place suction catheter, oral airway, and resuscitation bag in a location where they are easily reached if needed.	During a seizure, patients are at risk for hypoxia, vomiting, and pulmonary aspiration. Ready access ensures availability of suction in the event of a seizure. Oral airway and resuscitation bag ensure availability of emergency ventilation in the event of respiratory arrest.
9. Remove PPE, if used. Perform hand hygiene.	Removing PPE properly reduces the risk for infection transmission and contamination of other items. Hand hygiene prevents the spread of microorganisms.

Seizure Management

10. For patients with known seizures, be alert for the occurrence of an aura, if known. If the patient reports experiencing an aura, have the patient lie down.	Some patients report a warning or premonition before seizures occur; an aura can be a visual, auditory, or olfactory sensation that indicates a seizure is going to occur. Lying down prevents injury that might occur if the patient falls to the floor.
11. Once a seizure begins, close curtains around bed and close the door to the room, if possible.	Closing the door or curtain provides for patient privacy.
12. If the patient is seated, ease the patient to the floor.	Getting the patient to the floor prevents injury that might occur if the patient falls to the floor.
13. Remove patient's eyeglasses. Loosen any constricting clothing. Place something flat and soft, such as a folded blanket, under the head. Push aside furniture or other objects in area.	Removing objects and loosening clothing prevents possible injury. Blanket prevents injury from striking a hard surface (floor).
14. If the patient is in bed, remove the pillow and raise side rails.	Raised side rails prevents injury.
15. Do not restrain patient. Guide movements, if necessary. Do not try to insert	Guiding movements prevents injury. Restraint can injure the patient. Attempting to open the

ACTION	RATIONALE
anything in the patient's mouth or open jaws.	mouth and/or insert anything into the mouth can result in broken teeth, and injury to mouth, lips, or tongue.
16. If possible, place patient on the side with the head flexed forward, head of bed elevated 30 degrees. Begin administration of oxygen, based on facility policy. Clear airway using suction, as appropriate.	During a seizure, patients are at risk for hypoxia, vomiting, and pulmonary aspiration. This position allows the tongue to fall forward, and facilitates drainage of saliva and mucus and minimizes risk for aspiration. Oxygen supports the increased metabolism associated with neurologic and muscular hyperactivity. Patent airway is necessary to support ventilation.
17. Provide supervision throughout the seizure.	Supervision of the patient ensures safety.
18. Establish/maintain intravenous access as necessary. Administer medications, as appropriate, based on medical order and facility policy.	Pharmacologic therapy may be appropriate, based on patient history and medical diagnoses. Intravenous access is necessary to administer emergency medications.
19. After the seizure, place the patient in a side-lying position. Clear airway using suction, as appropriate.	Side-lying position facilitates drainage of secretions. Patent airway is necessary to support ventilation.
20. Monitor vital signs, oxygen saturation, and capillary glucose as appropriate.	Monitoring of parameters provides information for accurate assessment of patient status.
21. Allow the patient to sleep after the seizure. On awakening, orient and reassure the patient.	The patient will probably experience an inability to recall the seizure; patients may also experience confusion, anxiety, embarrassment, and/or fatigue after a seizure.
22. Remove PPE, if used. Perform hand hygiene.	Removing PPE properly reduces the risk for infection transmission and contamination of other items. Hand hygiene prevents the spread of microorganisms.

EVALUATION

- Patient remains free from injury.

DOCUMENTATION

- Document initiation of seizure precautions, including specific interventions put in place. Document if the beginning of the seizure was witnessed. If so, document noted circumstances before the seizure, such as visual, auditory, or olfactory stimuli, tactile stimuli, emotional or psychological disturbances, sleep, or hyperventilation. Note the occurrence of an aura; where the movements or stiffness began; gaze position and position of the head when the seizure began. Record the body part(s) and the type of movement(s) involved in the seizure. Document the pupil size; if eyes remained open during seizure; whether eyes or head turned to one side; presence or absence of repeated involuntary motor activity (e.g., repeated swallowing); incontinence of urine or stool; duration of seizure; presence of unconsciousness and duration; obvious paralysis or weakness of arms or legs after seizure; and inability to speak, movements, sleeping, and/or confusion after seizure. Document administration of oxygen, airway suction, safety measures, and administration of medications, if used. If the patient was injured during the seizure, document assessment of injury.

GENERAL CONSIDERATIONS

- Include patient and family/significant other teaching for patients with documented seizures, as well as those at risk for seizures. Teaching should include basic first aid management. Help person to lie down. Remove eyeglasses and loosen constrictive clothing. Clear the area around the person of anything hard or sharp. Place something flat and soft (e.g., a folded jacket) under the head. Turn the person gently on the side, if possible. Do not try to force anything into the patient's mouth. Stay with the person during the seizure. Remain calm. After the seizure, stay with the patient until consciousness is regained; reorient as necessary.
- Include guidelines for when to get emergency medical assistance. Patients' families and significant others should be instructed to call for emergency assistance if the seizure occurs in water; the person does not begin breathing after the seizure; if generalized tonic-clonic seizure lasts for more than 2 minutes; the person has one seizure right after another without regaining consciousness; or if the patient is injured during the seizure.

Skill · 150   **Assisting the Patient to Shave**

Some patients may need help with shaving when using a regular blade or may require that the nurse perform the shaving procedure for them completely. Patients with beards or mustaches may require nursing assistance to keep the beard and mustache clean. However, never trim or shave a patient's beard or mustache without the patient's consent. Female patients may require assistance with shaving underarm and leg hair, depending on the patient's personal preference and abilities. If available and permitted by the facility, electric shavers are usually recommended when the patient is receiving anticoagulant therapy or has a bleeding disorder, and are especially convenient for ill and bedridden patients.

EQUIPMENT

- Shaving cream
- Safety razor
- Towel
- Washcloth
- Bath basin
- Disposable gloves
- Additional PPE, as indicated
- Waterproof pad
- Aftershave or lotion (optional)

ASSESSMENT GUIDELINES

- Assess the patient's shaving preferences: frequency, time of day, and type of shaving products.
- Assess for any physical activity limitations. Assess patient for any bleeding problems. If patient is receiving any anticoagulant, such as heparin or warfarin (Coumadin), has received an antithrombolytic agent, or has a low platelet count, consider using an electric razor.
- Inspect the area to be shaved for any lesions or weeping areas.
- Assess the patient's ability to shave himself or herself or assist with the procedure.

NURSING DIAGNOSES

- Risk for Injury
- Bathing/Hygiene Self-Care Deficit
- Activity Intolerance
- Impaired Physical Mobility

OUTCOME IDENTIFICATION AND PLANNING

Expected outcomes may include:

- The patient will be clean, without evidence of hair growth or trauma to the skin.
- The patient tolerates shaving with minimal to no difficulty.
- The patient verbalizes feelings of improved self-esteem.

IMPLEMENTATION

ACTION	RATIONALE
1. Perform hand hygiene. Put on PPE, as indicated.	Hand hygiene and PPE prevent the spread of microorganisms. PPE is required based on transmission precautions.
2. Identify patient. Explain the procedure to the patient.	Identifying the patient ensures the right patient receives the intervention and helps prevent errors. Explanation facilitates cooperation.
3. Assemble equipment on overbed table within reach.	Organization facilitates performance of task.
4. Close curtains around bed and close the door to the room, if possible.	Provides for patient privacy.
5. Cover patient's chest with a towel or waterproof pad. Fill bath basin with warm (43°C to 46°C [110°F to 115°F]) water. Put on gloves. Moisten the area to be shaved with a washcloth.	Warm water is comfortable and relaxing for the patient. Gloves prevent the spread of microorganisms. Warm water softens the hair, making the process easier (MFMER, 2007c).
6. Dispense shaving cream into palm of hand. Apply cream to area to be shaved in a layer about 0.5 inch thick.	Using shaving cream helps to prevent skin irritation and prevents hair from pulling.
7. With one hand, pull the skin taut at the area to be shaved. Using a smooth stroke, begin shaving. *If shaving the face,* shave with the direction of hair growth in downward, short strokes (FIGURE 1). *If shaving a leg,* shave against the hair in upward, short strokes. *If shaving an underarm,* pull skin taut and use short, upward strokes.	The skin on the face is more sensitive and needs to be shaved with the direction of hair growth to prevent discomfort.

ACTION   RATIONALE

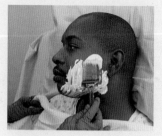

FIGURE 1 Shaving the face.

8. Wash off residual shaving cream.

Shaving cream can lead to irritation if left on the skin.

9. If patient requests, apply aftershave or lotion to area shaved.

Aftershave and lotion can reduce skin irritation.

10. Remove equipment and return patient to a position of comfort. Remove your gloves. Raise side rail and lower bed.

Promotes patient comfort and safety. Removing gloves properly reduces the risk for infection transmission and contamination of other items.

11. Remove additional PPE, if used. Perform hand hygiene.

Removing PPE properly reduces the risk for infection transmission and contamination of other items. Hand hygiene deters spread of microorganisms.

EVALUATION

• The patient exhibits a clean-shaven face without evidence of trauma, irritation, or redness.
• The patient verbalizes a positive body image.
• The patient reports an increase in comfort level.

DOCUMENTATION

• It is not usually necessary to document shaving a patient. However, if your skin assessment reveals any unusual findings, document your assessment and the procedure. If the patient or nurse breaks the skin while shaving, document the occurrence and your assessment of the patient.

GENERAL CONSIDERATIONS

• If the patient is brought to the facility with a full beard, do not shave the patient's beard without consent unless it is an emergency situation, such as insertion of an endotracheal tube. For this procedure, shave only the area needed and leave the rest of the beard.

Skill · 151   **Shampooing a Patient's Hair in Bed**

The easiest way to wash a patient's hair is to assist him or her in the shower, but not all patients can take showers. If the patient's hair needs to be washed but the patient is unable or not allowed to get out of bed, a bed shampoo can be performed. Shampoo caps are available, and are being used with increasing frequency. These commercially prepared, disposable caps contain a rinseless shampoo product. See the accompanying Skill Variation.

EQUIPMENT

• Water pitcher
• Warm water
• Shampoo
• Conditioner (optional)
• Disposable gloves
• Additional PPE, as indicated
• Protective pad for bed

• Shampoo board
• Bucket
• Towels
• Gown
• Comb or brush
• Blow dryer (optional)

ASSESSMENT GUIDELINES

• Assess the patient's hygiene preferences: frequency, time of day, and type of hygiene products.
• Assess eyes for any redness or drainage, which may indicate an eye infection or an allergic response. Assess for any physical activity limitations. Assess the patient's ability to get out of bed to have his or her hair washed. If the physician's orders allow it and patient is physically able to wash his or her hair in the shower, the patient may prefer to do so. If the patient cannot tolerate being out of bed or is not allowed to do so, perform a bed shampoo. Assess for any activity or positioning limitations.
• Inspect the patient's scalp for any cuts, lesions, or bumps. Note any flaking, drying, or excessive oiliness.

NURSING DIAGNOSES

• Activity Intolerance
• Impaired Physical Mobility

• Impaired Transfer Ability
• Disturbed Body Image

OUTCOME IDENTIFICATION AND PLANNING

Expected outcomes may include:
• The patient's hair will be clean.
• The patient will tolerate the shampoo with little to no difficulty.
• The patient will demonstrate an improved body image.
• The patient will verbalize an increase in comfort.

IMPLEMENTATION

ACTION	RATIONALE
1. Review the patient's chart for any limitations in physical activity or contraindications to the procedure.	Identifying limitations prevents patient discomfort and injury.
2. Perform hand hygiene. Put on PPE, as indicated.	Hand hygiene and PPE prevent the spread of microorganisms. PPE is required based on transmission precautions.
3. Identify the patient. Explain the procedure to the patient.	Patient identification validates the correct patient and correct procedure. Discussion and explanation help allay anxiety and prepare the patient for what to expect.
4. Assemble equipment on overbed table within reach.	Organization facilitates performance of task.
5. Close curtains around bed and close the door to the room, if possible.	Provides for patient privacy
6. Lower the head of the bed. Remove pillow and place protective pad under patient's head and shoulders.	A protective pad keeps the sheets from getting wet.
7. Fill the pitcher with warm water (43°C to 46°C [110°F to 115°F]). Position the patient at the top of the bed, in a supine position. Have the patient lift his or her head and place shampoo board underneath patient's head.	Warm water is comfortable and relaxing for the patient. It also stimulates circulation and provides for more effective cleaning. Padding the edge of the shampoo board may help increase patient comfort.

ACTION	RATIONALE
If necessary, pad the edge of the board with a small towel.	
8. Place bucket on floor underneath the drain of the shampoo board.	The bucket will catch the runoff water, preventing a mess on the floor.
9. Put on gloves. If the patient is able, have him or her hold a folded washcloth at the forehead. Pour a pitcher of warm water slowly over the patient's head, making sure that all hair is saturated. Refill pitcher if needed.	Gloves prevent the spread of microorganisms. A washcloth prevents water from running into the patient's eyes. By pouring slowly, more hair will become wet, and it is more soothing for the patient.
10. Apply a small amount of shampoo to the patient's hair. **Massage deep into the scalp, avoiding any cuts, lesions, or sore spots.**	Shampoo will help to remove dirt or oil.
11. Rinse with warm water (43°C to 46°C [110°F to 115°F]) until all shampoo is out of hair (FIGURE 1). Repeat shampoo, if necessary.	Shampoo left in hair may cause pruritus. If hair is still dirty, another shampoo treatment may be needed.

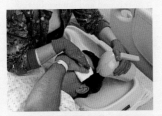

FIGURE 1 Rinsing shampoo from patient's head.

12. If patient has thick hair or requests it, apply a small amount of conditioner to hair and massage throughout. Avoid any cuts, lesions, or sore spots.	Conditioner eases tangles and moisturizes hair and scalp.
13. If bucket is small, empty before rinsing hair. Rinse with warm water (43°C to 6°C [110°F to 115°F]) until all conditioner is out of hair.	Bucket may overflow if not emptied. Conditioner left in hair may cause pruritus.

ACTION	RATIONALE
14. Remove shampoo board. Place towel around patient's hair.	This prevents the patient from getting cold.
15. Pat hair dry, avoiding any cuts, lesions, or sore spots. Remove protective padding but keep one dry protective pad under patient's hair.	Patting dry removes any excess water without damaging hair or scalp.
16. Gently brush hair, removing tangles, as needed.	Removing tangles helps hair to dry faster. Brushing hair improves patient's self-image.
17. Blow-dry hair on a cool setting if allowed and if patient wishes. If not, consider covering the patient's head with a dry towel, until hair is dry.	Blow-drying hair helps hair to dry faster and prevents patient from becoming chilled. Keeping the head covered prevents chilling while hair is drying.
18. Change patient's gown and remove protective pad. Replace pillow.	If patient's gown is damp, patient will become chilled. Protective pad is no longer needed once hair is dry.
19. Remove equipment and return patient to a position of comfort. Remove your gloves. Raise side rail and lower bed.	Promotes patient comfort and safety. Removing gloves properly reduces the risk for infection transmission and contamination of other items.
20. Remove additional PPE, if used. Perform hand hygiene.	Removing PPE properly reduces the risk for infection transmission and contamination of other items. Hand hygiene deters spread of microorganisms.

EVALUATION

- The patient's hair is clean.
- The patient verbalizes a positive body image.
- The patient reports an increase in comfort level.

DOCUMENTATION

- Record your assessment, significant observations, and unusual findings, such as bleeding or inflammation. Document any teaching done. Document procedure and patient response.

GENERAL CONSIDERATIONS

• If the patient has a spinal cord or neck injury, use of the shampoo board may be contraindicated. In this case, a makeshift protection area can be created to wash the patient's hair without using the board. Place a protective pad underneath the patient's head and shoulders. Roll a towel into the bottom of the protective pad and direct the roll into one area so that water will drain into the container.

Skill Variation | **Shampooing a Patient's Hair with a Shampoo Cap**

Shampoo caps are available and are being used with increasing frequency. These commercially prepared, disposable caps contain a rinseless shampoo product. The cap is warmed in the microwave or stored in a warmer until use. The cap is placed on the patient's head and the hair and scalp are massaged through the cap, to lather the shampoo. After shampooing for the manufacturer's suggested length of time, the cap is removed and discarded. The patient's hair is towel dried and styled.

1. Review chart for any limitations in physical activity or contraindications to the procedure.
2. Warm the cap in the microwave, according to the manufacturer's directions, or remove from the storage warmer.
3. Perform hand hygiene. Put on gloves and/or other PPE, as indicated.
4. Identify the patient. Explain the procedure to the patient.
5. Assemble equipment on overbed table within reach.

6. Close the curtains around bed and close door to room, if possible.
7. Place a towel across the patient's chest. Place the shampoo cap on the patient's head.
8. Massage the scalp and hair through the cap to lather the shampoo. Continue to massage according to the time frame specified by the manufacturer's directions (FIGURE A).
9. Remove and discard the shampoo cap.

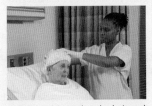

FIGURE A Massaging the hair and scalp.

10. Dry the patient's hair with a towel.
11. Remove the towel from the patient's chest.
12. Comb and style the hair.
13. Remove gloves and discard. Perform hand hygiene.

Skill · 152   **Applying a Sling**

A sling is a bandage that can provide support for an arm or immobilize an injured arm, wrist, or hand. Slings can be used to restrict movement of a fracture or dislocation and to support a muscle sprain. They may also be used to support a splint or secure dressings. Healthcare agencies usually use commercial slings. The sling should distribute the supported weight over a large area, not the back of the neck, to prevent pressure on the cervical spinal nerves.

EQUIPMENT
- Commercial arm sling
- ABD gauze pad
- Nonsterile gloves and/or other PPE, as indicated

ASSESSMENT GUIDELINES
- Assess the situation to determine the need for a sling. Assess the affected limb for pain and edema.
- Perform a neurovascular assessment of the affected extremity. Assess body parts distal to the site for cyanosis, pallor, coolness, numbness, tingling, swelling, and absent or diminished pulses.

NURSING DIAGNOSES
- Impaired Physical Mobility
- Acute Pain
- Risk for Impaired Skin Integrity
- Risk for Injury
- Dressing Self-Care Deficit
- Risk for Peripheral Neurovascular Dysfunction

OUTCOME IDENTIFICATION AND PLANNING
Expected outcomes may include:
- Patient's arm is immobilized.
- Patient maintains muscle strength and joint range of motion.
- Patient shows no evidence of contractures, venous stasis, thrombus formation, or skin breakdown.

IMPLEMENTATION

ACTION	RATIONALE
1. Review the medical record and nursing plan of care to determine the need for the use of a sling.	Reviewing the medical record and plan of care validates the correct patient and correct procedure and prevents injury.

ACTION	RATIONALE
2. Perform hand hygiene. Put on PPE, as indicated.	Hand hygiene and PPE prevent the spread of microorganisms. PPE is required based on transmission precautions.
3. Identify the patient. Explain the procedure to the patient.	Patient identification validates the correct patient and correct procedure. Discussion and explanation help allay anxiety and prepare the patient for what to expect.
4. Close curtains around the bed and close the door to the room, if possible. Place the bed at an appropriate and comfortable working height, if necessary.	Closing the door or curtain provides privacy. Proper bed height helps reduce back strain.
5. Assist the patient to a sitting position. Place the patient's forearm across the chest with the elbow flexed and the palm against the chest. Measure the sleeve length, if indicated.	Proper positioning facilitates sling application. Measurement ensures proper sizing of the sling and proper placement of the arm.
6. Enclose the arm in the sling, making sure the elbow fits into the corner of the fabric. Run the strap up the patient's back and across the shoulder opposite the injury, then down the chest to the fastener on the end of the sling (FIGURE 1).	This position ensures adequate support and keeps the arm out of a dependent position, preventing edema.

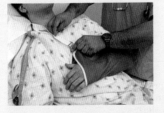

FIGURE 1 Placing the strap around the patient's neck.

ACTION	RATIONALE

7. Place the ABD pad under the strap, between the strap and the patient's neck. **Ensure that the sling and forearm are slightly elevated and at a right angle to the body (FIGURE 2).**

Padding prevents skin irritation and reduces pressure on the neck. Proper positioning ensures alignment, provides support, and prevents edema.

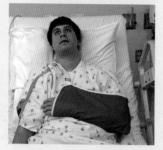

FIGURE 2 Patient with sling in place.

8. Place the bed in the lowest position, with the side rails up. Make sure the call bell and other necessary items are within easy reach.

Having the bed at proper height and leaving the call bell and other items within reach ensure patient safety.

9. Remove PPE, if used. Perform hand hygiene.

Removing PPE properly reduces the risk for infection transmission and contamination of other items. Hand hygiene prevents the spread of microorganisms.

10. Check the patient's level of comfort, arm positioning, and neurovascular status of the affected limb every 4 hours or according to facility policy. Assess the axillary and cervical skin frequently for irritation or breakdown.

Frequent assessment ensures patient safety, prevents injury, and provides early intervention for skin irritation and other complications.

EVALUATION

- Patient demonstrates extremity in proper alignment with adequate muscle strength and joint range of motion.
- Patient demonstrates proper use of sling.

• Patient remains free of complications, including contractures, venous stasis, thrombus formation, or skin breakdown.

DOCUMENTATION

• Document the time and date the sling was applied. Document the patient's response to the sling and the neurovascular status of the extremity.

GENERAL CONSIDERATIONS

• Be sure that the patient's wrist is enclosed in the sling. Do not allow it to hang out and down over the edge. This prevents pressure on nerves and blood vessels and prevents muscle contractures, deformity, and discomfort.
• Assess circulation and comfort at regular intervals.

Skill · 153   Collecting a Sputum Specimen for Culture

A sputum specimen comes from deep within the bronchi, not from the postnasal region. Sputum analysis is used to diagnose disease, test for drug sensitivity, and guide patient treatment. Sputum may be obtained to identify pathogenic organisms, determine if malignant cells are present, and assess for hypersensitivity states. A sputum specimen may be ordered if a bacterial, viral, or fungal infection of the pulmonary system is suspected. A sputum specimen can be collected by patient expectoration into a sterile container, by endotracheal suctioning, during bronchoscopy, and via transtracheal aspiration. Because secretions have accumulated during the night, it is desirable to collect an expectorated sputum specimen first thing in the morning when the patient rises, which aides in the collection process (Smeltzer et al., 2010). The following procedure describes collecting an expectorated sample. Collecting a sputum specimen by suctioning via an endotracheal tube is discussed in the Skill Variation at the end of this skill.

EQUIPMENT

• Sterile sputum specimen container
• Nonsterile gloves
• Goggles or safety glasses
• Additional PPE, as indicated
• Biohazard bag
• Appropriate label for specimen, based on facility policy and procedure

ASSESSMENT GUIDELINES

• Assess patient's lung sounds. Patients with a productive cough may have coarse, wheezing, or diminished lung sounds.

- Monitor oxygen saturation levels, because patients with excessive pulmonary secretions may have decreased oxygen saturation.
- Assess patient's level of pain. Consider administering pain medication before obtaining the sample, because the patient will have to cough.
- Assess the characteristics of the sputum: color, quantity, presence of blood, and viscosity.

NURSING DIAGNOSES

- Risk for Infection
- Acute Pain
- Ineffective Airway Clearance
- Impaired Gas Exchange

OUTCOME IDENTIFICATION AND PLANNING

Expected outcomes may include:
- Patient produces an adequate sample from the lungs.
- An uncontaminated specimen is obtained and sent to the laboratory promptly.
- Airway patency is maintained.
- Oxygen saturation increases.
- Patient demonstrates an understanding about the need for specimen collection.
- Patient demonstrates improved respiratory status.

IMPLEMENTATION

ACTION	RATIONALE
1. Bring necessary equipment to the bedside stand or over-bed table.	Bringing everything to the bedside conserves time and energy. Arranging items nearby is convenient, saves time, and avoids unnecessary stretching and twisting of muscles on the part of the nurse. Organization facilitates performance of tasks.
2. Perform hand hygiene and put on PPE, if indicated.	Hand hygiene and PPE prevent the transmission of microorganisms. PPE is required based on transmission precautions.
3. Identify the patient. Explain the procedure to the patient. If the patient might have pain with	Identifying the patient ensures the right patient receives the intervention and helps prevent errors. Discussion and explanation

ACTION	RATIONALE
coughing, administer pain medication, if ordered. If the patient can perform the task without assistance after instruction, leave the container at bedside with instructions to call the nurse as soon as specimen is produced.	help to allay some of the patient's anxiety and prepare the patient for what to expect. Pain relief facilitates compliance.
4. Check specimen label with the patient's identification bracelet. Label should include patient's name and identification number, time specimen was collected, route of collection, identification of the person obtaining the sample, and any other information required by agency policy.	Confirmation of patient identification information ensures specimen is labeled correctly for the right patient.
5. Close curtains around bed or close the door to the room, if possible.	Closing the curtain or door provides for patient privacy.
6. Put on disposable gloves and goggles.	The gloves and goggles prevent contact with blood and body fluids.
7. Adjust the bed to a comfortable working height, usually elbow height of the caregiver (VISN 8 Patient Safety Center, 2009). Lower side rail closest to you. Place patient in semi-Fowler's position. Have patient clear nose and throat and rinse mouth with water before beginning procedure.	Having the bed at the proper height prevents back and muscle strain. The semi-Fowler's position will help the patient to cough and expectorate the sputum specimen. Water will rinse the oral cavity of saliva and any food particles.
8. Instruct the patient to inhale deeply two or three times and cough with exhalation. If the patient has had abdominal surgery, assist the patient to splint abdomen.	The specimen will need to come from the lungs; saliva is not acceptable. Splinting helps to reduce the pain in the abdominal incision.

ACTION	RATIONALE
9. If the patient produces sputum, open the lid to the container and have the patient expectorate specimen into container.	The specimen needs to come from the lungs; saliva is not acceptable.
10. If patient believes he or she can produce more of the specimen, have the patient repeat the procedure.	This ensures that there is an adequate amount of specimen for analysis.
11. Close lid to container. Offer oral hygiene to the patient.	Closing the container prevents contamination of the specimen and possible infection transmission. Oral hygiene helps to remove pathogens from the oral cavity.
12. Remove equipment and return the patient to a position of comfort. Raise side rail and lower bed.	Repositioning promotes patient comfort. Raising rails promotes safety.
13. Remove goggles and gloves. Perform hand hygiene.	Removing gloves and goggles properly reduces the risk for infection transmission and contamination of other items. Hand hygiene reduces the transmission of microorganisms.
14. Place label on the container per facility policy. Place container in plastic, sealable biohazard bag.	Proper labeling of the specimen ensures the specimen is for the right patient. Packaging the specimen in a biohazard bag prevents the person transporting the container from coming in contact with the specimen.
15. Remove other PPE, if used. Perform hand hygiene.	Removing PPE properly reduces the risk for infection transmission and contamination of other items. Hand hygiene reduces the transmission of microorganisms.
16. Transport the specimen to the laboratory immediately. If immediate transport is not possible, check with laboratory personnel or policy manual whether refrigeration is contraindicated.	Timely transport ensures accurate results.

EVALUATION

- Patient expectorates sputum, and it is collected in a sterile container and sent to the laboratory as soon as possible.
- Patient maintains a patent airway.
- Patient's oxygen saturation level is within expected parameters.
- Patient demonstrates an understanding about the rationale for the specimen collection.

DOCUMENTATION

- Record the time the specimen was collected and sent, and the characteristics and amount of secretions. Document the tests for which the specimen was collected. Note the respiratory assessment pre- and postcollection. Note antibiotics administered in the past 24 hours on the laboratory request form, if required by the facility.

GENERAL CONSIDERATIONS

- Sputum specimens for acid-fast bacilli (AFB; to test for tuberculosis) should be collected for 3r days in a row, in the morning, before drinking eating, or smoking (Pennsylvania Department of Health, 2007).
- If patient understands directions and is able to cooperate, the specimen-collection container may be left at bedside for the patient to collect sputum when available. Instruct patient to call to inform staff as soon as sputum is produced, so it can be transported to laboratory in a timely manner.

Skill Variation | **Collecting Sputum Specimen via Endotracheal Suctioning**

1. Sputum specimens can be collected by suctioning an endotracheal tube or tracheostomy tube. A sterile collection receptacle is attached between the suction catheter and the suction tubing to trap sputum as it is removed from the patient's airway, before reaching the suction collection canister.

2. Refer to Skill 64 and/or 65 for the procedure for endotracheal suctioning.

3. After checking suction pressure, attach a sterile specimen trap to the suction tubing, taking care to avoid contaminating the open ends (see FIGURE A).

4. Continue with the suction procedure, taking care to handle the suction tubing and sputum trap with your nondominant hand.

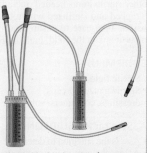

FIGURE A Suction trap for sputum collection.

(continued on page 806)

**Collecting Sputum Specimen via
Endotracheal Suctioning** *continued*

5. After first suction pass, if 1 to 2 mL of sputum has been obtained, disconnect specimen container, and set aside. If less than 1 mL has been collected, suction patient again, after waiting the appropriate amount of time for the patient to recover.

6. If secretions are extremely thick or tenacious, flush the catheter with a small amount (1 to 2 mL) of sterile normal saline to aid in moving the secretions into the trap.

7. Once sputum trap is removed, connect suction tubing to the suction catheter. The catheter may then be flushed with normal saline before suctioning again. Continue with suctioning procedure, if necessary.

8. When suctioning is completed, check specimen label with patient identification bracelet. Label should include patient's name and identification number, time specimen was collected, route of collection, and any other information required by agency policy. Place label on the container, per facility policy. Place container in plastic sealable biohazard bag and send to the laboratory immediately.

Skill · 154   **Adding Sterile Items to a Sterile Field**

A sterile field is created to provide a surgically aseptic workspace. It should be considered a restricted area. After establishing the sterile field, other sterile items needed, including solutions, are added. Items can be wrapped and sterilized within the agency or can be commercially prepared. Take care to ensure that nothing unsterile touches the field or other items in the field, including hands or clothes.

EQUIPMENT
- Sterile field
- Sterile gauze, forceps, dressings, containers, solutions, or other sterile supplies as needed
- PPE, as indicated

ASSESSMENT GUIDELINES
- Assess the situation to determine the necessity for creating a sterile field.
- Assess the area in which the sterile field is to be prepared. Move any unnecessary equipment out of the immediate vicinity.
- Identify additional supplies needed for the procedure.

NURSING DIAGNOSES

- Risk for Infection
- Ineffective Protection

OUTCOME IDENTIFICATION AND PLANNING

Expected outcomes may include:
- Sterile field is created without contamination.
- Patient remains free of exposure to potential infection-causing microorganisms.

IMPLEMENTATION

ACTION	RATIONALE
1. Perform hand hygiene and put on PPE, if indicated.	Hand hygiene and PPE prevent the spread of microorganisms. PPE is required based on transmission precautions.
2. Identify the patient. Explain the procedure to the patient.	Patient identification validates the correct patient and correct procedure. Discussion and explanation help allay anxiety and prepare the patient for what to expect.
3. Check that the sterile, packaged drape and supplies are dry and unopened. Also note expiration date, making sure that the date is still valid.	Moisture contaminates a sterile package. Expiration date indicates period that package remains sterile.
4. Select a work area that is waist level or higher.	Work area is within sight. Bacteria tend to settle, so there is less contamination above the waist.
5. Prepare sterile field as described in Skill 155 or Skill 156.	Proper technique maintains sterility.
6. Add sterile item:	
To Add an Agency-Wrapped and Sterilized Item	
a. Hold agency-wrapped item in the dominant hand, with top flap opening away	Only sterile surface and item are exposed before dropping onto sterile field.

ACTION	RATIONALE

from the body. With other hand, reach around the package and unfold top flap and both sides.

b. Keep a secure hold on the item through the wrapper with the dominant hand. Grasp the remaining flap of the wrapper closest to the body, taking care not to touch the inner surface of the wrapper or the item. Pull the flap back toward the wrist, so the wrapper covers the hand and wrist.

Only sterile surface and item are exposed before dropping onto sterile field.

c. Grasp all the corners of the wrapper together with the nondominant hand and pull back toward wrist, covering hand and wrist. Hold in place.

Only sterile surface and item are exposed before dropping onto sterile field.

d. Hold the item 6 inches above the surface of the sterile field and drop onto the field. Be careful to avoid touching the surface or other items or dropping onto the 1-inch border.

This prevents contamination of the field and inadvertent dropping of the sterile item too close to the edge or off the field. Any items landing on the 1-inch border are considered contaminated.

To Add a Commercially Wrapped and Sterilized Item

a. Hold package in one hand. Pull back top cover with other hand. Alternately, carefully peel the edges apart using both hands.

Contents remain uncontaminated by hands.

b. After top cover or edges are partially separated, hold the item 6 inches above the surface of the sterile field. Continue opening the package and

This prevents contamination of the field and inadvertent dropping of the sterile item too close to the edge or off the field. Any items landing on the 1-inch border are considered contaminated.

ACTION	RATIONALE

drop the item onto the field
(FIGURE 1). Be careful to
avoid touching the surface
or other items or dropping
onto the 1-inch border.

c. Discard wrapper.

A neat work area promotes proper
technique and avoid inadvertent
contamination of the field.

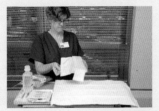

FIGURE 1 Dropping sterile item onto
sterile field.

To Add a Sterile Solution

a. Obtain appropriate solution and check expiration
date.

Once opened, a bottle should be
labeled with date and time. Solution remains sterile for 24 hours
once opened.

b. Open solution container
according to directions
and **place cap on table
away from the field with
edges up.**

Sterility of inside cap is
maintained.

c. Hold bottle outside the
edge of the sterile field
with the label side facing
the palm of your hand and
prepare to pour from a
height of 4 to 6 inches
(10 to 15 cm). The tip of
the bottle should never
touch a sterile container
or field.

Label remains dry, and solution
may be poured without reaching
across sterile field. Minimal
splashing occurs from that height.
Accidentally touching the tip of
the bottle to a container or dressing contaminates them both.

d. Pour required amount of
solution steadily into sterile container previously
added to sterile field and

A steady stream minimizes
the risk of splashing; moisture
contaminates sterile field.

ACTION	RATIONALE
positioned at side of the sterile field or onto dressings. **Avoid splashing any liquid.**	
e. Touch only the outside of the lid when recapping. Label solution with date and time of opening.	Solution remains uncontaminated and available for future use.
7. Continue with procedure as indicated.	
8. When procedure is completed, remove PPE, if used. Perform hand hygiene.	Removing PPE properly reduces the risk for infection transmission and contamination of other items. Hand hygiene prevents the spread of microorganisms.

EVALUATION

- Sterile field is prepared without contamination.
- Sterile supplies are not contaminated.
- Patient has remained free of exposure to potentially infectious microorganisms.

DOCUMENTATION

- It is not usually necessary to document the preparation of a sterile field. However, document the use of sterile technique for any procedure performed using sterile technique.

Skill · 155   **Preparing a Sterile Field Using a Commercially Prepared Sterile Kit or Tray**

A sterile field is created to provide a surgically aseptic workspace. It should be considered a restricted area. Commercially prepared sterile kits and trays are wrapped in a sterile wrapper that, once opened, becomes the sterile field. Sterile items and sterile gloved hands are the only objects allowed in the sterile field. If the area is breached, the entire sterile field is considered contaminated.

EQUIPMENT

- Commercially prepared sterile package
- Additional sterile supplies, such as dressings, containers, or solution, as needed
- PPE, as indicated

ASSESSMENT GUIDELINES

- Assess the situation to determine the necessity for creating a sterile field.
- Assess the area in which the sterile field is to be prepared. Move any unnecessary equipment out of the immediate vicinity.

NURSING DIAGNOSES

- Risk for Infection
- Ineffective Protection

OUTCOME IDENTIFICATION AND PLANNING

Expected outcomes may include:
- Sterile field is created without contamination.
- Contents of the package remain sterile.
- Patient remains free of exposure to potential infection-causing microorganisms.

IMPLEMENTATION

ACTION	RATIONALE
1. Perform hand hygiene and put on PPE, if indicated.	Hand hygiene and PPE prevent the spread of microorganisms. PPE is required based on transmission precautions.
2. Identify the patient. Explain the procedure to the patient.	Patient identification validates the correct patient and correct procedure. Discussion and explanation help allay anxiety and prepare the patient for what to expect.
3. Check that the packaged kit or tray is dry and unopened. Also note expiration date, making sure that the date is still valid.	Moisture contaminates a sterile package. Expiration date indicates period that package remains sterile.

ACTION	RATIONALE
4. Select a work area that is waist level or higher.	Work area is within sight. Bacteria tend to settle, so there is less contamination above the waist.
5. Open the outside cover of the package and remove the kit or tray. Place in the center of the work surface, with the topmost flap positioned on the far side of the package.	This allows sufficient room for the sterile field.
6. Reach around the package and grasp the outer surface of the end of the topmost flap, holding no more than 1 inch from the border of the flap. Pull open away from the body, keeping the arm outstretched and away from the inside of the wrapper (FIGURE 1). Allow the wrapper to lie flat on the work surface.	This maintains sterility of inside of wrapper, which is to become the sterile field. Outer surface of the wrapper is considered unsterile. Outer 1-inch border of the wrapper is considered contaminated.
7. Reach around the package and grasp the outer surface of the first side flap, holding no more than 1 inch from the border of the flap. Pull open to the side of the package, keeping the arm outstretched and away from the inside of the wrapper (FIGURE 2). Allow the wrapper to lie flat on the work surface.	This maintains sterility of inside of wrapper, which is to become the sterile field. Outer surface of the wrapper is considered unsterile. Outer 1-inch border of the wrapper is considered contaminated.

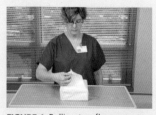

FIGURE 1 Pulling top flap open, away from body.

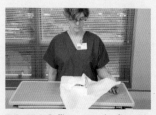

FIGURE 2 Pulling open the first side flap.

ACTION	RATIONALE
8. Reach around the package and grasp the outer surface of the remaining side flap, holding no more than 1 inch from the border of the flap. Pull open to the side of the package, keeping the arm outstretched and away from the inside of the wrapper (FIGURE 3). Allow the wrapper to lie flat on the work surface.	This maintains sterility of inside of wrapper, which is to become the sterile field. Outer surface of the wrapper is considered unsterile. Outer 1-inch of border of the wrapper is considered contaminated.
9. Stand away from the package and work surface. Grasp the outer surface of the remaining flap closest to the body, holding not more than 1 inch from the border of the flap. Pull the flap back toward the body, keeping arm outstretched and away from the inside of the wrapper (FIGURE 4). Keep this hand in place. Use other hand to grasp the wrapper on the underside (the side that is down to the work surface). Position the wrapper so that when flat, edges are on the work surface, and do not hang down over sides of work surface. Allow the wrapper to lie flat on the work surface.	This maintains sterility of inside of wrapper, which is to become the sterile field. Outer surface of the wrapper is considered unsterile. Outer 1-inch border of the wrapper is considered contaminated.

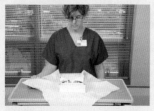

FIGURE 3 Pulling open the remaining side flap.

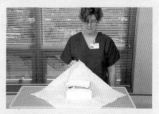

FIGURE 4 Pulling open flap closest to body.

ACTION	RATIONALE
10. The outer wrapper of the package has become a sterile field with the packaged supplies in the center. Do not touch or reach over the sterile field. Place additional sterile items on field as needed (see Skill 155). Continue with the procedure as indicated.	Sterility of the field and contents are maintained.
11. When procedure is completed, remove PPE, if used. Perform hand hygiene.	Removing PPE properly reduces the risk for infection transmission and contamination of other items. Hand hygiene prevents the spread of microorganisms.

EVALUATION
- Sterile field is prepared without contamination.
- Contents of the package remain sterile.
- Patient remains free of exposure to potential infection-causing microorganisms.

DOCUMENTATION
- It is not usually necessary to document the preparation of a sterile field. However, documentation should be recorded regarding the use of sterile technique for any procedure performed using sterile technique.

Skill · 156 | **Preparing a Sterile Field Using a Packaged Sterile Drape**

A sterile field is created to provide a surgically aseptic workspace. It should be considered a restricted area. A sterile drape may be used to establish a sterile field or to extend the sterile working area. The sterile drape should be waterproof on one side, with that side placed down on the work surface. After establishing the sterile field, other sterile items needed, including solutions, are added. Sterile items and sterile gloved hands are the only objects allowed in the sterile field.

EQUIPMENT
- Sterile wrapped drape
- Additional sterile supplies, such as dressings,

containers, or solution, as needed
- PPE, as indicated

ASSESSMENT GUIDELINES
- Assess the situation to determine the necessity for creating a sterile field.
- Assess the area in which the sterile field is to be prepared. Move any unnecessary equipment out of the immediate vicinity.

NURSING DIAGNOSES
- Risk for Infection
- Ineffective Protection

OUTCOME IDENTIFICATION AND PLANNING
Expected outcomes may include:
- Sterile field is created without contamination.
- Patient remains free of exposure to potential infection-causing microorganisms.

IMPLEMENTATION

ACTION	RATIONALE
1. Perform hand hygiene and put on PPE, if indicated.	Hand hygiene and PPE prevent the spread of microorganisms. PPE is required based on transmission precautions.
2. Identify the patient. Explain the procedure to the patient.	Patient identification validates the correct patient and correct procedure. Discussion and explanation help allay anxiety and prepare the patient for what to expect.
3. Check that packaged sterile drape is dry and unopened. Also note expiration date, making sure that the date is still valid.	Moisture contaminates a sterile package. Expiration date indicates period that package remains sterile.
4. Select a work area that is waist level or higher.	Work area is within sight. Bacteria tend to settle, so there is less contamination above the waist.

ACTION	RATIONALE
5. Open the outer covering of the drape. Remove sterile drape, lifting it carefully by its corners. Hold away from body and above the waist and work surface.	Outer 1 inch (2.5 cm) of drape is considered contaminated. Any item touching this area is also considered contaminated.
6. Continue to hold only by the corners. Allow the drape to unfold, away from your body and any other surface.	Touching the outer side of the wrapper maintains sterile field. Contact with any surface would contaminate the field.
7. Position the drape on the work surface with the mois-ture-proof side down. This would be the shiny or blue side. Avoid touching any other surface or object with the drape. If any portion of the drape hangs off the work surface, that part of the drape is considered contaminated.	Moisture-proof side prevents contamination of the field if it becomes wet. The moisture pen-etrates the sterile cloth or paper and carries organisms by capil-lary action to contaminate the field. A wet field is considered contaminated if the surface immediately below it is not sterile.
8. Place additional sterile items on field as needed. Refer to Skill 155. Continue with the procedure as indicated.	Sterility of the field is maintained.
9. When procedure is com-pleted, remove PPE, if used. Perform hand hygiene.	Removing PPE properly reduces the risk for infection transmis-sion and contamination of other items. Hand hygiene prevents the spread of microorganisms.

EVALUATION
• Sterile field is prepared without contamination.
• Patient has remained free of exposure to potentially infectious microorganisms.

DOCUMENTATION
• It is not usually necessary to document the preparation of a sterile field. However, document the use of sterile technique for any proce-dure performed using sterile technique.

Skill · 157   Collecting a Stool Specimen for Culture

A stool specimen may be ordered to screen for pathogenic organisms, such as *Clostridium difficile* or ova and parasites, electrolytes, fat, and leukocytes. The nurse is responsible for obtaining the specimen according to agency procedure, labeling the specimen, and ensuring that the specimen is transported to the laboratory in a timely manner. The institution's policy and procedure manual or laboratory manual identifies specific information about the amount of stool needed, the time frame during which stool is to be collected, and the type of specimen container to use. Usually, 1 inch (2.5 cm) of formed stool or 15 to 30 mL of liquid stool is sufficient. If portions of the stool include visible blood, mucus, or pus, include these with the specimen. Also be sure that the specimen is free of any barium or enema solution. Because a fresh specimen produces the most accurate results, send the specimen to the laboratory immediately. If this is not possible, refrigerate it unless contraindicated, such as when testing for ova and parasites. Refrigeration will affect parasites. Ova and parasites are best detected in warm stool. Some institutions require ova and parasite specimens to be placed in container filled with preservatives; check institutional policy.

EQUIPMENT
- Tongue blade (2)
- Clean specimen container (or container with preservatives for ova and parasites)
- Biohazard bag
- Nonsterile gloves
- Additional PPE, as indicated
- Appropriate label for specimen, based on facility policy and procedure

---

ASSESSMENT GUIDELINES
- Assess the patient's understanding of the need for the test and the requirements of the test.
- Assess the patient's understanding of the collection procedure and ability to cooperate.
- Ask the patient when his or her last bowel movement was, and check the patient's medical record for this information.

NURSING DIAGNOSES
- Deficient Knowledge
- Diarrhea
- Anxiety

OUTCOME IDENTIFICATION AND PLANNING

Expected outcomes may include:

• An uncontaminated stool sample is obtained, following collection guidelines, and transported to the laboratory within the recommended time frame, without adverse effect.
• Patient demonstrates ability to collect stool specimen.
• Specimen is obtained with minimal discomfort or anxiety.

IMPLEMENTATION

ACTION	RATIONALE
1. Gather necessary equipment to the bedside.	Organization facilitates performance of tasks.
2. Perform hand hygiene and put on PPE, if indicated.	Hand hygiene and PPE prevent the transmission of microorganisms. PPE is required based on transmission precautions.
3. Identify the patient. Discuss with the patient the need for a stool sample. Explain to the patient the process by which the stool will be collected, either from a bedpan, commode, or plastic receptacle in the toilet. Instruct patient to void first and not to discard toilet paper with stool. Tell the patient to call you as soon as a bowel movement is completed.	Identifying the patient ensures the right patient receives the intervention and helps prevent errors. Discussion and explanation help to allay some of the patient's anxiety and prepare the patient for what to expect. The patient should void first because the laboratory study may be inaccurate if the stool contains urine. Placing a container in the toilet or bedside commode aids in obtaining a clean stool specimen uncontaminated by urine.
4. Check specimen label with the patient's identification bracelet. Label should include patient's name and identification number, time specimen was collected, route of collection, identification of the person obtaining the sample, and any other information required by agency policy.	Confirmation of patient identification information ensures the specimen is labeled correctly for the right patient.

ACTION	RATIONALE
5. After the patient has passed a stool, put on gloves. Use the tongue blades to obtain a sample, free of blood or urine, and place it in the designated clean container.	The container does not have to be sterile, because stool is not sterile. To ensure accurate results, the stool should be free of urine or menstrual blood.
6. Collect as much of the stool as possible to send to the laboratory.	Different tests and laboratories require different amounts of stool. Collecting as much as possible helps to ensure that the laboratory has an adequate amount of specimen for testing.
7. Place lid on container. Dispose of used equipment per facility policy. Remove gloves and perform hand hygiene.	Proper disposal of equipment reduces the transmission of microorganisms. Removing gloves properly reduces the risk for infection transmission and contamination of other items. Hand hygiene deters the spread of microorganisms.
8. Place label on the container per facility policy. Place container in plastic sealable, biohazard bag.	Correct labeling is necessary to ensure accurate results. Packaging the specimen in a biohazard bag prevents the person transporting the container from coming in contact with stool.
9. Remove other PPE, if used. Perform hand hygiene.	Removing PPE properly reduces the risk for infection transmission and contamination of other items. Hand hygiene reduces the transmission of microorganisms.
10. Transport the specimen to the laboratory while stool is still warm. If immediate transport is impossible, check with laboratory personnel or policy manual whether refrigeration is contraindicated.	Most tests have better results with fresh stool. Different tests may require different preparation if the test is not immediately completed. Some tests will be compromised if the stool is refrigerated.

EVALUATION

* Stool sample is obtained following collection guidelines and transported to the laboratory within the recommended time frame, without adverse effect.
* Patient demonstrates accurate understanding of testing instructions.
* Specimen is obtained with minimal discomfort and embarrassment.

DOCUMENTATION

* Document amount, color, and consistency of stool obtained, time of collection, specific test for which the specimen was collected, and transport to laboratory.

GENERAL CONSIDERATIONS

* If patient is wearing an adult incontinence brief, the stool may be collected from the brief, as long as it is not contaminated with urine.
* Barium procedures and laxatives should be avoided for 1 week before specimen collection to ensure valid results.
* Specimen can be collected from an ostomy appliance. Apply a clean ostomy appliance and obtain sample as soon as patient passes stool into the appliance.
* If a timed stool test is ordered, such as fecal fat, the entire amount of stool produced for 24 to 72 hours is sent to the laboratory. Be sure to follow instructions for storage while collection is ongoing.

Skill · 158   **Testing Stool for Occult Blood**

Occult blood (hidden blood or blood that cannot be seen on gross examination) in the stool can be detected with simple screening tests. These tests, which may be performed quickly by nurses within an institution or by patients at home, use reagent substances to detect the enzyme peroxidase in the hemoglobin molecule. The Hematest and guaiac test are chemical tests commonly used to identify occult blood in the stool.

EQUIPMENT

* Nonsterile gloves; other PPE as indicated
* Wooden applicator
* Hemoccult testing card and developer
* Bedpan, or plastic collection receptacle for commode or toilet
* Biohazard bag
* Appropriate label for specimen, based on facility policy and procedure

ASSESSMENT GUIDELINES

- Assess the patient's understanding of the collection procedure and ability to cooperate, and for a history of gastrointestinal bleeding.
- Review prescribed restrictions for medications and diet, and evaluate patient compliance with required restrictions.
- Assess patient for any blood in the perineal area, including hemorrhoids, menstruation, urinary tract infection, or vaginal or rectal tears.

NURSING DIAGNOSES

- Deficient Knowledge
- Constipation
- Diarrhea
- Pain
- Anxiety
- Bowel Incontinence

OUTCOME IDENTIFICATION AND PLANNING

Expected outcomes may include:

- An uncontaminated stool sample is obtained, following collection guidelines, and transported to the laboratory within the recommended time frame, without adverse effect.
- Patient demonstrates an accurate understanding of testing instructions.
- Specimen is obtained with minimal discomfort or embarrassment.

IMPLEMENTATION

ACTION	RATIONALE
1. Bring necessary equipment to the bedside stand or over-bed table.	Bringing everything to the bedside conserves time and energy. Arranging items nearby is convenient, saves time, and avoids unnecessary stretching and twisting of muscles on the part of the nurse. Organization facilitates performance of tasks.
2. Perform hand hygiene and put on PPE, if indicated.	Hand hygiene and PPE prevent the transmission of microorganisms. PPE is required based on transmission precautions.

ACTION	RATIONALE

3. Identify the patient. Discuss with the patient the need for a stool sample. Explain to the patient the process by which the stool will be collected, either from a bedpan, commode, or plastic receptacle in the toilet.

Identifying the patient ensures the right patient receives the intervention and helps prevent errors. Discussion and explanation help to allay some of the patient's anxiety and prepare the patient for what to expect.

4. If sending the specimen to the laboratory, check specimen label with patient identification bracelet. Label should include patient's name and identification number, time specimen was collected, route of collection, identification of the person obtaining the sample, and any other information required by agency policy.

Facilities may allow point-of-service testing (at bedside or on unit) or specimen may have to be sent to laboratory for testing. Confirmation of patient identification information ensures the specimen is labeled correctly for the right patient.

5. Close curtains around bed or close the door to the room, if possible.

Closing the door or curtain provides for patient privacy.

6. Place the plastic collection receptacle in the toilet, if applicable. Assist the patient to the bathroom or onto the bedside commode, or assist the patient onto the bedpan. Instruct patient not to urinate or discard toilet paper with the stool.

Proper collection into an appropriate receptacle for stool prevents inaccurate results. Urine or toilet paper can contaminate the specimen, interfering with accurate results.

7. After the patient defecates, assist the patient out of the bathroom, off the commode, or remove the bedpan. Perform hand hygiene and put on disposable gloves.

Hand hygiene deters the spread of microorganisms. Gloves protect the nurse from microorganisms in feces.

ACTION	RATIONALE
8. With wooden applicator, apply a small amount of stool from the center of the bowel movement onto one window of the Hemoccult testing card. With opposite end of wooden applicator, obtain another sample of stool from another area and apply a small amount of stool onto second window of Hemoccult card (FIGURE 1).	Two separate areas of the same stool sample are tested in case there is trace blood from a hemorrhoid or fissure. By using opposite ends of the wooden applicator, cross-contamination is avoided.

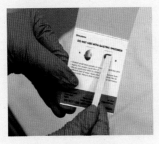

FIGURE 1 Applying stool to window of testing card.

ACTION	RATIONALE
9. Close flap over stool samples.	Closing the flap prevents contamination of the samples.
10. If sending to the laboratory, label the specimen card per facility policy. Place in a sealable plastic biohazard bag and send to the laboratory immediately.	Facilities may allow point-of-service testing (at bedside or on unit) or the specimen may have to be sent to the laboratory for testing. Correct labeling is necessary to ensure accurate results. Packaging the specimen in a biohazard bag prevents the person transporting the container from coming in contact with the specimen.
11. If testing at bedside, open flap on opposite side of card and place two drops of developer over each window	The developer will react with any blood in the stool. Following the manufacturer's instructions promotes accuracy of results.

ACTION	RATIONALE

and wait the time stated in the manufacturer's instructions.

12. Observe card for any blue areas (FIGURE 2).

Any blue coloring on the card indicates a positive test result for blood.

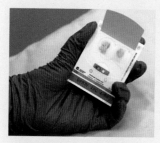

FIGURE 2 Observing windows on card for blue areas.

13. Discard Hemoccult testing slide appropriately, according to facility policy. Remove gloves and any other PPE, if used. Perform hand hygiene.

Removing PPE properly reduces the risk for infection transmission and contamination of other items. Hand hygiene and proper disposal of equipment reduces the transmission of microorganisms.

EVALUATION

- Stool sample is obtained following collection guidelines and transported to the laboratory within the recommended time frame, without adverse effect.
- Patient demonstrates an accurate understanding of testing instructions.
- Specimen is obtained with minimal discomfort and embarrassment.

DOCUMENTATION

- Document the method used to obtain the specimen and transport it to the laboratory. If testing is done by the nurse, document results and communication of results to the healthcare provider. Document significant assessment findings and stool characteristics.

GENERAL CONSIDERATIONS

- To ensure validity, the test should be repeated three to six times on different samples on different days.
- Specimen can be collected from an ostomy appliance. Apply a clean ostomy appliance and obtain a sample as soon as patient passes stool into the appliance.

Skill Variation — Performing a Digital Rectal Examination to Obtain a Stool Specimen for Occult Blood

1. Perform hand hygiene.

2. Identify the patient. Discuss with the patient the need for a stool sample. Explain to patient the process by which the stool will be collected, as a result of a digital rectal examination.

3. If sending the specimen to the laboratory, check the specimen label with the patient's identification bracelet. Label should include patient's name and identification number, time specimen was collected, route of collection, identification of the person obtaining the sample, and any other information required by agency policy.

4. Put on nonsterile gloves, and other PPE, as indicated.

5. Close curtains around bed or close the door to the room, if possible.

6. If the patient is able to stand, instruct the patient to bend over examination table or bed placed at a comfortable height. If patient is bedridden, place in Sims' or side-lying position.

7. **Generously lubricate 1 to 1.5 inches of finger with water-soluble lubricant to be inserted into anus to collect stool sample.**

8. Separate the buttocks with the nondominant hand. Ask patient to take a large, deep breath through the nose and exhale through the mouth. Gently insert lubricated finger of dominant hand 1 to 2 inches into the rectum while lightly palpating for any stool.

9. Remove finger. **Apply stool to one window of Hemoccult testing card. Apply stool to second window of Hemoccult testing card from different place on glove than first sample.**

10. Close flap over stool samples.

11. Depending on facility policy, actual testing of stool may take place at bedside or the specimen may be sent to the laboratory.

(continued on page 826)

Performing a Digital Rectal Examination to Obtain a Stool Specimen for Occult Blood *continued*

12. If sending to the laboratory, label the specimen card per facility policy. Place in sealable plastic biohazard bag and send to the laboratory immediately.

13. If testing at bedside, open flap on opposite side of card and place two drops of developer over each window and wait the time stated in the manufacturer's instructions.

14. Observe card for any blue areas.

15. Discard Hemoccult testing slide. Remove gloves and any other PPE, if used. Perform hand hygiene.

16. Document method used to obtain sample and testing results.

Skill · 159 **Suctioning the Nasopharyngeal and Oropharyngeal Airways**

Suctioning of the pharynx is indicated to maintain a patent airway and to remove saliva, pulmonary secretions, blood, vomitus, or foreign material from the pharynx. Suctioning helps a patient who cannot successfully clear his or her airway by coughing and expectorating. When performing suctioning, position yourself on the appropriate side of the patient. If you are right-handed, stand on the patient's right side; if left-handed, stand on the patient's left side. This allows for comfortable use of the dominant hand to manipulate the suction catheter.

EQUIPMENT

• Portable or wall suction unit with tubing
• A commercially prepared suction kit with an appropriate size catheter or
  • Sterile suction catheter with Y-port in the appropriate size (Adult: 10F to 16F)
• Sterile disposable container
• Sterile gloves
• Sterile water or saline
• Towel or waterproof pad
• Goggles and mask or face shield
• Disposable, clean gloves
• Water-soluble lubricant
• Additional PPE, as indicated

ASSESSMENT GUIDELINES

• Assess lung sounds. Patients who need to be suctioned may have wheezes, crackles, or gurgling present.

- Assess oxygenation saturation level. Oxygen saturation usually decreases when a patient needs to be suctioned.
- Assess respiratory status, including respiratory rate and depth. Patients may become tachypneic when they need to be suctioned. Assess the patient for signs of respiratory distress, such as nasal flaring, retractions, or grunting.
- Assess effectiveness of coughing and expectoration. Patients with an ineffective cough and who are unable to expectorate secretions may need to be suctioned.
- Assess for history of deviated septum, nasal polyps, nasal obstruction, nasal injury, epistaxis (nasal bleeding), or nasal swelling.

NURSING DIAGNOSES

- Ineffective Airway Clearance
- Impaired Gas Exchange
- Ineffective Breathing Pattern
- Risk for Aspiration

OUTCOME IDENTIFICATION AND PLANNING

Expected outcomes may include:
- Patient will exhibit improved breath sounds and a clear, patent airway.
- Patient will exhibit an oxygen saturation level within acceptable parameters.
- Patient will demonstrate a respiratory rate and depth within age-acceptable range.
- Patient will remain free of any signs of respiratory distress, including retractions, nasal flaring, or grunting.

IMPLEMENTATION

ACTION	RATIONALE
1. Bring necessary equipment to the bedside stand or over-bed table.	Bringing everything to the bedside conserves time and energy. Arranging items nearby is convenient, saves time, and avoids unnecessary stretching and twisting of muscles on the part of the nurse.
2. Perform hand hygiene and put on PPE, if indicated.	Hand hygiene and PPE prevent the spread of microorganisms. PPE is required based on transmission precautions.
3. Identify the patient.	Identifying the patient ensures the right patient receives the intervention and helps prevent errors.

ACTION	RATIONALE
4. Close curtains around bed and close the door to the room, if possible.	This ensures the patient's privacy.
5. Determine the need for suctioning. Verify the suction order in the patient's chart, if necessary. **For a postoperative patient, administer pain medication before suctioning.**	To minimize trauma to airway mucosa, suctioning should be done only when secretions have accumulated or adventitious breath sounds are audible. Some facilities require an order for naso- and oropharyngeal suctioning. Suctioning stimulates coughing, which is painful for patients with surgical incisions.
6. Explain what you are going to do and the reason for suctioning to the patient, even if the patient does not appear to be alert. Reassure the patient you will interrupt procedure if he or she indicates respiratory difficulty.	Explanation alleviates fears. Even if a patient appears unconscious, explain what is happening. Any procedure that compromises respiration is frightening for the patient.
7. Adjust bed to comfortable working height, usually elbow height of the caregiver (VISN 8 Patient Safety Center, 2009). Lower side rail closest to you. **If patient is conscious, place him or her in a semi-Fowler's position. If patient is unconscious, place him or her in the lateral position, facing you.** Move the bedside table close to your work area and raise it to waist height.	Having the bed at the proper height prevents back and muscle strain. A sitting position helps the patient to cough and makes breathing easier. Gravity also facilitates catheter insertion. The lateral position prevents the airway from becoming obstructed and promotes drainage of secretions. The bedside table provides a work surface and helps maintain sterility of objects on the work surface.
8. Place towel or waterproof pad across the patient's chest.	This protects bed linens.
9. **Adjust suction to appropriate pressure.** For a wall unit for an adult: 100–120 mm Hg (Roman, 2005); neonates: 60–80 mm Hg; infants: 80–100 mm Hg;	Higher pressures can cause excessive trauma, hypoxemia, and atelectasis.

ACTION

children: 80–100 mm Hg; adolescents: 80–120 mm Hg (Ireton, 2007).

For a portable unit for an adult: 10–15 cm Hg; neonates: 6–8 cm Hg; infants: 8–10 cm Hg; children: 8–10 cm Hg; adolescents: 8–10 cm Hg.

Put on a disposable, clean glove and occlude the end of the connecting tubing to check suction pressure. Place the connecting tubing in a convenient location.

10. Open sterile suction package using aseptic technique. The open wrapper or container becomes a sterile field to hold other supplies. Carefully remove the sterile container, touching only the outside surface. Set it up on the work surface and pour sterile saline into it.

11. Place a small amount of water-soluble lubricant on the sterile field, taking care to avoid touching the sterile field with the lubricant package.

12. Increase the patient's supplemental oxygen level or apply supplemental oxygen per facility policy or primary care provider order.

13. Put on face shield or goggles and mask. Put on sterile gloves. **The dominant hand will manipulate the catheter and must remain sterile. The nondominant hand is considered clean rather than sterile and will control the suction valve (Y-port) on the catheter.**

RATIONALE

Sterile normal saline or water is used to lubricate the outside of the catheter, minimizing irritation of mucosa during introduction. It is also used to clear the catheter between suction attempts.

Lubricant facilitates passage of the catheter and reduces trauma to mucous membranes.

Suctioning removes air from the patient's airway and can cause hypoxemia. Hyperoxygenation can help prevent suction-induced hypoxemia.

Handling the sterile catheter using a sterile glove helps prevent introducing organisms into the respiratory tract; the clean glove protects the nurse from microorganisms.

ACTION	RATIONALE
14. With dominant gloved hand, pick up sterile catheter. Pick up the connecting tubing with the nondominant hand and connect the tubing and suction catheter.	Sterility of the suction catheter is maintained.
15. Moisten the catheter by dipping it into the container of sterile saline. Occlude Y-tube to check suction.	Lubricating the inside of the catheter with saline helps move secretions in the catheter. Checking suction ensures equipment is working properly.
16. Encourage the patient to take several deep breaths.	Suctioning removes air from the patient's airway and can cause hypoxemia. Hyperventilation can help prevent suction-induced hypoxemia.
17. Apply lubricant to the first 2 to 3 inches of the catheter, using the lubricant that was placed on the sterile field.	Lubricant facilitates passage of the catheter and reduces trauma to mucous membranes.
18. Remove the oxygen delivery device, if appropriate. Do not apply suction as the catheter is inserted. Hold the catheter between your thumb and forefinger.	Using suction while inserting the catheter can cause trauma to the mucosa and remove oxygen from the respiratory tract. Correct distance for insertion ensures proper placement of the catheter. The general guideline for determining insertion distance for nasopharyngeal suctioning for an individual patient is to estimate the distance from the patient's earlobe to the nose.
19. Insert the catheter:	
a. For nasopharyngeal suctioning, gently insert catheter through the naris and along the floor of the nostril toward the trachea (FIGURE 1). Roll the catheter between your fingers to help advance it. Advance the catheter approximately 5″ to 6″ to reach the pharynx.	

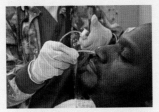

FIGURE 1 Inserting catheter through the naris.

b. For oropharyngeal suctioning, insert catheter through
the mouth, along the side of
the mouth toward the tra-
chea. Advance the catheter
3″ to 4″ to reach the pharynx. (For nasotracheal
suctioning, see the accompanying Skill Variation.)

20. **Apply suction by intermittently occluding the Y-port
on the catheter with the
thumb of your nondomi-
nant hand and gently rotating the catheter as it is
being withdrawn (FIGURE 2).
Do not suction for more
than 10 to 15 seconds at
a time.**

Turning the catheter as it is withdrawn minimizes trauma to the
mucosa. Suctioning for longer
than 10 to 15 seconds robs the
respiratory tract of oxygen,
which may result in hypoxemia.
Suctioning too quickly may be
ineffective at clearing all
secretions.

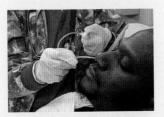

FIGURE 2 Suctioning nasopharynx.

21. Replace the oxygen-delivery
device using your nondominant hand, if appropriate, and
have the patient take several
deep breaths.

Suctioning removes air from the
patient's airway and can cause
hypoxemia. Hyperventilation can
help prevent suction-induced
hypoxemia.

ACTION	RATIONALE
22. Flush catheter with saline. Assess effectiveness of suctioning and repeat, as needed, and according to patient's tolerance. Wrap the suction catheter around your dominant hand between attempts.	Flushing clears catheter and lubricates it for next insertion. Reassessment determines the need for additional suctioning. Wrapping prevents inadvertent contamination of catheter.
23. **Allow at least a 30-second to 1-minute interval if additional suctioning is needed. No more than three suction passes should be made per suctioning episode. Alternate the nares, unless contraindicated, if repeated suctioning is required.** Do not force the catheter through the nares. Encourage the patient to cough and deep breathe between suctioning. Suction the oropharynx after suctioning the nasopharynx.	The interval allows for reventilation and reoxygenation of airways. Excessive suction passes contribute to complications. Alternating nares reduces trauma. Suctioning the oropharynx after the nasopharynx clears the mouth of secretions. More microorganisms are usually present in the mouth, so it is suctioned last to prevent transmission of contaminants.
24. When suctioning is completed, remove gloves from dominant hand over the coiled catheter, pulling them off inside-out. Remove glove from nondominant hand and dispose of gloves, catheter, and container with solution in the appropriate receptacle. Assist patient to a comfortable position. Raise bed rail and place bed in the lowest position.	This technique reduces transmission of microorganisms. Proper positioning with raised side rails and proper bed height provide for patient comfort and safety.
25. Turn off suction. Remove supplemental oxygen placed for suctioning, if appropriate. Remove face shield or goggles and mask. Perform hand hygiene.	Proper removal of PPE and hand hygiene reduces risk of transmission of microorganisms.

ACTION	RATIONALE
26. Offer oral hygiene after suctioning.	Respiratory secretions that are allowed to accumulate in the mouth are irritating to mucous membranes and unpleasant for the patient.
27. Reassess patient's respiratory status, including respiratory rate, effort, oxygen saturation, and lung sounds.	This assesses effectiveness of suctioning and the presence of complications.
28. Remove additional PPE, if used. Perform hand hygiene.	Removing PPE properly reduces the risk for infection transmission and contamination of other items. Hand hygiene prevents the spread of microorganisms.

EVALUATION

- Patient exhibits improved breath sounds and a clear and patent airway.
- Patient's oxygen saturation level is within acceptable parameters.
- Patient does not exhibit signs or symptoms of respiratory distress or complications.

DOCUMENTATION

- Document the time of suctioning, before and after intervention assessment, reason for suctioning, route used, and the characteristics and amount of secretions. Document patient teaching and patient response, if appropriate. If the patient coughs, document whether the cough is productive or nonproductive. If productive cough is present, include the characteristics of the sputum, including consistency, amount, and color.

Skill Variation   Nasotracheal Suctioning

Nasotracheal suctioning is indicated to maintain a patent airway and remove saliva, pulmonary secretions, blood, vomitus, or foreign material from the trachea. Tracheal suctioning can lead to hypoxemia, cardiac dysrhythmias, trauma, atelectasis, infection, bleeding, and pain. It is imperative to be diligent in maintaining aseptic technique and following facility guidelines and procedures to prevent potential hazards. When performing suctioning, position yourself on the appropriate side of the patient.

(continued on page 834)

Nasotracheal Suctioning *continued*

If you are right-handed, stand on the patient's right side; if left-handed, stand on the patient's left side. This allows for comfortable use of the dominant hand to manipulate the suction catheter. To perform nasotracheal suctioning:

1. Perform hand hygiene. Put on PPE, as indicated.

2. Identify the patient.

3. Determine the need for suctioning. For a postoperative patient, administer pain medication before suctioning.

4. Explain to the patient what you are going to do and the reason for doing it, even if the patient does not appear to be alert.

5. Adjust bed to a comfortable working position. Lower the side rail closest to you. If the patient is conscious, place him or her in a semi-Fowler's position. If the patient is unconscious, place him or her in the lateral position, facing you. Move the overbed table close to your work area and raise to waist height.

6. Place a towel or waterproof pad across the patient's chest.

7. Turn suction to appropriate pressure. Put on a disposable, clean glove and occlude the end of the connecting tubing to check suction pressure. Place the connecting tubing in a convenient location.

8. Open sterile suction package using aseptic technique. The open wrapper becomes a sterile field to hold other supplies. Carefully remove the sterile container, touching only the outside surface. Set it up on the work surface and pour sterile saline into it.

9. Place a small amount of water-soluble lubricant on the sterile field, taking care to avoid touching the sterile field with the lubricant package.

10. Increase the patient's supplemental oxygen level or apply supplemental oxygen per facility policy or physician order.

11. Put on face shield or goggles and mask. Put on sterile gloves. The dominant hand will manipulate the catheter and must remain sterile. The nondominant hand is considered clean rather than sterile and will control the suction valve.

12. With dominant gloved hand, pick up the sterile catheter. Pick up the connecting tubing with the nondominant hand and

(continued on page 835)

Nasotracheal Suctioning *continued*

connect the tubing and suction catheter.

13. Moisten the catheter by dipping it into the container of sterile saline. Occlude the Y-tube to check suction.

14. Encourage the patient to take several deep breaths.

15. Apply lubricant to the first 2 to 3 inches of the catheter, using the lubricant that was placed on the sterile field.

16. Remove the oxygen-delivery device, if appropriate. Do not apply suction as the catheter is inserted. Hold the catheter in your thumb and forefinger. Gently insert the catheter through the naris and along the floor of the nostril toward the trachea. Roll the catheter between your fingers to help advance it. Advance the catheter approximately 8 to 9 inches to reach the trachea. Resistance should not be met. If resistance is met, the carina or tracheal mucosa has been hit. Withdraw the catheter at least 12 inches before applying suction.

17. Apply suction by intermittently occluding the Y-port on the catheter with the thumb of your nondominant hand, and gently rotating the catheter as it is being withdrawn. **Do not suction for more than 10 to 15 seconds at a time.**

18. Replace the oxygen-delivery device using your nondominant hand and have the patient take several deep breaths.

19. Flush the catheter with saline. Assess effectiveness of suctioning and repeat as needed and according to patient's tolerance. Wrap the suction catheter around your dominant hand between attempts.

20. **Allow at least a 30-second to 1-minute interval if additional suctioning is needed. No more than three suction passes should be made per suctioning episode. Alternate the nares, unless contraindicated, if repeated suctioning is required. Do not force catheter through the nares. Encourage the patient to cough and deep breathe between suctioning. Suction the oropharynx after suctioning the trachea.**

21. When suctioning is completed, remove glove from dominant hand over the coiled catheter, pulling it off inside out. Remove glove from nondominant hand and dispose of gloves, catheter, and container with solution in the appropriate receptacle. Remove face shield or goggles and mask. Perform hand hygiene.

22. Turn off suction. Remove supplemental oxygen

(continued on page 836)

Nasotracheal Suctioning *continued*

placed for suctioning, if appropriate. Assist patient to a comfortable position.

23. Offer oral hygiene after suctioning.

24. Reassess patient's respiratory status, including respiratory rate, effort, oxygen saturation, and lung sounds.

25. Remove additional PPE, if used. Perform hand hygiene.

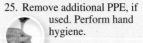

26. Document the time of suctioning, your before and after intervention assessment, the reason for suctioning, route used, and the characteristics and amount of secretions.

Skill · 160   Removing Surgical Staples

Surgical skin staples are made of stainless steel and are used to hold tissue and skin together. Staples decrease the risk of infection and allow faster wound closure. Surgical staples are removed when sufficient tensile strength has developed to hold the wound edges together during healing. The time frame for removal varies depending on the patient's age, nutritional status, and wound location. After skin staples are removed, adhesive wound closure strips are applied across the wound to keep the skin edges approximated as the wound continues to heal. Removal of surgical staples may be done by the primary care provider or by the nurse with a medical order.

EQUIPMENT
- Staple remover
- Gauze
- Wound cleansing agent, according to facility policy
- Clean disposable gloves
- Additional PPE, as indicated
- Adhesive wound closure strips
- Skin-protectant wipes

ASSESSMENT GUIDELINES
- Inspect the surgical incision and the surrounding tissue. Assess the appearance of the wound for the approximation of wound edges, the color of the wound and surrounding area, and signs of dehiscence. Note the stage of the healing process and the characteristics of any drainage.
- Assess the surrounding skin for color, temperature, and the presence of edema or ecchymosis.

NURSING DIAGNOSES

- Anxiety
- Acute Pain
- Impaired Skin Integrity
- Delayed Surgical Recovery
- Deficient Knowledge

OUTCOME IDENTIFICATION AND PLANNING

Expected outcomes may include:
- Patient's staples are removed without contaminating the incisional area, without causing trauma to the wound, and without causing the patient to experience pain or discomfort.
- Patient remains free of complications that would delay recovery.
- Patient verbalizes an understanding of the procedure.

IMPLEMENTATION

ACTION	RATIONALE
1. Review the medical orders for staple removal.	Reviewing the order and plan of care validates the correct patient and correct procedure.
2. Gather the necessary supplies and bring to the bedside stand or overbed table.	Preparation promotes efficient time management and an organized approach to the task. Bringing everything to the bedside conserves time and energy. Arranging items nearby is convenient, saves time, and avoids unnecessary stretching and twisting of muscles on the part of the nurse.
3. Perform hand hygiene and put on PPE, if indicated.	Hand hygiene and PPE prevent the spread of microorganisms. PPE is required based on transmission precautions.
4. Identify the patient.	Identifying the patient ensures that the right patient receives the intervention and helps prevent errors.
5. Close curtains around bed and close door to room, if possible. Explain what you	This ensures the patient's privacy. Explanation relieves anxiety and facilitates cooperation.

ACTION	RATIONALE
are going to do and why you are going to do it to the patient. Describe the sensation of staple removal as a pulling experience.	
6. Assess the patient for possible need for nonpharmacologic pain-reducing interventions or analgesic medication before beginning the procedure. Administer appropriate prescribed analgesic. Allow sufficient time for analgesic to achieve its effectiveness before beginning the procedure.	Pain is a subjective experience influenced by past experience. Wound care and dressing changes may cause pain for some patients.
7. Place a waste receptacle at a convenient location for use during the procedure.	Having a waste container handy means that the soiled dressing can be discarded easily, without the spread of microorganisms.
8. Adjust bed to comfortable working height, usually elbow height of the caregiver (VISN 8 Patient Safety Center, 2009).	Having the bed at the proper height prevents back and muscle strain.
9. Assist the patient to a comfortable position that provides easy access to the incision area. Use a bath blanket to cover any exposed area other than the incision. Place a waterproof pad under the incision site.	Patient positioning and use of a bath blanket provide for comfort and warmth. Waterproof pad protects underlying surfaces.
10. Put on clean gloves. Carefully and gently remove the soiled dressings. If there is resistance, use a silicone-based adhesive remover to help remove the tape. If any part of the dressing sticks to the underlying skin, use small amounts of sterile saline to help loosen and remove. Inspect the incision area.	Gloves protect the nurse from handling contaminated dressings. Cautious removal of the dressing is more comfortable for the patient and ensures that any drain present is not removed. A silicone-based adhesive remover allows for the easy, rapid, and painless removal without the associated problems of skin stripping (Rudoni, 2008; Stephen-Haynes, 2008). Sterile

ACTION	RATIONALE

saline moistens the dressing for easier removal and minimizes damage and pain.

11. Clean the incision using the wound cleanser and gauze, according to facility policies and procedures.

Incision cleaning prevents the spread of microorganisms and contamination of the wound.

12. Grasp the staple remover (FIGURE 1). Position the staple remover under the staple to be removed. Firmly close the staple remover. The staple will bend in the middle and the edges will pull up out of the skin.

Correct use of a staple remover prevents accidental injury to the wound and contamination of the incision area and resulting infection.

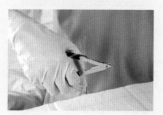

FIGURE 1 Grasping the staple remover.

13. Remove every other staple to be sure the wound edges are healed. If they are, remove the remaining staples as ordered. Dispose of staples in the sharps container.

Removing every other staple allows for inspection of the wound, while leaving an adequate number of staples in place to promote continued healing if the edges are not totally approximated.

14. If wound closure strips are to be applied, apply skin protectant to skin around incision. Do not apply to incision. Apply adhesive closure strips. Take care to handle the strips by the paper backing.

Skin protectant helps adherence of closure strips and prevents skin irritation. Adhesive wound closure strips provide additional support to the wound as it continues to heal. Handling by the paper backing avoids contamination.

15. Reapply the dressing, depending on the medical orders and facility policy.

A new dressing protects the wound. Some policies advise leaving the area uncovered.

ACTION	RATIONALE
16. Remove gloves and discard. Remove all remaining equipment; place the patient in a comfortable position, with side rails up and bed in the lowest position.	Proper removal of gloves prevents spread of microorganisms. Proper patient and bed positioning promotes safety and comfort.
17. Remove additional PPE, if used. Perform hand hygiene.	Removing PPE properly reduces the risk for infection transmission and contamination of other items. Hand hygiene prevents the spread of microorganisms.
18. Assess all wounds every shift. More frequent checks may be needed if the wound is more complex.	Checking drain ensures proper functioning and early detection of problems. Checking dressings ensures the assessment of changes in patient condition and timely intervention to prevent complications.

EVALUATION

• Patient exhibits an incision area that is clean, dry, and intact without staples.
• Patient's incision area is free of trauma and infection.
• Patient verbalizes little to no pain or discomfort during staple removal.
• Patient verbalizes an understanding of the procedure.

DOCUMENTATION

• Document the location of the incision and the assessment of the site. Include the appearance of the surrounding skin. Document cleansing of the site and staple removal. Record any skin care and the dressing applied, if appropriate. Note pertinent patient and family education and any patient reaction to this procedure, including patient's pain level and effectiveness of nonpharmacologic interventions or analgesia if administered.

GENERAL CONSIDERATIONS

• Encourage the patient to splint chest and abdominal wounds during activity, such as changing position, ambulation, coughing, and sneezing. This provides increased support for the skin and underlying tissues and can decrease discomfort.

Skill · 161 Removing Sutures

Skin sutures are used to hold tissue and skin together. Sutures may be black silk, synthetic material, or fine wire. Sutures are removed when sufficient tensile strength has developed to hold the wound edges together during healing. The time frame varies depending on the patient's age, nutritional status, and wound location. Frequently, after skin sutures are removed, adhesive wound closure strips are applied across the wound to give additional support as it continues to heal. The removal of sutures may be done by the primary care provider or by the nurse with a medical order.

EQUIPMENT

- Suture removal kit or forceps and scissors
- Gauze
- Wound cleansing agent, according to facility policy
- Clean disposable gloves
- Additional PPE, as indicated
- Adhesive wound closure strips
- Skin protectant wipes

ASSESSMENT GUIDELINES

- Inspect the surgical incision and the surrounding tissue. Assess the appearance of the wound for the approximation of wound edges, the color of the wound and surrounding area, presence of wound drainage noting color, volume, and odor, and for signs of dehiscence.
- Note the stage of the healing process and characteristics of any drainage.
- Assess the surrounding skin for color, temperature, and the presence of edema, maceration, or ecchymosis.

NURSING DIAGNOSES

- Anxiety
- Delayed Surgical Recovery
- Acute Pain
- Impaired Skin Integrity
- Deficient Knowledge

OUTCOME IDENTIFICATION AND PLANNING

Expected outcomes may include:
- Patient's sutures are removed without contaminating the incisional area, without causing trauma to the wound, and without causing the patient to experience pain or discomfort.
- Patient remains free of complications that would delay recovery.
- Patient verbalizes an understanding of the procedure.

IMPLEMENTATION

ACTION	RATIONALE
1. Review the medical orders for suture removal.	Reviewing the order and plan of care validates the correct patient and correct procedure.
2. Gather the necessary supplies and bring to the bedside stand or overbed table.	Preparation promotes efficient time management and an organized approach to the task. Bringing everything to the bedside conserves time and energy. Arranging items nearby is convenient, saves time, and avoids unnecessary stretching and twisting of muscles on the part of the nurse.
3. Perform hand hygiene and put on PPE, if indicated.	Hand hygiene and PPE prevent the spread of microorganisms. PPE is required based on transmission precautions.
4. Identify the patient.	Identifying the patient ensures that the right patient receives the intervention and helps prevent errors.
5. Close curtains around bed and close the door to room, if possible. Explain what you are going to do and why you are going to do it to the patient. Describe the sensation of suture removal as a pulling or slightly uncomfortable experience.	This ensures the patient's privacy. Explanation relieves anxiety and facilitates cooperation.
6. Assess the patient for possible need for nonpharmacologic pain-reducing interventions or analgesic medication before beginning the procedure. Administer appropriate prescribed analgesic. Allow sufficient time for analgesic to achieve its effectiveness before beginning the procedure.	Pain is a subjective experience influenced by past experience. Wound care and dressing changes may cause pain for some patients.

ACTION	RATIONALE
7. Place a waste receptacle at a convenient location for use during the procedure.	Having a waste container handy means that the soiled dressing can be discarded easily, without the spread of microorganisms.
8. Adjust bed to comfortable working height, usually elbow height of the caregiver (VISN 8 Patient Safety Center, 2009).	Having the bed at the proper height prevents back and muscle strain.
9. Assist the patient to a comfortable position that provides easy access to the incision area. Use a bath blanket to cover any exposed area other than the incision. Place a waterproof pad under the incision site.	Patient positioning and use of a bath blanket provide for comfort and warmth. Waterproof pad protects underlying surfaces.
10. Put on clean gloves. Carefully and gently remove the soiled dressings. If there is resistance, use a silicone-based adhesive remover to help remove the tape. If any part of the dressing sticks to the underlying skin, use small amounts of sterile saline to help loosen and remove it. Inspect the incision area.	Gloves protect the nurse from handling contaminated dressings. Cautious removal of the dressing is more comfortable for the patient and ensures that any drain present is not removed. A silicone-based adhesive remover allows for the easy, rapid, and painless removal without the associated problems of skin stripping (Rudoni, 2008; Stephen-Haynes, 2008). Sterile saline moistens the dressing for easier removal and minimizes damage and pain.
11. Clean the incision using the wound cleanser and gauze, according to facility policies and procedures.	Incision cleaning prevents the spread of microorganisms and contamination of the wound.
12. Using forceps, grasp the knot of the first suture and gently lift the knot up off the skin.	Raising the suture knot prevents accidental injury to the wound or skin when cutting.
13. Using the scissors, cut one side of the suture below the knot, close to the skin. Grasp the knot with the forceps and pull the cut suture through	Pulling the cut suture through the skin helps reduce the risk for contamination of the incision area and resulting infection.

ACTION	RATIONALE

the skin (FIGURE 1). **Avoid pulling the visible portion of the suture through the underlying tissue.**

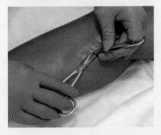

FIGURE 1 Using gloved hands to pull up on a suture with forceps and cutting the suture with sterile scissors.

14. Remove every other suture to be sure the wound edges are healed. If they are, remove the remaining sutures as ordered. Dispose of sutures according to facility policy.

Removing every other suture allows for inspection of the wound, while leaving adequate suture in place to promote continued healing if the edges are not totally approximated. Follow Standard Precautions in disposing of sutures.

15. If wound closure strips are to be applied, apply skin protectant to the skin around incision. **Do not apply to incision.** Apply adhesive closure strips. Take care to handle the strips by the paper backing.

Skin protectant helps adherence of closure strips and prevents skin irritation. Adhesive wound closure strips provide additional support to the wound as it continues to heal. Handling by the paper backing avoids contamination.

16. Reapply the dressing, depending on the medical orders and facility policy.

A new dressing protects the wound. Some policies advise leaving the area uncovered.

17. Remove gloves and discard. Remove all remaining equipment; place the patient in a comfortable position, with side rails up and bed in the lowest position.

Proper removal of gloves prevents spread of microorganisms. Proper patient and bed positioning promotes safety and comfort.

18. Remove additional PPE, if used. Perform hand hygiene.

Removing PPE properly reduces the risk for infection transmission and contamination of other items. Hand hygiene prevents the spread of microorganisms.

ACTION	RATIONALE
19. Assess all wounds every shift. More frequent checks may be needed if the wound is more complex.	Checking drain ensures proper functioning and early detection of problems. Checking dressings ensures the assessment of changes in patient condition and timely intervention to prevent complications.

EVALUATION

- Patient exhibits an incision area that is clean, dry, and intact without sutures.
- Patient's incision area is free of trauma and infection.
- Patient verbalizes little to no pain or discomfort during suture removal.
- Patient verbalizes an understanding of the procedure.

DOCUMENTATION

- Document the location of the incision and the assessment of the site. Include the appearance of the surrounding skin. Document cleansing of the site and suture removal. Record any skin care and the dressing applied, if appropriate. Note pertinent patient and family education and any patient reaction to this procedure, including patient's pain level and effectiveness of nonpharmacologic interventions or analgesia if administered.

GENERAL CONSIDERATIONS

- Encourage the patient to splint chest and abdominal wounds during activity, such as changing position, ambulation, coughing, and sneezing. This provides increased support for the skin and underlying tissues and can decrease discomfort.

Skill · 162 Assessing Body Temperature

Body temperature is the difference between the amount of heat produced by the body and the amount of heat lost to the environment, measured in degrees. To obtain an accurate measurement, the nurse must choose an appropriate site, the correct equipment, and the appropriate tool based on the patient's condition. If a temperature reading is obtained from a site other than the oral route, document the site used along with the measurement. If no site is listed with the documentation, it is generally assumed to be the oral route.

EQUIPMENT

- Digital, glass, or electronic thermometer, appropriate for site to be used
- Disposable probe covers
- Water-soluble lubricant for rectal temperature measurement
- Nonsterile gloves, if appropriate
- Additional PPE, as indicated
- Toilet tissue, if needed
- Pencil or pen, paper or flow sheet, computerized record

ASSESSMENT GUIDELINES

- Assess the patient to ensure that his or her cognitive functioning is intact and whether the patient can close his or her lips around the thermometer.
- Determine if the patient has a disease of the oral cavity; earache, significant ear drainage or a scarred tympanic membrane; scar tissue, open lesions or abrasions in the temporal areas.
- Determine if the patient has had surgery of the nose, mouth, or rectum; or has diarrhea or disease of the rectum.
- Ask the patient if he or she has recently smoked, has been chewing gum, or was eating and drinking.
- Check the patient's most recent platelet count.
- When taking a temporal artery temperature, assess for head coverings. Anything covering the area, such as a hat, hair, wigs, or bandages, would insulate the area, resulting in falsely high readings. Measure only the side of the head exposed to the environment. Do not measure temporal artery temperature over scar tissue, open lesions, or abrasions.

NURSING DIAGNOSES

- Risk for Trauma
- Hyperthermia
- Hypothermia
- Risk for Imbalanced Body Temperature
- Ineffective Thermoregulation

OUTCOME IDENTIFICATION AND PLANNING

Expected outcomes may include:
- The patient's temperature is assessed accurately without injury
- Patient experiences minimal discomfort.

IMPLEMENTATION

ACTION	RATIONALE
1. Check medical order or nursing care plan for frequency of measurement and route.	Assessment and measurement of vital signs at appropriate intervals provide important data

ACTION	RATIONALE
More frequent temperature measurement may be appropriate based on nursing judgment.	about the patient's health status. Bringing everything to the bedside conserves time and energy. Arranging items nearby is convenient, saves time, and avoids unnecessary stretching and twisting of muscles on the part of the nurse.
Bring necessary equipment to the bedside stand or overbed table.	
2. Perform hand hygiene and put on PPE, if indicated.	Hand hygiene and PPE prevent the spread of microorganisms. PPE is required based on transmission precautions.
3. Identify the patient.	Identifying the patient ensures the right patient receives the intervention and helps prevent errors.
4. Close curtains around bed and close the door to the room if possible. Discuss procedure with patient and assess the patient's ability to assist with the procedure.	This ensures the patient's privacy. Explanation relieves anxiety and facilitates cooperation. Dialogue encourages patient participation and allows for individualized nursing care.
5. Ensure the electronic or digital thermometer is in working condition.	Improperly functioning thermometer may not give an accurate reading.
6. Put on gloves if appropriate or indicated.	Gloves prevent contact with blood and body fluids. Gloves are usually not required for an oral, axillary, or tympanic temperature measurement, unless contact with blood or body fluids is anticipated. Gloves should be worn for rectal temperature measurement.
7. Select the appropriate site based on previous assessment data.	This ensures safety and accuracy of measurement.
8. Follow the steps as outlined below for the appropriate type of thermometer.	

ACTION	RATIONALE

9. When measurement is completed, remove gloves, if worn. Remove additional PPE, if used. Perform hand hygiene.

Removing PPE properly reduces the risk for infection transmission and contamination of other items. Hand hygiene prevents the spread of microorganisms.

Measuring a Tympanic Membrane Temperature

10. If necessary, push the "on" button and wait for the "ready" signal on the unit.

For proper function, the thermometer must be turned on and warmed up.

11. Attach tympanic probe covering.

Use of the covering deters the spread of microorganisms.

12. **Insert the probe snugly into the external ear using gentle but firm pressure, angling the thermometer toward the patient's jaw line. Pull pinna up and back to straighten the ear canal in an adult (FIGURE 1).**

If the probe is not inserted correctly, the patient's temperature may be noted as lower than normal.

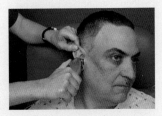

FIGURE 1 Thermometer in patient's ear canal with pinna pulled up and back.

13. Activate the unit by pushing the trigger button. The reading is immediate (usually within 2 seconds). Note the reading.

The digital thermometer must be activated to record the temperature.

14. Discard the probe cover in an appropriate receptacle by pushing the probe-release button or use rim of cover to remove from probe. Replace the thermometer in its charger, if necessary.

Discarding the probe cover ensures that it will not be reused accidentally on another patient. Proper disposal prevents the spread of microorganisms. If necessary, the thermometer should stay on the charger so that it is ready to use at all times.

ACTION	RATIONALE

Assessing Oral Temperature

10. Remove the electronic unit from the charging unit, and remove the probe from within the recording unit.

Electronic unit must be taken into the patient's room to assess the patient's temperature. On some models, by removing the probe the machine is already turned on.

11. Cover thermometer probe with disposable probe cover and slide it on until it snaps into place.

Using a cover prevents contamination of the thermometer probe.

12. **Place the probe beneath the patient's tongue in the posterior sublingual pocket (FIGURE 2). Ask the patient to close his or her lips around the probe.**

When the probe rests deep in the posterior sublingual pocket, it is in contact with blood vessels lying close to the surface.

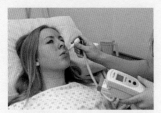

FIGURE 2 Inserting thermometer under the tongue in the posterior sublingual pocket.

13. **Continue to hold the probe until you hear a beep. Note the temperature reading.**

If left unsupported, the weight of the probe tends to pull it away from the correct location. The signal indicates the measurement is completed. The electronic thermometer provides a digital display of the measured temperature.

14. Remove the probe from the patient's mouth. Dispose of the probe cover by holding the probe over an appropriate receptacle and pressing the probe release button.

Disposing of the probe cover ensures that it will not be reused accidentally on another patient. Proper disposal prevents spread of microorganisms.

15. Return the thermometer probe to the storage place within the unit. Return the

The thermometer needs to be recharged for future use. If necessary, the thermometer should

ACTION	RATIONALE
electronic unit to the charging unit, if appropriate.	stay on the charger so that it is ready to use at all times.

Assessing Rectal Temperature

ACTION	RATIONALE
10. Adjust bed to comfortable working height, usually elbow height of the care giver (VISN 8 Patient Safety Center, 2009). Put on nonsterile gloves.	Having the bed at the proper height prevents back and muscle strain. Gloves prevent contact with contaminants and body fluids.
11. Assist the patient to a side-lying position. Pull back the covers sufficiently to expose only the buttocks.	The side-lying position allows the nurse to visualize the buttocks. Exposing only the buttocks keeps the patient warm and maintains his or her dignity.
12. Remove the rectal probe from within the recording unit of the electronic thermometer. Cover the probe with a disposable probe cover and slide it into place until it snaps in place.	Using a cover prevents contamination of the thermometer.
13. **Lubricate about 1 inch of the probe with a water-soluble lubricant.**	Lubrication reduces friction and facilitates insertion, minimizing the risk of irritation or injury to the rectal mucous membranes.
14. Reassure the patient. Separate the buttocks until the anal sphincter is clearly visible.	If not placed directly into the anal opening, the thermometer probe may injure adjacent tissue or cause discomfort.
15. **Insert the thermometer probe into the anus about 1.5 inches in an adult or 1 inch in a child (FIGURE 3).**	Depth of insertion must be adjusted based on the patient's age. Rectal temperatures are not normally taken in an infant, but may be indicated. Refer to the Special Considerations section at the end of the skill.
16. Hold the probe in place until you hear a beep, then carefully remove the probe. Note the temperature reading on the display.	If left unsupported, movement of the probe in the rectum could cause injury and/or discomfort. The signal indicates the measurement is completed. The electronic thermometer provides a digital display of the measured temperature.

ACTION

RATIONALE

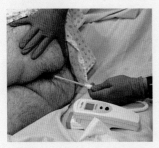

FIGURE 3 Inserting thermometer into the anus.

17. Dispose of the probe cover by holding the probe over an appropriate waste receptacle and pressing the release button.

Proper probe cover disposal reduces risk of microorganism transmission.

18. Using toilet tissue, wipe the anus of any feces or excess lubricant. Dispose of the toilet tissue. Remove gloves and discard them.

Wiping promotes cleanliness. Disposing of the toilet tissue avoids transmission of microorganisms.

19. Cover the patient and help him or her to a position of comfort.

Ensures patient comfort.

20. Place the bed in the lowest position; elevate rails as needed.

These actions provide for the patient's safety.

21. Return the thermometer to the charging unit.

The thermometer needs to be recharged for future use.

Assessing Axillary Temperature

10. Move the patient's clothing to expose only the axilla.

The axilla must be exposed for placement of the thermometer. Exposing only the axilla keeps the patient warm and maintains his or her dignity.

11. Remove the probe from the recording unit of the electronic thermometer. Place a disposable probe cover on by sliding it on and snapping it securely.

Using a cover prevents contamination of the thermometer probe.

ACTION	RATIONALE
12. **Place the end of the probe in the center of the axilla (FIGURE 4). Have the patient bring the arm down and close to the body.**	The deepest area of the axilla provides the most accurate measurement; surrounding the bulb with skin surface provides a more reliable measurement.

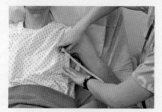

FIGURE 4 Placing thermometer in center of axilla.

ACTION	RATIONALE
13. Hold the probe in place until you hear a beep, and then carefully remove the probe. Note the temperature reading.	Axillary thermometers must be held in place to obtain an accurate temperature.
14. Cover the patient and help him or her to a position of comfort.	Ensures patient comfort.
15. Dispose of the probe cover by holding the probe over an appropriate waste receptacle and pushing the release button.	Discarding the probe cover ensures that it will not be reused accidentally on another patient.
16. Place the bed in the lowest position and elevate rails as needed. Leave the patient clean and comfortable.	Low bed position and elevated side rails provide for patient safety.
17. Return the electronic thermometer to the charging unit.	Thermometer needs to be recharged for future use.

Assessing Temporal Artery Temperature

ACTION	RATIONALE
10. Brush the patient's hair aside if covering the temporal artery area.	Anything covering the area, such as a hat, hair, wigs, or bandages, would insulate the area, resulting in falsely high readings. Measure only the side of the head exposed to the environment.

ACTION	RATIONALE
11. Apply a probe cover.	Using a cover prevents contamination of the thermometer probe.
12. Hold the thermometer like a remote control device, with your thumb on the red 'ON' button. Place the probe flush on the center of the forehead, with the body of the instrument sideways (not straight up and down), so it is not in the patient's face.	Allows for easy use of the device and reading of the display. Holding the instrument straight up and down could be intimidating for the patient, particularly young patients and/or those with alterations in mental status.
13. Depress the 'ON' button. Keep the button depressed throughout the measurement.	
14. Slowly slide the probe straight across the forehead, midline, to the hair line (FIGURE 5). The thermometer will click; fast clicking indicates a rise to a higher temperature, slow clicking indicates the instrument is still scanning, but not finding any higher temperature.	Midline on the forehead, the temporal artery is less than two millimeters below the skin; whereas at the side of the face, the temporal artery is much deeper. Measuring there would result in falsely low readings.

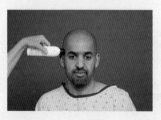

FIGURE 5 Sliding the probe across the forehead to the hairline.

15. Brush hair aside if covering ear, exposing the area of the neck under the ear lobe. Lift the probe from the forehead and touch on the neck just behind the ear lobe, in the depression just below the mastoid (FIGURE 6).	Sweat causes evaporative cooling of the skin on the forehead, possibly leading to a falsely low reading. During diaphoresis, the area on the head behind the ear lobe exhibits high blood flow necessary for the arterial measurement; it is a double check for the thermometer.

ACTION	RATIONALE

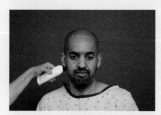

FIGURE 6 Touching the probe behind the ear.

16. Release the button and read the thermometer measurement.

17. Hold the thermometer over a waste receptacle. Gently push the probe cover with your thumb against the proximal edge to dispose of probe cover.

Discarding the probe cover ensures that it will not be reused accidentally on another patient.

18. Instrument will automatically turn off in 30 seconds, or press and release the power button.

Turns thermometer off.

EVALUATION
- Patient's temperature is assessed accurately without injury.
- Patient experiences minimal discomfort.

DOCUMENTATION
- Record temperature on paper, flow sheet, or computerized record. Report abnormal findings to the appropriate person. Identify the site of assessment if other than oral.

GENERAL CONSIDERATIONS
- When using a tympanic thermometer, make sure to insert the probe into the ear canal sufficiently tightly to seal the opening to ensure an accurate reading.
- Nonmercury glass thermometers used for oral readings commonly have long, thin bulbs. Those for rectal readings have a blunt bulb to prevent injury. See the accompanying Skill Variation for information on assessing temperature with a nonmercury glass thermometer.
- Axillary temperatures are generally about one degree less than oral temperatures; rectal temperatures are generally about one degree higher.

- If the patient smoked, chewed gum, or consumed hot or cold food or fluids, 30 minutes before taking an oral temperature to allow the oral tissues to return to baseline temperature.
- Nasal oxygen is not thought to affect oral temperature readings. Oral temperatures should not be assessed for patients receiving oxygen by mask. Removal of the mask for the time period required for assessment could result in a serious drop in the patient's blood oxygen level.
- If the patient's axilla has been recently washed, wait 15 to 30 minutes before taking an axillary temperature to allow the skin to return to baseline temperature.
- A dirty probe lens and cone on the temporal artery thermometer can cause a falsely low reading. If the lens is not shiny in appearance, clean the lens and cone with an alcohol prep or swab moistened in alcohol.

Skill · 163 Applying and Caring for a Patient Using a TENS Unit

Transcutaneous electrical nerve stimulation (TENS) is a noninvasive technique for providing pain relief that involves the electrical stimulation of large-diameter fibers to inhibit the transmission of painful impulses carried over small-diameter fibers. The TENS unit consists of a battery-powered portable unit, lead wires, and cutaneous electrode pads that are applied to or around the painful area. It is most beneficial when used to treat pain that is localized, and requires an order from the primary healthcare provider. The TENS unit may be applied intermittently throughout the day or worn for extended periods.

EQUIPMENT
- TENS unit
- Electrodes
- Electrode gel (if electrodes are not pregelled)
- Tape (if electrodes are not self-adhesive)
- Pain assessment tool and/or scale
- Skin cleanser and water
- Towel and washcloth
- PPE, as indicated

ASSESSMENT GUIDELINES
- Review the patient's medical record and plan of care for specific instructions related to TENS therapy, including the order and conditions indicating the need for therapy.
- Review the patient's history for conditions that might contraindicate therapy, such as pacemaker insertion, cardiac monitoring, or electrocardiography.

- Determine the location of electrode placement in consultation with the ordering practitioner and on the patient's report of pain.
- Assess the patient's understanding of TENS therapy and the rationale for its use.
- Inspect the skin of the area designated for electrode placement for irritation, redness, or breakdown.
- Assess the patient's pain and level of discomfort using an appropriate assessment tool. Assess the characteristics of any pain. Assess for other symptoms that often occur with the pain, such as headache or restlessness. Ask the patient what interventions have and have not been successful in the past to promote comfort and relieve pain.
- Assess the patient's vital signs.
- Check the patient's medication administration record for the time an analgesic was last administered.
- Assess the patient's response to a particular intervention to evaluate the effectiveness and presence of adverse effect.
- Check the unit to ensure proper functioning and review the manufacturer's instructions for use.

NURSING DIAGNOSES
- Acute Pain
- Risk for Impaired Skin Integrity
- Chronic Pain
- Deficient Knowledge
- Anxiety
- Ineffective Coping
- Risk for Injury

OUTCOME IDENTIFICATION AND PLANNING
Expected outcomes may include:
- Patient verbalizes decreased discomfort and pain, without experiencing any injury or skin irritation or breakdown.
- Patient displays decreased anxiety, improved coping skills, and an understanding of the therapy and the reason for its use.

IMPLEMENTATION

ACTION

1. Perform hand hygiene and put on PPE, if indicated.

RATIONALE

Hand hygiene and PPE prevent the spread of microorganisms. PPE is required based on transmission precautions.

ACTION	RATIONALE
2. Identify the patient.	Identifying the patient ensures the right patient receives the intervention and helps prevent errors.
3. Show the patient the device, and explain the function of the device and the reason for its use.	Explanation encourages patient understanding and cooperation and reduces apprehension.
4. Assess the patient's pain, using an appropriate assessment tool and measurement scale.	Accurate assessment is necessary to guide treatment/relief interventions and evaluate the effectiveness of pain control measures.
5. Inspect the area where the electrodes are to be placed. Clean the patient's skin, using skin cleanser and water. Dry the area thoroughly.	Inspection ensures that the electrodes will be applied to intact skin. Cleaning and drying help ensure that electrodes will adhere.
6. Remove the adhesive backing from the electrodes and apply them to the specified location. **If the electrodes are not pregelled, apply a small amount of electrode gel to the bottom of each electrode.** If the electrodes are not self-adhering, tape them in place.	Application to the proper location enhances the success of the therapy. Gel is necessary to promote conduction of the electrical current.
7. **Check the placement of the electrodes; leave at least a 2-inch (5 cm) space (about the width of one electrode) between them.**	Proper spacing is necessary to reduce the risk of burns due to the proximity of the electrodes.
8. **Check the controls on the TENS unit to make sure that they are off.** Connect the wires to the electrodes (if not already attached) and plug them into the unit.	Having controls off prevents flow of electricity. This connection completes the electrical circuit necessary to stimulate the nerve fibers.
9. Turn on the unit and adjust the intensity setting to the	Using the lowest setting at first introduces the patient to the

ACTION	RATIONALE
lowest intensity and determine if the patient can feel a tingling, burning, or buzzing sensation. Then adjust the intensity to the prescribed amount or the setting most comfortable for the patient. Secure the unit to the patient.	sensations. Adjusting the intensity is necessary to provide the proper amount of stimulation.
10. Set the pulse width (duration of each pulsation) as indicated or recommended.	The pulse width determines the depth and width of the stimulation.
11. Assess the patient's pain level during therapy.	Pain assessment helps evaluate the effectiveness of therapy.
a. If intermittent use is ordered, turn off the unit after the specified duration of treatment and remove the electrodes. Provide skin care to the area.	TENS therapy can be ordered for intermittent or continuous use. Skin care reduces the risk for irritation and breakdown.
b. If continuous therapy is ordered, periodically remove the electrodes from the skin (after turning off the unit) to inspect the area and clean the skin, according to facility policy. Reapply electrodes and continue therapy. Change electrodes according to manufacturer's directions.	Periodic removal of electrodes allows for skin assessment. Skin care reduces the risk for irritation and breakdown. Reapplication ensures continued therapy.
12. When therapy is discontinued, turn the unit off and remove the electrodes. Clean the patient's skin. Clean the unit and replace the batteries.	Turning the unit off and removing electrodes when therapy is discontinued reduces the risk of injury to the patient. Cleaning the unit and replacing the batteries ensure that the unit is ready for future use.
13. Remove PPE, if used. Perform hand hygiene.	Removing PPE properly reduces the risk for infection transmission and contamination of other items. Hand hygiene prevents transmission of microorganisms.

EVALUATION

- Patient verbalizes pain relief.
- Patient remains free of signs and symptoms of skin irritation and breakdown and injury.
- Patient reports decreased anxiety and increased ability to cope with pain.
- Patient verbalizes information related to the functioning of the unit and reasons for its use.

DOCUMENTATION

- Document the date and time of application. Document the initial pain assessment and skin assessment. Record electrode placement location, intensity and pulse width, and therapy duration. Document pain assessments during therapy and patient's response. Record time of removal or therapy discontinuation.

GENERAL CONSIDERATIONS

- Never place electrodes over the carotid sinus nerves, laryngeal or pharyngeal muscles, the eyes, or the uterus of a pregnant woman.
- Do not use TENS when the etiology of the pain is unknown because it may mask a new pathology.
- Whenever electrodes are being repositioned or removed, first turn off the unit.

Skill · 164   Providing Tracheostomy Care

The nurse is responsible for either replacing a disposable inner cannula or cleaning a nondisposable inner cannula. The inner cannula requires replacement or cleaning to prevent accumulation of secretions that can interfere with respiration and occlude the airway. Because soiled tracheostomy dressings place the patient at risk for the development of skin breakdown and infection, regularly change dressings and tracheostomy collar or ties. Use gauze dressings that are not filled with cotton to prevent aspiration of foreign bodies (e.g., lint or cotton fibers) into the trachea. Clean the skin around a tracheostomy to prevent buildup of dried secretions and skin breakdown. Exercise care when changing the tracheostomy collar or ties to prevent accidental decannulation or expulsion of the tube. Have an assistant hold the tube in place during the changing of a collar. When changing a tracheostomy tie, keep the soiled tie in place until a clean one is securely attached. Agency policy and patient condition determine specific procedures and schedules, but a newly inserted tracheostomy may require attention every 1 to 2 hours. Because the respiratory tract is sterile and the tracheostomy provides a direct opening, meticulous care using aseptic technique is necessary.

EQUIPMENT

- Disposable gloves
- Sterile gloves
- Goggles and mask or face shield
- Additional PPE, as indicated
- Sterile normal saline
- Sterile cup or basin
- Sterile cotton-tipped applicators
- Sterile gauze sponges
- Disposable inner cannula, appropriate size for patient
- Sterile suction catheter and glove set
- Commercially prepared tracheostomy or drain dressing
- Commercially prepared tracheostomy holder
- Plastic disposal bag
- Additional nurse

ASSESSMENT GUIDELINES

- Assess for signs and symptoms of the need to perform tracheostomy care, which include soiled dressings and holder or ties, secretions in the tracheostomy tube, and diminished airflow through the tracheostomy, or in accordance with facility policy.
- Assess insertion site for any redness or purulent drainage; if present, these may signify an infection.
- Assess patient for pain. If tracheostomy is new, pain medication may be needed before performing tracheostomy care.
- Assess lung sounds and oxygen saturation levels. Lung sounds should be equal in all lobes, with an oxygen saturation level greater than 93%. If tracheostomy is dislodged, lung sounds and oxygen saturation level will diminish.
- Inspect the area on the posterior portion of the neck for any skin breakdown that may result from irritation or pressure from tracheostomy holder or ties.

NURSING DIAGNOSES

- Impaired Skin Integrity
- Risk for Infection
- Risk for Aspiration
- Ineffective Airway Clearance

OUTCOME IDENTIFICATION AND PLANNING

Expected outcomes may include:
- Patient will exhibit a tracheostomy tube and site free from drainage, secretions, and skin irritation or breakdown.
- Patient's oxygen saturation levels will be within acceptable parameters.
- Patient will have no evidence of respiratory distress.

IMPLEMENTATION

ACTION	RATIONALE
1. Bring necessary equipment to the bedside stand or over-bed table.	Bringing everything to the bedside conserves time and energy. Arranging items nearby is convenient, saves time, and avoids unnecessary stretching and twisting of muscles on the part of the nurse.
2. Perform hand hygiene and put on PPE, if indicated.	Hand hygiene and PPE prevent the spread of microorganisms. PPE is required based on transmission precautions.
3. Identify the patient.	Identifying the patient ensures the right patient receives the intervention and helps prevent errors.
4. Close curtains around bed and close the door to the room, if possible.	This ensures the patient's privacy.
5. Determine the need for tracheostomy care. **Assess patient's pain and administer pain medication, if indicated.**	If the tracheostomy is new, pain medication may be needed before performing tracheostomy care.
6. Explain what you are going to do and the reason to the patient, even if the patient does not appear to be alert. Reassure the patient you will interrupt the procedure if he or she indicates respiratory difficulty.	Explanation alleviates fears. Even if the patient appears unconscious, the nurse should explain what is happening. Any procedure that compromises respiration is frightening for the patient.
7. Adjust bed to comfortable working position, usually elbow height of the caregiver (VISN 8 Patient Safety Center, 2009). Lower side rail closest to you. **If the patient is conscious, place him or her in a semi-Fowler's position. If patient is**	Having the bed at the proper height prevents back and muscle strain. A sitting position helps the patient to cough and makes breathing easier. Gravity also facilitates catheter insertion. The lateral position prevents the airway from becoming obstructed and promotes drainage of secretions.

ACTION	RATIONALE
unconscious, place him or her in the lateral position, facing you. Move the overbed table close to your work area and raise it to waist height. Place a trash receptacle within easy reach of work area.	The overbed table provides a work surface and maintains sterility of objects on it. Trash receptacle within reach prevents reaching over sterile field or turning back to field to dispose of trash.
8. Put on face shield or goggles and mask. Suction tracheostomy, if necessary. If tracheostomy has just been suctioned, remove soiled site dressing and discard before removal of gloves used to perform suctioning.	Personnel protective equipment prevents contact with contaminants. Suctioning removes secretions to prevent occluding outer cannula while the inner cannula is removed.

Cleaning the Tracheostomy: Disposable Inner Cannula

(See the accompanying Skill Variation for steps for cleaning a nondisposable inner cannula.)

ACTION	RATIONALE
9. Carefully open the package with the new disposable inner cannula, taking care not to contaminate the cannula or the inside of the package. Carefully open the package with the sterile cotton-tipped applicators, taking care not to contaminate them. Open sterile cup or basin and fill ½ inch deep with saline. Open the plastic disposable bag and place within reach on the work surface.	Inner cannula must remain sterile. Saline and applicators will be used to clean the tracheostomy site. Plastic disposable bag will be used to discard removed inner cannula.
10. Put on disposable gloves.	Gloves protect against exposure to blood and body fluids.
11. Remove the oxygen source if one is present. Stabilize the outer cannula and faceplate of the tracheostomy with	Stabilizing baseplate prevents trauma to, and pain from, stoma. Releasing the lock permits removal of the inner cannula.

ACTION	RATIONALE

your nondominant hand. Grasp the locking mechanism of the inner cannula with your dominant hand. Press the tabs and release the lock (FIGURE 1). Gently remove inner cannula and place in disposal bag. If not already removed, remove site dressing and dispose of in the trash.

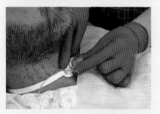

FIGURE 1 Releasing lock on inner cannula.

12. Discard gloves and put on sterile gloves. Pick up the new inner cannula with your dominant hand; stabilize the faceplate with our nondominant hand and gently insert the new inner cannula into the outer cannula. Press the tabs to allow the lock to grab the outer cannula (FIGURE 2). Reapply oxygen source, if needed.

Sterile gloves are necessary to prevent contamination of the new inner cannula. Locking to outer cannula secures the inner cannula in place. Maintains oxygen supply to the patient.

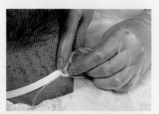

FIGURE 2 Locking new inner cannula in place.

ACTION	RATIONALE

Applying Clean Dressing and Holder
(See accompanying Skill Variations for steps for an alternate site dressing if a commercially prepared sponge is not available and to secure a tracheostomy with a tracheostomy ties/tape instead of a collar.)

13. Remove oxygen source, if necessary. Dip cotton-tipped applicator or gauze sponge in cup or basin with sterile saline and clean stoma under faceplate. **Use each applicator or sponge only once, moving from stoma site outward.**

Saline is nonirritating to tissue. Cleansing from stoma outward and using each applicator only once promotes aseptic technique.

14. Pat skin gently with dry 4 × 4 gauze sponge.

Gauze removes excess moisture.

15. Slide commercially prepared tracheostomy dressing or prefolded non–cotton-filled 4 × 4-dressing under the faceplate.

Lint or fiber from a cut cotton-filled gauze pad can be aspirated into the trachea, causing respiratory distress, or can embed in the stoma and cause irritation or infection.

16. Change the tracheostomy holder:

a. **Obtain the assistance of a second individual to hold the tracheostomy tube in place while the old collar is removed and the new collar is placed.**

Holding the tracheostomy tube in place ensures that the tracheostomy will not inadvertently be expelled if the patient coughs or moves.

Doing so provides attachment for one side of the faceplate.

b. Open the package for the new tracheostomy collar.

Allows access to the new collar.

c. Both nurses should put on clean gloves.

Gloves prevent contact with blood, body fluids, and contaminants.

d. One nurse holds the faceplate while the other pulls up the Velcro tabs. Gently remove the collar.

Holding the tracheostomy tube in place ensures that the tracheostomy will not inadvertently be expelled if the patient

ACTION	RATIONALE

coughs or moves. Pulling up the Velcro tabs loosens the collar.

e. The first nurse continues to hold the tracheostomy faceplate.

Prevents accidental extubation.

f. The other nurse places the collar around the patient's neck and inserts first one tab, then the other, into the openings on the faceplate and secures the Velcro tabs on the tracheostomy holder (FIGURE 3).

Securing the Velcro tabs holds the tracheostomy in place and prevents accidental expulsion of the tracheostomy tube.

g. Check the fit of the tracheostomy collar. You should be able to fit one finger between the neck and the collar. Check to make sure that the patient can flex neck comfortably. Reapply oxygen source, if necessary.

Allowing one finger-breadth under collar permits neck flexion that is comfortable and ensures that collar will not compromise circulation to the area. Maintains oxygen supply to the patient.

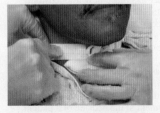

FIGURE 3 Securing tabs on tracheostomy holder.

17. Remove gloves. Assist patient to a comfortable position. Raise the bed rail and place the bed in the lowest position.

Removing PPE properly reduces the risk for infection transmission and contamination of other items. Ensures patient comfort. Proper positioning with raised side rails and proper bed height provide for patient comfort and safety.

18. Remove face shield or goggles and mask. Remove additional PPE, if used. Perform hand hygiene.

Removing PPE properly reduces the risk for infection transmission and contamination of other items. Hand hygiene prevents the spread of microorganisms.

ACTION	RATIONALE
19. Reassess patient's respiratory status, including respiratory rate, effort, oxygen saturation, and lung sounds.	Assessments determine the effectiveness of interventions and the presence of complications.

EVALUATION

- Patient exhibits a tracheostomy tube and site that are free from drainage, secretions, and skin irritation or breakdown.
- Patient's oxygen saturation level is within acceptable parameters.
- Patient is without evidence of respiratory distress.
- Patient verbalizes that site is free of pain and exhibits no evidence of skin breakdown on the posterior portion of the neck.

DOCUMENTATION

- Document pre- and postassessments, including site assessment, presence of pain, lung sounds, and oxygen saturation levels. Document presence of skin breakdown that may result from irritation or pressure from the tracheostomy collar. Document care given.

GENERAL CONSIDERATIONS

- One nurse working alone should always place new tracheostomy ties in place before removing old ties to prevent accidental extubation of the tracheostomy. If it is necessary to remove old ties first, obtain the assistance of a second person to hold the tracheostomy tube in place while the old tie is removed and the new tie is replaced.
- Emergency equipment should be easily accessible at the bedside. Keep a bag-valve mask, oxygen, the obturator from the current tracheostomy, spare tracheostomy of the same size, spare tracheostomy one size smaller, and suction equipment at the bedside of a patient with an endotracheal tube at all times.
- If the patient is currently using a tracheostomy without a cuff, keep a spare tracheostomy of the same size with a cuff at the bedside for emergency use.

Skill Variation	Cleaning a Nondisposable Inner Cannula

Some tracheostomies use nondisposable inner cannulas, requiring the nurse to clean the inner cannula. Aseptic technique is maintained during the procedure. Additional equipment includes the following: sterile tracheostomy cleaning

(continued on page 867)

Cleaning a Nondisposable Inner Cannula *continued*

kit, if available, or three sterile basins, sterile brush/pipe cleaners, and sterile cleaning solutions (hydrogen peroxide and normal saline solution).

1. Bring necessary equipment to the bedside stand or overbed table.

2. Perform hand hygiene and put on PPE, if indicated.

3. Identify the patient.

4. Close curtains around bed and close the door to the room, if possible.

5. Determine the need for tracheostomy care. Assess the patient's pain and administer pain medication, if indicated. Explain what you are going to do and the reason for doing it to the patient, even if the patient does not appear to be alert. Reassure the patient that you will interrupt the procedure if he or she indicates respiratory difficulty.

6. Adjust the bed to a comfortable working position, usually elbow height of the caregiver (VISN 8 Patient Safety Center, 2009). Lower the side rail closest to you. **If the patient is conscious, place him or her in a semi-Fowler's position. If the patient is unconscious, place him or her in the lateral position, facing you.** Move the overbed table close to your work area and raise it to waist height. Place a trash receptacle within easy reach of the work area.

7. Put on face shield or goggles and mask. Suction tracheostomy, if necessary. If tracheostomy has just been suctioned, remove soiled site dressing and discard before removal of gloves used to perform suctioning.

8. Prepare supplies: Open the tracheostomy care kit and separate basins, touching only the edges. If kit is not available, open three sterile basins. Fill one basin ½ inch deep with hydrogen peroxide or half hydrogen peroxide and half saline, based on facility policy. Fill other two basins ½ inch with saline. Open sterile brush or pipe cleaners, cotton-tipped applicators, and gauze pads, if they are not already available in the cleaning kit.

9. Put on disposable gloves.

10. Remove the oxygen source if one is present. If not already removed, remove site dressing and dispose of it in the trash. Stabilize the outer cannula and faceplate of the tracheostomy with your nondominant hand. Rotate the inner cannula in

(continued on page 868)

Cleaning a Nondisposable Inner Cannula *continued*

a counterclockwise motion with your dominant hand to release the lock (FIGURE 4).

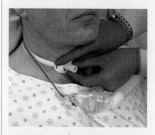

FIGURE 4 Rotating inner cannula while stabilizing outer cannula.

11. Continue to hold the faceplate. Gently remove the inner cannula and carefully drop it in the basin with the hydrogen peroxide. Replace the oxygen source over the outer cannula.

12. Discard gloves and put on sterile gloves. Remove the inner cannula from the soaking solution. Moisten the brush or pipe cleaner in saline and insert into tube, using a back-and-forth motion to clean.

13. Agitate the cannula in saline solution. Remove and it tap against the inner surface of the basin. Place on sterile gauze pad. If secretions have accumulated in the outer cannula during cleaning of inner cannula, suction outer cannula using sterile technique.

14. Stabilize the outer cannula and faceplate with nondominant hand. Replace inner cannula into outer cannula with dominant hand. Turn clockwise and check that the inner cannula is secure (FIGURE 5). Reapply oxygen source, if needed.

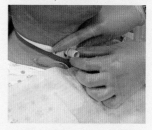

FIGURE 5 Replacing inner cannula.

15. Continue with site care as detailed above.

Skill Variation **Using Alternate Site Dressing When Commercially Prepared Sponge is Not Available**

If a commercially prepared site dressing or drain sponge is not available, do not cut a gauze sponge to use at the tracheostomy site. Cutting the gauze can cause loose fibers, which can become lodged in the stoma, causing irritation or infection. Loose fibers could also be inhaled into the trachea, causing respiratory distress.

1. Identify the patient.

(continued on page 869)

Using Alternate Site Dressing When Commercially Prepared Sponge is Not Available *continued*

2. Determine the need for tracheostomy care. Assess the patient's pain and administer pain medication, if indicated.

3. Explain what you are going to do and the reason for doing it to the patient, even if the patient does not appear to be alert. Reassure the patient that you will interrupt the procedure if he or she indicates respiratory difficulty.

4. Perform hand hygiene.

5. Adjust bed to a comfortable working position. Lower side rail closest to you. If the patient is conscious, place him or her in a semi-Fowler's position. If the patient is unconscious, place him or her in the lateral position, facing you. Move the overbed table close to your work area and raise it to waist height. Place a trash receptacle within easy reach of the work area.

6. Remove oxygen source. Dip cotton-tipped applicator or gauze sponge in second basin with sterile saline and clean stoma under faceplate. Use each applicator or sponge only once, moving from stoma site outward.

7. Pat skin gently with dry 4 × 4 gauze sponge.

8. Fold two gauze sponges on the diagonal, to form triangles. Slide one triangle under the faceplate on each side of the stoma, with the longest side of the triangle against the tracheostomy tube.

Skill Variation   Securing a Tracheostomy With Ties/Tape

A tracheostomy may be secured in place using twill ties or tape. One nurse working alone should always place new tracheostomy ties in place before removing old ties to prevent accidental extubation of the tracheostomy. If it is necessary to remove old ties first, obtain the assistance of a second person to hold the tracheostomy tube in place while the old tie is removed and the new tie is replaced.

1. Bring necessary equipment to the bedside stand or overbed table.

2. Perform hand hygiene and put on PPE, if indicated.

3. Identify the patient.

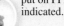

(continued on page 870)

Securing a Tracheostomy With Ties/Tape *continued*

4. Close curtains around bed and close the door to the room, if possible. Determine the need for tracheostomy care. Assess the patient's pain and administer pain medication, if indicated. Explain what you are going to do and the reason for doing it to the patient, even if the patient does not appear to be alert. Reassure the patient that you will interrupt the procedure if he or she indicates respiratory difficulty.

5. Adjust bed to comfortable working position, usually elbow height of the caregiver (VISN 8 Patient Safety Center, 2009). Lower side rail closest to you. **If patient is conscious, place him or her in a semi-Fowler's position. If patient is unconscious, place him or her in the lateral position, facing you.** Move the overbed table close to your work area and raise it to waist height. Place a trash receptacle within easy reach of the work area.

6. Put on clean gloves. If another nurse is assisting, both nurses should put on clean gloves.

7. Cut a piece of the tape twice the length of the neck circumference plus 4 inches. Trim ends of tape on the diagonal.

8. Insert one end of the tape through the faceplate opening alongside the old tie. Pull through until both ends are an even length (FIGURE 6).

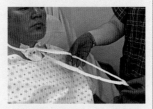

FIGURE 6 Pulling tape through faceplate opening alongside old tie.

9. Slide both ends of the tape under the patient's neck and insert one end through remaining opening on other side of faceplate. Pull snugly and tie ends in double square knot. You should be able to fit one finger between the neck and the ties. Check to make sure the patient can flex his or her neck comfortably.

10. Carefully cut and remove old ties. Reapply oxygen supply, if necessary.

11. Continue with care as detailed above.

Skill · 165   Suctioning the Tracheostomy: Open System

Suctioning through a tracheostomy is indicated to maintain a patent airway. Tracheal suctioning can lead to hypoxemia, cardiac dysrhythmias, trauma, atelectasis, infection, bleeding, and pain. It is imperative to be diligent in maintaining aseptic technique and following facility guidelines and procedures to prevent potential hazards. Suctioning frequency is based on clinical assessment to determine the need for suctioning.

The purpose of suctioning is to remove secretions that are not accessible to bypassed cilia, so the recommendation is to insert the catheter only as far as the end of the tracheostomy tube is recommended. Catheter contact and suction cause tracheal mucosal damage, loss of cilia, edema, and fibrosis, as well as increasing the risk of infection and bleeding for the patient. Insertion of the suction catheter to a predetermined distance, no more than 1 cm past the length of the tracheostomy tube, avoids contact with the trachea and carina, reducing the effects of tracheal mucosal damage (Ireton, 2007; Pate, 2004; Pate & Zapata, 2002).

Note: In-line, closed suction systems are available to suction mechanically ventilated patients. The use of closed suction catheter systems may avoid some of the infection control issues and other complications associated with open suction techniques. The closed suctioning procedure is the same for patients with tracheostomy tubes and endotracheal tubes connected to mechanical ventilation. See Skill 65.

EQUIPMENT
- Portable or wall suction unit with tubing
- A commercially prepared suction kit with an appropriate-size catheter (See General Considerations) or
  - Sterile suction catheter with Y-port in the appropriate size
- Sterile disposable container
- Sterile gloves
- Towel or waterproof pad
- Goggles and mask or face shield
- Additional PPE, as indicated
- Disposable, clean gloves
- Resuscitation bag connected to 100% oxygen

ASSESSMENT GUIDELINES
- Assess lung sounds. Patients who need to be suctioned may have wheezes, crackles, or gurgling present.
- Assess oxygenation saturation level. Oxygen saturation usually decreases when a patient needs to be suctioned.
- Assess respiratory status, including respiratory rate and depth. Patients may become tachypneic when they need to be suctioned.
- Additional indications for suctioning via a tracheostomy tube include secretions in the tube, acute respiratory distress, and frequent or sustained coughing.

- Assess for pain and the potential to cause pain during the intervention. Perform individualized pain management in response to the patient's needs (Arroyo-Novoa, et al., 2007). If the patient has had abdominal surgery or other procedures, administer pain medication before suctioning.
- Assess appropriate suction catheter depth.

NURSING DIAGNOSES

- Ineffective Airway Clearance
- Risk for Aspiration
- Ineffective Breathing Pattern
- Impaired Gas Exchange

OUTCOME IDENTIFICATION AND PLANNING

Expected outcomes may include:
- Patient will exhibit improved breath sounds and a clear, patent airway.
- Patient will exhibit an oxygen saturation level within acceptable parameters.
- Patient will demonstrate a respiratory rate and depth within age-acceptable range.
- Patient will remain free of any signs of respiratory distress.

IMPLEMENTATION

ACTION	RATIONALE
1. Bring necessary equipment to the bedside stand or over-bed table.	Bringing everything to the bedside conserves time and energy. Arranging items nearby is convenient, saves time, and avoids unnecessary stretching and twisting of muscles on the part of the nurse.
2. Perform hand hygiene and put on PPE, if indicated.	Hand hygiene and PPE prevent the spread of microorganisms. PPE is required based on transmission precautions.
3. Identify the patient.	Identifying the patient ensures the right patient receives the intervention and helps prevent errors.
4. Close curtains around bed and close the door to the room, if possible.	This ensures the patient's privacy.

ACTION	RATIONALE
5. Determine the need for suctioning. Verify the suction order in the patient's chart. **Assess for pain or the potential to cause pain. Administer pain medication, as prescribed, before suctioning.**	To minimize trauma to airway mucosa, suctioning should be done only when secretions have accumulated or adventitious breath sounds are audible. Suctioning can cause moderate to severe pain for patients. Individualized pain management is imperative (Arroyo-Novoa, et al., 2007). Suctioning stimulates coughing, which is painful for patients with surgical incisions.
6. Explain to the patient what you are going to do and the reason or doing it, even if the patient does not appear to be alert. Reassure the patient you will interrupt the procedure if he or she indicates respiratory difficulty.	Explanation alleviates fears. Even if the patient appears unconscious, the nurse should explain what is happening. Any procedure that compromises respiration is frightening for the patient.
7. Adjust bed to comfortable working position, usually elbow height of the caregiver (VISN 8, 2009). Lower side rail closest to you. **If patient is conscious, place him or her in a semi-Fowler's position. If patient is unconscious, place him or her in the lateral position, facing you.** Move the overbed table close to your work area and raise to waist height.	Having the bed at the proper height prevents back and muscle strain. A sitting position helps the patient to cough and makes breathing easier. Gravity also facilitates catheter insertion. The lateral position prevents the airway from becoming obstructed and promotes drainage of secretions. The overbed table provides a work surface and maintains sterility of objects on it.
8. Place towel or waterproof pad across the patient's chest.	This protects bed linens and the patient.
9. **Turn suction to appropriate pressure.** For a wall unit for an adult: 100 to 120 mm Hg (Roman, 2005); neonates: 60 to 80 mm Hg; infants: 80 to 100 mm Hg; children: 80 to 100 mm Hg;	Higher pressures can cause excessive trauma, hypoxemia, and atelectasis. Glove prevents contact with blood and body fluids. Checking pressure ensures equipment is working properly. Allows for an

ACTION	RATIONALE
adolescents: 80 to 120 mm Hg (Ireton, 2007).	organized approach to procedure.
For a portable unit for an adult: 10 to 15 cm Hg; neonates: 6 to 8 cm Hg; infants 8 to 10 cm Hg; children 8 to 10 cm Hg; adolescents: 8 to 10 cm Hg.	
Put on a disposable, clean glove and occlude the end of the connecting tubing to check suction pressure. Place the connecting tubing in a convenient location. If using a resuscitation bag, place resuscitation bag connected to oxygen within convenient reach.	
10. Open sterile suction package using aseptic technique. The open wrapper or container becomes a sterile field to hold other supplies. Carefully remove the sterile container, touching only the outside surface. Set it up on the work surface and pour sterile saline into it.	Sterile normal saline or water is used to lubricate the outside of the catheter, minimizing irritation of mucosa during introduction. It is also used to clear the catheter between suction attempts.
11. Put on face shield or goggles and mask. Put on sterile gloves. **The dominant hand will manipulate the catheter and must remain sterile. The nondominant hand is considered clean rather than sterile and will control the suction valve (Y-port) on the catheter.**	Handling the sterile catheter using a sterile glove helps prevent introducing organisms into the respiratory tract; the clean glove protects the nurse from microorganisms.
12. With dominant gloved hand, pick up sterile catheter. Pick up the connecting tubing with the nondominant hand and connect the tubing and suction catheter.	Sterility of the suction catheter is maintained.

ACTION	RATIONALE
13. Moisten the catheter by dipping it into the container of sterile saline, unless it is a silicone catheter. Occlude Y-tube to check suction.	Lubricating the inside of the catheter with saline helps move secretions in the catheter. Silicone catheters do not require lubrication. Checking ensures equipment is working properly.
14. Using your nondominant hand and a manual resuscitation bag, hyperventilate the patient, delivering three to six breaths or use the 'sigh' mechanism on a mechanical ventilator.	Hyperoxygenation and hyperventilation aid in preventing hypoxemia during suctioning.
15. Open the adapter on the mechanical ventilator tubing or remove oxygen delivery setup with your nondominant hand.	This exposes the tracheostomy tube without contaminating sterile gloved hand.
16. Using your dominant hand, gently and quickly insert catheter into trachea. **Advance the catheter to the predetermined length. Do not occlude the Y-port when inserting catheter.**	Catheter contact and suction cause tracheal mucosal damage, loss of cilia, edema, and fibrosis, as well as increasing the risk of infection and bleeding for the patient. Insertion of the suction catheter to a predetermined distance, no more than 1 cm past the length of the endotracheal tube, avoids contact with the trachea and carina, reducing the effects of tracheal mucosal damage (Ireton, 2007; Pate, 2004; Pate & Zapata, 2002). If resistance is met, the carina or tracheal mucosa has been hit. Withdraw the catheter at least ½ inch before applying suction. Suctioning when inserting the catheter increases the risk for trauma to airway mucosa and the risk of hypoxemia.
17. Apply suction by intermittently occluding the Y-port on the catheter with the thumb of your nondominant	Turning the catheter as it is withdrawn minimizes trauma to the mucosa. Suctioning for longer than 10 to 15 seconds robs the

ACTION	RATIONALE

hand, and gently rotate the catheter as it is being withdrawn (FIGURE 1). **Do not suction for more than 10 to 15 seconds at a time.**

respiratory tract of oxygen, which may result in hypoxemia. Suctioning too quickly may be ineffective at clearing all secretions.

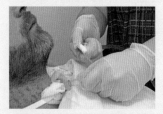

FIGURE 1 Applying intermittent suction while withdrawing catheter.

18. Hyperventilate the patient using your nondominant hand and a manual resuscitation bag, delivering three to six breaths. Replace the oxygen delivery device, if applicable, using your nondominant hand and have the patient take several deep breaths. If the patient is mechanically ventilated, close the adapter on the mechanical ventilator tubing and use the 'sigh' mechanism on a mechanical ventilator.

Suctioning removes air from the patient's airway and can cause hypoxemia. Hyperventilation can help prevent suction-induced hypoxemia.

19. Flush catheter with saline. Assess effectiveness of suctioning and repeat, as needed, and according to patient's tolerance. Wrap the suction catheter around your dominant hand between attempts.

Flushing clears the catheter and lubricates it for next insertion. Reassessment determines need for additional suctioning. Prevents inadvertent contamination of catheter.

20. **Allow at least a 30-second to 1-minute interval if additional suctioning is needed. No more than three suction passes should be made per suctioning episode. Encourage patient to cough and**

The interval allows for reventilation and reoxygenation of airways. Excessive suction passes contribute to complications. Alternating nares reduces trauma. Clears the mouth of secretions. More microorganisms are

ACTION	RATIONALE
deep breathe between suctionings. Suction the oropharynx after suctioning the trachea. Do not reinsert in the tracheostomy after suctioning the mouth.	usually present in the mouth, so it is suctioned last to prevent transmission of contaminants.
21. When suctioning is completed, remove gloves from dominant hand over the coiled catheter, pulling it off inside out. Remove glove from nondominant hand and dispose of gloves, catheter, and container with solution in the appropriate receptacle. Assist patient to a comfortable position. Raise bed rail and place bed in the lowest position.	This technique reduces transmission of microorganisms. Ensures patient comfort. Proper positioning with raised side rails and proper bed height provides for patient comfort and safety.
22. Turn off suction. Remove supplemental oxygen placed for suctioning, if appropriate. Remove face shield or goggles and mask. Perform hand hygiene.	Removing PPE properly reduces the risk for infection transmission and contamination of other items. Hand hygiene prevents transmission of microorganisms.
23. Offer oral hygiene after suctioning.	Respiratory secretions that are allowed to accumulate in the mouth are irritating to mucous membranes and unpleasant for the patient.
24. Reassess the patient's respiratory status, including respiratory rate, effort, oxygen saturation, and lung sounds.	These assess effectiveness of suctioning and the presence of complications.
25. Remove additional PPE, if used. Perform hand hygiene.	Removing PPE properly reduces the risk for infection transmission and contamination of other items. Hand hygiene prevents the spread of microorganisms.

EVALUATION
- Patient exhibits improved breath sounds and a clear and patent airway.
- The patient's oxygen saturation level is within acceptable parameters.
- Patient does not exhibit signs or symptoms of respiratory distress or complications.

DOCUMENTATION
- Document the time of suctioning, pre- and postintervention assessment, reason for suctioning, and the characteristics and amount of secretions.

GENERAL CONSIDERATIONS
- Determine the size catheter to use by the size of the tracheostomy. The external diameter of the suction catheter should not exceed half of the internal diameter of the tracheostomy. Larger catheters can contribute to trauma and hypoxemia.
- Emergency equipment should be easily accessible at the bedside. Keep bag-valve mask, oxygen, and suction equipment at the bedside of a patient with a tracheostomy tube at all times.

Skill · 166   **Caring for a Patient in Halo Traction**

Halo traction provides immobilization to patients with spinal cord injury. Halo traction consists of a metal ring that fits over the patient's head, connected with skull pins into the skull, and metal bars that connect the ring to a vest that distributes the weight of the device around the chest. It immobilizes the head and neck after traumatic injury to the cervical vertebrae and allows early mobility.

Nursing responsibilities include reassuring the patient, maintaining the device, monitoring neurovascular status, monitoring respiratory status, promoting exercise, preventing complications from the therapy, preventing infection by providing pin-site care, and providing teaching to ensure compliance and self-care. Pin-site care is performed frequently in the first 48 to 72 hours after application, when drainage may be heavy. Thereafter, pin-site care may be done daily or weekly. Dressings are often applied for the first 48 to 72 hours, and then sites may be left open to air. There is little research evidence on which to base the management of pin sites (Baird-Holmes & Brown, 2005; Walker, 2007). Pin-site care varies based on physician and facility policy. Refer to specific patient medical orders and facility guidelines.

EQUIPMENT

- Basin of warm water
- Bath towels
- Medicated skin powder or cornstarch, per physician order or facility policy
- Sterile applicators
- Cleansing solution, usually sterile normal saline or chlorhexidine, per physician order or facility policy
- Sterile gauze or dressing, per order or policy
- Antimicrobial ointment, per physician's order or facility policy
- Analgesic, per physician's order
- Clean gloves, if appropriate, for bathing under the vest
- Sterile gloves for performing pin care, depending on facility policy
- Additional PPE, as indicated

ASSESSMENT GUIDELINES

- Review the patient's medical record, medical orders, and nursing plan of care to determine the type of device being used and prescribed care.
- Assess the halo traction device to ensure proper function and position.
- Perform respiratory, neurologic, and skin assessments.
- Inspect the pin insertion sites for inflammation and infection, including swelling, cloudy or offensive drainage, pain, or redness.
- Assess the patient's knowledge regarding the device and self-care activities and responsibilities, and his or her feelings related to treatment.

NURSING DIAGNOSES

- Anxiety
- Risk for Falls
- Disturbed Body Image
- Ineffective Coping
- Deficient Knowledge
- Risk for Infection
- Risk for Injury
- Impaired Physical Mobility
- Acute Pain
- Impaired Skin Integrity
- Self-Care Deficit (toileting, bathing, dressing)
- Disturbed Sleep Pattern

OUTCOME IDENTIFICATION AND PLANNING

Expected outcomes may include:
- Patient maintains cervical alignment.
- Patient shows no evidence of infection.
- Patient is free from complications, such as respiratory impairment, orthostatic hypotension, and skin breakdown.
- Patient experiences relief from pain.
- Patient is free from injury.

IMPLEMENTATION

ACTION	RATIONALE
1. Review the medical record and the nursing plan of care to determine the type of device being used and prescribed care.	Reviewing the medical record and care plan validates the correct patient and correct procedure.
2. Gather the necessary supplies and bring to the bedside stand or overbed table.	Preparation promotes efficient time management and an organized approach to the task. Bringing everything to the bedside conserves time and energy. Arranging items nearby is convenient, saves time, and avoids unnecessary stretching and twisting of muscles on the part of the nurse.
3. Perform hand hygiene and put on PPE, if indicated.	Hand hygiene and PPE prevent the spread of microorganisms. PPE is required based on transmission precautions.
4. Identify the patient.	Identifying the patient ensures the right patient receives the intervention and helps prevent errors.
5. Close curtains around bed and close the door to the room, if possible. Explain what you are going to do and why you are going to do it to the patient.	This ensures the patient's privacy. Explanation relieves anxiety and facilitates cooperation.
6. Assess the patient for possible need for nonpharmacologic pain-reducing interventions or analgesic medication before beginning. Administer appropriate prescribed analgesic. Allow sufficient time for analgesic to achieve its effectiveness before beginning the procedure.	Pain is a subjective experience influenced by past experience. Pin care may cause pain for some patients.

ACTION	RATIONALE
7. Place a waste receptacle at a convenient location for use during the procedure.	Having a waste container handy means that the soiled dressing may be discarded easily, without the spread of microorganisms.
8. Adjust bed to comfortable working height, usually elbow height of the caregiver if the patient will remain in bed (VISN 8, 2009). Alternatively, have the patient sit up, if appropriate.	Having the bed at the proper height prevents back and muscle strain.
9. Assist the patient to a comfortable position that provides easy access to the head. Place a waterproof pad under the head if patient is lying down.	Patient positioning provides for comfort. Waterproof pad protects underlying surfaces.
10. Monitor vital signs and perform a neurologic assessment, including level of consciousness, motor function, and sensation, per facility policy. This is usually at least every 2 hours for 24 hours, or possibly every hour for 48 hours.	Changes in the neurologic assessment could indicate spinal cord trauma, which would require immediate intervention.
11. Remove the patient's shirt or gown. Examine the halo vest unit every 8 hours for stability, secure connections, and check positioning. Make sure the patient's head is centered in the halo without neck flexion or extension. Check each bolt for loosening.	Removal of clothing from torso allows visualization of, and access to, appropriate areas. Assessment ensures correct function of the device and patient safety.
12. Check the fit of the vest. With the patient in a supine position, you should be able to insert one or two fingers under the jacket at the shoulder and chest.	Checking the fit prevents compression on the chest, which could interfere with respiratory status.

ACTION	RATIONALE
13. Put on nonsterile gloves, if appropriate. Wash the patient's chest and back daily. Loosen the bottom Velcro straps.	Gloves prevent contact with blood and body fluids. Daily cleaning prevents skin breakdown and allows assessment. Loosening the straps allows access to the chest and back.
14. Wring out a bath towel soaked in warm water. Pull the towel back and forth in a drying motion beneath the front. Do not use soap or lotion under the vest.	Using an overly wet towel could lead to skin maceration and breakdown. Soaps and lotions can cause skin irritation.
15. Thoroughly dry the skin in the same manner with a dry towel. Inspect the skin for tender, reddened areas or pressure spots. Lightly dust the skin with a prescribed medicated powder or cornstarch.	Drying and using powder or cornstarch, which helps absorb moisture, prevent skin breakdown.
16. Turn the patient on his or her side, less than 45 degrees if lying supine, and repeat the process on the back. Close the Velcro straps. Assist the patient with putting on a new shirt, if desired.	Doing so prevents skin breakdown. Soaps and lotions can cause skin irritation.
17. Perform a respiratory assessment. Check for respiratory impairment, such as absence of breath sounds, the presence of adventitious sounds, reduced inspiratory effort, or shortness of breath.	The halo vest limits chest expansion, which could lead to alterations in respiratory function. Pulmonary embolus is a common complication associated with spinal cord injury.
18. Assess the pin sites for redness; tenting of the skin; prolonged or purulent drainage; swelling; and bowing, bending, or loosening of the pins. Monitor body temperature.	Pin sites provide an entry for microorganisms. Assessment allows for early detection and prompt intervention should problems arise.
19. Perform pin-site care. (See Skills 169 and 170.)	Pin-site care reduces the risk of infection and subsequent osteomyelitis.

ACTION	RATIONALE
20. Depending on physician order and facility policy, apply the antimicrobial ointment to pin sites and apply a dressing.	Antimicrobial ointment helps prevent infection. Dressing provides protection and helps contain any drainage.
21. Remove gloves and dispose of them appropriately. Raise rails, as appropriate, and place the bed in the lowest position. Assist patient to a comfortable position.	Disposing of gloves reduces the risk of microorganism transmission. Rails assist with patient positioning. Proper bed height ensures patient safety.
22. Remove additional PPE, if used. Perform hand hygiene.	Removing PPE properly reduces the risk for infection transmission and contamination of other items. Hand hygiene prevents the spread of microorganisms.

EVALUATION

- Patient maintains cervical alignment.
- Patient shows no evidence of infection.
- Patient is free from complications, such as respiratory impairment, orthostatic hypotension, and skin breakdown.
- Patient experiences relief from pain.
- Patient is free from injury.

DOCUMENTATION

- Document the time, date, and type of device in place. Document the skin assessment, pin-site assessment, personal hygiene, and pin-site care. Document the patient's response to the device and the neurologic assessment and respiratory assessment.

GENERAL CONSIDERATIONS

- Wrenches specific for the vest should always be kept at the bedside for emergency removal of the anterior portion of the vest should it be necessary to perform CPR.
- Patient teaching to prevent injury is very important. Patients need to learn to turn slowly and refrain from bending forward to avoid falls.
- Stress to the frame could cause spine misalignment and straining or tearing of the skin.

Skill · 167 **Caring for a Patient in Skeletal Traction**

Skeletal traction provides pull to a body part by attaching weight directly to the bone, using pins, screws, wires, or tongs. It is used to immobilize a body part for prolonged periods. This method of traction is used to treat fractures of the femur, tibia, and cervical spine. Nursing responsibilities related to skeletal traction include maintaining the traction, maintaining body alignment, monitoring neurovascular status, promoting exercise, preventing complications from the therapy and immobility, and preventing infection by providing pin site care. Pin site care is performed frequently in the first 48 to 72 hours after application, when drainage may be heavy. Thereafter, pin site care may be done daily or weekly. Dressings are often applied for the first 48 to 72 hours, and then sites may be left open to air. There is little research evidence on which to base the management of skeletal pin sites (Baird Holmes & Brown, 2005). Skeletal pin site care varies based on primary care provider and facility policy. Refer to specific patient medical orders and facility guidelines.

EQUIPMENT
- Sterile gloves
- Sterile applicators
- Cleansing agent for pin care, usually sterile normal saline or chlorhexidine, per physician order or facility policy
- Sterile container
- Antimicrobial ointment, if ordered
- Foam, nonstick, or gauze dressing, per medical order or facility policy
- Additional PPE, as indicated

ASSESSMENT GUIDELINES
- Review the patient's medical record and nursing plan of care to determine the type of traction, traction weight, and line of pull. Assess the traction equipment to ensure proper function, including inspecting the ropes for fraying and proper positioning.
- Assess the patient's body alignment. Perform a skin assessment and neurovascular assessment. Inspect the pin insertion sites for inflammation and infection, including swelling, cloudy or offensive drainage, pain, or redness.
- Assess for complications of immobility, including alterations in respiratory function, constipation, alterations in skin integrity, alterations in urinary elimination, and muscle weakness, contractures, thrombophlebitis, pulmonary embolism, and fatigue.

NURSING DIAGNOSES
- Impaired Skin Integrity
- Risk for Injury
- Ineffective Airway Clearance

- Anxiety
- Risk for Constipation
- Deficient Knowledge
- Impaired Bed Mobility
- Acute Pain
- Impaired Physical Mobility
- Risk for Infection
- Self-Care Deficit (Toileting, Bathing, or Dressing)
- Impaired Gas Exchange

OUTCOME IDENTIFICATION AND PLANNING

Expected outcomes may include:
- Traction is maintained with the appropriate counterbalance.
- Patient is free from complications of immobility and infection.
- Patient maintains proper body alignment.
- Patient reports an increased level of comfort.
- Patient is free from injury.

IMPLEMENTATION

ACTION	RATIONALE
1. Review the medical record and the nursing plan of care to determine the type of traction being used and the prescribed care.	Reviewing the medical record and plan of care validates the correct patient and correct procedure.
2. Perform hand hygiene. Put on PPE, as indicated.	Hand hygiene and PPE prevent the spread of microorganisms. PPE is required based on transmission precautions.
3. Identify the patient. Explain the procedure to the patient, emphasizing the importance of maintaining counterbalance, alignment, and position.	Patient identification validates the correct patient and correct procedure. Discussion and explanation help allay anxiety and prepare the patient for what to expect.
4. Perform a pain assessment and assess for muscle spasm. Administer prescribed medications in sufficient time to allow for the full effect of the analgesic and/or muscle relaxant.	Assessing for pain and administering analgesics promote patient comfort.

ACTION	RATIONALE
5. Close curtains around bed and close the door to the room, if possible. Place the bed at an appropriate and comfortable working height.	Closing the door or curtains provides for privacy. Proper bed height prevents back and muscle strain.
6. Ensure the traction apparatus is attached securely to the bed. Assess the traction setup, including application of the ordered amount of weight. Be sure that the weights hang freely, not touching the bed or the floor.	Proper traction application reduces the risk of injury by promoting accurate counterbalance and function of the traction.
7. Check that the ropes move freely through the pulleys. Check that all knots are tight and are positioned away from the pulleys. Pulleys should be free from the linens.	Free ropes and pulleys ensure accurate counterbalance and function of the traction.
8. Check the alignment of the patient's body, as prescribed.	Proper alignment maintains an effective line of pull and prevents injury.
9. Perform a skin assessment. Pay attention to pressure points, including the ischial tuberosity, popliteal space, Achilles' tendon, sacrum, and heel.	Skin assessment provides early intervention for skin irritation, impaired tissue perfusion, and other complications.
10. Perform a neurovascular assessment. Assess the extremity distal to the traction for edema and peripheral pulses. Assess the temperature and color and compare with the unaffected limb. Check for pain, inability to move body parts distal to the traction, pallor, and abnormal sensations. Assess for indicators of deep-vein thrombosis, including calf tenderness, and swelling.	Neurovascular assessment aids in early identification and allows for prompt intervention should compromised circulation and oxygenation of tissues develop.

ACTION	RATIONALE
11. Assess the site at and around the pins for redness, edema, and odor. Assess for skin tenting, prolonged or purulent drainage, elevated body temperature, elevated pin site temperature, and bowing or bending of the pins.	Pin sites provide a possible entry for microorganisms. Skin inspection allows for early detection and prompt intervention should complications develop.
12. Provide pin site care.	Performing pin site care prevents crusting at the site that could lead to fluid buildup, infection, and osteomyelitis.
a. Using sterile technique, open the applicator package and pour the cleansing agent into the sterile container.	Using sterile technique reduces the risk for transmission of microorganisms.
b. Put on the sterile gloves.	Gloves prevent contact with blood and/or body fluids.
c. Place the applicators into the solution.	
d. Clean the pin site starting at the insertion area and working outward, away from the pin site (FIGURE 1).	Cleaning from the center outward ensures movement from the least to most contaminated area.
e. Use each applicator once. Use a new applicator for each pin site.	Using an applicator once reduces the risk of transmission of microorganisms.

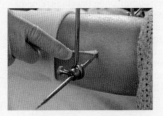

FIGURE 1 Cleaning around pin sites with normal saline on an applicator.

ACTION	RATIONALE
13. Depending on the primary care provider order and facility policy, apply the antimicrobial ointment to pin sites and apply a dressing.	Antimicrobial ointment helps reduce the risk of infection. A dressing aids in protecting the pin sites from contamination and will contain any drainage.
14. Remove gloves and any other PPE, if used. Perform hand hygiene.	Removing PPE properly decreases the risk for infection transmission and contamination of other items. Hand hygiene prevents the spread of microorganisms.
15. Perform range-of-motion exercises on all joint areas, unless contraindicated. Encourage the patient to cough and deep breathe every 2 hours.	Range-of-motion exercises promote joint mobility. Coughing and deep breathing reduce the risk of respiratory complications related to immobility.

EVALUATION

• Patient demonstrates maintenance of skeletal traction with pin sites free of infection.
• Patient maintains proper body alignment and joint function.
• Patient verbalizes pain relief.
• Patient remains free of injury.

DOCUMENTATION

• Document the time, date, type of traction, and the amount of weight used. Include the skin and pin site assessments, and pin site care. Document the patient's response to the traction and the neurovascular status of the extremity.

GENERAL CONSIDERATIONS

• If mechanical looseness or early signs of infection (swelling, cloudy or offensive drainage, pain, or redness) are present, increase the frequency of pin site care (Baird Holmes & Brown, 2005).
• Assess the patient for chronic conditions, such as diabetes mellitus, peripheral vascular disease, and chronic obstructive pulmonary disease, which can significantly increase a patient's risk for complications when skeletal traction is in use.
• Never remove the weights from skeletal traction unless a life-threatening situation occurs. Removal of the weights interferes with therapy and can result in injury to the patient.
• Inspect the pin sites for inflammation and evidence of infection at least every 8 hours. Prevention of osteomyelitis is of utmost importance.

Skin · 168 **Applying Skin Traction and Caring for a Patient in Skin Traction**

Traction is the application of a pulling force to a part of the body. It is used to reduce fractures, treat dislocations, correct or prevent deformities, improve or correct contractures, or decrease muscle spasms. The affected body part is immobilized by pulling with equal force on each end of the injured area, mixing traction and countertraction. Weights provide the pulling force or traction. The use of additional weights or positioning the patient's body weight against the traction pull provides the countertraction. Skin traction is applied directly to the skin, exerting indirect pull on the bone. The force may be applied using adhesive or nonadhesive traction tape or a boot, belt, or halter. Skin traction immobilizes a body part intermittently. Nursing care for skin traction includes setting up the traction, applying the traction, monitoring the application and patient response, and preventing complications from the therapy and immobility.

EQUIPMENT
- Bed with traction frame and trapeze
- Weights
- Velcro straps or other straps
- Rope and pulleys
- Boot with footplate
- Elastic antiembolism stocking, as appropriate
- Nonsterile gloves and/or other PPE, as indicated
- Skin cleansing supplies

ASSESSMENT GUIDELINES
- Assess the patient's medical record and the nursing plan of care to determine the type of traction, traction weight, and line of pull.
- Assess the traction equipment to ensure proper function, including inspecting the ropes for fraying and proper positioning.
- Assess the patient's body alignment. Perform a skin and neurovascular assessments. Assess for complications of immobility, including alterations in respiratory function, skin integrity, urinary and bowel elimination, and muscle weakness, contractures, thrombophlebitis, pulmonary embolism, and fatigue.

NURSING DIAGNOSES
- Risk for Injury
- Ineffective Airway Clearance
- Anxiety
- Risk for Constipation
- Impaired Gas Exchange
- Deficient Knowledge
- Impaired Bed Mobility
- Acute Pain
- Impaired Physical Mobility

• Risk for Impaired Skin Integrity
• Self-Care Deficit (Bathing, Feeding, Dressing, or Toileting)

OUTCOME IDENTIFICATION AND PLANNING

Expected outcomes may include:
• Traction is maintained with the appropriate counterbalance.
• Patient is free from complications of immobility.
• Patient maintains proper body alignment.
• Patient reports an increased level of comfort.
• Patient is free from injury.

IMPLEMENTATION

ACTION	RATIONALE
1. Review the medical record and the nursing plan of care to determine the type of traction being used and care for the affected body part.	Reviewing the medical record and plan of care validates the correct patient and correct procedure.
2. Perform hand hygiene. Put on PPE, as indicated.	Hand hygiene and PPE prevent the spread of microorganisms. PPE is required based on transmission precautions.
3. Identify the patient. Explain the procedure to the patient, emphasizing the importance of maintaining counterbalance, alignment, and position.	Patient identification validates the correct patient and correct procedure. Discussion and explanation help allay anxiety and prepare the patient for what to expect.
4. Perform a pain assessment and assess for muscle spasm. Administer prescribed medications in sufficient time to allow for the full effect of the analgesic and/or muscle relaxant.	Assessing pain and administering analgesics promote patient comfort.
5. Close curtains around bed and close the door to the room, if possible. Place the bed at an appropriate and comfortable working height.	Closing the door or curtains provides for privacy. Proper bed height prevents back and muscle strain.

ACTION	RATIONALE

Applying Skin Traction

6. Ensure the traction apparatus is attached securely to the bed. Assess the traction setup.

Assessment of traction setup and weights promotes safety.

7. Check that the ropes move freely through the pulleys. Check that all knots are tight and are positioned away from the pulleys. Pulleys should be free from the linens.

Checking ropes and pulleys ensures that weight is being applied correctly, promoting accurate counterbalance and function of the traction.

8. Place the patient in a supine position with the foot of the bed elevated slightly. The patient's head should be near the head of the bed and in alignment.

Proper patient positioning maintains proper counterbalance and promotes safety.

9. Cleanse the affected area. Place the elastic stocking on the affected limb as appropriate.

Skin care aids in preventing skin breakdown. Use of elastic anti-embolism stocking prevents edema and neurovascular complications.

10. Place the traction boot over the patient's leg (FIGURE 1). Be sure the patient's heel is in the heel of the boot. Secure the boot with the straps.

The boot provides a means for attaching traction; proper application ensures proper pull.

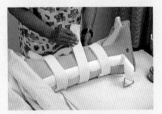

FIGURE 1 Applying the traction boot with an elastic stocking in place on the leg.

11. Attach the traction cord to the footplate of the boot. Pass the rope over the pulley fastened at the end of the bed. Attach the weight to the hook on the rope, usually 5 to 10 pounds for an adult.

Attachment of weight applies the pull for the traction. Gently releasing the weight prevents a quick pull on the extremity and possible injury and pain. Properly hanging weights and correct patient positioning ensure accurate

ACTION	RATIONALE
Gently let go of the weight. **The weight should hang freely, not touching the bed or the floor.**	counterbalance and function of the traction.
12. **Check the patient's alignment with the traction.**	Proper alignment is necessary for proper counterbalance and ensures patient safety.
13. **Check the boot for placement and alignment. Make sure the line of pull is parallel to the bed and not angled downward.**	Misalignment causes ineffective traction and may interfere with healing. A properly positioned boot prevents pressure on the heel.
14. Place the bed in the lowest position that still allows the weight to hang freely.	Proper bed positioning ensures effective application of traction without patient injury.
15. Remove PPE, if used. Perform hand hygiene.	Removing PPE properly decreases the risk for infection transmission and contamination of other items. Hand hygiene prevents the spread of microorganisms.

Caring for a Patient With Skin Traction

16. Perform a skin-traction assessment per facility policy. This assessment includes checking the traction equipment, examining the affected body part, maintaining proper body alignment, and performing skin and neurovascular assessments.	Assessment provides information to determine proper application and alignment, thereby reducing the risk for injury. Misalignment causes ineffective traction and may interfere with healing.
17. Remove the straps every 4 hours per the physician's order or facility policy. Check bony prominences for skin breakdown, abrasions, and pressure areas. Remove the boot per physician's order or facility policy every 8 hours. Put on gloves and wash, rinse, and thoroughly dry the skin.	Removing the straps provides assessment information for early detection and prompt intervention of potential complications should they arise. Washing the area enhances circulation to skin; thorough drying prevents skin breakdown. Using gloves prevents transfer of microorganisms.

ACTION	RATIONALE
18. Assess the extremity distal to the traction for edema, and assess peripheral pulses. Assess the temperature, color, and capillary refill, and compare with the unaffected limb. Check for pain, inability to move body parts distal to the traction, pallor, and abnormal sensations. Assess for indicators of deep-vein thrombosis, including calf tenderness, and swelling.	Doing so helps detect signs of abnormal neurovascular function and allows for prompt intervention. Assessing neurovascular status determines the circulation and oxygenation of tissues. Pressure within the traction boot may increase with edema.
19. Replace the traction and remove gloves and dispose of them appropriately.	Replacing traction is necessary to provide immobilization and facilitate healing. Proper disposal of gloves prevents the transmission of microorganisms.
20. Check the boot for placement and alignment. **Make sure the line of pull is parallel to the bed and not angled downward.**	Misalignment causes ineffective traction and may interfere with healing. A properly positioned boot prevents pressure on the heel.
21. **Ensure the patient is positioned in the center of the bed, with the affected leg aligned with the trunk of the patient's body.**	Misalignment interferes with the effectiveness of traction and may lead to complications.
22. Examine the weights and pulley system. **Weights should hang freely, off the floor and bed. Knots should be secure. Ropes should move freely through the pulleys. The pulleys should not be constrained by knots (FIGURE 2).**	Checking the weights and pulley system ensures proper application and reduces the risk for patient injury from traction application.

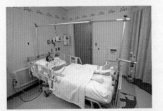

FIGURE 2 Skin traction in place.

ACTION	RATIONALE
23. Perform range-of-motion exercises on all unaffected joint areas, unless contraindicated. Encourage the patient to cough and deep breathe every 2 hours.	Range-of-motion exercises maintain joint function. Coughing and deep breathing help to reduce the risk for respiratory complications related to immobility.
24. Raise the side rails. Place the bed in the lowest position that still allows the weight to hang freely.	Raising the side rails promotes patient safety. Proper bed positioning ensures effective application of traction without patient injury.
25. Remove PPE, if used. Perform hand hygiene.	Removing PPE properly decreases the risk for infection transmission and contamination of other items. Hand hygiene prevents the spread of microorganisms.

EVALUATION

- Patient demonstrates proper body alignment with traction applied and maintained with appropriate counterbalance.
- Patient verbalizes pain relief.
- Patient remains free of injury.

DOCUMENTATION

- Document the time, date, type, amount of weight used, and the site where the traction was applied. Include the skin assessment and care provided before application. Document the patient's response to the traction and the neurovascular status of the extremity.

GENERAL CONSIDERATIONS

- Unless contraindicated, encourage the patient to do active flexion–extension ankle exercise and calf-pumping exercises at regular intervals to decrease venous stasis.
- Be alert for pressure on peripheral nerves with skin traction. Take care with Buck's traction to avoid pressure on the peroneal nerve at the point where it passes around the neck of the fibula just below the knee.
- Assess patients who are in traction for extended periods for development of helplessness, isolation, confinement, and loss of control. Diversional activities, therapeutic communication, and frequent visits by staff and significant others are an important part of care.

Skill · 169   **Transferring a Patient From the Bed to a Chair**

Before performing the transfer, identify any restrictions related to the patient's condition and determine how activity levels may be affected. FIGURE 1, Safe Patient Handling Algorithm 1, can assist in making decisions about safe patient handling and movement. Using assistance, appropriate lifting and repositioning devices, good body mechanics, and correct technique are important to avoid injuries to yourself and the patient.

Algorithm 1: Transfer to and From: Bed to Chair, Chair to Toilet, Chair to Chair, or Car to Chair

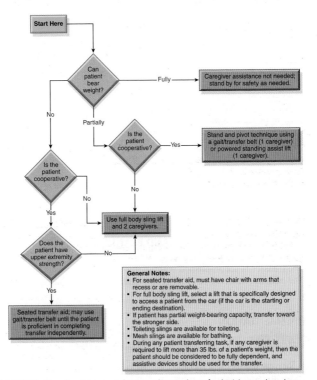

FIGURE 1 Step-by-step procedure used to make safe decisions related to transferring a patient to and from bed to chair, chair to toilet, chair to car, or car to chair. (From VISN 8 Patient Safety Center. [2009]. *Safe patient handling and movement algorithms.* Tampa, FL: Author. Available at http://www.VISN8.med.va.gov/patientsafetycenter/safePtHandling/default.asp. Accessed April 23, 2010.)

EQUIPMENT

- Chair or wheelchair
- Gait belt
- Stand-assist aid, if available
- Additional staff person to assist
- Blanket to cover the patient in the chair
- Nonsterile gloves and/or other PPE, as indicated

ASSESSMENT GUIDELINES

- Assess the situation to determine the need to get the patient out of bed. Review the medical record and nursing plan of care for conditions that may influence the patient's ability to move or to be transferred.
- Assess for tubes, IV lines, incisions, or equipment that may alter the positioning procedure.
- Assess the patient's level of consciousness, ability to understand and follow directions, and ability to assist with the transfer.
- Assess the patient's weight and your strength to determine the number of caregivers required to assist with the activity. Determine if there is a need for bariatric equipment.
- Assess the patient's comfort level; if needed, medicate as ordered with analgesics.
- If the patient is able to bear only partial weight, consider a second staff person to assist. If the patient is unable to bear even partial weight, or is uncooperative, use a full-body sling lift to move patient.

NURSING DIAGNOSES

- Activity Intolerance
- Acute Pain
- Anxiety
- Risk for Impaired Skin Integrity
- Risk for Falls
- Impaired Transfer Ability

OUTCOME IDENTIFICATION AND PLANNING

Expected outcomes may include:
- The transfer is accomplished without injury to patient or nurse.
- The patient remains free of any complications of immobility.

IMPLEMENTATION

ACTION

RATIONALE

1. Review the medical record and nursing plan of care for conditions that may influence the patient's ability to move or to be positioned. Assess for tubes, intravenous lines,

Reviewing the medical record and plan of care validates the correct patient and correct procedure. Identification of limitations and ability and use of an algorithm helps to prevent injury and

ACTION	RATIONALE
incisions, or equipment that may alter the positioning procedure. Identify any movement limitations. Consult patient handling algorithm, if available, to plan appropriate approach to moving the patient. Check equipment for proper functioning.	aids in determining best plan for patient movement.
2. Perform hand hygiene and put on PPE, if indicated.	Hand hygiene and PPE prevent the spread of microorganisms. PPE is required based on transmission precautions.
3. Identify the patient. Explain the procedure to the patient.	Patient identification validates the correct patient and correct procedure. Discussion and explanation help allay anxiety and prepare the patient for what to expect.
4. If needed, move equipment to make room for the chair. Close curtains around bed and close the door to the room, if possible.	A clear pathway from the bed to the chair facilitates the transfer. Closing the door or curtain provides for privacy.
5. Place the bed in the lowest position. Raise the head of the bed to a sitting position, or as high as the patient can tolerate.	Proper bed height and positioning facilitate the transfer. The amount of energy needed to move from a sitting position or elevated position to a sitting position is decreased.
6. **Make sure the bed brakes are locked. Put the chair next to the bed, facing the foot of the bed. If available, lock the brakes of the chair. If the chair does not have brakes, brace the chair against a secure object.**	Locking brakes or bracing the chair prevents movement during transfer and increases stability and patient safety.
7. Encourage the patient to make use of a stand-assist aid, either freestanding or attached to the side of the	Encourages independence, reduces strain for staff, and decreases risk for patient injury.

ACTION	RATIONALE
bed, if available, to move to the side of the bed and to a side-lying position, facing the side of the bed on which the patient will sit.	
8. Lower the side rail, if necessary, and stand near the patient's hips. Stand with your legs shoulder width apart with one foot near the head of the bed, slightly in front of the other foot.	The nurse's center of gravity is placed near the patient's greatest weight to assist the patient to a sitting position safely.
9. Encourage the patient to make use of the stand-assist device. Assist the patient to sit up on the side of the bed; ask the patient to swing his or her legs over the side of the bed. At the same time, pivot on your back leg to lift the patient's trunk and shoulders. Keep your back straight; avoid twisting.	Gravity lowers the patient's legs over the bed. The nurse transfers weight in the direction of motion and protects his or her back from injury.
10. **Stand in front of the patient, and assess for any balance problems or complaints of dizziness. Allow the patient's legs to dangle a few minutes before continuing.**	Standing in front of the patient prevents falls or injuries from orthostatic hypotension. The sitting position facilitates transfer to the chair and allows the circulatory system to adjust to a change in position.
11. Assist the patient to put on a robe and nonskid footwear.	Robe provides warmth and privacy. Nonskid soles reduce the risk for falling.
12. Wrap the gait belt around the patient's waist, based on assessed need and facility policy.	Gait belts improve the caregiver's grasp, reducing the risk of musculoskeletal injuries to staff and the patient. Provides firmer grasp for the caregiver if patient should lose his or her balance.
13. Stand facing the patient. Spread your feet about shoulder width apart and flex your hips and knees.	This position provides stability and allows for smooth movement using the legs' large muscle groups.

ACTION	RATIONALE

14. Ask the patient to slide his or her buttocks to the edge of the bed until the feet touch the floor. Position yourself as close as possible to the patient, with your foot positioned on the outside of the patient's foot. If a second staff person is assisting, have him or her assume a similar position.

Doing so provides balance and support.

15. Encourage the patient to make use of the stand-assist device. If necessary, have second staff person grasp gait belt on opposite side. Using the gait belt, assist the patient to stand (FIGURE 2). Rock back and forth while counting to three. **On the count of three, use your legs (not your back) to help raise the patient to a standing position.** If indicated, brace your front knee against the patient's weak extremity as he or she stands. Assess the patient's balance and leg strength. If the patient is weak or unsteady, return the patient to bed.

Holding at the gait belt prevents injury to the patient. Bracing your knee against a weak extremity prevents a weak knee from buckling and the patient from falling. Assessing balance and strength helps to identify the need for additional assistance to prevent falling.

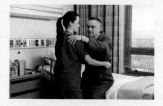

FIGURE 2 Assisting the patient to stand using the gait belt.

16. Pivot on your back foot and assist the patient to turn until the patient feels the chair against his or her legs.

This action ensures proper positioning before sitting.

ACTION	RATIONALE
17. Ask the patient to use an arm to steady him- or herself on the arm of the chair while slowly lowering to a sitting position. Continue to brace the patient's knees with your knees and hold the gait belt. Flex your hips and knees when helping the patient sit in the chair.	The patient uses his or her own arm for support and stability. Flexing hips and knees uses major muscle groups to aid in movement and reduce strain on the nurse's back.
18. Assess the patient's alignment in the chair. Remove gait belt, if desired. Depending on patient comfort, it could be left in place to use when returning to bed. Cover with a blanket, if needed. Make sure the call bell and other necessary items are within easy reach.	Assessment promotes comfort; blanket provides warmth and privacy; having the call bell readily available helps promote safety.
19. Clean transfer aids per facility policy, if not indicated for single patient use. Remove gloves and any other PPE, if used. Perform hand hygiene.	Proper cleaning of equipment between patient use prevents the spread of microorganisms. Removing PPE properly reduces the risk for infection transmission and contamination of other items. Hand hygiene prevents the spread of microorganisms.

EVALUATION

• The patient is transferred to the chair without injury to patient or nurse.
• The patient exhibits no signs and symptoms of problems or complications related to immobility.

DOCUMENTATION

• Document the activity, including the length of time the patient sat in the chair, any other pertinent observations, and the patient's tolerance of and reaction to the activity. Document the use of transfer aids and number of staff required for transfer.

GENERAL CONSIDERATIONS

- Transfer of a patient to a chair or toilet can be accomplished using a powered stand-assist and repositioning lift, if available. These devices can be used with patients who have weight-bearing ability on at least one leg and who can follow directions and are cooperative. A simple sling is placed around the patient's back and under the arms. The patient rests feet on the device's footrest and places his or her hands on the handle. The device mechanically assists the patient to stand, without any lifting by the nurse. Once the patient is standing, the device can be wheeled to a chair, the toilet, or bed. Some devices have removable footrests and can be used as a walker. Some have scales incorporated into the device that can be used to weigh the patient.
- Patients who are unable to bear partial weight or full weight or who are uncooperative should be transferred using a full-body sling lift.
- The transfer of patients is often delegated to unlicensed personnel. Before moving patients, all personnel need to complete instructions and must be able to provide return demonstrations of transfer skills. Before the transfer, communicate clearly any mobility restrictions or special care needs.

Skill · 170 Transferring a Patient From the Bed to a Stretcher

Considerable care must be taken when moving someone from a bed to a stretcher or from a stretcher to a bed to prevent injury to the patient or staff. Refer to FIGURE 1, Safe Patient Handling Algorithm 2, to help in making decisions about safe patient handling and movement. Using assistance, appropriate lifting and repositioning devices, good body mechanics, and correct technique are important to avoid injuries to yourself and to the patient. Be familiar with the proper way to use lateral-assist devices, based on the manufacturer's directions.

EQUIPMENT

- Transport stretcher
- Friction-reducing sheet
- Lateral-assist device, such as a transfer board, roller board, or mechanical lateral-assist device, if available
- Bath blanket
- Regular blanket
- At least two assistants, depending on the patient's condition
- Nonsterile gloves and/or other PPE, as indicated

ASSESSMENT GUIDELINES

- Review the medical record and nursing plan of care for conditions that may influence the patient's ability to move or to be transferred.

Algorithm 2: Lateral Transfer to and From: Bed to Stretcher, Trolley

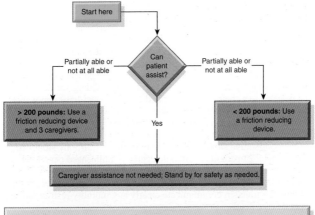

General Notes:
- Surfaces should be even for all lateral patient moves.
- For patients with Stage 3 or 4 pressure ulcers, care must be taken to avoid shearing force.
- During any patient transferring task, if any caregiver is required to lift more than 35 pounds of a patient's weight, then the patient should be considered to be fully dependent and assistive devices should be used for the transfer.

FIGURE 1 Step-by-step procedure used to make safe decisions related to transferring a patient from bed to stretcher/trolley. (From VISN 8 Patient Safety Center. [2009]. *Safe patient handling and movement algorithms.* Tampa, FL: Author. Available at http://www.visn8.med.va.gov/patientsafetycenter/safePtHandling/default.asp.) Accessed April 23, 2010.

- Assess for tubes, IV lines, incisions, or equipment that may alter the positioning procedure.
- Assess the patient's level of consciousness, ability to understand and follow directions, and ability to assist with moving.
- Assess the patient's weight and your strength to determine the number of caregivers required to assist with the activity. Determine if there is a need for bariatric equipment.
- Assess the patient's comfort level; if needed, medicate as ordered with analgesics.

NURSING DIAGNOSES
- Activity Intolerance
- Acute Pain
- Anxiety
- Risk for Impaired Skin Integrity
- Risk for Falls
- Impaired Transfer Ability

OUTCOME IDENTIFICATION AND PLANNING

Expected outcomes may include:
• Patient is transferred without injury to patient or nurse.

IMPLEMENTATION

ACTION	RATIONALE
1. Review the medical record and nursing plan of care for conditions that may influence the patient's ability to move or to be positioned. Assess for tubes, intravenous lines, incisions, or equipment that may alter the positioning procedure. Identify any movement limitations. Consult patient handling algorithm, if available, to plan appropriate approach to moving the patient. Check equipment for proper functioning.	Reviewing the order and plan of care validates the correct patient and correct procedure. Identification of limitations and ability and use of an algorithm and properly functioning equipment helps to prevent injury and aids in determining best plan for patient movement.
2. Perform hand hygiene and put on PPE, if indicated.	Hand hygiene and PPE prevent the spread of microorganisms. PPE is required based on transmission precautions.
3. Identify the patient. Explain the procedure to the patient.	Patient identification validates the correct patient and correct procedure. Discussion and explanation help allay anxiety and prepare the patient for what to expect.
4. Close curtain around bed and close the door to the room, if possible. Adjust the head of the bed to a flat position or as low as the patient can tolerate. Raise the bed to a height that is even with the transport stretcher (VISN 8, 2009). Lower the side rails, if in place.	Closing the door or curtain provides privacy. Proper bed height and lowering side rails makes transfer easier and decreases the risk for injury.

ACTION	RATIONALE
5. Place the bath blanket over the patient and remove the top covers from underneath.	Bath blanket provides privacy and warmth.
6. If a friction-reducing transfer sheet is not in place under the patient, place one under the patient's midsection. Have patient fold arms against chest and move chin to chest. Use the friction-reducing sheet to move the patient to the side of the bed where the stretcher will be placed. Alternately, place a lateral-assist device under the patient. Follow manufacturer's directions for use.	A friction-reducing sheet supports the patient's weight, reduces friction during the lift, and provides for a secure hold. A transfer board or other lateral-assist device makes it easier to move the patient and minimizes the risk for injury to the patient and nurses.
7. Position the stretcher next to (and parallel to) the bed. **Lock the wheels on the stretcher and the bed.**	Positioning equipment makes the transfer easier and decreases the risk for injury. Locking the wheels keeps the bed and stretcher from moving.
8. Two nurses should stand on the stretcher side of the bed. A third nurse should stand on the side of the bed without the stretcher.	Team coordination provides for patient safety during transfer.
9. Use the friction-reducing sheet to roll the patient away from the stretcher. Slide the transfer board across the space between the stretcher and the bed, partially under the patient (FIGURE 2). Roll the patient onto his or her back so that the patient is partially on the transfer board.	The transfer board or other lateral-assist device reduces friction, easing the workload to move patient.

ACTION

RATIONALE

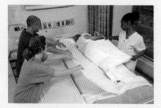

FIGURE 2. Sliding transfer board partially under patient.

10. The nurse on the side of the bed without the stretcher should grasp the friction-reducing sheet at the head and chest areas of the patient. One nurse on the stretcher side of the bed should grasp the friction-reducing sheet at the head and chest, and the other nurse at the chest and leg areas of the patient.

Doing so evenly supports the patient.

11. **At a signal given by one of the nurses, have the nurses standing on the stretcher side of the bed pull the friction-reducing sheet. At the same time, the nurse (or nurses) on the other side push, transferring the patient's weight toward the transfer board, and pushing the patient from the bed to the stretcher.**

Working in unison distributes the work of moving the patient and facilitates the transfer.

12. Once the patient is transferred to the stretcher, remove the transfer board, and secure the patient until the side rails are raised. Raise the side rails. To ensure the patient's comfort, cover the patient with a blanket and remove the bath blanket from underneath. Leave the friction-reducing sheet in place for the return transfer.

Side rails promote safety; blanket promotes comfort and warmth.

ACTION	RATIONALE
13. Clean transfer aids per facility policy, if not indicated for single patient use. Remove gloves and any other PPE, if used. Perform hand hygiene.	Proper cleaning of equipment between patient use prevents the spread of microorganisms. Removing PPE properly reduces the risk for infection transmission and contamination of other items. Hand hygiene prevents the spread of microorganisms.

EVALUATION
- Patient is transferred to the stretcher without injury to patient or nurse.

DOCUMENTATION
- Document the time and method of transport, and patient's destination, according to facility policy. Document the use of transfer aids and number of staff required for transfer.

GENERAL CONSIDERATIONS
- Some mechanical lateral-transfer aids are motorized and others use a hand crank. If a mechanical lateral-assist device is used, follow the manufacturer's directions for safe movement of the patient. Be familiar with weight restrictions for individual pieces of equipment.
- Keep in mind that the transfer of patients is often delegated to unlicensed personnel. Before moving patients, all personnel need to complete instructions about this skill and must be able to provide return demonstrations of transfer skills. When a patient is being transferred, communicate clearly any mobility restrictions or special care needs.

Skill · 171   Transferring a Patient Using a Powered Full-Body Sling Lift

When it has been determined through the use of a transfer assessment and/or the patient cannot bear any weight, use a powered full-body sling lift device to move them up in or out of bed, into and out of a chair, and to a commode or stretcher. A full-body sling is placed under the patient's body, including head and torso, and then the sling is attached to the lift. The device slowly lifts the patient. Some devices can be lowered to the floor to pick up a patient who has fallen. These devices are available on portable bases and ceiling-mounted tracks. Each manufacturer's device is slightly different, so review the instructions for your particular device.

EQUIPMENT

- Powered full-body sling lift
- Sheet or pad to cover the sling, if sling is not dedicated to only one patient
- Chair or wheelchair, as appropriate
- One or more caregivers for assistance, based on assessment
- Nonsterile gloves and/or other PPE, as indicated

ASSESSMENT GUIDELINES

- Assess the situation to determine the need to use the lift. Review the medical record and nursing plan of care for conditions that may influence the patient's ability to move or to be positioned.
- Assess for tubes, IV lines, incisions, or equipment that may alter the positioning procedure.
- Assess the patient's level of consciousness, ability to understand and follow directions, and ability to assist with moving.
- Assess the patient's weight and your strength to determine the number of caregivers required to assist with the activity. Determine if there is a need for bariatric equipment.
- Assess the patient's comfort level; if needed, medicate as ordered with analgesics.

NURSING DIAGNOSES

- Activity Intolerance
- Impaired Skin Integrity
- Risk for Injury
- Risk for Impaired Skin Integrity
- Acute Pain
- Impaired Bed Mobility
- Chronic Pain

OUTCOME IDENTIFICATION AND PLANNING

Expected outcomes may include:
- Patient remains free from injury and maintains proper body alignment during movement.
- Transfer is accomplished without injury to patient or nurse.
- Patient reports improved comfort.
- Patient's skin is clean, dry, and intact, without any redness, irritation, or breakdown.

IMPLEMENTATION

ACTION	RATIONALE
1. Review the medical record and nursing plan of care for conditions that may influence the patient's ability to move or to be positioned. Assess for tubes, intravenous lines, incisions, or equipment that may alter the positioning procedure. Identify any movement limitations. Consult patient handling algorithm, if available, to plan appropriate approach to moving the patient. Check equipment for proper functioning.	Reviewing the order and plan of care validates the correct patient and correct procedure. Identification of limitations and ability and use of an algorithm and properly functioning equipment help to prevent injury and aid in determining best plan for patient movement.
2. Perform hand hygiene and put on PPE, if indicated.	Hand hygiene and PPE prevent the spread of microorganisms. PPE is required based on transmission precautions.
3. Identify the patient. Explain the procedure to the patient.	Patient identification validates the correct patient and correct procedure. Discussion and explanation help allay anxiety and prepare the patient for what to expect.

Using Full Body Sling to Reposition Patient in Bed

4. Close curtains around bed or close the door to the room, if possible. Place the bed at an appropriate and comfortable working height, usually elbow height of the caregiver (VISN, 2009). Adjust the head of the bed to a flat position or as low as the patient can tolerate.	Closing the door or curtain provides for privacy. Proper bed height helps reduce back strain while you are performing the procedure. Flat positioning helps to decrease the gravitational pull of the upper body and assists in placement of sling.
5. Remove all pillows from under the patient. Leave one at the head of the bed, leaning upright against the headboard.	Removing pillows from under the patient facilitates movement; placing a pillow at the head of the bed prevents accidental head injury against the top of the bed.

ACTION	RATIONALE
6. Position at least one nurse on either side of the bed, and lower both side rails.	Proper positioning and lowering the side rails facilitate moving the patient and minimize strain on the nurses.
7. Place cover sheet on sling surface. Place sling under patient.	Protects sling surface and reduces transmission of microorganisms on sling.
8. Roll the base of the lift under the side of the bed nearest to the chair. **Center the frame over the patient. Using the base-adjustment lever, widen the stance of the device base. Lock the wheels of the lift.**	Positions the lift for safe use. Locking wheels prevents accidental movement of lift.
9. Position one nurse and the other caregiver at the patient's midsection on opposite sides of the bed. If necessary, additional staff can support the patient's legs.	Positioning in this manner provides assistance and reduces risk for injury.
10. Crank or engage the mechanism to raise the sling, with the patient, up off the bed. Raise the patient just high enough to clear the bed surface.	Decreased friction.
11. Guide the sling and relocate the patient to the appropriate place at the head of the bed.	Repositions patient in correct position in bed.
12. Release the sling slowly or activate the lowering device on the lift and slowly lower the patient to the bed surface.	Promotes safety and reduces patient anxiety.
13. Remove the sling or leave in place for future use, based on facility policy.	Facilitates future use.
14. Assist the patient to a comfortable position and readjust the pillows and supports as needed. Raise the side rails. Place the bed in the lowest position.	Promotes patient comfort and safety.

ACTION	RATIONALE

15. Clean transfer aids per facility policy, if not indicated for single patient use. Remove gloves or other PPE, if used. Perform hand hygiene.

Proper cleaning of equipment between patient use prevents the spread of microorganisms. Removing PPE properly reduces the risk for infection transmission and contamination of other items. Hand hygiene prevents the spread of microorganisms.

Transferring a Patient Using a Powered Full-Body Sling Lift

16. If needed, move the equipment to make room for the chair. Close the door or draw the curtains.

Moving equipment out of the way provides a clear path and facilitates the transfer. Closing the door or curtain provides for privacy.

17. Adjust the bed to a comfortable working height, usually elbow height of the caregiver (VISN 8, 2009). **Lock the bed brakes.**

Having the bed at the proper height prevents back and muscle strain. Locking the brakes prevents bed movement and ensures patient safety.

18. Lower the side rail, if in use, on the side of the bed you are working. If the sling is for use with more than one patient, place a cover or pad on the sling. Place the sling evenly under the patient. Roll the patient to one side and place half of the sling with the sheet or pad on it under the patient from shoulders to mid-thigh. Raise the rail and move to the other side. Lower the rail, if necessary. Roll the patient to the other side and pull the sling under the patient. Raise the side rail.

Lowering the side rail prevents strain on the nurse's back. Covering the sling prevents transmission of microorganisms. Some facilities, such as long-term care institutions, provide each patient with own transport sling. Rolling the patient positions the patient on the sling with minimal movement. Even distribution of the patient's weight in the sling provides for patient comfort and safety.

19. Bring the chair to the side of the bed. **Lock the wheels, if present.**

Bringing the chair close to the bed minimizes the distance needed for transfer. Locking the wheels prevents chair movement and ensures patient safety.

ACTION	RATIONALE
20. Lower the side rail on the chair side of the bed. **Roll the base of the lift under the side of the bed nearest to the chair. Center the frame over the patient. Lock the wheels of the lift.**	Lowering the rail allows for ease of transfer. Doing so reduces the distance necessary for transfer. Centering the frame helps maintain the balance of the lift. Locking the lift's wheels prevents the lift from rolling.
21. Using the base-adjustment lever, widen the stance of the base.	A wider stance provides greater stability and prevents tipping.
22. Lower the arms close enough to attach the sling to the frame.	Lowering the arms is necessary to allow for the attachment of the sling's hooks.
23. Place the strap or chain hooks through the holes of the sling (FIGURE 1). Short straps attach behind the patient's back and long straps attach at the other end. Check the patient to make sure the hooks are not pressing into the skin. Some lifts have straps on the sling that attach to hooks on the frame. Check the manufacturer's instructions for each lift.	Connecting the straps or chains permits attachment of the sling to the lift. Checking the patient's skin for pressure from the hooks prevents injury.

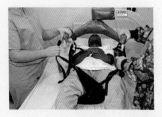

FIGURE 1 Connecting the straps to the lift.

ACTION	RATIONALE
24. Check all equipment, lines, and drains attached to the patient so that they are not interfering with the device. Have the patient fold his or her arms across the chest.	Ensuring that equipment and lines are free of the device prevents dislodgement and possible injury.

ACTION	RATIONALE
25. With a person standing on each side of the lift, tell the patient that he or she will be lifted from the bed. Support injured limbs as necessary. Engage the pump to raise the patient about 6 inches above the bed.	Having the necessary persons available provides for safety. Supporting injured limbs helps maintain stability. Informing the patient about what will occur reassures the patient and reduces fear.
26. Unlock the wheels of the lift. **Carefully wheel the patient straight back and away from the bed.** Support the patient's limbs as needed.	Moving in this manner promotes stability and safety.
27. Position the patient over the chair with the base of the lift straddling the chair (FIGURE 2). Lock the wheels of the lift.	Proper positioning of the patient and device promotes stability and safety.

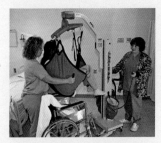

FIGURE 2 Positioning the patient in the sling over the chair.

ACTION	RATIONALE
28. Gently lower the patient to the chair until the hooks or straps are slightly loosened from the sling or frame. Guide the patient into the chair with your hands as the sling lowers.	Gently lowering the patient in this manner places the patient fully in the chair and reduces the risk for injury.
29. Disconnect the hooks or strap from the frame. Keep the sling in place under the patient.	Disconnecting the hooks or straps allows the patient to be supported by the chair and promotes comfort. The sling will need to be reattached to the lift to move the patient back to bed.
30. Adjust the patient's position, using pillows if necessary.	Pillows and proper alignment provide for patient safety and

ACTION	RATIONALE
Check the patient's alignment in the chair. Cover the patient with a blanket if necessary. Place the call bell within reach. When it is time for the patient to return to bed, reattach the hooks or straps and reverse the steps.	comfort. Reattaching the hooks or straps allows the lift to support the patient for transfer back to bed.
31. Clean transfer aids per facility policy, if not indicated for single patient use. Remove gloves or other PPE, if used. Perform hand hygiene.	Proper cleaning of equipment between patient use prevents the spread of microorganisms. Removing PPE properly reduces the risk for infection transmission and contamination of other items. Hand hygiene prevents the spread of microorganisms.

EVALUATION

- Patient is moved up in bed without injury and maintains proper body alignment.
- Transfer is accomplished without injury to patient or nurse.
- Patient is comfortable.
- Patient demonstrates intact skin without evidence of any breakdown.

DOCUMENTATION

- Many facilities provide areas on the bedside flow sheet to document repositioning. Document the time of the patient's change of position, use of supports, and any pertinent observations, including skin assessment. Document the patient's tolerance of the position change. Document the use of the sling and lift to facilitate movement. Document the activity, transfer, any observations, the patient's tolerance of the procedure, and the length of time in the chair. Document the use of transfer aids and number of staff required for transfer.

GENERAL CONSIDERATIONS

- The transfer of patients is often delegated to unlicensed personnel. Before moving patients, all personnel need complete instructions and must be able to provide return demonstrations of transfer skills. Before the transfer, communicate clearly any mobility restrictions or special care needs.

- When moving a patient with a leg or foot problem, such as a cast, wound, or fracture, one assistant should be assigned to lift and move that extremity.
- Calculate the body mass index (BMI) for patients weighing over 300 pounds. If BMI exceeds 50, institute bariatric algorithms and use bariatric equipment.

Skill · 172 Assisting a Patient With Turning in Bed

The nurse needs to use knowledge of correct body alignment and assistive devices to turn the patient in bed. FIGURE 1, Safe Patient Handling Algorithm 4, can help you make decisions about safe patient handling and movement. Mastering and using these techniques will help you maintain a turn schedule to prevent complications for a patient who is immobile. If a patient requires logrolling, please refer to Skill 97, Logrolling a Patient. During any patient-handling task, if any caregiver is required to lift more than 35 pounds of a patient's weight, consider the patient to be fully dependent and use assistive devices.

EQUIPMENT

- Friction-reducing sheet or draw sheet
- Bed surface that inflates to aid in turning
- Pillows or other supports to help the patient maintain the desired position after turning
- and to maintain correct body alignment for the patient
- Additional caregivers to assist, based on assessment
- Nonsterile gloves, if indicated; other PPE as indicated

ASSESSMENT GUIDELINES

- Check the medical record for any conditions or orders that will limit mobility. Assess for any precautions or activity restrictions for the patient.
- Perform a pain assessment before the time for the activity. If the patient reports pain, administer the prescribed medication in sufficient time to allow for the full effect of the analgesic.
- Assess the patient's ability to assist with moving, the need for assistive devices, and the need for a second or third individual to assist with the activity. Determine if there is a need for bariatric equipment.
- Assess the patient's skin for signs of irritation, redness, edema, or blanching.

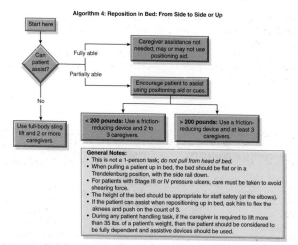

FIGURE 1 Step-by-step procedure or algorithm used to outline safe technique for repositioning a patient in bed. (From VISN 8 Patient Safety Center. [2009]. *Safe patient handling and movement algorithms.* Tampa, FL: Author. Available at http://www.visn8.med.va.gov/patientsafetycenter/safePtHandling/default.asp). Accessed April 23, 2010.

NURSING DIAGNOSES

- Activity Intolerance
- Acute Pain
- Risk for Activity Intolerance
- Chronic Pain
- Fatigue
- Risk for Impaired Skin Integrity
- Risk for Injury
- Impaired Skin Integrity
- Impaired Bed Mobility

OUTCOME IDENTIFICATION AND PLANNING

Expected outcomes may include:
- The activity takes place without injury to patient or nurse.
- The patient is comfortable and in proper body alignment.

IMPLEMENTATION

ACTION	RATIONALE
1. Review the physician's orders and nursing plan of care for patient activity. Iden-	Checking the physician's order and plan of care validates the correct patient and correct procedure.

ACTION	RATIONALE
tify any movement limitations and the ability of the patient to assist with turning. Consult patient handling algorithm, if available, to plan appropriate approach to moving the patient.	Identification of limitations and ability and use of an algorithm helps to prevent injury and aids in determining best plan for patient movement.
2. Gather any positioning aids or supports, if necessary.	Having aids readily available promotes efficient time management.
3. Perform hand hygiene. Put on PPE, as indicated.	Hand hygiene and PPE prevent the spread of microorganisms. PPE is required based on transmission precautions.
4. Identify the patient. Explain the procedure to the patient.	Patient identification validates the correct patient and correct procedure. Discussion and explanation help allay anxiety and prepare the patient for what to expect.
5. Close the curtains around bed and close the door to the room, if possible. Position at least one nurse on either side of the bed. Place pillows, wedges, or any other support to be used for positioning within easy reach. Place the bed at an appropriate and comfortable working height, usually elbow height of the caregiver (VISN 8, 2009). Lower both side rails.	Closing the door or curtain provides privacy. Proper bed height helps reduce back strain while performing the procedure. Proper positioning and lowering the side rails facilitate moving the patient and minimize strain on the nurses.
6. If not already in place, position a friction-reducing sheet under the patient.	Sheets aid in preventing shearing and reducing friction and the force required to move the patient.
7. Using the friction-reducing sheet, move the patient to the edge of the bed, opposite the side to which he or she will be turned. Raise the side rails.	With this placement, the patient will be on the center of the bed after turning is accomplished. Raising side rails ensures patient safety.
8. If the patient is able, have the patient grasp the side rail on	Encourages the patient to assist as much as possible with the

ACTION	RATIONALE

the side of the bed toward which he or she is turning. Alternately, place the patient's arms across his or her chest and cross his or her far leg over the leg nearest you.

movement. This facilitates the turning motion and protects the patient's arms during the turn.

9. If available, activate the bed mechanism to inflate the side of the bed behind the patient's back.

Activating the turn mechanism inflates the side of the bed for approximately 10 seconds, aiding in propelling the patient to turn, and reducing the work required by the nurse. This helps avoid straining the nurse's lower back.

10. **The nurse on the side of the bed toward which the patient is turning should stand opposite the patient's center with his or her feet spread about shoulder width and with one foot ahead of the other. Tighten your gluteal and abdominal muscles and flex your knees. Use your leg muscles to do the pulling. The other nurse should position his or hands on the patient's shoulder and hip, assisting to roll the patient to the side. Instruct the patient to pull on the bed rail at the same time. Use the friction-reducing sheet to gently pull the patient over on his or her side (FIGURE 2).**

The nurse is in a stable position with good body alignment and prepared to use large muscle masses to turn the patient. These maneuvers support the patient's body and makes use of the nurse's weight to assist with turning.

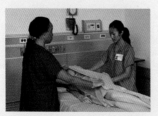

FIGURE 2 Working together to position patient on her side. (*Photo by B. Proud.*)

ACTION	RATIONALE
11. Use a pillow or other support behind the patient's back. Pull the shoulder blade forward and out from under the patient.	Pillow will provide support and help the patient maintain the desired position. Positioning the shoulder blade removes pressure from the bony prominence.
12. Make the patient comfortable and position in proper alignment, using pillows or other supports under the leg and arm, as needed. Readjust the pillow under the patient's head. Elevate the head of the bed as needed for comfort.	Positioning in proper alignment with supports ensures that the patient will be able to maintain the desired position and will be comfortable.
13. **Place the bed in the lowest position, with the side rails up. Make sure the call bell and other necessary items are within easy reach.**	Adjusting the bed height ensures patient safety.
14. Clean transfer aids, per facility policy, if not indicated for single patient use. Remove gloves and other PPE, if used. Perform hand hygiene.	Proper cleaning of equipment between patient use prevents the spread of microorganisms. Removing PPE properly reduces the risk for infection transmission and contamination of other items. Hand hygiene prevents the spread of microorganisms.

EVALUATION

- The patient is turned and repositioned without injury to patient or nurse.
- The patient demonstrates proper body alignment and verbalizes comfort.

DOCUMENTATION

- Many facilities provide areas on the bedside flow sheet to document repositioning. Be sure to document the time of the patient's change of position, use of supports, and any pertinent observations, including skin assessment. Document the patient's tolerance of the position change. Document aids used to facilitate movement.

Skill · 173 Assisting With the Use of a Urinal

Male patients confined to bed usually prefer to use the urinal for voiding. Often, male patients prefer to use the urinal at the bedside as a matter of convenience. The use of a urinal in the standing position facilitates emptying of the bladder. Patients who are unable to stand alone may benefit from assistance when voiding into a urinal. If the patient is unable to stand, the urinal may be used in bed. Patients may also use a urinal in the bathroom to facilitate measurement of urinary output. Many patients find it embarrassing to use the urinal. Promote comfort and normalcy as much as possible, while respecting the patient's privacy. Provide skin care and perineal hygiene after urinal use and maintain a professional manner.

EQUIPMENT
- Urinal with end cover (usually attached)
- Toilet tissue
- Clean gloves
- Additional PPE, as indicated

ASSESSMENT GUIDELINES
- Assess the patient's normal elimination habits. Determine why the patient needs to use a urinal, such as a physician's order for strict bed rest or immobilization.
- Assess the patient's degree of limitation and ability to help with activity. Assess for activity limitations, such as hip surgery or spinal injury, which would contraindicate certain actions by the patient.
- Check for the presence of drains, dressings, intravenous fluid infusion sites/equipment, traction, or any other devices that could interfere with the patient's ability to help with the procedure or that could become dislodged.
- Assess the characteristics of the urine and the patient's skin.

NURSING DIAGNOSES
- Impaired Physical Mobility
- Deficient Knowledge
- Impaired Urinary Elimination
- Functional Urinary Incontinence
- Toileting Self-Care Deficit

OUTCOME IDENTIFICATION AND PLANNING
Expected outcomes may include:
- Patient is able to void with assistance.
- Patient maintains continence.
- Patient demonstrates how to use the urinal.
- Patient maintains skin integrity.

IMPLEMENTATION

ACTION	RATIONALE
1. Review the patient's chart for any limitations in physical activity.	Activity limitations may contraindicate certain actions by the patient.
2. Bring urinal and other necessary equipment to the bedside stand or overbed table.	Bringing everything to the bedside conserves time and energy. Arranging items nearby is convenient, saves time, and avoids unnecessary stretching and twisting of muscles on the part of the nurse.
3. Perform hand hygiene and put on PPE, if indicated.	Hand hygiene and PPE prevent the spread of microorganisms. PPE is required based on transmission precautions.
4. Identify the patient.	Identifying the patient ensures the right patient receives the intervention and helps prevent errors.
5. Close the curtains around the bed and close the door to the room if possible. Discuss procedure with patient and assess the patient's ability to assist with the procedure, as well as personal hygiene preferences.	This ensures the patient's privacy. This discussion promotes reassurance and provides knowledge about the procedure. Dialogue encourages patient participation and allows for individualized nursing care.
6. Put on gloves.	Gloves prevent exposure to blood and body fluids.
7. Assist the patient to an appropriate position as necessary: standing at the bedside; lying on one side or back, sitting in bed with the head elevated, or sitting on the side of the bed.	These positions facilitate voiding and emptying of the bladder.
8. If the patient remains in the bed, fold the linens just enough to allow for proper placement of the urinal.	Folding back the linen in this manner minimizes unnecessary exposure while still allowing the nurse to place the urinal.

ACTION	RATIONALE

9. If the patient is not standing, have him spread his legs slightly. **Hold the urinal close to the penis and position the penis completely within the urinal. Keep the bottom of the urinal lower than the penis. If necessary, assist the patient to hold the urinal in place.**

Slight spreading of the legs allows for proper positioning of the urinal. Placing penis completely within the urinal and keeping the bottom lower than the penis avoids urine spills.

10. Cover the patient with the bed linens.

Covering promotes warmth and privacy.

11. Place call bell and toilet tissue within easy reach. Have a receptacle, such as plastic trash bag, handy for discarding tissue. Ensure the bed is in the lowest position. Leave patient if it is safe to do so. Use side rails appropriately.

Falls can be prevented if the patient does not have to reach for items he or she needs. Placing the bed in the lowest position promotes patient safety. Leave the patient alone, if possible, promotes self-esteem and shows respect for privacy. Side rails assist the patient in repositioning.

12. Remove gloves and additional PPE, if used. Perform hand hygiene.

Proper removal of PPE reduces transmission of microorganisms. Hand hygiene deters the spread of microorganisms.

Removing the Urinal

13. Perform hand hygiene. Put on gloves and additional PPE, as indicated.

Hand hygiene and PPE prevent the spread of microorganisms. Gloves prevent exposure to blood and body fluids. PPE is required based on transmission precautions.

14. Pull back the patient's bed linens just enough to remove the urinal. Remove the urinal. Cover the open end of the urinal. Place on the bedside chair. If patient needs assistance with hygiene, wrap tissue around the hand several times, and wipe patient clean. Place tissue in receptacle.

Covering the end of the urinal helps to prevent the spread of microorganisms.

ACTION	RATIONALE
15. Return the patient to a comfortable position. Make sure the linens under the patient are dry. Remove your gloves and ensure that the patient is covered.	Proper positioning promotes patient comfort. Removing contaminated gloves prevents spread of microorganisms.
16. Ensure patient call bell is in reach.	Promotes patient safety.
17. Offer patient supplies to wash and dry his hands, assisting as necessary.	Washing hands after using the urinal helps prevent the spread of microorganisms.
18. Put on clean gloves. Empty and clean the urinal, measuring urine in graduated container, as necessary. Discard trash receptacle with used toilet paper per facility policy. Remove gloves and perform hand hygiene.	Gloves prevent exposure to blood and body fluids. Measurement of urine volume is required for accurate intake and output records. Hand hygiene helps prevent the spread of microorganisms.
19. Remove additional PPE, if used. Perform hand hygiene.	Removing PPE properly reduces the risk for infection transmission and contamination of other items. Hand hygiene prevents the spread of microorganisms.

EVALUATION

- Patient voids using the urinal.
- Patient remains dry.
- Patient does not experience episodes of incontinence.
- Patient demonstrates measures to assist with using the urinal.
- Patient does not experience impaired skin integrity.

DOCUMENTATION

- Document the patient's tolerance of the activity. Record the amount of urine voided on the intake and output record, if appropriate. Document any other assessments, such as unusual urine characteristics or alterations in the patient's skin.

GENERAL CONSIDERATIONS

- Urinal should not be left in place for extended periods of time because pressure and irritation to the patient's skin can result. If

patient is unable to use alone or with assistance, consider other interventions, such as commode or external condom catheter.
* It may be necessary to assist patients who have difficulty holding the urinal in place, such as those with limited upper extremity movement or alteration in mentation, to prevent spillage of urine.
* The urinal may also be used standing or sitting at the bedside or in the patient's bathroom, if patient is able to do so.

Skill · 174   Catheterizing the Female Urinary Bladder

Urinary catheterization is the introduction of a catheter (tube) through the urethra into the bladder for the purpose of withdrawing urine. Urinary catheterization is considered the most common cause of nosocomial infections (infections acquired in a hospital). Therefore, catheterization should be avoided whenever possible. When it is deemed necessary, it should be performed using aseptic technique.

Intermittent urethral catheters, or straight catheters, are used to drain the bladder for shorter periods (5 to 10 minutes). If a catheter is to remain in place for continuous drainage, an indwelling urethral catheter is used. Indwelling catheters are also called retention or Foley catheters. The indwelling urethral catheter is designed so that it does not slip out of the bladder. A balloon is inflated to ensure that the catheter remains in the bladder once it is inserted. The following procedure reviews insertion of an indwelling catheter. The procedure for an intermittent catheter follows as a Skill Variation.

EQUIPMENT
* Sterile catheter kit that contains:
  * Sterile gloves
  * Sterile drapes (one of which is fenestrated [having a window-like opening])
  * Sterile catheter (Use the smallest appropriate-size catheter, usually a 14F to 16F catheter with a 5- to 10-mL balloon [Mercer Smith, 2003; Newman, 2008]).
  * Antiseptic cleansing solution and cotton balls or gauze squares; antiseptic swabs
  * Lubricant
* Forceps
* Prefilled syringe with sterile water (sufficient to inflate indwelling catheter balloon)
* Sterile basin (usually base of kit serves as this)
* Sterile specimen container (if specimen is required)
* Flashlight or lamp
* Waterproof, disposable pad
* Sterile, disposable urine collection bag and drainage tubing (may be connected to catheter in catheter kit)
* Velcro leg strap or tape

- Disposable gloves
- Additional PPE, as indicated
- Washcloth and warm water to perform perineal hygiene

before and after catheterization

ASSESSMENT GUIDELINES

- Assess the patient's normal elimination habits.
- Assess the patient's degree of limitations and ability to help with activity. Assess for activity limitations, such as hip surgery or spinal injury, which would contraindicate certain actions by the patient.
- Assess for the presence of any other conditions that may interfere with passage of the catheter or contraindicate insertion of the catheter, such as urethral strictures or bladder cancer.
- Check for the presence of drains, dressings, intravenous fluid infusion sites/equipment, traction, or any other devices that could interfere with the patient's ability to help with the procedure or that could become dislodged.
- Assess bladder fullness before performing procedure, either by palpation or with a handheld bladder ultrasound device.
- Question patient about any allergies, especially to latex and iodine.
- Ask the patient if she has ever been catheterized. If she had an indwelling catheter previously, ask why and for how long it was used. The patient may have urethral strictures, which may make catheter insertion more difficult.
- Assess the characteristics of the urine and the patient's skin.

NURSING DIAGNOSES

- Impaired Urinary Elimination
- Risk for Infection
- Urinary Retention
- Risk for Impaired Skin Integrity
- Risk for Injury

OUTCOME IDENTIFICATION AND PLANNING

Expected outcomes may include:
- Patient's urinary elimination will be maintained, with a urine output of at least 30 mL/hour.
- Patient's bladder will not be distended.
- Patient's skin remains clean, dry, and intact, without evidence of irritation or breakdown.
- Patient verbalizes an understanding of the purpose for and care of the catheter, as appropriate.

IMPLEMENTATION

ACTION	RATIONALE
1. Review the patient's chart for any limitations in physical activity. Confirm the medical order for indwelling catheter insertion.	Physical limitations may require adaptations in performing the skill. Verifying the medical order ensures that the correct intervention is administered to the right patient.
2. Bring the catheter kit and other necessary equipment to the bedside. Obtain assistance from another staff member, if necessary.	Bringing everything to the bedside conserves time and energy. Arranging items nearby is convenient, saves time, and avoids unnecessary stretching and twisting of muscles on the part of the nurse. Assistance from another person may be required to perform the intervention safely.
3. Perform hand hygiene and put on PPE, if indicated.	Hand hygiene and PPE prevent the spread of microorganisms. PPE is required based on transmission precautions.
4. Identify the patient.	Identifying the patient ensures the right patient receives the intervention and helps prevent errors.
5. Close curtains around bed and close the door to the room, if possible. Discuss the procedure with the patient and assess the patient's ability to assist with the procedure. Ask the patient if she has any allergies, especially to latex or iodine.	This ensures the patient's privacy. This discussion promotes reassurance and provides knowledge about the procedure. Dialogue encourages patient participation and allows for individualized nursing care. Some catheters and gloves in kits are made of latex. Some antiseptic solutions contain iodine.
6. Provide good lighting. Artificial light is recommended (use of a flashlight requires an assistant to hold and position it). Place a trash receptacle within easy reach.	Good lighting is necessary to see the meatus clearly. A readily available trash receptacle allows for prompt disposal of used supplies and reduces the risk of contaminating the sterile field.

ACTION	RATIONALE
7. Adjust the bed to a comfortable working height, usually elbow height of the caregiver (VISN 8, 2009). Stand on the patient's right side if you are right-handed, patient's left side if you are left-handed.	Having the bed at the proper height prevents back and muscle strain. Positioning allows for ease of use of dominant hand for catheter insertion.
8. Assist the patient to a dorsal recumbent position with knees flexed, feet about 2 feet apart, with her legs abducted. Drape patient. Alternately, the Sims', or lateral, position can be used. Place the patient's buttocks near the edge of the bed with her shoulders at the opposite edge and her knees drawn toward her chest. Allow the patient to lie on either side, depending on which position is easiest for the nurse and best for the patient's comfort. Slide waterproof pad under patient.	Proper positioning allows adequate visualization of the urinary meatus. Embarrassment, chilliness, and tension can interfere with catheter insertion; draping the patient will promote comfort and relaxation. The Sims' position may allow better visualization and be more comfortable for the patient, especially if hip and knee movements are difficult. The smaller area of exposure is also less stressful for the patient. The waterproof pad will protect bed linens from moisture.
9. Put on clean gloves. Clean the perineal area with washcloth, skin cleanser, and warm water, using a different corner of the washcloth with each stroke. Wipe from above orifice downward toward sacrum (front to back). Rinse and dry. Remove gloves. Perform hand hygiene again.	Gloves reduce the risk of exposure to blood and body fluids. Cleaning reduces microorganisms near the urethral meatus and provides an opportunity to visualize the perineum and landmarks before the procedure. Hand hygiene reduces the spread of microorganisms.
10. Prepare urine drainage setup if a separate urine collection system is to be used. Secure to bed frame according to manufacturer's directions.	This facilitates connection of the catheter to the drainage system and provides for easy access.

ACTION	RATIONALE
11. Open sterile catheterization tray on a clean overbed table using sterile technique.	Placement of equipment near the work site increases efficiency. Sterile technique protects patient and prevents transmission of microorganisms.
12. Put on sterile gloves. Grasp upper corners of drape and unfold drape without touching unsterile areas. Fold back a corner on each side to make a cuff over gloved hands. Ask patient to lift her buttocks and slide sterile drape under her with gloves protected by cuff.	The drape provides a sterile field close to the meatus. Covering the gloved hands will help keep the gloves sterile while placing the drape.
13. Based on facility policy, position the fenestrated sterile drape. Place a fenestrated sterile drape over the perineal area, exposing the labia.	The drape expands the sterile field and protects against contamination. Use of a fenestrated drape may limit visualization and is considered optional by some practitioners and/or facility policies.
14. Place sterile tray on drape between patient's thighs.	This provides easy access to supplies.
15. Open all the supplies. Fluff cotton balls in tray before pouring antiseptic solution over them. Alternately, open package of antiseptic swabs. Open specimen container if specimen is to be obtained.	It is necessary to open all supplies and prepare for the procedure while both hands are sterile.
16. Lubricate 1 to 2 inches of catheter tip.	Lubrication facilitates catheter insertion and reduces tissue trauma.
17. With thumb and one finger of nondominant hand, spread labia and identify meatus. **Be prepared to maintain separation of labia with one hand until catheter is inserted and urine is flowing well and continuously.** If the patient is in the side-lying	Smoothing the area immediately surrounding the meatus helps to make it visible. Allowing the labia to drop back into position may contaminate the area around the meatus, as well as the catheter. The nondominant hand is now contaminated.

ACTION	RATIONALE

position, lift the upper buttock and labia to expose the urinary meatus.

18. Use the dominant hand to pick up a cotton ball or antiseptic swab. **Clean one labial fold, top to bottom (from above the meatus down toward the rectum), then discard the cotton ball. Using a new cotton ball/swab for each stroke, continue to clean the other labial fold, then directly over the meatus.**

Moving from an area where there is likely to be less contamination to an area where there is more contamination helps prevent the spread of microorganisms. Cleaning the meatus last helps reduce the possibility of introducing microorganisms into the bladder.

19. With your uncontaminated, dominant hand, place the drainage end of the catheter in receptacle. If the catheter is preattached to sterile tubing and drainage container (closed drainage system), position catheter and setup within easy reach on sterile field. Ensure that clamp on drainage bag is closed.

This facilitates drainage of urine and minimizes risk of contaminating sterile equipment.

20. **Using your dominant hand, hold the catheter 2 to 3 inches from the tip and insert slowly into the urethra. Advance the catheter until there is a return of urine (approximately 2 to 3 inches [4.8 to 7.2 cm]). Once urine drains, advance catheter another 2 to 3 inches (4.8 to 7.2 cm). Do not force catheter through urethra into bladder.** Ask patient to breathe deeply, and rotate catheter gently if slight resistance is met as catheter reaches external sphincter.

The female urethra is about 1.5 to 2.5 inches (3.6 to 6.0 cm) long. Applying force on the catheter is likely to injure mucous membranes. The sphincter relaxes and the catheter can enter the bladder easily when the patient relaxes. Advancing an indwelling catheter an additional 2 to 3 inches (4.8 to 7.2 cm) ensures placement in the bladder and facilitates inflation of the balloon without damaging the urethra.

ACTION	RATIONALE
21. Hold the catheter securely at the meatus with your non-dominant hand. Use your dominant hand to inflate the catheter balloon. Inject entire volume of sterile water supplied in prefilled syringe.	Bladder or sphincter contraction could push the catheter out. The balloon anchors the catheter in place in the bladder. Manufacturer provides appropriate amount of sterile water for the size of catheter in the kit; as a result, use entire syringe provided in the kit.
22. Pull gently on catheter after balloon is inflated to feel resistance.	Improper inflation can cause patient discomfort and malpositioning of catheter.
23. Attach catheter to drainage system if not already pre-attached.	Closed drainage system minimizes the risk for microorganisms being introduced into the bladder.
24. Remove equipment and dispose of it according to facility policy. Discard syringe in sharps container. Wash and dry the perineal area as needed.	Proper disposal prevents the spread of microorganisms. Placing syringe in sharps container prevents reuse. Cleaning promotes comfort and appropriate personal hygiene.
25. Remove gloves. **Secure catheter tubing to the patient's inner thigh with Velcro leg strap or tape.** Leave some slack in catheter for leg movement.	Proper attachment prevents trauma to the urethra and meatus from tension on the tubing. Whether to tape the drainage tubing over or under the leg depends on gravity flow, patient's mobility, and comfort of the patient.
26. Assist the patient to a comfortable position. Cover the patient with bed linens. Place the bed in the lowest position.	Positioning and covering provides warmth and promotes comfort.
27. Secure drainage bag below the level of the bladder. Check that drainage tubing is not kinked and that movement of side rails does not interfere with catheter or drainage bag.	This facilitates drainage of urine and prevents the backflow of urine.
28. Put on clean gloves. Obtain urine specimen immediately,	Catheter system is sterile. Obtaining specimen immediately

ACTION	RATIONALE
if needed, from drainage bag. Label specimen. Send urine specimen to the laboratory promptly or refrigerate it.	allows access to sterile system. Keeping urine at room temperature may cause microorganisms, if present, to grow and distort laboratory findings.
29. Remove gloves and additional PPE, if used. Perform hand hygiene.	Removing PPE properly reduces the risk for infection transmission and contamination of other items. Hand hygiene prevents the spread of microorganisms.

EVALUATION

- Catheter is inserted using sterile technique, results in the immediate flow of urine, and the bladder is not distended.
- Patient does not experience trauma, reports little to no pain on insertion, and the perineal area remains clean and dry.

DOCUMENTATION

- Document the type and size of catheter and balloon inserted, as well as the amount of fluid used to inflate the balloon. Document the patient's tolerance of the activity. Record the amount of urine obtained through the catheter and any specimen obtained. Document any other assessments, such as unusual urine characteristics or alterations in the patient's skin. Record urine amount on intake and output record, if appropriate.

GENERAL CONSIDERATIONS

- In the past, pretesting of the catheter balloon was recommended to prevent insertion of a defective catheter. Most catheter manufacturers in the U.S. no longer recommend pretesting because the balloons are pretested during the manufacturing process. Pretesting silicone balloons is not recommended; the silicone can form a cuff or crease in the balloon area that can cause trauma to the urethra during catheter insertion (Mercer Smith, 2003)
- Be familiar with facility policy and/or primary practitioner guidelines for the maximum amount of urine to remove from bladder at the time of insertion.
- If patient is unable to lift buttocks or maintain required position for the procedure, the assistance of another staff member may be necessary to place the drape under the patient and to help the patient maintain the required position.

- Supplies can be opened and prepared on the overbed table, moving the tray onto the bed just before cleansing the patient.
- If there is not an immediate flow of urine after the catheter has been inserted, several measures may prove helpful:
  - Have the patient take a deep breath, which helps to relax the perineal and abdominal muscles.
  - Rotate the catheter slightly, because a drainage hole may be resting against the bladder wall.
  - Raise the head of the patient's bed to increase pressure in the bladder area.
  - Assess the patient's intake to ensure adequate fluid intake for urine production.
  - Assess the catheter and drainage tubing for kinks and occlusion.
- If the catheter cannot be advanced, have the patient take several deep breaths. Rotate the catheter half a turn and try to advance. If you are still unable to advance, remove the catheter. Notify the primary care provider.
- Some catheter kits do not contain the catheter. This allows you to select a catheter and balloon size separately.

Skill Variation   Intermittent Female Urethral Catheterization

1. Check the medical record 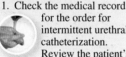 for the order for intermittent urethral catheterization. Review the patient's chart for any limitations in physical activity. Bring the catheter kit and other necessary equipment to the bedside. Obtain assistance from another staff member, if necessary. Perform hand hygiene. Put on PPE, as indicated, based on transmission precautions.

2. Identify the patient. Discuss the procedure with the patient and assess the patient's ability to assist with the procedure. Ask the patient if she has any allergies, especially to latex or iodine.

3. Close curtains around bed and close the door to the room, if possible.

4. Provide good lighting. Artificial light is recommended (use of a flashlight requires an assistant to hold and position it). Place a trash receptacle within easy reach.

5. Raise the bed to a comfortable working height. Stand on the patient's right side if you are right-handed, patient's left side if you are left-handed.

6. Put on disposable gloves. Assist the patient to dorsal recumbent position with knees flexed, feet about 2 feet apart, with her legs abducted. Drape patient. Alternately, use the Sims',

(continued on page 932)

Intermittent Female Urethral Catheterization continued

or lateral, position. Place the patient's buttocks near the edge of the bed with her shoulders at the opposite edge and her knees drawn toward her chest. Slide waterproof drape under patient.

7. Put on clean gloves. Clean the perineal area with washcloth, skin cleanser, and warm water, using a different corner of the washcloth with each stroke. Wipe from above the orifice downward toward the sacrum (front to back). Rinse and dry. Remove gloves. Perform hand hygiene again.

8. Open sterile catheterization tray on a clean overbed table using sterile technique.

9. Put on sterile gloves. Grasp upper corners of drape and unfold drape without touching unsterile areas. Fold back a corner on each side to make a cuff over gloved hands. Ask patient to lift her buttocks and slide sterile drape under her with gloves protected by cuff.

10. Place a fenestrated sterile drape over the perineal area, exposing the labia, if appropriate.

11. Place sterile tray on drape between patient's thighs.

12. Open all the supplies. Fluff cotton balls in tray before pouring antiseptic solution over them. Alternately, open package of antiseptic swabs. Open specimen container if specimen is to be obtained.

13. Lubricate 1 to 2 inches of catheter tip.

14. With thumb and one finger of nondominant hand, spread labia and identify meatus. If the patient is in the side-lying position, lift the upper buttock and labia to expose the urinary meatus. Be prepared to maintain separation of labia with one hand until catheter is inserted and urine is flowing well and continuously.

15. Use the dominant hand to pick up a cotton ball. Clean one labial fold, top to bottom (from above the meatus down toward the rectum), then discard the cotton ball. Using a new cotton ball for each stroke, continue to clean the other labial fold, then directly over the meatus.

16. With the uncontaminated, dominant hand, place drainage end of catheter in receptacle. If a specimen is required, place the end into the specimen container in the receptacle.

17. Using the dominant hand, hold the catheter 2 to 3 inches from the tip and insert slowly into the urethra. Advance the catheter until there is a return of

(continued on page 933)

Intermittent Female Urethral Catheterization *continued*

urine (approximately 2 to 3 inches [4.8 to 7.2 cm]). Do not force the catheter through the urethra into the bladder. Ask the patient to breathe deeply, and rotate the catheter gently if slight resistance is met as the catheter reaches external sphincter.

18. Hold the catheter securely at the meatus with the nondominant hand while the bladder empties. If a specimen is being collected, remove the drainage end of the tubing from the specimen container after required amount is obtained and allow urine to flow into receptacle. Set specimen container aside and place lid on container.

19. Allow the bladder to empty. Withdraw catheter slowly and smoothly after urine has stopped flowing.

Remove equipment and dispose of it according to facility policy. Discard syringe in sharps container to prevent reuse. Wash and dry the perineal area as needed.

20. Remove gloves. Assist the patient to a comfortable position. Cover the patient with bed linens. Place the bed in the lowest position.

21. Put on clean gloves. Secure the container lid and label specimen. Send urine specimen to the laboratory promptly or refrigerate it.

22. Remove gloves and additional PPE, if used. Perform hand hygiene.

23. Intermittent catheterization in the home is performed using clean technique.

Note: The bladder's natural resistance to the microorganisms normally found in the home makes sterile technique unnecessary. Catheters are washed, dried, and stored for repeated use.

Skill · 175   **Catheterizing the Male Urinary Bladder**

Urinary catheterization is the introduction of a catheter (tube) through the urethra into the bladder for the purpose of withdrawing urine. Catheterization is considered the most common cause of nosocomial infections (infections acquired in a hospital). Therefore, catheterization should be avoided whenever possible. When it is deemed necessary, it should be performed using aseptic technique.

Intermittent urethral catheters, or straight catheters, are used to drain the bladder for shorter periods. If a catheter is to remain in place for continuous drainage, an indwelling urethral catheter is used. Indwelling catheters are also called *retention* or *Foley* catheters. The indwelling urethral catheter is designed so that it does not slip out of the bladder. A balloon is inflated to ensure that the catheter remains in the bladder once it is inserted.

The following procedure reviews insertion of an indwelling catheter into the male urinary bladder. The procedure for an intermittent catheter of a male bladder follows as a Skill Variation.

EQUIPMENT

- Sterile catheter kit that contains:
  - Sterile gloves
  - Sterile drapes (one of which is fenestrated [having a window-like opening])
  - Sterile catheter (Use the smallest appropriate-size catheter, usually a 14F to 16F catheter with a 5- to 10-mL balloon [Mercer Smith, 2003; Newman, 2008]).
- Antiseptic cleansing solution and cotton balls or gauze squares; antiseptic swabs
- Lubricant
- Forceps
- Prefilled syringe with sterile water (sufficient to
inflate indwelling catheter balloon)
  - Sterile basin (usually base of kit serves as this)
  - Sterile specimen container (if specimen is required)
- Flashlight or lamp
- Waterproof, disposable pad
- Sterile disposable urine collection bag and drainage tubing (may be connected to catheter in catheter kit)
- Velcro leg strap or tape
- Disposable gloves
- Additional PPE, as indicated
- Washcloth and warm water to perform perineal hygiene before and after catheterization

ASSESSMENT GUIDELINES

- Assess the patient's normal elimination habits.
- Assess the patient's degree of limitations and ability to help with activity. Assess for activity limitations, such as hip surgery or spinal injury, which would contraindicate certain actions by the patient.
- Assess for the presence of any other conditions that may interfere with passage of the catheter or contraindicate insertion of the catheter, such as urethral strictures or bladder cancer.
- Check for the presence of drains, dressings, intravenous fluid infusion sites/equipment, traction, or any other devices that could interfere with the patient's ability to help with the procedure or that could become dislodged.
- Assess bladder fullness before performing the procedure, either by palpation or with a handheld bladder ultrasound device, and question patient about any allergies, especially to latex and iodine.
- Ask the patient if he has ever been catheterized. If he had an indwelling catheter previously, ask why and for how long it was used. The

patient may have urethral strictures, which may make catheter insertion more difficult. If the patient is 50 years of age or older, ask if he has had any prostate problems. Prostate enlargement typically is noted around the age of 50 years.

• Assess the characteristics of the urine and the patient's skin.

NURSING DIAGNOSES

• Impaired Urinary Elimination
• Urinary Retention
• Risk for Infection
• Risk for Impaired Skin Integrity
• Risk for Injury

OUTCOME IDENTIFICATION AND PLANNING

Expected outcomes may include:
• Patient's urinary elimination will be maintained, with a urine output of at least 30 mL/hour, and the patient's bladder will not be distended.
• Patient's skin remains clean, dry, and intact, without evidence of irritation or breakdown.
• Patient verbalizes an understanding of the purpose for, and care of, the catheter, as appropriate.

IMPLEMENTATION

ACTION	RATIONALE
1. Review chart for any limitations in physical activity. Confirm the medical order for indwelling catheter insertion.	Physical limitations may require adaptations in performing the skill. Verifying the medical order ensures that the correct intervention is administered to the right patient.
2. Bring catheter kit and other necessary equipment to the bedside. Obtain assistance from another staff member, if necessary.	Bringing everything to the bedside conserves time and energy. Arranging items nearby is convenient, saves time, and avoids unnecessary stretching and twisting of muscles on the part of the nurse. Assistance from another person may be required to perform the intervention safely.
3. Perform hand hygiene and put on PPE, if indicated.	Hand hygiene and PPE prevent the spread of microorganisms. PPE is required based on transmission precautions.

ACTION	RATIONALE
4. Identify the patient.	Identifying the patient ensures the right patient receives the intervention and helps prevent errors.
5. Close curtains around bed and close the door to the room, if possible. Discuss the procedure with the patient and assess patient's ability to assist with the procedure. Ask the patient if he has any allergies, especially to latex or iodine.	This ensures the patient's privacy. This discussion promotes reassurance and provides knowledge about the procedure. Dialogue encourages patient participation and allows for individualized nursing care. Some catheters and gloves in kits are made of latex. Some antiseptic solutions contain iodine.
6. Provide good lighting. Artificial light is recommended (use of a flashlight requires an assistant to hold and position it). Place a trash receptacle within easy reach.	Good lighting is necessary to see the meatus clearly. A readily available trash receptacle allows for prompt disposal of used supplies and reduces the risk of contaminating the sterile field.
7. Adjust the bed to a comfortable working height, usually elbow height of the caregiver (VISN 8, 2009). Stand on the patient's right side if you are right-handed, patient's left side if you are left-handed.	Having the bed at the proper height prevents back and muscle strain. Positioning allows for ease of use of dominant hand for catheter insertion.
8. Position the patient on his back with thighs slightly apart. Drape the patient so that only the area around the penis is exposed. Slide waterproof pad under patient.	This prevents unnecessary exposure and promotes warmth. The waterproof pad will protect bed linens from moisture.
9. Put on clean gloves. Clean the genital area with washcloth, skin cleanser, and warm water. Clean the tip of the penis first, moving the washcloth in a circular motion from the meatus outward. Wash the shaft of the	Gloves reduce the risk of exposure to blood and body fluids. Cleaning the penis reduces microorganisms near the urethral meatus. Hand hygiene reduces the spread of microorganisms.

ACTION	RATIONALE
penis using downward strokes toward the pubic area. Rinse and dry. Remove gloves. Perform hand hygiene again.	
10. Prepare urine drainage setup if a separate urine collection system is to be used. Secure to bed frame according to manufacturer's directions.	This facilitates connection of the catheter to the drainage system and provides for easy access.
11. Open sterile catheterization tray on a clean overbed table, using sterile technique.	Placement of equipment near worksite increases efficiency. Sterile technique protects patient and prevents spread of microorganisms.
12. Put on sterile gloves. Open sterile drape and place on patient's thighs. Place fenestrated drape with opening over penis.	This maintains a sterile working area.
13. Place catheter set on or next to patient's legs on sterile drape.	Sterile setup should be arranged so that the nurse's back is not turned to it, nor should it be out of the nurse's range of vision.
14. Open all the supplies. Fluff cotton balls in tray before pouring antiseptic solution over them. Alternately, open package of antiseptic swabs. Open specimen container if specimen is to be obtained. Remove cap from syringe prefilled with lubricant.	It is necessary to open all supplies and prepare for the procedure while both hands are sterile.
15. Place drainage end of catheter in receptacle. If the catheter is preattached to sterile tubing and drainage container (closed drainage system), position catheter and setup within easy reach on sterile field. Ensure that clamp on drainage bag is closed.	This facilitates drainage of urine and minimizes risk of contaminating sterile equipment.

ACTION	RATIONALE
16. Lift penis with nondominant hand. Retract foreskin in uncircumcised patient. **Be prepared to keep this hand in this position until catheter is inserted and urine is flowing well and continuously. Using the dominant hand and the forceps, pick up a cotton ball or antiseptic swab. Using a circular motion, clean the penis, moving from the meatus down the glans of the penis. Repeat this cleansing motion two more times, using a new cotton ball/swab each time. Discard each cotton ball/swab after one use.**	The hand touching the penis becomes contaminated. Cleansing the area around the meatus and under the foreskin in the uncircumcised patient helps prevent infection. Moving from the meatus toward the base of the penis prevents bringing microorganisms to the meatus.
17. Hold penis with slight upward tension and perpendicular to patient's body. Use the dominant hand to pick up the lubricant syringe. **Gently insert tip of syringe with lubricant into urethra and instill the 10 mL of lubricant** (Society of Urologic Nurses and Associates, 2005c).	The lubricant causes the urethra to distend slightly and facilitates passage of the catheter without traumatizing the lining of the urethra (Mercer Smith, 2003; Society of Urologic Nurses and Associates, 2005c). If the prepackaged kit does not contain a syringe with lubricant, the nurse may need assistance in filling a syringe while keeping the lubricant sterile. Some institutions use lidocaine jelly for lubrication before insertion of the catheter. The jelly comes prepackaged in a sterile syringe and serves a dual purpose of lubricating and numbing the urethra. A medical order is necessary for the use of lidocaine jelly.
18. Use the dominant hand to pick up the catheter and hold it an inch or two from the tip. Ask patient to bear down as if voiding. **Insert catheter**	Bearing down eases the passage of the catheter through the urethra. The male urethra is about 20 cm long. Having the patient take deep breaths or twisting the

ACTION	RATIONALE

tip into meatus. Ask the patient to take deep breaths. Advance the catheter to the bifurcation or "Y" level of the ports. Do not use force to introduce the catheter. If the catheter resists entry, ask patient to breathe deeply and rotate catheter slightly.

catheter slightly may ease the catheter past resistance at the sphincters. Advancing an indwelling catheter to the bifurcation ensures its placement in the bladder and facilitates inflation of the balloon without damaging the urethra.

19. Hold the catheter securely at the meatus with your non-dominant hand. Use your dominant hand to inflate the catheter balloon. **Inject the entire volume of sterile water supplied in the pre-filled syringe. Once the balloon is inflated, the catheter may be gently pulled back into place. Replace foreskin over catheter. Lower penis.**

Bladder or sphincter contraction could push out the catheter. The balloon anchors the catheter in place in the bladder. Manufacturer provides appropriate amount of solution for the size of catheter in the kit; as a result, use entire syringe provided in the kit.

20. Pull gently on catheter after balloon is inflated to feel resistance.

Improper inflation can cause patient discomfort and malpositioning of catheter.

21. Attach catheter to drainage system, if necessary.

Closed drainage system minimizes the risk for microorganisms being introduced into the bladder.

22. Remove equipment and dispose of it according to facility policy. Discard syringe in sharps container. Wash and dry the perineal area, as needed.

Proper disposal prevents the spread of microorganisms. Placing syringe in sharps container prevents reuse. Promotes comfort and appropriate personal hygiene.

23. Remove gloves. Secure catheter tubing to the patient's inner thigh or lower abdomen (with the penis directed toward the patient's chest) with Velcro leg strap or tape. Leave some slack in catheter for leg movement.

Proper attachment prevents trauma to the urethra and meatus from tension on the tubing. Whether to take the drainage tubing over or under the leg depends on gravity flow, patient's mobility, and comfort of the patient.

ACTION	RATIONALE
24. Assist the patient to a comfortable position. Cover the patient with bed linens. Place the bed in the lowest position.	Positioning and covering provides warmth and promotes comfort.
25. Secure drainage bag below the level of the bladder. Check that drainage tubing is not kinked and that movement of side rails does not interfere with catheter or drainage bag.	This facilitates drainage of urine and prevents the backflow of urine.
26. Put on clean gloves. Obtain urine specimen immediately, if needed, from drainage bag. Label specimen. Send urine specimen to the laboratory promptly or refrigerate it.	Catheter system is sterile. Obtaining specimen immediately allows access to sterile system. Keeping urine at room temperature may cause microorganisms, if present, to grow and distort laboratory findings.
27. Remove gloves and additional PPE, if used. Perform hand hygiene.	Removing PPE properly reduces the risk for infection transmission and contamination of other items. Hand hygiene prevents the spread of microorganisms.

EVALUATION

• Urinary catheter is inserted using sterile technique; it results in the immediate flow of urine, and the bladder is not distended.
• Patient does not experience trauma, reports little to no pain on insertion, and the perineal area remains clean and dry.

DOCUMENTATION

• Document the type and size of catheter and balloon inserted, as well as the amount of fluid used to inflate the balloon. Document the patient's tolerance of the activity. Record the amount of urine obtained through the catheter and any specimen obtained. Document any other assessments, such as unusual urine characteristics or alterations in the patient's skin. Record urine amount on intake and output record, if appropriate.

GENERAL CONSIDERATIONS

- In the past, pretesting of the catheter balloon was recommended to prevent insertion of a defective catheter. Most catheter manufacturers in the United States no longer recommend pretesting because the balloons are pretested during the manufacturing process. Pretesting silicone balloons is not recommended; the silicone can form a cuff or crease in the balloon area that can cause trauma to the urethra during catheter insertion (Mercer Smith, 2003).

- Be familiar with facility policy and/or primary practitioner guidelines for the maximum amount of urine to remove from bladder at the time of insertion.

- Supplies can be opened and prepared on the overbed table, moving the tray onto the bed just before cleansing the patient.

- If there is not an immediate flow of urine after the catheter has been inserted, several measures may prove helpful:
  - Have the patient take a deep breath, which helps to relax the perineal and abdominal muscles.
  - Rotate the catheter slightly, because a drainage hole may be resting against the bladder wall.
  - Raise the head of the patient's bed to increase pressure in the bladder area.
  - Assess the patient's intake to ensure adequate fluid intake for urine production.
  - Assess the catheter and drainage tubing for kinks and occlusion.
  - Urethral strictures, false passages, prostatic enlargement, and postsurgical bladder-neck contractures can make urethral catheterization difficult and may require the services of a urologist. With any question to the location of the catheter, such as no return of urine, do not inflate the balloon. Remove the catheter and notify the physician (Society of Urologic Nurses and Associates, 2005c).

- If the catheter cannot be advanced, having the patient take several deep breaths may be helpful. Rotate the catheter half a turn, and try to advance it. If you are still unable to advance it, remove the catheter. Notify the physician.

- Some catheter kits do not contain the catheter. This allows you to select a catheter and balloon size separately.

- If resistance is met while inserting a catheter and rotating does not help, the catheter is never forced. Enlargement of the prostate gland is commonly seen in men over age 50. A special crook-tipped catheter, called a Coude catheter, inserted by the physician or advanced practice nurse, may be required to maneuver past the prostate gland.

Skill Variation — Intermittent Male Urethral Catheterization

1. Check the medical record for the order for intermittent urethral catheterization. Review chart for any limitations in physical activity. Bring the catheter kit and other necessary equipment to bedside. Obtain assistance from another staff member, if necessary. Perform hand hygiene. Put on PPE, as indicated, based on transmission precautions.

2. Identify the patient. Discuss the procedure with the patient and assess his ability to assist with the procedure. Discuss any allergies with the patient, especially to iodine and latex.

3. Close curtains around bed and close the door to the room, if possible.

4. Provide good lighting. Artificial light is recommended. Place a trash receptacle within easy reach.

5. Raise the bed to a comfortable working height. Stand on the patient's right side if you are right-handed, patient's left side if you are left-handed.

6. Position patient on his back with thighs slightly apart. Drape patient so that only the area around the penis is exposed. Slide waterproof pad under patient.

7. Put on clean gloves. Clean the genital area with washcloth, skin cleanser, and warm water. Clean the tip of the penis first, moving the washcloth in a circular motion from the meatus outward. Wash the shaft of the penis using downward strokes toward the pubic area. Rinse and dry. Remove gloves. Perform hand hygiene again.

8. Open sterile catheterization tray on a clean overbed table using sterile technique.

9. Put on sterile gloves. Open sterile drape and place on patient's thighs. Place fenestrated drape with opening over penis.

10. Place catheter set on or next to patient's legs on sterile drape.

11. Open all the supplies. Fluff cotton balls in tray before pouring antiseptic solution over them. Alternately, open package of antiseptic swabs. Open specimen container if specimen is to be obtained.

12. Remove cap from syringe prefilled with lubricant.

13. Lift penis with nondominant hand. Retract foreskin in uncircumcised patient. Be prepared to keep this hand in this position until catheter is inserted and urine is flowing well and continuously.

(continued on page 943)

Intermittent Male Urethral Catheterization *continued*

14. Using the dominant hand and the forceps, pick up a cotton ball or antiseptic swab. Using a circular motion, clean the penis, moving from the meatus down the glans of the penis. Repeat this cleansing motion two more times, using a new cotton ball/swab each time. Discard each cotton ball/swab after one use.

15. Hold penis with slight upward tension and perpendicular to patient's body. Use the dominant hand to pick up the lubricant syringe. Gently insert tip of syringe with lubricant into urethra and instill the 10 mL of lubricant.

16. With the uncontaminated, dominant hand, place drainage end of catheter in receptacle. If a specimen is required, place the end into the specimen container in the receptacle.

17. Use the dominant hand to pick up the catheter and hold it an inch or two from the tip. Ask the patient to bear down as if voiding. Insert catheter tip into meatus. Ask the patient to take deep breaths as you advance the catheter 6 to 8 inches (14.4 to 19.2 cm) or until urine flows.

18. Hold the catheter securely at the meatus with the non-dominant hand while the bladder empties. If a specimen is being collected, remove the drainage end of the tubing from the specimen container after the required amount is obtained and allow urine to flow into receptacle. Set specimen container aside.

19. Allow the bladder to empty. Withdraw catheter slowly and smoothly after urine has stopped flowing. Remove equipment and dispose of it according to facility policy. Discard syringe in sharps container to prevent reuse. Wash and dry the genital area as needed. Replace foreskin in forward position if necessary.

20. Remove gloves. Assist the patient to a comfortable position. Cover the patient with bed linens. Place the bed in the lowest position.

21. Put on clean gloves. Cover and label the specimen. Send the urine specimen to the laboratory promptly or refrigerate it.

22. Remove gloves and additional PPE, if used. Perform hand hygiene.

Note: Intermittent catheterization in the home is performed using clean technique. The bladder's natural resistance to the microorganisms normally found in the home makes sterile technique unnecessary. Catheters are washed, dried, and stored for repeated use.

Skill · 176   **Performing Intermittent Closed Catheter Irrigation**

Indwelling catheters at times require irrigation, or flushing, with solution to restore or maintain the patency of the drainage system. Sediment or debris, as well as blood clots, might block the catheter, preventing the flow of urine out of the catheter. Irrigations might also be used to instill medications that will act directly on the bladder wall. Irrigating a catheter through a closed system is preferred to opening the catheter because opening the catheter could lead to contamination and infection.

EQUIPMENT

- Sterile basin or container
- Sterile irrigating solution (at room temperature or warmed to body temperature)
- 30- to 60-mL syringe (with 18- or 19-gauge blunt-end needle, if catheter access port is not a needleless system)
- Clamp for drainage tubing
- Bath blanket
- Disposable gloves
- Additional PPE, as indicated
- Waterproof pad

ASSESSMENT GUIDELINES

- Check the medical record for an order to irrigate the catheter, including the type and amount of solution to use for the irrigation.
- Assess catheter drainage and amount of urine in drainage bag.
- Assess for bladder fullness, either by palpation or with a handheld bladder ultrasound device.
- Assess for signs of adverse effects, which may include pain, bladder spasm, bladder distension/fullness, or lack of drainage from the catheter.

NURSING DIAGNOSES

- Impaired Urinary Elimination
- Risk for Infection

OUTCOME IDENTIFICATION AND PLANNING

Expected outcomes may include:
- Patient exhibits the free flow of urine through the catheter.
- Patient's bladder is not distended.
- Patient remains free from pain.
- Patient remains free of any signs and symptoms of infection.

IMPLEMENTATION

ACTION	RATIONALE
1. Confirm the order for catheter irrigation in the medical record.	Verifying the medical order ensures that the correct intervention is administered to the right patient.
2. Bring necessary equipment to the bedside.	Bringing everything to the bedside conserves time and energy. Arranging items nearby is convenient, saves time, and avoids unnecessary stretching and twisting of muscles on the part of the nurse.
3. Perform hand hygiene and put on PPE, if indicated.	Hand hygiene and PPE prevent the spread of microorganisms. PPE is required based on transmission precautions.
4. Identify the patient.	Identifying the patient ensures the right patient receives the intervention and helps prevent errors.
5. Close curtains around bed and close the door to the room, if possible. Discuss the procedure with patient.	This ensures the patient's privacy. This discussion promotes reassurance and provides knowledge about the procedure. Dialogue encourages patient participation and allows for individualized nursing care.
6. Adjust bed to comfortable working height, usually elbow height of the caregiver (VISN 8, 2009).	Having the bed at the proper height prevents back and muscle strain.
7. Put on gloves. Empty the catheter drainage bag and measure the amount of urine, noting the amount and characteristics of the urine. Remove gloves.	Gloves prevent contact with blood and body fluids. Emptying the drainage bag allows for accurate assessment of drainage after the irrigation solution is instilled. Assessment of urine provides a baseline for future comparison. Proper removal of PPE prevents transmission of microorganisms.

ACTION	RATIONALE
8. Assist patient to comfortable position and expose the access port on catheter setup. Place waterproof pad under catheter and aspiration port. Remove catheter from device or tape anchoring catheter to the patient.	This provides adequate visualization. Waterproof pad protects patient and bed from leakage. Removing the catheter from the anchoring device or tape allows for manipulation of the catheter.
9. Open supplies, using aseptic technique. Pour sterile solution into sterile basin. Aspirate the prescribed amount of irrigant (usually 30 to 60 mL) into sterile syringe. Put on gloves.	Use of aseptic technique ensures sterility of irrigating fluid and prevents spread of microorganisms. Gloves prevent contact with blood and body fluids.
10. **Cleanse the access port on catheter with antimicrobial swab.**	Cleaning the port reduces the risk of introducing organisms into the closed urinary system.
11. Clamp or fold catheter tubing below the access port.	This directs the irrigating solution into the bladder, preventing flow into the drainage bag.
12. Attach the syringe to the access port on the catheter using a twisting motion (FIGURE 1). **Gently instill solution into catheter.**	Gentle irrigation prevents damage to bladder lining. Instillation of fluid dislodges material blocking the catheter.

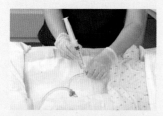

FIGURE 1 Attaching the syringe to the access port on catheter using a twisting motion.

ACTION	RATIONALE
13. Remove syringe from access port. **Unclamp or unfold tubing and allow irrigant and urine to flow into the drainage bag. Repeat procedure, as necessary.**	Gravity aids drainage of urine and irrigant from the bladder.

ACTION	RATIONALE
14. Remove gloves. Secure catheter tubing to the patient's inner thigh or lower abdomen (if a male patient) with anchoring device or tape. Leave some slack in the catheter for leg movement.	Proper attachment prevents trauma to the urethra and meatus from tension on the tubing. Whether to take the drainage tubing over or under the leg depends on gravity flow and patient's mobility and comfort.
15. Assist the patient to a comfortable position. Cover the patient with bed linens. Place the bed in the lowest position.	Positioning and covering provide warmth and promote comfort. Lowering bed contributes to patient safety.
16. Secure drainage bag below the level of the bladder. Check that drainage tubing is not kinked and that movement of side rails does not interfere with catheter or drainage bag.	This facilitates drainage of urine and prevents the backflow of urine.
17. Remove equipment and discard syringe in appropriate receptacle. Remove gloves and additional PPE, if used. Perform hand hygiene.	Proper disposal of equipment prevents transmission of microorganisms. Removing PPE properly reduces the risk for infection transmission and contamination of other items. Hand hygiene prevents the spread of microorganisms.
18. Assess patient's response to the procedure and the quality and amount of drainage after the irrigation.	This provides an accurate assessment of the patient's response to the procedure.

EVALUATION

- Patient exhibits the free flow of urine through the catheter, and the irrigant and urine are returned into the drainage bag.
- Patient's bladder is not distended.
- Patient remains free from pain.
- Patient remains free of any signs and symptoms of infection.

DOCUMENTATION

- Document baseline assessment of patient. Document the amount and type of irrigation solution used and the amount and characteristics of drainage returned after the procedure. Document the ease of irrigation and the patient's tolerance of the procedure. Record urine amount emptied from the drainage bag before the procedure and the amount of irrigant used on intake and output record. Subtract irrigant amount from the urine output when totaling output to provide an accurate recording of urine output.

GENERAL CONSIDERATIONS

• If irrigant is a medication intended for action in the bladder, be aware of specific dwell time included in the order or determined by the action of the medication. Allow the appropriate amount of time to lapse before unclamping the drainage tubing after instillation of irrigant.

Skill · 177   **Removing an Indwelling Catheter**

Removal of an indwelling catheter is performed using clean technique. Take care to prevent trauma to the urethra during the procedure. Completely deflate the catheter balloon before catheter removal to avoid irritation and damage to the urethra and meatus. The patient may experience burning or irritation the first few times he/she voids after removal, due to urethral irritation. If the catheter was in place for more than a few days, decreased bladder muscle tone and swelling of the urethra may cause the patient to experience difficulty voiding or an inability to void. Monitor the patient for urinary retention. It is important to encourage adequate oral fluid intake to promote adequate urinary output. Check facility policy regarding the length of time the patient is allowed to accomplish successful voiding after catheter removal.

EQUIPMENT

• Syringe sufficiently large to accommodate the volume of solution used to inflate the balloon (balloon size/inflation volume is printed on the balloon inflation valve on the catheter at the bifurcation)
• Waterproof, disposable pad
• Disposable gloves
• Additional PPE, as indicated
• Washcloth and warm water to perform perineal hygiene after catheter removal

ASSESSMENT GUIDELINES

• Check the medical record for an order to remove the catheter.
• Assess for discharge or encrustation around the urethral meatus.
• Assess urine output, including color and current amount, in drainage bag.

NURSING DIAGNOSES
- Impaired Urinary Elimination
- Urinary Retention
- Risk for Injury

OUTCOME IDENTIFICATION AND PLANNING
Expected outcomes may include:
- Catheter will be removed without difficulty and with minimal patient discomfort.
- Patient voids without discomfort after catheter removal.
- Patient voids a minimum of 250 mL of urine within 6 to 8 hours of catheter removal.
- Patient's skin remains clean, dry, and intact, without evidence of irritation or breakdown.
- Patient verbalizes an understanding of the need to maintain adequate fluid intake, as appropriate.

IMPLEMENTATION

ACTION	RATIONALE
1. Confirm the order for catheter removal in the medical record.	Verifying the medical order ensures that the correct intervention is administered to the right patient.
2. Bring necessary equipment to the bedside.	Bringing everything to the bedside conserves time and energy. Arranging items nearby is convenient, saves time, and avoids unnecessary stretching and twisting of muscles on the part of the nurse.
3. Perform hand hygiene and put on PPE, if indicated.	Hand hygiene and PPE prevent the spread of microorganisms. PPE is required based on transmission precautions.
4. Identify the patient.	Identifying the patient ensures the right patient receives the intervention and helps prevent errors.
5. Close curtains around the bed and close the door to the	This ensures the patient's privacy. This discussion promotes

ACTION	RATIONALE

room, if possible. Discuss the procedure with the patient and assess the patient's ability to assist with the procedure.

reassurance and provides knowledge about the procedure. Dialogue encourages patient participation and allows for individualized nursing care.

6. Adjust bed to comfortable working height, usually elbow height of the caregiver (VISN 8, 2009). Stand on the patient's right side if you are right-handed, patient's left side if you are left-handed.

Having the bed at the proper height prevents back and muscle strain. Positioning allows for ease of use of dominant hand for catheter removal.

7. Position the patient as for catheter insertion. Drape the patient so that only the area around the catheter is exposed. Slide waterproof pad between the female patient's legs or over the male patient's thighs.

Positioning allows access to site. Draping prevents unnecessary exposure and promotes warmth. The waterproof pad will protect bed linens from moisture and serve as a receptacle for the used catheter after removal.

8. Remove the leg strap, tape, or other device used to secure the catheter to the patient's thigh or abdomen.

This action permits removal of catheter.

9. **Insert the syringe into the balloon inflation port. Allow water to come back by gravity (Mercer Smith, 2003). Alternately, aspirate the entire amount of sterile water used to inflate the balloon (FIGURE 1). Refer to**

Removal of sterile water deflates the balloon to allow for catheter removal. All of the sterile water must be removed to prevent injury to the patient. Aspiration by pulling on the syringe plunger may result in collapse of the inflation lumen; contribute to the

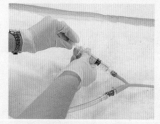

FIGURE 1 Removing fluid from balloon.

ACTION	RATIONALE
manufacturer's instructions for deflation. Do not cut the inflation port.	formation of creases, ridges, or cuffing at the balloon area; and increase the catheter balloon diameter size on deflation, resulting in difficult removal and urethral trauma (Mercer Smith, 2003).
10. Ask the patient to take several slow deep breaths. **Slowly and gently remove the catheter.** Place it on the waterproof pad and wrap it in the pad.	Slow deep breathing helps to relax the sphincter muscles. Slow gentle removal prevents trauma to the urethra. Using a waterproof pad prevents contact with the catheter.
11. Wash and dry the perineal area, as needed.	Cleaning promotes comfort and appropriate personal hygiene.
12. Remove gloves. Assist the patient to a comfortable position. Cover the patient with bed linens. Place the bed in the lowest position.	These actions provide warmth and promote comfort and safety.
13. Put on clean gloves. Remove equipment and dispose of it according to facility policy. Note characteristics and amount of urine in drainage bag.	Proper disposal prevents the spread of microorganisms. Observing the characteristics ensures accurate documentation.
14. Remove gloves and additional PPE, if used. Perform hand hygiene.	Removing PPE properly reduces the risk for infection transmission and contamination of other items. Hand hygiene prevents the spread of microorganisms.

EVALUATION

• Catheter is removed without difficulty and with minimal patient discomfort.
• Patient voids without discomfort after catheter removal.
• Patient voids a minimum of 250 mL of urine within 6 to 8 hours of catheter removal.
• Patient's skin remains clean, dry, and intact, without evidence of irritation or breakdown.
• Patient verbalizes an understanding of the need to maintain adequate fluid intake, as appropriate.

DOCUMENTATION

• Document the type and size of catheter removed and the amount of fluid removed from the balloon Document the patient's tolerance of the procedure. Record the amount of urine in the drainage bag. Note the time the patient is due to void. Document any other assessments, such as unusual urine characteristics or alterations in the patient's skin. Record urine amount on intake and output record, if appropriate.

GENERAL CONSIDERATIONS

• Have alternate toileting measures available, as necessary, based on patient assessment. A bedside commode, urinal, or bedpan may be necessary if the patient is unable to get to the bathroom.
• Refer to facility policy and manufacturer's recommendation regarding balloon deflation. Aspiration by pulling on the syringe plunger may result in collapse of the inflation lumen; contribute to the formation of creases, ridges, or cuffing at the balloon area; and increase the catheter balloon diameter size on deflation, resulting in difficult removal and urethral trauma (Mercer Smith, 2003).

Skill · 178 **Caring for a Suprapubic Urinary Catheter**

A suprapubic catheter may be used for long-term continuous urinary drainage. This type of catheter is surgically inserted through a small incision above the pubic area. Suprapubic bladder drainage diverts urine from the urethra when injury, stricture, prostatic obstruction, or gynecologic or abdominal surgery has compromised the flow of urine through the urethra. A suprapubic catheter is often preferred over indwelling urethral catheters for long-term urinary drainage. Suprapubic catheters are associated with decreased risk of contamination with organisms from fecal material, elimination of damage to the urethra, a higher rate of patient satisfaction, and lower risk of catheter-associated urinary tract infections. The drainage tube is secured with sutures or tape. Care of the patient with a suprapubic catheter includes skin care around the insertion site; care of the drainage tubing and drainage bag is the same as for an indwelling catheter.

EQUIPMENT

• Washcloth
• Gentle soap or skin cleanser
• Disposable gloves
• Additional PPE, as indicated
• Velcro tube holder or tape to secure tube
• Drainage sponge (if necessary)
• Plastic trash bag
• Sterile cotton-tipped applicators and sterile saline solution (if the patient has a new suprapubic catheter)

ASSESSMENT GUIDELINES

• Assess the suprapubic catheter and bag, observing the condition of the catheter and the drainage bag connected to the catheter, and the product style. If a dressing is in place at the insertion site, assess the dressing for drainage.
• Inspect the site around the suprapubic catheter, looking for drainage, erythema, or excoriation.
• Assess the method used to secure the catheter in place. If sutures are present, assess for intactness.
• Assess the characteristics of the urine in the drainage bag.
• Assess the patient's knowledge of caring for a suprapubic catheter.

NURSING DIAGNOSES

• Impaired Urinary Elimination
• Risk for Impaired Skin Integrity
• Risk for Infection
• Deficient Knowledge

OUTCOME IDENTIFICATION AND PLANNING

Expected outcomes may include:
• Patient's skin remains clean, dry, and intact, without evidence of irritation or breakdown.
• Patient verbalizes an understanding of the purpose for, and care of, the catheter, as appropriate.
• Patient's urinary elimination is maintained, with a urine output of at least 30 mL/hour, and the patient's bladder is not distended.

IMPLEMENTATION

ACTION	RATIONALE
1. Bring necessary equipment to the bedside stand or over-bed table.	Bringing everything to the bedside conserves time and energy. Arranging items nearby is convenient, saves time, and avoids unnecessary stretching and twisting of muscles on the part of the nurse.
2. Perform hand hygiene and put on PPE, if indicated.	Hand hygiene and PPE prevent the spread of microorganisms. PPE is required based on transmission precautions.

ACTION	RATIONALE

3. Identify the patient.

Identifying the patient ensures the right patient receives the intervention and helps prevent errors.

4. Close curtains around bed and close the door to the room, if possible. Explain what you are going to do, and why you are going to do it, to the patient. Encourage the patient to observe or participate, if possible.

This ensures the patient's privacy. Explanation relieves anxiety and facilitates cooperation. Discussion promotes cooperation and helps to minimize anxiety. Having the patient observe or assist encourages self-acceptance.

5. Adjust bed to comfortable working height, usually elbow height of the caregiver (VISN 8, 2009). Assist patient to a supine position. Place waterproof pad under the patient at the stoma site.

Having the bed at the proper height prevents back and muscle strain. The supine position is usually the best way to gain access to the suprapubic urinary catheter. A waterproof pad protects linens and patient from moisture.

6. Put on clean gloves. Gently remove old dressing, if one is in place. Place dressing in trash bag. Remove gloves. Perform hand hygiene.

Gloves protect the nurse from blood, body fluids, and microorganisms. Proper disposal of contaminated dressing and hand hygiene deter the spread of microorganisms.

7. Assess the insertion site and surrounding skin.

Any changes in assessment could indicate potential infection.

8. Wet washcloth with warm water and apply skin cleanser. **Gently cleanse around suprapubic exit site.** Remove any encrustations. If this is a new suprapubic catheter, use sterile cotton-tipped applicators and sterile saline to clean the site until the incision has healed. **Moisten the applicators with the saline and clean in circular motion from the insertion site outward.**

Using a gentle soap or cleanser helps to protect the skin. The exit site is the most common area of skin irritation with a suprapubic catheter. If encrustations are left on the skin, they provide a medium for bacteria and an area of skin irritation.

ACTION	RATIONALE
9. Rinse area of all cleanser. Pat dry.	If left on the skin, soap can cause irritation. The skin needs to be kept dry to prevent any irritation.
10. If the exit site has been draining, place small drain sponge around the catheter to absorb any drainage. Be prepared to change this sponge throughout the day, depending on the amount of drainage. Do not cut a 4 × 4 gauze to make a drain sponge.	A small amount of drainage from the exit site is normal. The sponge needs to be changed when it becomes soiled to prevent skin irritation and breakdown. The fibers from the cut 4 × 4 gauze may enter the exit site and cause irritation or infection.
11. Remove gloves. Form a loop in tubing and anchor the tubing on the patient's abdomen.	Anchoring the catheter and tubing absorbs any tugging, preventing tension on and irritation to the skin or bladder.
12. Assist the patient to a comfortable position. Cover the patient with bed linens. Place the bed in the lowest position.	Positioning and covering provide warmth and promote comfort. Bed in lowest position promotes patient safety.
13. Put on clean gloves. Remove or discard equipment and assess the patient's response to the procedure.	Gloves prevent contact with blood and body fluids. The patient's response may indicate acceptance of the catheter or the need for health teaching.
14. Remove gloves and additional PPE, if used. Perform hand hygiene.	Removing PPE properly reduces the risk for infection transmission and contamination of other items. Hand hygiene prevents the spread of microorganisms.

EVALUATION

- Patient's skin remains clean, dry, and intact, without evidence of irritation or breakdown.
- Patient verbalizes an understanding of the purpose for, and care of, the catheter, as appropriate.
- Patient's urinary elimination is maintained, with a urine output of at least 30 mL/hour.
- Patient's bladder is not distended.

DOCUMENTATION

- Document the appearance of catheter exit site and surrounding skin, urine amount and characteristics, as well as patient's reaction to the procedure.

GENERAL CONSIDERATIONS

- Depending on the patient's situation, he/she may have both a suprapubic and indwelling urethral catheter. Urine will drain from both catheters; usually, drainage from the suprapubic catheter is the larger volume.
- If suprapubic catheter is not draining into bag but, instead, has a valve at the end of the catheter, open the valve at least every 6 hours (or more frequently depending on the order in the medical record or institutional policy) to drain the urine from the bladder.

Skill · 179   **Collecting a Urine Specimen (Clean Catch, Midstream) for Urinalysis and Culture**

Collecting a urine specimen for urinalysis and culture is an assessment measure to determine the characteristics of a patient's urine. A voided urine specimen for culture is collected midstream to provide a specimen that most closely reflects the characteristics of the urine being produced by the body. If the patient is able to understand and follow the procedure, the patient may collect the sample on his or her own, after explanation and instruction. The procedure for obtaining a specimen for urinalysis from an infant or young child is outlined in the accompanying skill variation.

EQUIPMENT

- Moist cleansing towelettes or soap, water, and washcloth
- Nonsterile gloves
- Additional PPE, as indicated
- Sterile specimen container
- Biohazard bag
- Appropriate label for specimen, based on facility policy and procedure

ASSESSMENT GUIDELINES

- After verifying the order for specimen collection in the medical record, review the medical record for information about any medications that the patient is taking, because medications may affect the results of the test.
- Assess for any signs and symptoms of a urinary tract infection, such as burning, pain (dysuria), or frequency.

- Assess the patient's ability to cooperate with the collection process. Determine the need for assistance to obtain specimen correctly.

NURSING DIAGNOSES
- Impaired Urinary Elimination
- Anxiety
- Deficient Knowledge

OUTCOME IDENTIFICATION AND PLANNING
Expected outcomes may include:
- An adequate amount of urine is obtained from the patient without contamination.
- An uncontaminated specimen is obtained and sent to the laboratory promptly.
- The patient exhibits minimal anxiety during specimen collection.
- The patient demonstrates the ability to collect a clean urine specimen.

IMPLEMENTATION

ACTION	RATIONALE
1. Bring necessary equipment to the bedside stand or over-bed table.	Bringing everything to the bedside conserves time and energy. Arranging items nearby is convenient, saves time, and avoids unnecessary stretching and twisting of muscles on the part of the nurse. Organization facilitates performance of tasks.
2. Perform hand hygiene and put on PPE, if indicated.	Hand hygiene and PPE prevent the transmission of microorganisms. PPE is required based on transmission precautions.
3. Identify the patient. Explain the procedure to the patient. If the patient can perform the task without assistance after instruction, leave the container at bedside with instructions to call the nurse as soon as a specimen is produced.	Identifying the patient ensures the right patient receives the intervention and helps prevent errors. Discussion and explanation help to allay some of the patient's anxiety and prepare the patient for what to expect.
4. Have patient perform hand hygiene, if performing self-collection.	Hand hygiene prevents the transmission of microorganisms.

ACTION	RATIONALE
5. Check the specimen label with the patient's identification bracelet. Label should include patient's name and identification number, time specimen was collected, route of collection, identification of the person obtaining sample, and any other information required by agency policy.	Confirmation of patient identification information ensures the specimen is labeled correctly for the right patient.
6. Close curtains around bed or close the door to the room, if possible.	Closing the door or curtain provides for patient privacy.
7. Put on unsterile gloves. Assist the patient to the bathroom, or onto the bedside commode or bedpan. Instruct the patient not to defecate or discard toilet paper into the urine.	Gloves reduce the transmission of microorganisms. Stool and/or toilet paper may contaminate the specimen.
8. Instruct the female patient to separate the labia for cleaning of the area and during collection of urine. Female patients should use the towelettes or wet washcloth to clean each side of the urinary meatus, then the center over the meatus, from front to back, using a new wipe or a clean area of the washcloth for each stroke (FIGURE 1). Male patients should use a towelette to clean the tip of the penis, wiping in a circular motion away from the urethra. Instruct uncircumcised male patient to retract the foreskin before cleaning and during collection (FIGURE 2).	Cleaning the perineal area or penis reduces the risk for contamination of the specimen.

RATIONALE

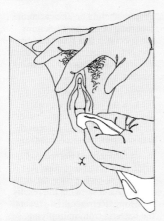

FIGURE 1 Cleaning female perineum. Separating labia and cleansing from front to back.

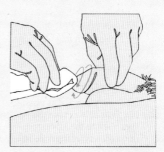

FIGURE 2 Cleaning male genitalia. Wiping in a circular motion away from urethra.

9. **Have patient void a small amount of urine into the toilet, bedpan, or commode. The patient should then stop urinating briefly, then void into collection container. Collect specimen (10 to 20 mL is sufficient) and then finish voiding. Do not touch the inside of the container or the lid.**	Collecting a midstream specimen ensures that fresh urine is analyzed. Some urine may have collected in the urethra from the last void. By voiding a little before collecting the specimen, the specimen will contain only fresh urine.
10. Place lid on container. If necessary, transfer the specimen to appropriate containers for ordered test, according to facility policy.	Placing the lid on the container helps to keep the specimen clean and prevents spills.
11. Assist the patient from the bathroom, off the commode, or off the bedpan. Provide perineal care, if necessary.	Perineal care promotes patient comfort and hygiene.
12. Remove gloves and perform hand hygiene.	Removing gloves and goggles properly reduces the risk for infection transmission and contamination of other items. Hand hygiene reduces the transmission of microorganisms.

ACTION	RATIONALE
13. Place label on the container per facility policy. Place container in plastic, sealable biohazard bag.	Proper labeling ensures accurate reporting of results. Packaging the specimen in a biohazard bag prevents the person transporting the container from coming in contact with urine.
14. Remove other PPE, if used. Perform hand hygiene.	Removing PPE properly reduces the risk for infection transmission and contamination of other items. Hand hygiene reduces the transmission of microorganisms.
15. Transport the specimen to the laboratory as soon as possible. If unable to take the specimen to the laboratory immediately, refrigerate it.	If not refrigerated immediately, urine may act as a culture medium, allowing bacteria to multiply and skewing the results of testing. Refrigeration prevents the bacteria from multiplying.

EVALUATION

• An adequate amount of urine is obtained from the patient without contamination.
• An uncontaminated specimen is obtained and sent to the laboratory promptly.
• The patient exhibits minimal anxiety during specimen collection.
• The patient demonstrates the ability to collect a clean urine specimen.

DOCUMENTATION

• Document that the specimen was sent to the laboratory. Note the characteristics of the urine, including odor, amount (if known), color, and clarity. Include any significant patient assessments, such as patient complaints of burning or pain on urination.

GENERAL CONSIDERATIONS

• For many urine tests, such as a urinalysis, drug testing, or diabetes testing, the specimen does not need to be sterile and does not need to be collected as a midstream specimen. However, in the case of urinalysis, if the specimen shows nitrates and white blood cells, a culture of a urine specimen may be ordered.
• Because the first voiding of the day contains the highest bacterial counts, this sample should be collected whenever possible.
• Urine specimens may also be obtained by direct urethral catheterization. Refer to Skill 180.

| **Skill Variation** | **Obtaining a Bagged Urine Specimen for Urinalysis from an Infant or Young Child** |

1. Identify the patient. Explain the steps to a young child, if old enough, and to the parents. Talk to the child at the child's level, stressing that no pain will be involved.

2. Perform hand hygiene and put on nonsterile gloves.

3. Remove the diaper or underwear. Perform thorough perineal care with soap and water: for girls, spread labia and cleanse area; for boys, retract foreskin if intact and cleanse glans of penis. Pat skin dry.

4. Remove paper backing from adhesive faceplate. Apply faceplate over labia or over penis. Gently push faceplate so that seal forms on skin (FIGURE A).

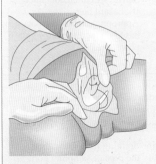

FIGURE A Applying infant urine collection bag.

5. Apply clean diaper or underwear over bag to help prevent dislodgement. Remove gloves and perform hand hygiene. Check bag every 15 minutes to see whether the child has voided.

6. As soon as the patient has voided, perform hand hygiene and put on nonsterile gloves. Gently remove bag by pushing skin away from bag. Transfer urine to appropriate container.

7. Perform perineal care and reapply diaper or clothing.

8. Remove gloves. Perform hand hygiene.

9. Check specimen label with the patient's identification bracelet. Label should include patient's name and identification number, time specimen was collected, route of collection, and any other information required by agency policy. Place label on the container per facility policy. Place container in plastic sealable biohazard bag.

10. Transport the specimen to the laboratory as soon as possible. If unable to take the specimen to the laboratory immediately, refrigerate it.

11. If voiding does not occur within 15 minutes after applying the bag, remove

(continued on page 962)

Obtaining a Bagged Urine Specimen for Urinalysis from an Infant or Young Child   *continued*

the bag and reapply it following the same cleaning routine. **Check the bag every 15 minutes until the patient voids** (Dulczak, 2005).

12. If the collection bag falls off or does not adhere completely, remove the bag, perform perineal care, and apply a new collection bag.

Skill · 180   **Obtaining a Urine Specimen From an Indwelling Urinary Catheter**

Indwelling catheter drainage tubes have special sampling ports in the tubing for removal of urine for testing. Some ports require the use of a needle or blunt cannula to access the sampling port; others are needleless systems. The drainage tubing below the access port may be bent back on itself or clamped so that urine collects near the port, unless contraindicated, based on the patient's condition. Do not open the drainage system to obtain urine specimens. Urine specimens should never be taken from the catheter drainage bag because the urine is not fresh.

EQUIPMENT

- 10-mL sterile syringe
- 18-gauge needle or blunt cannula, if needed, based on specific catheter use
- Nonsterile gloves
- Additional PPE, as indicated
- Sterile specimen container
- Biohazard bag
- Appropriate label for specimen, based on facility policy and procedure

ASSESSMENT GUIDELINES

- After verifying the order for specimen collection in the medical record, review the medical record for information about any medications that the patient is taking, because medications may affect the results of the test.
- Assess the characteristics of the urine draining from the catheter.
- Inspect the catheter tubing to identify the type of sampling port.

NURSING DIAGNOSES

- Impaired Urinary Elimination
- Anxiety
- Deficient Knowledge

OUTCOME IDENTIFICATION AND PLANNING

Expected outcomes may include:

- An adequate amount of urine is obtained from the patient without contamination.
- An uncontaminated specimen is obtained and sent to the laboratory promptly.
- The patient exhibits minimal anxiety during specimen collection.
- The patient demonstrates an understanding of the reason for the specimen.

IMPLEMENTATION

ACTION	RATIONALE
1. Bring necessary equipment to the bedside stand or over-bed table.	Bringing everything to the bedside conserves time and energy. Arranging items nearby is convenient, saves time, and avoids unnecessary stretching and twisting of muscles on the part of the nurse. Organization facilitates performance of tasks.
2. Perform hand hygiene and put on PPE, if indicated.	Hand hygiene and PPE prevent the transmission of microorganisms. PPE is required based on transmission precautions.
3. Identify the patient. Explain the procedure to the patient.	Identifying the patient ensures the right patient receives the intervention and helps prevent errors. Explanation provides reassurance and promotes cooperation.
4. Check the specimen label with the patient's identification bracelet. Label should include patient's name and identification number, time specimen was collected, route of collection, identification of person obtaining the sample, and any other information required by agency policy.	Confirmation of patient identification information ensures the specimen is labeled correctly for the right patient.
5. Close curtains around bed and close the door to the room, if possible.	Closing curtain or door provides for patient privacy.
6. Put on unsterile gloves.	Gloves reduce the transmission of microorganisms.

ACTION	RATIONALE
7. Clamp the catheter drainage tubing or bend it back on itself distal to the port. If an insufficient amount of urine is present in the tubing, allow the tubing to remain clamped up to 30 minutes to collect a sufficient amount of urine, unless contraindicated (Fischbach & Dunning, 2006). Remove lid from specimen container, keeping the inside of the container and lid free from contamination.	Clamping the tubing ensures the collection of an adequate amount of fresh urine. Clamping for an extended period of time leads to overdistention of the bladder. Clamping may be contraindicated based on the patient's condition (e.g., after bladder surgery). The container needs to remain sterile so as not to contaminate the urine.
8. **Cleanse aspiration port with alcohol wipe and allow port to air dry.**	Cleaning with alcohol deters entry of microorganisms when the needle punctures the port.
9. Insert the needle or blunt-tipped cannula into the port, or attach the syringe to the aspiration port. Slowly aspirate enough urine for specimen (usually 10 mL is adequate; check facility requirements) (FIGURE 1). Remove needle, blunt-tipped cannula, or syringe from port. Engage the needle guard. **Unclamp the drainage tubing.**	Using a blunt-tipped needle prevents a needlestick. Collecting urine from the port ensures that the specimen will contain fresh urine. Unclamping catheter drainage tubing prevents overdistention of and injury to the patient's bladder.

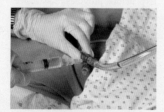

FIGURE 1 Inserting the needle in aspiration port and slowly aspirating urine into syringe.

10. If a needle or blunt-tipped cannula was used on the syringe, remove from the syringe before emptying the urine from the syringe into the specimen cup. Place the needle into sharps collection container. **Slowly inject**	**Forcing urine through the needle breaks up cells and impedes accurate results of microscopic urinalysis. Safe disposal of sharps prevents accidental injury.** If the urine is injected quickly into the container, it may splash out of the

ACTION	RATIONALE
urine in the syringe into specimen container. Replace lid on container. Dispose of syringe appropriately.	container or into the nurse's eyes. Proper disposal of equipment prevents injury and transmission of microorganisms.
11. Remove gloves and perform hand hygiene.	Removing gloves properly reduces the risk for infection transmission and contamination of other items. Hand hygiene reduces the transmission of microorganisms.
12. Place label on the container per facility policy. Place container in plastic sealable biohazard bag.	Proper labeling ensures accurate reporting of results. Packaging the specimen in a biohazard bag prevents the person transporting the container from coming in contact with the specimen.
13. Remove other PPE, if used. Perform hand hygiene.	Removing PPE properly reduces the risk for infection transmission and contamination of other items. Hand hygiene reduces the transmission of microorganisms.
14. Transport the specimen to the laboratory as soon as possible. If unable to take the specimen to laboratory immediately, refrigerate it.	If not refrigerated immediately, urine may act as a culture medium, allowing bacteria to multiply and skewing the results of testing. Refrigeration prevents the bacteria from multiplying.

EVALUATION

- An adequate amount of urine is obtained from the patient without contamination.
- An uncontaminated specimen is obtained and sent to the laboratory promptly.
- The patient exhibits minimal anxiety during specimen collection.
- The patient demonstrates understanding about the reason for the specimen.

DOCUMENTATION

- Document the method used to obtain the specimen, type of specimen sent, and characteristics of urine. Note any significant patient assessments. Record urine volume on intake and output record, if appropriate.

GENERAL CONSIDERATIONS

- It is very important to remove the clamp from the drainage tubing as soon as the specimen is collected, unless there is a specific order to leave clamped, to prevent overdistention of the patient's bladder and injury.

Skill · 181   **Caring for a Patient with an External Ventriculostomy (Intraventricular Catheter–Closed Fluid-Filled System)**

An external ventriculostomy is one method used to monitor intracranial pressure (ICP). It is part of a system that includes an external drainage system and an external transducer. This device is inserted into a ventricle of the brain, most commonly the nondominant lateral ventricle, through a hole drilled into the skull. The dura is incised or punctured, and the catheter is passed through the cerebral tissue into the ventricle (Arbour, 2004). The ventriculostomy can be used to measure the ICP, to drain cerebrospinal fluid (CSF), such as removing excess fluid associated with hydrocephalus, or to decrease the volume in the cranial vault, thereby decreasing the ICP, and to instill medications. ICP measurement is used to calculate cerebral perfusion pressure (CPP), an estimate of the adequacy of cerebral blood supply. CPP is the pressure difference across the brain. It is the difference between the incoming systemic mean arterial pressure (MAP) and the ICP. It is calculated by finding the difference between the MAP and the ICP (Blissitt, 2006).

EQUIPMENT
- Flashlight
- PPE, as indicated
- Ventriculostomy setup

ASSESSMENT GUIDELINES
- Assess the color of the fluid draining from the ventriculostomy. Normal CSF is clear or straw colored. Cloudy CSF may suggest an infection. Red or pink CSF may indicate bleeding.
- Assess vital signs, because changes in vital signs can reflect a neurologic problem.
- Assess the patient's pain level. The patient may be experiencing pain at the ventriculostomy insertion site.
- Assess the patient's level of consciousness. If the patient is awake, assess for his or her orientation to person, place, and time. If the patient's level of consciousness is decreased, note the patient's ability to respond and to be aroused. Inspect pupil size and response to light. Pupils should be equal and round and should react to light bilaterally. Any changes in level of consciousness or pupillary response may suggest a neurologic problem. If the patient can move the extremities, assess strength of hands and feet. A change in strength or a difference in strength on one side compared with the other may indicate a neurologic problem.

NURSING DIAGNOSES
- Risk for Injury
- Pain

• Activity Intolerance
• Risk for Infection
• Risk for Ineffective Cerebral Tissue Perfusion

OUTCOME IDENTIFICATION AND PLANNING

Expected outcomes may include:
• Patient maintains intracranial pressure at less than 10 to 15 mm Hg (Arbour, 2004) and cerebral perfusion pressure at 60 to 90 mm Hg (Hickey, 2009).
• Patient is free from infection.
• Patient is free from pain.
• Patient/significant others understand the need for the ventriculostomy.

IMPLEMENTATION

ACTION	RATIONALE
1. Review the medical orders for specific information about ventriculostomy parameters.	The nurse needs to know the most recent order for the height of the ventriculostomy. For example, if the healthcare practitioner has ordered that the ventriculostomy is to be at 10 cm, this means the patient's ICP must rise above 10 cm before the ventriculostomy will drain CSF.
2. Gather the necessary supplies and bring to the bedside stand or overbed table.	Preparation promotes efficient time management and an organized approach to the task. Bringing everything to the bedside conserves time and energy. Arranging items nearby is convenient, saves time, and avoids unnecessary stretching and twisting of muscles on the part of the nurse.
3. Perform hand hygiene and put on PPE, if indicated.	Hand hygiene and PPE prevent the spread of microorganisms. PPE is required based on transmission precautions.
4. Identify the patient.	Identifying the patient ensures the right patient receives the intervention and helps prevent errors.

ACTION	RATIONALE

5. Close curtains around bed and close the door to the room, if possible. Explain what you are going to do and why you are going to do it to the patient.

This ensures the patient's privacy. Explanation relieves anxiety and facilitates cooperation.

6. Assess patient for any changes in neurologic status.

Patients with ventriculostomies are at risk for problems with the neurologic system.

7. **Assess the height of the ventriculostomy system to ensure that the stopcock is at the level of midpoint between the outer canthus of the patient's eye and the tragus of the patient's ear or external auditory canal (Littlejohns, 2005), using carpenter level, bubble-line level, or laser level, according to facility policy.** Adjust the height of the system if needed. **Move the drip chamber to the ordered height.** Assess the amount of CSF in the drip chamber if the ventriculostomy is draining.

For measurements to be accurate, the stopcock must be at the level of the foramen of Monro, which is the actual level for measurements. If the transducer and extraventricular drain (EVD) are not referenced to the foramen of Monro correctly, using a carpenter level, bubble-line level, or laser level, there can be a significant error (March, 2005). If the ventriculostomy is used just to measure the ICP and not to drain the CSF, the stopcock will be turned off to the drip chamber. If the ventriculostomy is to drain CSF, the nurse must turn the stopcock off to the drip chamber. After the ICP value is obtained, remember to turn the stopcock back off to the transducer so that CSF is allowed to drain.

8. **Zero the transducer.** Turn stopcock off to the patient. Remove the cap from the transducer, being careful not to touch the end of the cap. Press and hold the calibration button on the monitor until the monitor beeps. Return the cap to the transducer. **Turn the stopcock off to the drip chamber to obtain an ICP reading. After obtaining a reading, turn the stopcock off to the transducer.**

The readings would not be considered accurate if the transducer had not been recently zeroed. If the stopcock is not turned off to the patient, when opened to room air, CSF will flow out of the stopcock. The end of the cap must remain sterile to prevent an infection. The stopcock must be off to the drip chamber (open to the transducer) to obtain an ICP. If the ventriculostomy is to drain CSF, the nurse must turn the

ACTION	RATIONALE
	stopcock off to the drip chamber. After the ICP value is obtained, remember to turn the stopcock back off to the transducer so that CSF is allowed to drain into the drip chamber.
9. **Adjust the ventriculostomy height to prevent too much drainage, too little drainage, or inaccurate ICP readings.**	If the patient's head is lower than the ventriculostomy, the drainage of CSF will slow or stop. If the patient's head is higher than the ventriculostomy, the drainage of CSF will increase. Any ICP readings taken when the ventriculostomy is not level with the outer canthus of the eye would be inaccurate.
10. Care for the insertion site according to the institution's policy. Assess the site for any signs of infection, such as purulent drainage, redness, or warmth. Ensure the catheter is secured at site per facility policy.	Site care varies, possibly ranging from leaving the site open to air to applying antibiotic ointment and gauze. Securing the catheters after insertion prevents dislodgement and breakage of the device.
11. Calculate the CPP, if necessary. Calculate the difference between the systemic MAP and the ICP.	CPP is an estimate of the adequacy of the blood supply to the brain.
12. Remove PPE, if used. Perform hand hygiene.	Removing PPE properly reduces the risk for infection transmission and contamination of other items. Hand hygiene prevents the spread of microorganisms.
13. Assess ICP, MAP, and CPP at least hourly.	Frequent assessment provides valuable indicators for identifying subtle trends that may suggest developing problems.

EVALUATION

- Patient demonstrates a CPP and an ICP within identified parameters.
- Patient remains free from infection.
- Patient understands the need for the ventriculostomy.
- Patient reports no pain.

DOCUMENTATION

- Document the amount and color of CSF. Record the ICP and CPP measurement readings. Document pupil status; motor strength bilaterally; orientation to time, person, and place; level of consciousness; vital signs; pain; appearance of insertion site; and height of ventriculostomy.

GENERAL CONSIDERATIONS

- Secure the catheters according to facility policy after insertion and use care when moving patients to prevent dislodgement and breakage of these devices (March, 2005).
- Keep in mind that several independent nursing activities, such as turning and positioning, have been shown to increase ICP. Take precautions when caring for patients with ICP monitoring to manage factors known to increase ICP. Turn and position the patient in proper body alignment, avoiding angulation of body parts. Extreme hip flexion or flexion of upper legs can increase intra-abdominal pressure, leading to increased ICP. Use logrolling. Maintain the neck in neutral position at all times to avoid neck vein compression, which can interfere with venous return. Maintain the head of the bed in the flat position or elevated to 30 degrees, depending on medical orders and facility procedure. Avoid noxious stimuli, using soft voices or music and a gentle touch. Plan care to avoid grouping activities and procedures known to increase ICP. Bathing, turning, and other routine care often have a cumulative effect to increase ICP when performed in succession. Allow rest periods between procedures and carefully assess the patient's response to interventions (Hickey, 2009; Hockenberry & Wilson, 2009).

Skill · 182   **Collecting a Wound Culture**

A wound culture may be ordered to identify the causative organism of an infected wound. Identifying the invading microorganism will provide useful information to select the most appropriate therapy. A nurse or other primary healthcare provider can perform a wound culture. Maintaining strict asepsis is crucial so that only the pathogen present in the wound is isolated. It is essential to use the correct swab, based on the tests ordered, to collect a specimen to isolate aerobic and/or anaerobic organisms.

EQUIPMENT

- A sterile Culturette kit (aerobic or anaerobic) with swab, or a culture tube with individual sterile swabs
- Sterile gloves
- Clean disposable gloves
- Additional PPE, as indicated

- Plastic bag or appropriate waste receptacle
- Patient label for the sample tube
- Biohazard specimen bag
- Bath blanket (if necessary to drape the patient)

- Supplies to clean the wound and reapply a sterile dressing after obtaining the culture

ASSESSMENT GUIDELINES

- Assess the situation to determine the need for wound culture. Confirm any medical orders relevant to obtaining a wound culture, as well as wound care, and/or any wound care included in the nursing plan of care.
- Assess the patient's level of comfort and the need for analgesics before obtaining the wound culture.
- Inspect the wound and the surrounding tissue. Assess the location, appearance of the wound, stage (if appropriate), drainage, and types of tissue present in the wound. Measure the wound. Note the stage of the healing process and characteristics of any drainage.
- Assess the surrounding skin for color, temperature, and edema, ecchymosis, or maceration.

NURSING DIAGNOSES

- Acute Pain
- Impaired Tissue Integrity
- Impaired Skin Integrity
- Disturbed Body Image
- Delayed Surgical Recovery

OUTCOME IDENTIFICATION AND PLANNING

Expected outcomes may include:
- Culture is obtained without evidence of contamination, without exposing the patient to additional pathogens, and without causing discomfort for the patient.

IMPLEMENTATION

ACTION	RATIONALE
1. Review the medical orders for obtaining a wound culture.	Reviewing the order and plan of care validates the correct patient and correct procedure.
2. Gather the necessary supplies and bring to the bedside stand or overbed table.	Preparation promotes efficient time management and an organized approach to the task. Bringing everything to the bedside conserves time and energy.

ACTION	RATIONALE
	Arranging items nearby is convenient, saves time, and avoids unnecessary stretching and twisting of muscles on the part of the nurse.
3. Perform hand hygiene and put on PPE, if indicated.	Hand hygiene and PPE prevent the spread of microorganisms. PPE is required based on transmission precautions.
4. Identify the patient.	Identifying the patient ensures that the right patient receives the intervention and helps prevent errors.
5. Close curtains around bed and close door to room if possible. Explain what you are going to do and why you are going to do it to the patient.	This ensures the patient's privacy. Explanation relieves anxiety and facilitates cooperation.
6. Assess the patient for possible need for nonpharmacologic pain-reducing interventions or analgesic medication before obtaining the wound culture. Administer appropriate prescribed analgesic. Allow sufficient time for analgesic to achieve its effectiveness before beginning the procedure.	Pain is a subjective experience influenced by past experience. Wound care and dressing changes can cause pain for some patients.
7. Place an appropriate waste receptacle within easy reach for use during the procedure.	Having the waste container handy means that soiled materials can be discarded easily, without the spread of microorganisms.
8. Adjust bed to comfortable working height, usually elbow height of the caregiver (VISN 8, 2009).	Having the bed at the proper height prevents back and muscle strain.

ACTION	RATIONALE
9. Assist the patient to a comfortable position that provides easy access to the wound. If necessary, drape the patient with the bath blanket to expose only the wound area. Place a waterproof pad under the wound site. Check the culture label against the patient's identification bracelet.	Patient positioning and use of a bath blanket provide for comfort and warmth. Checking the culture label with the patient's identification ensures the correct patient and the correct procedure.
10. If a dressing is in place on the wound, put on clean gloves. Carefully and gently remove the soiled dressings. If there is resistance, use a silicone-based adhesive remover to help remove the tape. If any part of the dressing sticks to the underlying skin, use small amounts of sterile saline to help loosen and remove.	Gloves protect the nurse from handling contaminated dressings. Cautious removal of the dressing is more comfortable for the patient and ensures that any drain present is not removed. A silicone-based adhesive remover allows for the easy, rapid, and painless removal without the associated problems of skin stripping (Rudoni, 2008; Stephen-Haynes, 2008). Sterile saline moistens the dressing for easier removal and minimizes damage and pain.
11. After removing the dressing, note the presence, amount, type, color, and odor of any drainage on the dressings. Place soiled dressings in the appropriate waste receptacle.	The presence of drainage should be documented. Discarding dressings appropriately prevents the spread of microorganisms.
12. Assess the wound for appearance, stage, the presence of eschar, granulation tissue, epithelialization, undermining, tunneling, necrosis, sinus tract, and drainage. Assess the appearance of the surrounding tissue. Measure the wound.	This information provides evidence about the wound healing process and/or the presence of infection.
13. Remove gloves and put them in the receptacle.	Discarding gloves prevents the spread of microorganisms.

ACTION	RATIONALE
14. Set up a sterile field, if indicated, and wound cleaning supplies. Put on the sterile gloves. Alternately, clean gloves (clean technique) may be used when cleaning a chronic wound.	Sterile gloves maintain surgical asepsis. Clean technique is appropriate when cleaning chronic wounds.
15. Clean the wound. (Refer to Skill 55.) Alternately, irrigate the wound, as ordered or required. (Refer to Skill 183.)	Cleaning the wound removes previous drainage and wound debris, which could introduce extraneous organisms into the collected specimen, resulting in inaccurate results.
16. Dry the surrounding skin with gauze dressings. Put on clean gloves.	Moisture provides a medium for growth of microorganisms. Excess moisture can contribute to skin irritation and breakdown. The use of a culture swab does not require immediate contact with the skin or wound, so clean gloves are appropriate to protect the nurse from contact with blood and/or body fluids.
17. Twist the cap to loosen the swab on the Culturette tube, or open the separate swab and remove the cap from the culture tube. **Keep the swab and inside of the culture tube sterile.**	Supplies are ready to use and within easy reach, and aseptic technique is maintained.
18. If contact with the wound is necessary to separate wound margins to permit insertion of the swab deep into the wound, put a sterile glove on one hand to manipulate the wound margins. Clean gloves may be appropriate for contact with pressure ulcers and chronic wounds.	If contact with the wound is necessary to collect the specimen, a sterile glove is necessary to prevent contamination of the wound.
19. **Carefully insert the swab into the wound. Press and rotate the swab several times over the wound**	Cotton tip absorbs wound drainage. Contact with skin could introduce extraneous organisms into the collected specimen,

ACTION	RATIONALE

surfaces. Avoid touching the swab to intact skin at the wound edges (FIGURE 1). Use another swab if collecting a specimen from another site.

resulting in inaccurate results. Using another swab at a different site prevents cross-contamination of the wound.

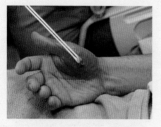

FIGURE 1 Swabbing the wound.

20. Place the swab back in the culture tube. **Do not touch the outside of the tube with the swab.** Secure the cap. Some swab containers have an ampule of medium at the bottom of the tube. It might be necessary to crush this ampule to activate. Follow the manufacturer's instructions for use.

The outside of the container is protected from contamination with microorganisms, and the sample is not contaminated with organisms not in the wound. Surrounding the swab with culture medium is necessary for accurate culture results.

21. Remove gloves and discard them accordingly.

Removing gloves properly reduces the risk for infection transmission and contamination of other items.

22. Put on gloves. Place a dressing on the wound, as appropriate, based on medical orders and/or the nursing plan of care. Remove gloves.

Wound dressings protect, absorb drainage, provide a moist environment, and promote wound healing. Removing gloves properly reduces the risk for infection transmission and contamination of other items.

23. After securing the dressing, label dressing with date and time. Remove all remaining equipment; place the patient

Recording date and time provides communication and demonstrates adherence to plan of care. Proper patient and bed

ACTION	RATIONALE
in a comfortable position, with side rails up and bed in the lowest position.	positioning promotes safety and comfort.
24. Label the specimen according to your institution's guidelines and send it to the laboratory in a biohazard bag.	Proper labeling ensures proper identification of the specimen.
25. Remove PPE, if used. Perform hand hygiene.	Removing PPE properly reduces the risk for infection transmission and contamination of other items. Hand hygiene prevents the spread of microorganisms.

EVALUATION

• Patient's wound is cultured without evidence of contamination, and the patient remains free of exposure to additional pathogens.

DOCUMENTATION

• Document the location of the wound, the assessment of the wound, including type of tissue present, presence of necrotic tissue, stage (if appropriate) and characteristics of drainage. Include the appearance of the surrounding skin. Document cleansing of the wound and the obtaining of the culture. Record any skin care and/or dressing applied. Note pertinent patient and family education and any patient reaction to this procedure, including patient's pain level and effectiveness of nonpharmacologic interventions or analgesia if administered.

GENERAL CONSIDERATIONS

• Guidelines from the Wound, Ostomy, Continence Nurses Society (WOCN) and National Pressure Ulcer Advisory Panel (NPUAP) recommend that clean gloves may be used to treat chronic wounds and pressure ulcers as long as the infection-control procedures are followed. The *no-touch technique* may be used within these guidelines. Clean gloves are used to handle dressing material. Irrigants and dressings are sterile. The wound is redressed by picking up dressing materials by the corner and placing the untouched side over the wound (NPUAP, 2007b; Wooten & Hawkins, 2005).

ACTION	RATIONALE
are going to do and why you are going to do it to the patient.	
6. Assess the patient for possible need for nonpharmacologic pain-reducing interventions or analgesic medication before wound care and/or dressing change. Administer appropriate prescribed analgesic. Allow sufficient time for analgesic to achieve its effectiveness before beginning the procedure.	Pain is a subjective experience influenced by past experience. Wound care and dressing changes may cause pain for some patients.
7. Place a waste receptacle or bag at a convenient location for use during the procedure.	Having a waste container handy means the soiled dressing can be discarded easily, without the spread of microorganisms.
8. Adjust bed to comfortable working height, usually elbow height of the caregiver (VISN 8, 2009).	Having the bed at the proper height prevents back and muscle strain.
9. Assist the patient to a comfortable position that provides easy access to the wound area. Position the patient so the irrigation solution will flow from the clean end of the wound toward the dirtier end. Use the bath blanket to cover any exposed area other than the wound. Place a waterproof pad under the wound site.	Patient positioning and use of a bath blanket provide for comfort and warmth. Gravity directs the flow of liquid from the least contaminated to the most contaminated area. Waterproof pad protects underlying surfaces.
10. Put on a gown, mask, and eye protection.	Using personal protective equipment such as gowns, masks, and eye protection is part of Standard Precautions. A gown protects clothes from contamination should splashing occur. Goggles protect mucous membranes of eyes from contact with irrigant fluid or wound drainage.

ACTION	RATIONALE
11. Put on clean gloves. Carefully and gently remove the soiled dressings. If there is resistance, use a silicone-based adhesive remover to help remove the tape. If any part of the dressing sticks to the underlying skin, use small amounts of sterile saline to help loosen and remove.	Gloves protect the nurse from handling contaminated dressings. Cautious removal of the dressing is more comfortable for the patient and ensures that any drain present is not removed. A silicone-based adhesive remover allows for the easy, rapid and painless removal without the associated problems of skin stripping (Rudoni, 2008; Stephen-Haynes, 2008). Sterile saline moistens the dressing for easier removal and minimizes damage and pain.
12. After removing the dressing, note the presence, amount, type, color, and odor of any drainage on the dressings. Place soiled dressings in the appropriate waste receptacle.	Document the presence of drainage. Discarding dressings appropriately prevents the spread of microorganisms.
13. Assess the wound for appearance, stage, the presence of eschar, granulation tissue, epithelialization, undermining, tunneling, necrosis, sinus tract, and drainage. Assess the appearance of the surrounding tissue. Measure the wound.	This information provides evidence about the wound healing process and/or the presence of infection.
14. Remove your gloves and put them in the receptacle.	Discarding gloves prevents the spread of microorganisms.
15. Set up a sterile field, if indicated, and the wound cleaning supplies. Pour warmed sterile irrigating solution into the sterile container. Put on the sterile gloves. Alternately, clean gloves (clean technique) may be used when irrigating a chronic wound.	Using warmed solution prevents chilling of the patient and may minimize patient discomfort. Sterile technique and gloves maintain surgical asepsis. Clean technique is appropriate for irrigating chronic wounds.
16. Position the sterile basin below the wound to collect the irrigation fluid.	Patient and bed linens are protected from contaminated fluid.

ACTION	RATIONALE
17. Fill the irrigation syringe with solution. Using your nondominant hand, gently apply pressure to the basin against the skin below the wound to form a seal with the skin.	The solution will collect in the basin and prevent the irrigant from running down the skin. Patient and bed linens are protected from contaminated fluid.
18. Gently direct a stream of solution into the wound (FIGURE 1). Keep the tip of the syringe at least 1 inch above the upper tip of the wound. When using a catheter tip, insert it gently into the wound until it meets resistance. Gently flush all wound areas.	Debris and contaminated solution flow from the least contaminated to most contaminated area. High-pressure irrigation flow can cause patient discomfort as well as damage granulation tissue. A catheter tip allows the introduction of irrigant into a wound with a small opening or one that is deep.

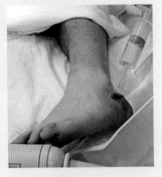

FIGURE 1 Irrigating wound with a gentle stream of solution. Solution drains into collection container.

ACTION	RATIONALE
19. Watch for the solution to flow smoothly and evenly. When the solution from the wound flows out clear, discontinue irrigation.	Irrigation removes exudate and debris.
20. Dry the surrounding skin with gauze dressings.	Moisture provides a medium for growth of microorganisms. Excess moisture can contribute to skin irritation and breakdown.
21. Apply a skin protectant to the surrounding skin.	A skin protectant prevents skin irritation and breakdown.

ACTION	RATIONALE
22. Apply a new dressing to the wound. (See Skills 55, 56, 58.)	Dressings absorb drainage, protect the wound, and promote healing.
23. Remove and discard gloves. Apply tape, Montgomery straps, or roller gauze to secure the dressings. Alternately, many commercial wound products are self-adhesive and do not require additional tape.	Tape or other securing products are easier to apply after gloves have been removed. Proper disposal of gloves prevents the spread of microorganisms.
24. After securing the dressing, label it with date and time. Remove all remaining equipment; place the patient in a comfortable position, with side rails up and bed in the lowest position.	Recording date and time provides communication and demonstrates adherence to plan of care. Proper patient and bed positioning promotes safety and comfort.
25. Remove remaining PPE. Perform hand hygiene.	Removing PPE properly reduces the risk for infection transmission and contamination of other items. Hand hygiene prevents the spread of microorganisms.
26. Check all wound dressings every shift. More frequent checks may be needed if the wound is more complex or dressings become saturated quickly.	Checking dressings ensures the assessment of changes in patient condition and timely intervention to prevent complications.

EVALUATION

- Wound irrigation is completed without contamination and trauma.
- Patient verbalizes little to no pain or discomfort.
- Patient verbalizes understanding of the need for irrigation.
- Patient's wound continues to show signs of progression of healing.

DOCUMENTATION

- Document the location of the wound and that the dressing was removed. Record assessment of the wound, including evidence of granulation tissue, presence of necrotic tissue, stage (if appropriate), and characteristics of drainage. Include the appearance of the surrounding skin. Document the irrigation of the wound and solution used. Record the type of dressing that was applied. Note pertinent patient and family education and any patient reaction to this procedure, including patient's pain level and effectiveness of nonpharmacologic interventions or analgesia if administered.

GENERAL CONSIDERATIONS

- Guidelines from the Wound, Ostomy, Continence Nurses Society (WOCN) and National Pressure Ulcer Advisory Panel (NPUAP) recommend that clean gloves may be used to treat chronic wounds and pressure ulcers as long as the infection-control procedures are followed. The *no-touch technique* may be used within these guidelines. Clean gloves are used to handle dressing material. Irrigants and dressings are sterile. The wound is redressed by picking up dressing materials by the corner and placing the untouched side over the wound (NPUAP, 2007b; Wooten & Hawkins, 2005).
- Many products are available to treat chronic and pressure ulcers. Treatment varies based on facility policy, nursing protocol, clinical specialist referrals, and primary care provider's orders.

Bibliography

American Diabetes Association. (2004). Insulin administration: Position statement. *Diabetes Care, 27*(Supplement 1), S106–S1069.

American Dietetic Association (ADA). (2008). Position of the American Dietetic Association: Ethical and legal issues in nutrition, hydration, and feeding. *Journal of the American Dietetic Association, 108*(5), 873–882.

Annersten, M., & Willman, A. (2005). Performing subcutaneous injections: A literature review. *Worldviews on Evidence-Based Nursing, 2*(3), 122–130.

Arbique, J., & Arbique, D. (2007). I.V. rounds. Reducing the risk of nerve injuries. *Nursing, 37*(11), 20–21.

Arbour, R. (2004). Intracranial hypertension. Monitoring and nursing assessment. *Critical Care Nurse, 24*(5), 19–32.

Armed with the facts. (2008). *Nursing, 38*(6), 10.

Baird Holmes, S., & Brown, S. (2005). National Association of Orthopaedic Nurses. Guidelines for orthopaedic nursing: Skeletal pin site care. *Orthopaedic Nursing, 24*(2), 99–107.

Bernardini, J., Bender, F., Florio, T., et al. (2005). Randomized, double-blind trial of antibiotic exit site cream for prevention of exit site infection in peritoneal dialysis patients. *Journal of the American Society of Nephrology, 16*(2), 539–545.

Bhanushali, M., & Helmers, S. (2008). Diagnosis and acute management of seizure in adults. *Hospital Physician, 44*(11), 37–42, 48.

Blissitt, P. (2006). Hemodynamic monitoring in the care of the critically ill neuroscience patient. *AACN Advanced Critical Care, 17*(3), 327–340.

Booker, R. (2008a). Pulse oximetry. *Nursing Standard, 22*(30), 39–41.

Booker, R. (2008b). Simple spirometry measurement. *Nursing Standard, 22*(32), 35–39.

Bourgault, A., Ipe, L., Weaver, J., et al. (2007). Development of evidence-based guidelines and critical care nurses' knowledge of enteral feeding. *Critical Care Nurse, 27*(4), 17–29.

Brown, A., & Butcher, M. (2005). A guide to emollient therapy. *Nursing Standard, 19*(24), 68–75.

Caffrey, R. (2003). Diabetes under control: Are all syringes created equal? *American Journal of Nursing, 103*(6), 46–49.

Castle, N. (2007). Resuscitation of patients during pregnancy. *Emergency Nurse, 15*(2), 20–22.

Centers for Disease Control and Prevention (CDC). (2009). *The Pink Book: Appendices. Epidemiology and prevention of vaccine preventable diseases.* (11th ed.). Appendix D. Vaccine administration. Vaccine administration guidelines. Available at www.cdc.gov/vaccines/pubs/pinkbook/pink-appendx.htm#appd. Accessed July 2, 2009.

Centers for Disease Control and Prevention (CDC). (2008a). Injection safety FAQs for providers. Available at www.cdc.gov/ncidod/dhqp/InjectionSafetyFAQs. html. Accessed June 20, 2009.

Centers for Disease Control and Prevention (CDC). (2008b). Injection safety information for providers. Available at www.cdc.gov/ncidod/dhqp/ps_providerInfo. html. Accessed June 20, 2009.

Centers for Disease Control and Prevention (CDC). (2008c). Needle length and injection site of intramuscular injections. Available at www.cdc.gov/vaccines/ ed/encounter08/Downloads.Table%207.pdf. Accessed June 20, 2009.

Centers for Disease Control and Prevention (CDC). (2007). National immuniza-
tion program. Vaccine administration. (Slide presentation). Available at
www.cdc.gov/vaccines/ed/vpd2007/download/slides/admin-images.ppt. Accessed June 23, 2009.

Centers for Disease Control and Prevention. (2004a). Guidance for the selection
and use of personal protective equipment (PPE) in healthcare settings. (Slide
presentation). Available at www.cdc.gov/ncidod/dhqp/ppe.html. Accessed
June 10, 2009.

Centers for Disease Control and Prevention. (2004b). Sequence for donning and
removing personal protective equipment (PPE). Poster. Available at www.cdc.
gov/ncidod/dhqp/ppe.html. Accessed June 10, 2009.

Charous, S. (2008). Use of the ON-Q pain pump management system in the head
and neck: Preliminary report. *Otolaryngology-Head and Neck Surgery, 138*(1),
110–112.

Craig, K. (2005). How to provide transcutaneous pacing. *Nursing, 35*(10), 52–53.

DeMeulenaere, S. (2007). Pulse oximetry: Uses and limitations. *The Journal for
Nurse Practitioners, 3*(5), 312–317.

Del Monte, L. (2006). *Medtronic. Noninvasive pacing: What you should
know.* Educational Series. Redmond, WA: Medtronic Emergency Response
Systems, Inc.

Ferguson, A., (2005). Blood glucose monitoring. *Nursing Times 101*(38), 28–29.

Fernandez, M., Burns, K., Calhoun, B., et al. (2007). Evaluation of a new pulse
oximeter sensor. *American Journal of Critical Care, 16*(2), 146–152.

Fischbach, F., & Dunning M. (2009). *A Manual of Laboratory and Diagnostic
Tests.* (8th ed.). Philadelphia, PA: Wolters Kluwer Health/Lippincott Williams
& Wilkins.

Fischbach, F., & Dunning M. (2009). *A Manual of Laboratory and Diagnostic
Tests.* (8th ed.). Philadelphia, PA: Wolters Kluwer/Lippincott Williams &
Wilkins.

Flori, L. (2007). Don't throw in the towel: Tips for bathing a patient who has dementia.
Nursing, 37(7), 22–23.

Friesner, S., Curry, D., & Moddeman, G. (2006). Comparison of two pain-management
strategies during chest tube removal: Relaxation exercise with opioids and
opioids alone. *Issues in Pain Management, 35*(4), 269–276.

Gray-Micelli, D. (2008). Hartford Institute for Geriatric Nursing. FALLS. Nursing
standard of practice protocol: Fall Prevention. Available at www.consultgerirn.
org/topics/falls/want_to_know_more. Accessed March 5, 2009.

Halm, M. (2007). To strip or not to strip? Physiological effects of chest tube manipulation. *American Journal of Critical Care, 16*(6), 609–612.

Hadaway, L. (2006). Technology of flushing vascular access devices. *Journal of
Infusion Nursing. 29*(3), 137–145.

Haynes, J. (2007). The ear as an alternative site for a pulse oximeter finger clip
sensor. *Respiratory Care, 52*(6), 727–729.

Hendrich, A. (2007). Predicting patient falls. *American Journal of Nursing,
107*(11), 50–58.

Hess, C. (2008). *Skin & Wound Care.* (6th ed.). Philadelphia, PA: Wolters Kluwer
Health/Lippincott Williams & Wilkins.

Hickey, J. (2009). *The Clinical Practice of Neurological and Neurosurgical
Nursing.* (6th ed.). Philadelphia, PA: Wolters Kluwer Health/Lippincott Williams & Wilkins.

Hockenberry, M., & Wilson, D. (2009). *Wong's Essentials of Pediatric Nursing.*
(8th ed.). St. Louis, MO: Elsevier Mosby.

Holman, C., Roberts, S., & Nicol, M. (2005). Practice update: Clinical skills with older people. Promoting oral hygiene. *Nursing Older People, 16*(10), 37–38.

Hudson, T., Dukes, S., & Reilly, K. (2006). Use of local anesthesia for arterial punctures. *American Journal of Critical Care, 15*(6), 595–599.

Infection Control Today (ICT). (2005). Chlorhexidine: The preferred skin antiseptic. Available at www.infectioncontroltoday.com/articles/406/406_521feat4.html. Accessed March 2, 2009.

Infusion Nurses Society. (2006). Infusion nursing standards of practice. *Journal of Infusion Nursing, 29*(1S), S1–S92.

Ireton, J. (2007). Tracheostomy suction: A protocol for practice. *Paediatric Nursing, 19*(10), 14–18.

I.V. Rounds. Comparing short peripheral cannula insertion sites. (2008). *Nursing, 38*(5), 60.

Jevon, P. (2007a). Cardiac monitoring: Part 1. Electrocardiography (ECG). *Nursing Times, 103*(1), 26–27.

Jevon, P. (2007b). Cardiac monitoring: Part 2. Recording a 12-lead ECG. *Nursing Times, 103*(2), 26–27.

Jevon, P. (2007c). Cardiac monitoring: Part 3. External pacing. *Nursing Times, 103*(3), 26–27.

The Joanna Briggs Institute. (2004). Clinical effectiveness of different approaches to peritoneal dialysis catheter exit-site care. *Best*Practice, *8*(1), 1–7.

The Joint Commission. (2008). Speak Up. What you should know about pain management. Available at www.jointcommission.org/PatientSafety/SpeakUp. Accessed on December 27, 2007.

Karadag, A., Mentes, B., & Ayaz, S. (2005). Colostomy irrigation: Results of 25 cases with particular reference to quality of life. *Journal of Clinical Nursing, 14*(4), 479–485.

Kratz, A. (2008). Use of the acute confusion protocol: A research utilization project. *Journal of Nursing Care Quality, 23*(4), 331–337.

Kyle, T. (2008). *Essentials of Pediatric Nursing.* Philadelphia, PA: Wolters Kluwer Health/Lippincott Williams & Wilkins.

Kwekkeboom, K., Hau, H., Wanta, B., et al. (2008). Patients' perceptions of the effectiveness of guided imagery and progressive muscle relaxation interventions used for cancer pain. *Complementary Therapies in Clinical Practice, 14*(3), 185–194.

Lannefors, L. (2006). Inhalation therapy: Practical considerations for nebulisation therapy. *Physical Therapy Reviews, 11*(1), 21–27.

Lavery, I. (2005). Peripheral intravenous therapy: Key risks and implications for practice. *Nursing Standard, 19*(46), 55–64.

Lavery, I., & Ingram, P. (2005). Venipuncture: Best practice. *Nursing Standard, 19*(49), 55–65.

Liu, S., Ridhman, J., Thirlby, R., et al. (2006). Efficacy of continuous wound catheters delivering local anesthetic for postoperative analgesia: a quantitative and qualitative systemic review of randomized controlled trial. *Journal of the American College of Surgeons, 203*(6), 914–932.

Lynch, D., Ferraro, M., Krol, J., et al. (2005). Continuous passive motion improves shoulder joint integrity following stroke. *Clinical Rehabilitation, 19*(6), 594–599.

MacCulloch, P., Gardner, T., & Bonner, A. (2007). Comprehensive fall prevention programs across settings: A review of the literature. *Geriatric Nursing, 28*(5), 306–311.

March, Karen. (2005). Intracranial pressure monitoring: Why monitor? *AACN Clinical Issues: Advanced Practice in Acute & Critical Care, 16*(4), 456–475.

Malli, S. (2005). Device safety. Keep a close eye on vacuum-assisted wound closure. *Nursing, 35*(7), 25.

Masoorli, S. (2007). Nerve injuries related to vascular access insertion and assessment. *Journal of Infusion, 30*(6), 346–350.

Mayo Clinic. (2007). *How to choose and use a walker.* Available at www.mayoclinic.com/health/walker/HA00060. Accessed July 3, 2008.

Mercer Smith, J. (2003). Indwelling catheter management: From habit-based to evidence-based practice. *Ostomy Wound Management, 49*(12), 34–45.

McCaffery, M., & Pasero, C. (1999). *Pain clinical manual* (2nd ed.). St. Louis: Mosby.

McClave, S., Lukan, J., Stefater, J., et al. (2005). Poor validity of residual volumes as a marker for risk of aspiration in critically ill patients. *Critical Care Medicine, 33*(2), 324–330.

Metheny, N. (2008). Residual volume measurement should be retained in enteral feeding protocols. *American Journal of Critical Care, 17*(1), 62–64.

Mincer, A. (2007). Assistive devices for the adult patient with orthopaedic dysfunction: why physical therapists choose what they do. *Orthopaedic Nursing, 26*(4), 226–233.

Moore, T. (2007). Respiratory assessment in adults. *Nursing Standard, 21*(49), 48–56.

Nadzam, D. (2008). Joint Commission Resources. Preventing patient falls. Available at www.jcrinc.com/Preventing-Patient-Falls/. Accessed February 25, 2009.

National Cancer Institute (NCI). (2008). Gastrointestinal complications (PDQ). Constipation. Available at www.cancer.gov/cancertopics/pdq/supportivecare/gastrointestinalcomplications/HealthProfessional/page3#Section_5. Accessed October 28, 2008.

Padula, C., Kenny, A., Olanchon, C., et al. (2004). Enteral feedings: What the evidence says: Avoid contamination of feedings and its sequelae with this research-based protocol. *American Journal of Nursing, 104*(7), 62–69.

Pennsylvania Department of Health (PA Dept. of Health). Bureau of Laboratories. (2007). Sputum collection for tuberculosis. Available at www.dsf.health.state.pa.us/health/lib/health/labs/sputum_collection_directions.pdf. Accessed August 22, 2008.

Pickering, T. (2005) Measure of blood pressure in and out of the office. *Journal of Clinical Hypertension 7*(2), 123–129.

Pickering, T., Hall, J., Appel, L., et al. (2004). American Heart Association Scientific Statement. Recommendations for blood pressure measurement in humans and experimental animals. Part 1: Blood pressure measurement in humans: A statement for professionals from the subcommittee of professional and public education of the American Heart Association Council on High Blood Pressure Research. Available at http://hyper.ahajournals.org/cgi/content/full/45/1/142. Accessed August 5, 2010.

Preston, G. (2008). An overview of topical negative pressure therapy in wound care. *Nursing Standard, 23*(7), 62–68.

Redmond, A., & Doherty, E. (2005). Peritoneal dialysis. *Nursing Standard, 19*(40), 55–65.

Roman, M. (2005). Tracheostomy tubes. *MEDSURG Nursing, 14*(2), 143–144.

Rubin, B., & Durotoye, L. (2004). How do patients determine that their metered-dose inhaler is empty? *Chest, 126*(4), 1134–1137.

Rudoni, C. (2008). A service evaluation of the use of silicone-based adhesive remover. *British Journal of Nursing, Stoma Care Supplement, 17*(2), S4, S6, S8–S9.

Rushing, J. (2004). How to administer a subcutaneous injection. *Nursing, 34*(6), 32.

Sander, N., Fusco-Walker, S. Harder, J., et al. (2006). Dose counting and the use of pressurized metered-dose inhalers: running on empty. *Annals of Allergy, Asthma & Immunology, 97*(1), 34–38.

Scales, K. (2008). A practical guide to venepuncture and blood sampling. *Nursing Standard, 22*(29), 29–36.

Schaffer, S., & Yucha, C. (2004). Relaxation & pain management: The relaxation response can play a role in managing chronic and acute pain. *American Journal of Nursing, 104*(8), 75–82.

Sanofi Aventis. (2007). A 6-step guide for the self-administration of Lovenox. Available at www.lovenox.com/hcp/dosingAdministration/lovenoxSelfAdministration.aspx. Accessed June 21, 2009.

Sinclair, J. (2002). Servo-control for maintaining abdominal skin temperature at 36C in low birth weight infants. *Cochrane Database of Systematic Reviews.* Issue 1. Article No.:CD001074.DOE 10.1002/14651858.CD001074. Accessed March 12, 2008.

Smeltzer, S., Bare, B., Hinkle, J., et al. (2010). *Brunner & Suddarth's Textbook of Medical-Surgical Nursing.* (12th ed.). Philadelphia, PA: Wolters Kluwer Health/Lippincott Williams & Wilkins.

Smith, B., & Hannum, F. (2008). Optimizing IV therapy in the elderly. *Advance for Nurses, 10*(18), 27–28.

Society of Urologic Nurses and Associates. (2005c). Male urethral catheterization: Clinical practice guideline. Available at suna.org/resources/maleCatheterization. pdf. Accessed November 15, 2005.

Stephen-Haynes, J., & Thompson, G. (2007). The different methods of wound debridement. *British Journal of Community Nursing, 12*(6), Wound Care: S6, S8–S10, S12-4.

Stevens, E. (2005). Bladder ultrasound: Avoiding unnecessary catheterizations. *MEDSURG Nursing, 14*(4), 249–253.

Sullivan, B. (2008). Nursing management of patients with a chest drain. *British Journal of Nursing, 17*(6), 388–393.

Swann, J. (2008). Fall prevention is everyone's responsibility. *Nursing & Residential Care, 10*(6), 294–298.

Thompson, G. (2008). An overview of negative pressure wound therapy (NPWT). *Wound Care, 13*(6), Wound Care: S23–S4, S26, S28–S30.

Toedter Williams, N. (2008). Medication administration through enteral feeding tubes. *American Journal of Health-System Pharmacy, 65*(24), 2347–2357.

Tracy, S., Dufault, M., Kogut, S., et al. (2006). Translating best practices in non-drug postoperative pain management. *Nursing Research, 55*(2), S57–S67.

Usichenko, T., Pavlovic, D., Foellner, S., et al. (2004). Reducing venipuncture pain by a cough trick: A randomized crossover volunteer study. *Anesthesia & Analgesia, 98*(2), 343–345.

VISN 8 Patient Safety Center. (2009). *Safe Patient Handling and Movement Algorithms.* Tampa, FL: Author. Available at http://www.visn8.va.gov/patientsafetycenter/safePtHandling/default.asp. Accessed April 23, 2010.

VISN 8 Patient Safety Center. (2007). *Safe Patient Handling Nursing School Curriculum Module.* Tampa, FL: Author. Available at http://www.visn8.med.va.gov/PatientSafetyCenter/safePtHandling/SPHMToolkit_Final.DOC

VISN 8 Patient Safety Center. (2005). *Patient Care Ergonomics Resource Guide: Safe Patient Handling and Movement.* Tampa, FL: Available at: http://www. visn8.med.va.gov/patientsafetycenter/safePtHandling/default.as.

Voegeli, D. (2008a). Care or harm: Exploring essential components in skin care regimens. *British Journal of Nursing, 17*(1), 24–30.

Voegeli, D. (2008b). The effect of washing and drying practices on skin barrier function. *Journal of Wound, Ostomy & Continence Nursing, 35*(1), 84–90.

Voegeli, D. (2007). The role of emollients in the care of patients with dry skin. *Nursing Standard, 22*(7), 62, 64–68.

Watkins, P. (2008). Using emollients to restore and maintain skin integrity. *Nursing Standard, 22*(41), 51–58, 60.

Weber, J., & Kelly, J. (2007). *Health Assessment in Nursing.* (3rd ed.). Philadelphia: Wolters Kluwer Health/Lippincott Williams & Wilkins.